15

Eat Yourself Slim

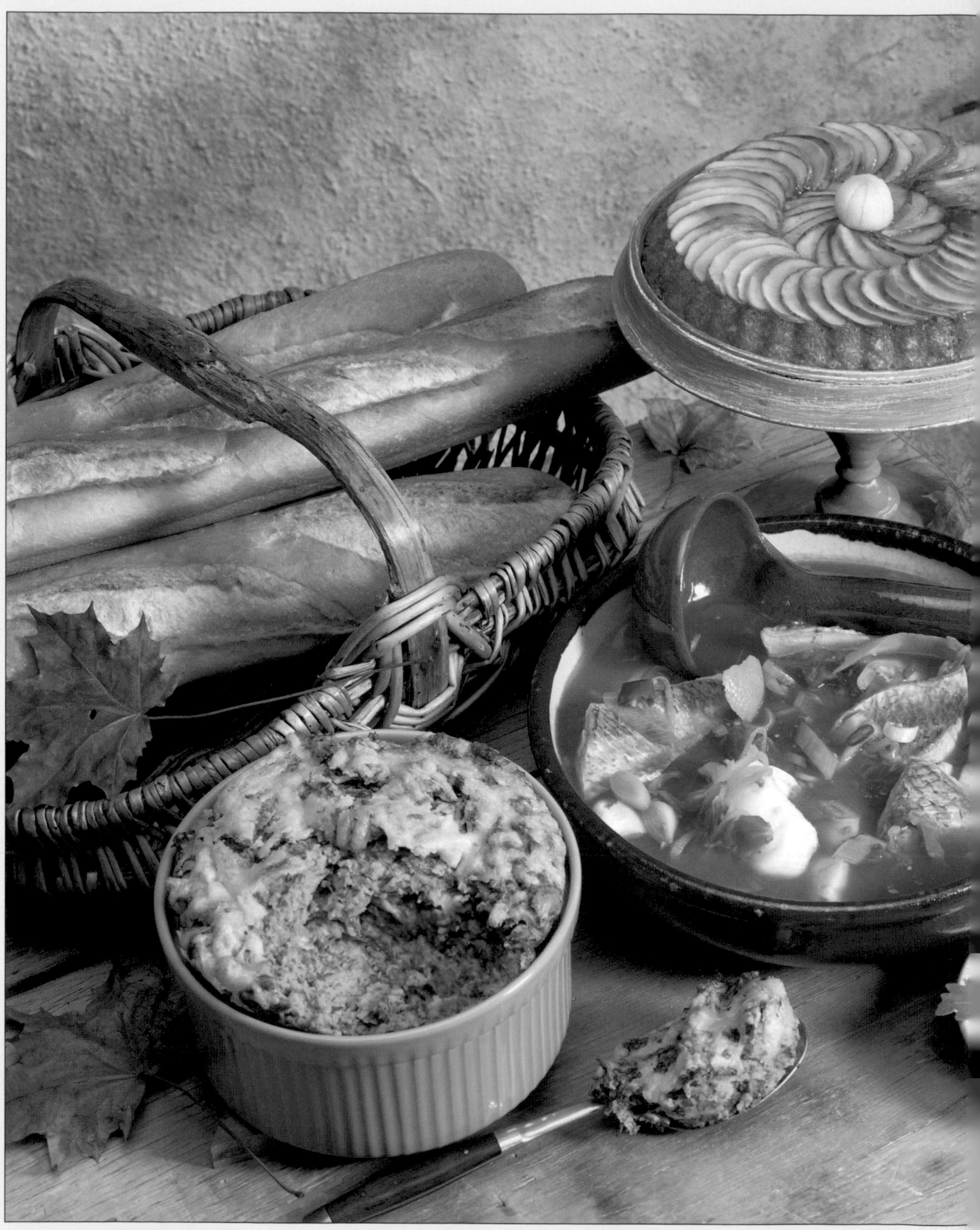

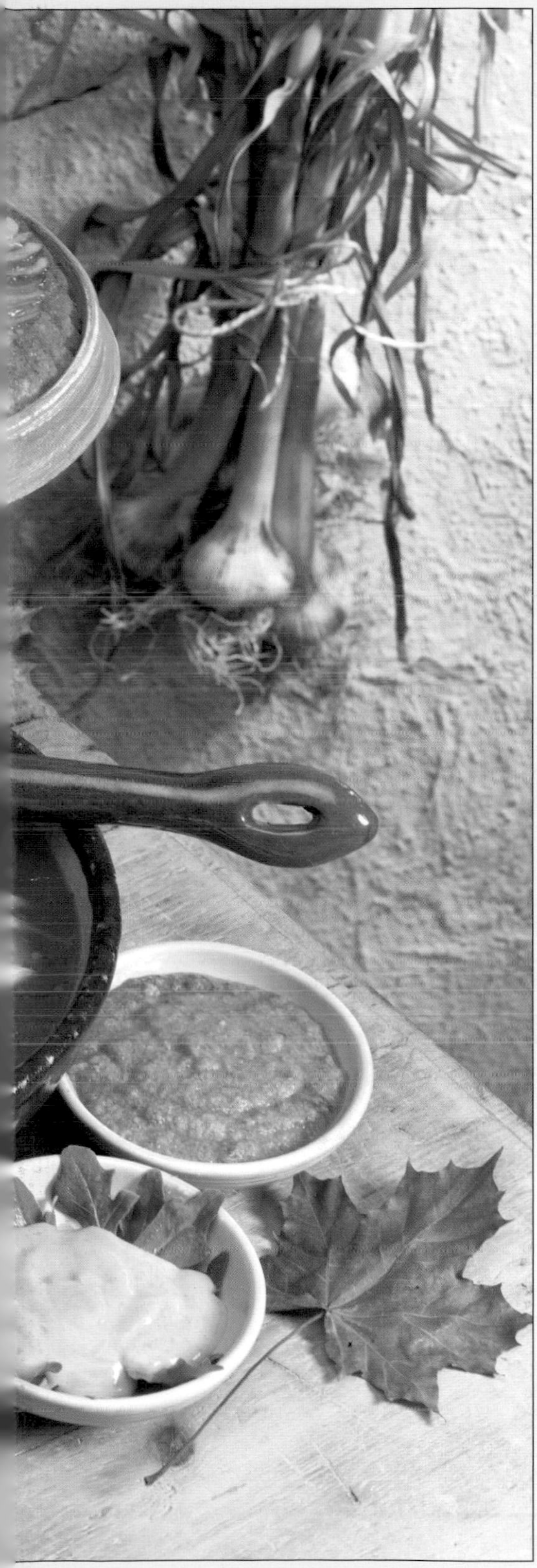

Eat Yourself Slim

Rosemary Conley

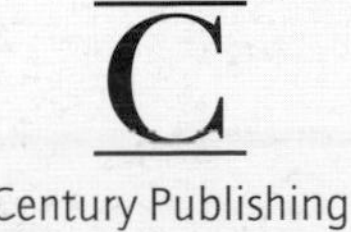

Century Publishing

Published by Century in 2001

3 5 7 9 10 8 6 4 2

First published in the United Kingdom in 2001 by Century
Random House UK Limited
20 Vauxhall Bridge Road, London SW1V 2SA

Random House Australia (Pty) Limited
20 Alfred Street, Milsons Point, Sydney,
New South Wales 2061, Australia

Random House New Zealand Limited
18 Poland Road, Glenfield
Auckland 10, New Zealand

Random House (Pty) Limited
Endulini, 5a Jubilee Road, Parktown 2193, South Africa

The Random House Group Limited Reg. No. 954009
www.randomhouse.co.uk

A CIP catalogue record for this book is available from the British Library

Papers used by Random House UK Limited are natural, recyclable products made from wood grown in sustainable forests. The manufacturing processes conform to the environmental regulations of the country of origin

ISBN 0 7126 1549 0

Photography by Peter Barry
Food styling by Dean Simpole-Clarke
Designed by Roger Walker

Printed and bound in Great Britain by
Butler & Tanner Ltd, Frome and London

Also by Rosemary Conley

Rosemary Conley's Hip and Thigh Diet
Rosemary Conley's Complete Hip and Thigh Diet
Rosemary Conley's Inch Loss Plan
Rosemary Conley's Hip and Thigh Diet Cookbook
(with Patricia Bourne)
Rosemary Conley's Metabolism Booster Diet
Rosemary Conley's Whole Body Programme
Rosemary Conley's New Hip and Thigh Diet Cookbook
(with Patricia Bourne)
Shape Up for Summer
Rosemary Conley's Beach Body Plan
Rosemary Conley's Flat Stomach Plan
Be Slim! Be Fit!
Rosemary Conley's Complete Flat Stomach Plan
Rosemary Conley's New Body Plan
Rosemary Conley's New Inch Loss Plan
Rosemary Conley's Low Fat Cookbook
Rosemary Conley's Red Wine Diet
Rosemary Conley's Low Fat Cookbook Two

IMPORTANT
If you have a medical condition or are pregnant, the diet described in this book should not be followed without first consulting your doctor. All guidelines and warnings should be read carefully, and the author and publisher cannot accept responsibility for injuries or damage arising out of a failure to comply with the same.

Contents

Acknowledgements

This is my 25th book and I am only too aware that without the help of my wonderful team this latest volume would not now be in your hands.

So, a huge thank you to Dean Simpole-Clarke for creating, yet again, so many delicious, mouthwatering low-fat recipes and for recreating them so beautifully for the photographs, also to photographer Peter Barry for his expertise in illustrating the food so clearly.

Also, thank you so much to my assistant Melody Patterson who worked tirelessly for months, drawing together the various elements of the book, putting them into a readable format and for completing the nutritional analysis of every recipe and menu suggestion. My PA Louise Jones was a great help too, particularly when it came to proof reading. Thank you, Lou.

Special thanks must go to my editor, Jan Bowmer, who has, once again, provided her expertise in making this book a workable, logical volume for you, the reader, to follow. Her meticulous attention to detail never ceases to amaze me.

Thank you to Dr Susan Jebb for her invaluable help and expertise in checking that the advice and facts we give you are correct and appropriate.

To my publishers Century I say a big thank you and to art director Dennis Barker and designer Roger Walker. Also to Andy McKillop who encouraged me to write the book, and to Ron Beard for selling it so enthusiastically, through his sales team, to the retailers.

Last, but by no means least, I want to say thank you to the members of Rosemary Conley Diet and Fitness Clubs for completing the questionnaires on the effectiveness of this diet and to Ally Evans, who worked so hard in collating these results into a useable format. You did a brilliant job, Ally. Thank you.

Foreword

For many years Rosemary Conley has endeavoured to help people put their good intentions into practice with low-fat eating plans, combined with exercise, to maximise weight loss and promote good health. This approach worked because in the past most low-fat foods contained fewer calories than their high-fat equivalents. However, advances in food processing and food technology mean that today some low-fat foods contain just as many calories as the high-fat varieties. To lose weight successfully you need to cut fat *and* calories.

This book combines an individualised, calorie-controlled eating plan, together with a wealth of new low-fat recipes to make it easier and more interesting to plan your meals. Using these ideas, you can cook healthy food for the whole family, while choosing the right portions to help you cut calories and lose weight.

Dr Susan Jebb
Deputy Chair of the Association for the Study of Obesity

Useful Information

Weight conversions

All weights are given in imperial and metric. All conversions are approximate. Use only one set of measures and do not mix the two. The table below shows the conversions used.

Ounce (oz)	*Pound (lb)*	*Gram (g)*
1		25
2		50
3		75
4	1/4	115
5		150
6		175
7		200
8	1/2	225
16	1	450
	1 1/2	675
	2	900

Liquid measures

1 tablespoon	=	3 teaspoons	=	1/2fl oz	=	15ml
2 tablespoons	=	6 teaspoons	=	1fl oz	=	30ml
4 tablespoons	=	1/4 cup	=	2fl oz	=	50ml
5 tablespoons	=	1/3 cup	=	2 1/2fl oz	=	75ml
8 tablespoons	=	1/2 cup	=	4fl oz	=	120ml
10 tablespoons	=	2/3 cup	=	5fl oz	=	150ml (1/4 pint)
12 tablespoons	=	3/4 cup	=	6fl oz	=	175ml
16 tablespoons	=	1 cup	=	8fl oz	=	250ml (1/2 US pint)

Note: A UK pint contains 20fl oz

American cup measures can be convenient to use, especially when making large quantities. However, although the volume remains the same, the weight may vary, as illustrated opposite.

Imperial	*American*
Flour	*Flour*
plain and self-raising	all purpose
1oz	1/4 cup
4oz	1 cup
Cornflour	*Cornstarch*
1oz	1/4 cup
generous 2oz	1/2 cup
4 1/2 oz	1 cup
Sugar (granulated/caster)	*Sugar (granulated)*
4oz	1/2 cup
7 1/2 oz	1 cup
Sugar (icing)	*Sugar (confectioner's)*
1oz	1/4 cup
4 1/2 oz	1 cup
Sugar (soft brown)	*Sugar (light and dark brown)*
4oz	1/2 cup firmly packed
8oz	1 cup firmly packed

Useful measures

1 egg	56ml	2fl oz
1 egg white	28ml	1fl oz
2 rounded tablespoons breadcrumbs	30g	1oz
2 level teaspoons gelatine	8g	1/4oz

1oz (25g) granular aspic sets 600ml (1 pint).
1/2oz (15g) powdered gelatine or 4 leaves sets 600ml (1 pint).

All spoon measures are level unless otherwise stated.

Wine quantities

Average serving	*ml*	*fl oz*
1 glass wine	90ml	3fl oz
1 glass port or sherry	60ml	2fl oz
1 glass liqueur	30ml	1fl oz

Oven temperature conversions

Celsius (Centigrade)	*Fahrenheit*	*Gas Mark*	*Definition*
130	250	½	very cool
140	275	1	cool
150	300	2	warm
170	325	3	moderate
180	350	4	moderate
190	375	5	moderately hot
200	400	6	hot
220	425	7	hot
230	450	8	very hot
240	475	9	very hot

Abbreviations

oz	ounce
lb	pound
kg	kilogram
fl oz	fluid ounce
ml	millilitre
C	Celsius (Centigrade)
F	Fahrenheit
kcal	kilocalorie (calorie)

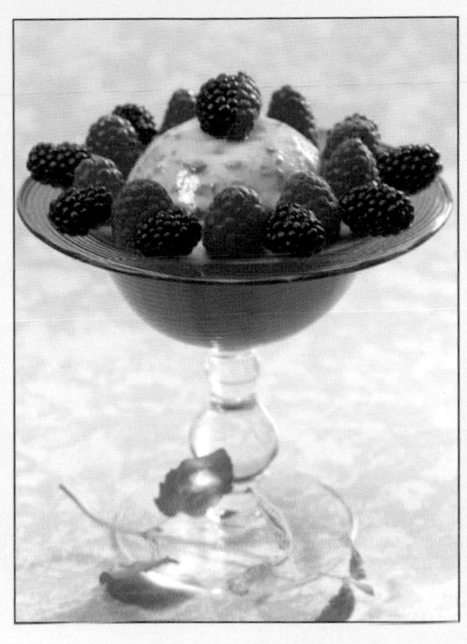

Equipment and terms

British	American
baking tin	baking pan
base	bottom
cocktail stick	toothpick
dough or mixture	batter
frying pan	skillet
greaseproof paper	waxed paper
grill/grilled	broil/broiled
knock back dough	punch back dough
liquidiser	blender
muslin	cheesecloth
pudding basin	ovenproof bowl
stoned	pitted
top and tail (gooseberries)	clean (gooseberries)
whip/whisk	beat/whip

Ingredients

British	American
aubergine	egg plant
bacon rashers	bacon slices
bicarbonate of soda	baking soda
black cherries	bing cherries
boiling chicken	stewing chicken
broad beans	fava or lima beans
capsicum pepper	sweet pepper
cauliflower florets	cauliflowerets
celery stick	celery stalk
stock cube	bouillon cube
chicory	belgium endive
chilli	chile pepper

British	*American*
cooking apple	baking apple
coriander	cilantro
cornflour	cornstarch
courgette	zucchini
crystallised ginger	candied ginger
curly endive	chicory
demerara sugar	light brown sugar
essence	extracts
fresh beetroot	raw beets
gelatine	gelatin
head celery	bunch celery
icing	frosting
icing sugar	confectioner's sugar
plain flour	all purpose flour
root ginger	ginger root
self-raising flour	all purpose flour sifted with baking powder
soft brown sugar	light brown sugar
spring onion	scallion
stem ginger	preserved ginger
sultanas	seedless white raisins
wholemeal	wholewheat

Introduction

This is a diet book and a low-fat cookbook, rolled into one.

I have included a tried and tested, incredibly effective diet combined with a selection of sumptuous recipes to keep your taste buds satisfied as you lose your unwanted weight, or to keep you slim if you have already achieved your goal.

The principle of the diet is somewhat different from any of my other diets as it includes an optional, daily high-fat treat which can be saved up for a bigger treat if you want to. Also the diet is based on your own personal daily calorie allowance which you will be able to calculate for yourself.

Over the last 20 months, the principle of the Eat Yourself Slim diet has been followed by members of Rosemary Conley Diet and Fitness Clubs across the UK. Around 300,000 women (and some men) have followed it and undeniably proved its effectiveness.

After they had followed the diet for six months, I asked 600 members, selected at random, to complete a questionnaire. I wanted to know the diet's effectiveness since I was now including an optional high-fat treat each day.

All my previous diet plans had strictly excluded anything high in fat. Also how did everyone feel about being a calorie counter again after shying away from them for years?

What about inch loss – was this diet as effective in that area? How did the dieters get on with their personal calorie allowance? Did they find it easy to follow?

I needn't have worried. The results were fantastic! Out of those questioned, 98 per cent said the diet was easy to follow, 78 per cent said it was the most effective diet they had ever followed and 76 per cent said they had lost more inches than ever before!

The weekly weight losses for all 600 members questioned were added together and divided by 600 to arrive at an average weekly weight loss figure. Many dieters had been on the diet for many months, some for a somewhat shorter period of time. Nevertheless, the average loss across all 600 worked out at 1.7lb per week. This is incredible when you realise that some people have only a small amount to lose and that it was taken over a wide time scale.

When asked if they lost weight faster on this diet, 67 per cent said they did, 27 per cent said that the progress was about the same with only 6 per cent saying 'no'.

When asked if they were happy with their inch loss, 1 per cent said they were disappointed, 1 per cent said they were not very happy, 17 per cent were happy, 31 per cent were very happy and 50 per cent were delighted.

Seventy-seven per cent said they were happy to count calories and 94 per cent were pleasantly surprised at how many calories they were allowed.

This book, which accompanies my TV series by the same name, offers you an extended version of the original diet plan used by our Rosemary Conley Diet and Fitness Club members. You will also find plenty of motivational tips to keep you going until you reach your weight-loss goal – and keep it off in the long term.

I have tried to give you the ultimate guide to help you achieve a trim and healthy body. If you combine the diet with some extra physical activity, you'll maximise your weight-loss progress. So enjoy the journey and revel in your ultimate success.

To encourage you, here are some comments from just a few of the trial dieters:

'This plan is definitely the one for me, as it's normal good food that's easy to buy, cook, prepare, etc. and very tasty to eat!'

Kimberley Fay, Milton Keynes

'This diet is my favourite. So uncomplicated, so much choice and good to eat. Easy to adapt for my husband. Not so much a diet but a new way of life.'

Janet West, Huddersfield

'I have never felt this good in a long time and the weight loss has given me tremendous confidence.'

Allison Baines, Co. Durham

'I can't begin to describe the changes I feel about myself – apart from the excellent weight loss I feel so much more positive. I don't feel like I'm dieting – more like at last I'm in control of my size and health.'

H.C., Surrey

'I have tried other diets, but this is the best one I have ever done. I can't believe the number of inches I have lost with the weight.'

Susan Fox, Hampshire

'I like the idea of the diet being based on your basal metabolic rate because it makes it more personal as everybody is different. My caloric allowance is very sufficient and I feel I am getting plenty to eat and do not get the urge to "snack" between meals.'

Angela Howard, Oxfordshire

'I'm losing more weight than expected. I have to pinch myself to believe it!'

Michelle Cardy, Cornwall

'I have been much more successful on this diet. I feel great and have experienced a total change in my attitude to food and exercise, which has improved my work and social life enormously!'

L.H., Dundee

'What I like about it is the fact that the calorie allowance is connected to how much you weigh. In my case, because I weighed a lot, I was pleasantly surprised by how much I was allowed initially. Also, whenever I get a new allowance I feel proud because it means that I am right on my way, so cutting down on calories doesn't seem to be such a big scare any more.'

Julie Knoblich, Essex

'I have found this diet so easy. I have never been very successful before, but this time the weight just fell off and I'm managing to keep it fairly constant.'

Laura Knight, East Sussex

Why 'Eat Yourself Slim'?

Thirty years ago I started my first slimming club, having realised that the only way to lose weight successfully was to eat more than most diets recommended. In those days doctors handed out 1,000-calorie diet sheets, which were impossible to stick to. There just wasn't enough food to eat. I conquered my own overweight problem by giving myself more calories – and sticking to it.

In 1986 I had to follow a low-fat diet because of a gallstone problem. Without realising it, my body changed shape, shedding fat from areas I had tried to slim down since puberty – namely my hips and thighs. I always have been the ultimate pear shape.

Millions of women and some men have become slimmer and healthier since they too changed to low-fat eating.

Despite many other diets being published and promoted from various corners of the world, there is no shadow of a doubt that if you want to lose weight fast and yet healthily, if you want to be lean and energetic, there is no better way than to eat a calorie-controlled, low-fat diet and combine it with increased physical activity.

Becoming more active need only mean walking for 30 minutes, three times a week – not having to run a marathon! I am always delighted though to hear how those who hate the thought of exercise at the beginning become great fans of it later.

Often we 'hate' exercise because we 'fear' it. We think: 'I'm not going to be able to go to a class – I'm not coordinated and I might pass out'. 'Imagine the embarrassment!' 'I couldn't possibly go for a jog – everyone would laugh at me!' or 'If you think I'm going to show off my fat in public, think again!'

But you are not alone. We all felt like that – I know I did. Once we get started we find we *can* cope, but to make sure that we can, the exercise has to be at *our* level. Personally I hate running, but I love walking. I hate swimming, but I love working out to music in an aerobics class – but at a *moderate level*. I have no inclination to workout at a mega level – it would be too exhausting – so I don't do it. Find *your* level and progress at your *own* pace, then hopefully you will keep doing it.

While I was asking some of the members of our classes for their responses to the new diet plan, I decided to ask them about their attitude towards exercise. Had it changed since they joined our classes? These were the results:

Of the 600 women questioned 25 per cent admitted to not enjoying exercise before attending a Rosemary Conley Diet and Fitness class. When asked how they felt now, having attended classes for some time, only 4 per cent still didn't enjoy it. So why the big turn around? They realised they could do the exercise (our classes cater for all capabilities and all of our instructors are specially trained to modify exercises when necessary), they enjoyed the friendships of fellow members just like them and, as the weeks went by, they became fitter and could do more when *they* felt they could. As their fear diminished their confidence grew and this will happen to you too.

If you don't exercise already you need to start. It doesn't have to be awful. You can exercise in so many different ways – sporting activities, just walking or gardening (mowing the lawn is great exercise), working out at an exercise class (see inside back cover for details of where our classes are held), working out to a fitness video (click on to our website for details of several of mine), join a gym, play physical games with the children, swim – there are so many things you can do. Some cost money, but lots don't.

So what is the optimum way of losing weight?

The secret of successful, long-term, weight loss is to try to make your body believe it isn't dieting. You can achieve this by eating sufficient calories to meet your bodily needs yet few enough to affect a weight loss. It means you shouldn't starve yourself or miss out on delicious food, because if you are happy with what you are eating, you are less likely to cheat, and that is what this book is all about.

First you will be able to calculate your individual calorie allowance from the tables on pages 19–20, which are based on your sex, age and weight. Next you can choose from the many low-fat, calorie-counted menu suggestions listed, including some fabulous recipes from expert chef Dean Simpole-Clarke, with whom I have worked on TV for several years. Dean totally understands my low-fat philosophy.

Plus, for the first time in one of my diet books, you are allowed a 150-calorie daily treat which is exempt from my 4% fat rule. And for anyone not familiar with the 4% fat rule, all of my diets are based on the consumption of foods that contain 4% or less fat with the exception of oily fish, which is included, as it is vital for good health.

So why, after all these years of promoting low fat have I relented and allowed a 150-calorie high-fat treat? Well, just as 30 years ago I realised that dieters lost more weight by having a higher calorie allowance because they could stick to it, two years ago I realised that many of my low-fat dieters just couldn't find the willpower to never ever eat chocolate, Häagen-Dazs or Pringles without feeling so guilty that they broke the diet completely. So, a compromise was created and, having since then tried out this theory in our Clubs, I have proved beyond a shadow of a doubt that allowing a daily treat (which can be saved up if you wish) does not adversely affect weight and fat loss but greatly increases the level of adherence to the diet.

Never have we experienced such weight-loss successes at our Clubs as we have since the introduction of this new diet (which in the classes we called the New You Plan). The key to your success is keeping to your personal calorie allowance, making sure that the calories you eat are low fat except for your treat, and that you try to increase your activity levels within your everyday lifestyle. You can still have a glass of wine or other alcoholic drink, and, depending on how many calories you have to spend, these may be taken within or outside of your treat allowance. For example, if your daily allowance is 1700 kcal, you could have 1 unit of alcohol (e.g. 1 glass of wine) in addition to your 150 kcal treat because you have sufficient calories left to enable you to eat plenty of nutritious foods to keep your body healthy. If, on the other hand, you had a daily allowance of only 1300, then to get sufficient nutrients into the body you would have to take your unit of alcohol as part of your 150-kcal treat allowance.

As you lose each stone recalculate your calorie allowance to ensure maximum progress. As your body gets smaller it needs less fuel to feed it, so your calorie requirement reduces.

How to work out your optimum calorie allowance

Basal Metabolic Rate (BMR) Table

Women aged 18–29			**Women aged 30–59**			**Women aged 60–74**		
Body Weight			*Body Weight*			*Body Weight*		
Stones	*Kilos*	*BMR*	*Stones*	*Kilos*	*BMR*	*Stones*	*Kilos*	*BMR*
7	45	1147	7	45	1208	7	45	1048
7.5	48	1194	7.5	48	1233	7.5	48	1073
8	51	1241	8	51	1259	8	51	1099
8.5	54	1288	8.5	54	1285	8.5	54	1125
9	57	1335	9	57	1311	9	57	1151
9.5	60.5	1382	9.5	60.5	1337	9.5	60.5	1176
10	64	1430	10	64	1373	10	64	1202
10.5	67	1477	10.5	67	1389	10.5	67	1228
11	70	1524	11	70	1414	11	70	1254
11.5	73	1571	11.5	73	1440	11.5	73	1279
12	76	1618	12	76	1466	12	76	1305
12.5	80	1665	12.5	80	1492	12.5	80	1331
13	83	1712	13	83	1518	13	83	1357
13.5	86	1760	13.5	86	1544	13.5	86	1382
14	89	1807	14	89	1570	14	89	1408
14.5	92	1854	14.5	92	1595	14.5	92	1434
15	95.5	1901	15	95.5	1621	15	95.5	1460
15.5	99	1948	15.5	99	1647	15.5	99	1485
16	102	1995	16	102	1673	16	102	1511
16.5	105	2043	16.5	105	1699	16.5	105	1537
17	108	2090	17	108	1725	17	108	1563
17.5	111	2137	17.5	111	1751	17.5	111	1588
18	115	2184	18	115	1776	18	115	1614
18.5	118	2231	18.5	118	1802	18.5	118	1640
19	121	2278	19	121	1828	19	121	1666
19.5	124	2325	19.5	124	1854	19.5	124	1691
20	127	2373	20	127	1880	20	127	1717

Basal Metabolic Rate (BMR) Table

Men aged 18–29			**Men aged 30–59**			**Men aged 60–74**		
Body Weight			*Body Weight*			*Body Weight*		
Stones	*Kilos*	*BMR*	*Stones*	*Kilos*	*BMR*	*Stones*	*Kilos*	*BMR*
7	45	1363	7	45	1384	7	45	1232
7.5	48	1411	7.5	48	1421	7.5	48	1270
8	51	1459	8	51	1457	8	51	1307
8.5	54	1507	8.5	54	1494	8.5	54	1345
9	57	1555	9	57	1530	9	57	1383
9.5	60.5	1602	9.5	60.5	1567	9.5	60.5	1421
10	64	1650	10	64	1603	10	64	1459
10.5	67	1698	10.5	67	1640	10.5	67	1497
11	70	1746	11	70	1676	11	70	1535
11.5	73	1794	11.5	73	1713	11.5	73	1573
12	76	1842	12	76	1749	12	76	1611
12.5	80	1890	12.5	80	1786	12.5	80	1649
13	83	1938	13	83	1822	13	83	1687
13.5	86	1986	13.5	86	1859	13.5	86	1725
14	89	2034	14	89	1895	14	89	1763
14.5	92	2082	14.5	92	1932	14.5	92	1801
15	95.5	2129	15	95.5	1968	15	95.5	1839
15.5	99	2177	15.5	99	2005	15.5	99	1877
16	102	2225	16	102	2041	16	102	1915
16.5	105	2273	16.5	105	2078	16.5	105	1953
17	108	2321	17	108	2114	17	108	1991
17.5	111	2369	17.5	111	2151	17.5	111	2028
18	115	2417	18	115	2187	18	115	2066
18.5	118	2465	18.5	118	2224	18.5	118	2104
19	121	2513	19	121	2260	19	121	2142
19.5	124	2561	19.5	124	2297	19.5	124	2180
20	127	2609	20	127	2333	20	127	2218

The secret of long-term success

There's no better feeling when you're trying to lose weight than a waistband that's now loose (such a relief from when your stomach hung over it), trousers that have fresh air between your leg and the fabric (so much more comfortable than that feeling of material being superglued to your legs), and your top showing an attractive and feminine bustline rather than a bosom that resembles an oversized pillow being squeezed into a too small pillowcase!

Following this calorie-controlled, low-fat diet will definitely enable you to lose weight. Taking regular exercise is guaranteed to help to tone up your body and speed up your weight loss. However, even a diet combined with exercise is still not enough to achieve long-term success. You need to change your *mindset* towards food and activity in general.

This change in attitude needs you to create some positive, and remove some negative, habits *as well as* following the diet and taking regular exercise.

Place a tick alongside the statements opposite if they apply to you.

None of these actions constitutes a major sin on its own; they're just 'little extras' compared with going to the sweet counter and buying a Mars bar and a Snickers and eating them both.

- ☐ 'I always eat everything on my plate.' (*I was* made *to do that as a child.*)
- ☐ 'With their permission, I eat other family members' leftovers at the table.' (*Shame to waste it.*)
- ☐ 'I sometimes eat leftovers while walking to the kitchen.' (*If no one sees me it doesn't count!*)
- ☐ 'I eat leftovers while alone in the kitchen.' (*Think of the starving millions.*)
- ☐ 'I lick the spoon from the trifle/dessert before washing it up.' (*Saves messing up the washing up water.*)
- ☐ 'I like to level off the remaining trifle/dessert before placing in the fridge.' (*To make it look tidier.*)
- ☐ 'I keep levelling off remaining trifle/dessert over next day or so.' (*To check that it hasn't 'gone off'.*)
- ☐ 'I occasionally slice off a sliver of cheese from the fridge when I'm feeling peckish.' (*Sometimes more than a sliver.*)
- ☐ 'I eat occasional sweets or chocolates when offered by a friend.' (*I don't want to appear holier-than-thou.*)
- ☐ 'I eat ingredients during preparation of a recipe and lick the spoon afterwards.' (*To check that it tastes OK.*)

But I bet you put a tick in more than one box. If you ticked more than seven you might as well have had the Mars bar! By these seemingly harmless actions you are effectively sabotaging your chances of success on your weight-loss campaign. One by one, try and break all these negative habits.

So now to some positive actions and activities which take little effort but have a big effect:

- Stop leaving things at the bottom of the stairs – take them up every time.
- When the TV commercials come on, get up and do something (not get food though). Go upstairs for something, wash up, dry up, put washing in, walk dog for 2 minutes, walk around garden.
- When shopping, always use the stairs not the lift or elevator. If you must use the elevator, walk up it.
- Park further away from the door when going shopping or at the gym/pool/class.
- Make a list of your exercise programme for each week. Pin it on a noticeboard and tick off each activity as you do it . Don't beat yourself up if you don't do it all. Any is better than none.
- Go walking in your lunch break – even browsing round the shops is activity.
- Stand up when making phone calls, rather than sitting down.
- Look at housework as a workout not a chore. Vacuuming, sweeping, cleaning windows are great fat burners.
- Play active games with your children (or borrow someone else's) and have fun while you burn those calories.
- Washing and polishing your car, mowing the lawn or cutting the hedge are great forms of calorie-burning exercise. Include them in your workout schedule.

So, if you work towards stopping the habits on the first list and incorporate some of the activities in the second, you'll be amazed how positively your body will respond. Follow the diet strictly and the results will be better than ever before. You *can* lose weight . You *will* lose weight but, to do it, you need the right attitude. Remember these phrases – say them out loud. 'Every extra mouthful of food I eat means I'll lose less weight' and 'Every bit of extra activity I do – no matter now small – will speed up my weight loss.' Go on, just do it!

Are you a yo-yo dieter?

One minute you have the willpower of a saint and you know that this time you're going to really stick to the diet, exercise three times a week and see fantastic results. Then, for no particular reason, you find yourself devouring a chocolate bar – or two – as though they had just been washed up on a desert island and you hadn't eaten proper food for a month! You can't eat it fast enough, it doesn't seem to touch the sides, and before you know it, down goes bar number two!

Then horror strikes. It suddenly dawns on you what you've done. You suddenly remember you're trying to lose weight. It was almost as though you didn't decide to eat the chocolate – it just found its way into your mouth. You feel gutted. You can't believe you've just done it!

'Am I going mad, perhaps?' you ask yourself. You decide you must be. You say to yourself: 'How can this sensible, intelligent, rational woman who has a responsible job, whom people respect, behave like an irresponsible idiot?'

Well, take heart, because you, and millions of women just like you, go through exactly the same emotion time and time again. It isn't about intelligence, or irresponsibility, or uselessness. It is a pain in the backside fact of life, that when you are trying to lose weight you are vulnerable. As normal, regular human beings we are open to temptation. As soon as we make some restrictions on our food intake, that 'forbidden fruit' appeals all the more. When Eve was in the Garden of Eden she could have anything she wanted except off one particular tree. So what does she do? She chooses to eat from the forbidden tree. Why? Because she was tempted, and we are no different today.

When we go on a diet we tell ourselves that we can't eat this and that (but we enjoy those things!) and that we need to exercise (but we don't like getting hot and sweaty!), so we are telling our brain: 'I've got to do all these things I don't like – and I'll probably feel hungry too – just to get slimmer! In a weak moment we throw in the towel and 'eat from the forbidden tree' because it seems like a good idea at the time. Why? Because we've told our brain only negative messages, only the disadvantages of going on a diet and fitness programme, instead of positive ones. Positive messages are words like, 'When I lose weight I'll be wearing size 12 instead of a size 18. I'll be able to join in my child's sports day without being an embarrassment. My husband will think I look more attractive – I will have so much more energy. I will look younger and feel 10 times healthier. I'll be able to wear all those clothes in the wardrobe that I've not been able to wear for ages.'

Just because you've been a yo-yo dieter in the past, doesn't mean you have to be so for ever. I used to be one and I've cured myself by eating three substantial, low-fat meals a day. I cured myself by making the rule, that if I had a binge I wouldn't skip the next meal in an attempt to cancel it. It worked. I would eat my normal, low-fat, calorie-controlled meal and put the binge behind me. One binge doesn't matter, but three binges do! Don't beat yourself up about it. You're human. You're bound to have bad days – we all do. Don't use them as an excuse to pack it in.

So, draw a line under your dieting history now. Decide today that this is a brand new start and this time, you will do it! And you can!

Facts about food and how the Eat Yourself Slim Diet works

As a guideline, I recommend you select foods with 4% or less fat – that's up to 4 grams of fat for every 100 grams of product, though there are some exceptions such as oily fish.

The 4% fat guideline is an extremely simple and effective rule of thumb, with no need to count or add up fat grams. It has been proved that following a calorie-controlled, low-fat diet is unquestionably the safest and most effective way to lose fat from the body and therefore lose weight. It really, really works.

Let me explain how. Compared with other foods such as carbohydrates and proteins, fat in the diet is very easily stored as fat on the body.

Too much fat in the diet has been proven to be harmful to health. Too little fat can be unhealthy, too, which is why we recommend you eat between 23 and 40 grams of fat a day while you are losing your excess weight but no more than 70 grams when maintaining a healthy weight. My eating plan will help you achieve this.

Get to know the nutrition labels on the packaging of all the foods that you buy. Most nutrition panels will give the quantities per 100g of product and some will give the nutrition details per serving. On the left-hand side will be the words like Energy, Protein, Carbohydrate and so on. Energy means the number of calories that the product yields and this is the figure that you need to be mindful of as far as the serving size is concerned. You have calculated your personal calorie allowance, and every item of food that you eat needs to be included in this. The only other column on the nutrition panel that you really need to look at is under 'fat' and it doesn't matter whether it's saturated or unsaturated since, as far as gaining or losing weight is concerned, fat is fat. Under the 100g column you need to select foods with 4% or less fat and this will ensure that you are following a low-fat diet. In this diet I allow you to have a 150-calorie treat that is exempt of the 4g fat rule.

If you follow the 4% rule for the rest of your food, the fat grams will look after themselves. So just keep an eye on the daily calorie intake. It is easy to eat too many low-fat foods and consequently eat too many calories and then weight loss can be very slow or non-existent. I want you to lose your weight as fast as it's healthy to do so, so calories are crucial. The total fat grams per serving are not important and I would strongly suggest that you do not get into the habit of counting fat grams as well as calories. You just don't need to.

I have created a selection of everyday meals from which you can choose to eat what you like best. All the calories have been counted for you, so you simply need to look under the different calorie headings as to whether you want a 200-calorie breakfast or one that contains 250 calories, and so on. If you stick to the calorie allowance that you have calculated from the tables on pages 19–20, you will definitely lose weight and, if you combine your eating plan with increased physical activity, you will lose weight even faster.

Each day I recommend that you eat breakfast, lunch and dinner and also consume 450ml (3/4 pint) of skimmed or semi-skimmed milk. Also, of course, in your total calorie allowance there's your special treat allowance of 150 calories to consider, which can be taken daily if you wish or saved up for a special occasion each week. However, don't carry it over to the next week.

Each day your daily intake should include five portions of fruit and/or vegetables. Fruit can be eaten with or between meals but remember to include the calories in your daily total.

This eating plan has been designed to work for anyone, whatever your personal circumstances or preference for food. Just select your favourite meals from the variety of menus listed. You can easily plan ahead if you wish. Losing weight has never been easier.

If you know you will be dining out in the evening, you can save up some calories by choosing lower-calorie options for breakfast and lunch and use up your day's treat allowance too. Alternatively, you might have saved up a previous day's treat so that you can relax and indulge yourself with a clear conscience.

I understand that losing weight isn't straightforward because it can be a struggle to maintain sufficient willpower. Some people find it almost impossible to stick unfalteringly to a weight-reducing eating plan. We all need a safety valve. We need to feel we can indulge legitimately if we have a serious craving for something, without feeling we've ruined all our hard work.

As you know, each day you are allowed 150 calories as a treat. Now, while you are free to select any high-fat treat you wish within the 150-calorie allowance, it is important to understand that if you select treats that fall *within* the 4% fat rule you are likely to lose your excess weight and inches even more quickly. Depending on your personal calorie allowance, all or part of this daily treat can be taken as a dessert after your main meal or at any other time. If you wish you could also take your treat as an alcoholic drink, providing of course that you keep within the calorie allowance. Furthermore, these treat calories can be saved up over a week and used for bigger treats. So if you desperately want to eat a cream cake or even a Mars bar you can just save up a few days' worth of treats. The same applies to alcohol. If your weekends are very sociable, save up your treat allowance and enjoy a few drinks with your friends.

You might well ask: 'But will I still lose weight if I choose treats with more than 4% fat?' Well, providing you don't exceed your daily calorie allowance and you use your treat allowance accurately, yes you definitely will. But if you relax your portion sizes, nibble extras in between meals and are rather casual about your treats, you may not. Losing weight is a matter of physics. If we eat fewer calories than our body uses for energy, it's inevitable that we will lose weight. It's rather like a bank account. Every time we spend money our bank balance reduces. If we overspend we have to draw on our savings to make up the difference. It's the same with our bodies. If we spend more energy than we take in in the form of food, we draw on our savings of fat stored around our body to make up the difference.

You may also ask: 'How is it that I have to follow the 4% fat rule for the rest of the diet but not for my treat. Surely that will cause me to gain weight fast?' Providing you stick to the calorie allowance for your daily treat you can't do much damage when you balance it out against the low-fat food you are eating throughout the rest of the day. If you save up your treats for a special occasion, it means you will have gone without them on other days so it all balances out. I must stress, though, that it is better to spread them out if you can.

Basic nutrition

We need to eat a variety of foods to obtain the nutrients we need for good health. I find it easier to think of nutrients as falling into two categories – tangible and intangible. Tangible nutrients are carbohydrates, proteins and fats. Minerals and vitamins fall into the intangible category because they are found *within* carbohydrates, proteins and fats. The key to good nutrition is getting the balance right. Eating too much of one thing can be as bad as eating too little of another. Here are some basic nutritional guidelines.

Carbohydrates

Carbohydrates include foods such as bread, potatoes, rice, cereals, pasta, as well as fruit and vegetables. These foods provide bulk in the diet and will only be stored as fat on the body if eaten in great excess. One gram of carbohydrate yields 4 calories. Carbohydrate should feature as the largest component in every meal, as out of all the food groups, it is the most important supplier of energy, and 60% of the calories we consume each day should come from this food group.

Proteins

Proteins include foods such as meat, fish and poultry, eggs, cheese and milk. Their primary use is to help the body grow and to renew and repair existing tissue. It should be eaten in moderation, forming about 15% of our daily calorie intake. Too much protein can be harmful because it has to be metabolised by the kidneys, so high-protein diets are neither healthy nor recommended. If we eat more protein than we need, the excess cannot be stored by the body. Instead, part of the protein will be excreted from the body and the remainder will be used to provide energy, therefore delaying the burning of fat.

Fats

Fats include foods such as oil, butter, margarine, cream and lard. Fat is also found in varying amounts in other foods, such as cakes, biscuits, pastry and confectionery. It is a concentrated form of energy that is efficiently stored by the body for emergencies and also supplies some valuable nutrients for health. Fat contains 9 calories per gram, which is more than twice the number of calories contained in one gram of carbohydrate or protein.

On a weight-reducing diet women should allow between 23 and 40 grams per day, while men should allow between 38 and 50 grams. When seeking to maintain weight, rather than trying to lose it, the maximum fat intake should not exceed 70 grams per day for women and 100 grams per day for men.

A small amount of fat is necessary for good health, and oily fish such as salmon, mackerel and herrings contain essential fatty acids that are particularly beneficial. I recommend that you eat one portion of oily fish each week.

Minerals

There are many minerals, all of which play an important role in helping us achieve good health. In most cases, a varied and healthy diet will ensure we are not missing out. However, there are two important minerals – calcium and iron – which require special mention. Since dairy products are the richest source of calcium, and red meat is the richest source of iron, on a low-fat diet it is particularly important to make sure you are taking in sufficient amounts. If you consume 450ml (3/4 pint) of skimmed or semi-skimmed milk plus a small pot of yogurt (150g/5oz) each day and eat red meat four times a week, you will probably meet your needs.

We need calcium to help maintain our bones and teeth and we need iron to make haemoglobin, which carries oxygen around the body in the red blood cells. Too little iron, and we become anaemic. Too little calcium, and we reduce the strength of our bones and risk osteoporosis. The tables on pages 30 and 31 will help you check if you are getting enough of each nutrient. If you're not, you need to amend your diet accordingly.

Please note, these tables are intended as a rough guide only, since the iron and calcium content of foods may differ slightly with different cuts of meat and different brands of cereals, especially if they have been fortified.

Vitamins

Vitamins fall into two categories: fat-soluble and water-soluble. Vitamins A, D, E and K are fat-soluble and do not need to be consumed daily, since the body is able to store them. However, the B complex vitamins and vitamin C are water-soluble. Since these cannot be stored by the body, they need to be consumed daily. Each vitamin has its own special function and all are essential for good health.

Even though my diets are designed to be healthy and balanced, I do recommend you take a multivitamin tablet daily, just to make doubly sure you have all the vitamins you need. This will ensure that you always get all the micronutrients your body needs.

These days much attention has been focused on the antioxidant vitamins (vitamins A, C, and E). These vitamins help to zap the free radicals that occur naturally in the body. For thousands of years, the balance between antioxidants and free radicals in the body has been just fine, naturally. But now, with increased pollution, radiation from microwaves, TVs and computers and even electric light bulbs, as well as increased exposure to stress, the body is producing more free radicals. These are the bad guys. To neutralise them, we need to increase the number of antioxidants (the good guys) by eating more of the foods that contain the ACE vitamins. They're easy to spot because many of these vitamins are found in brightly coloured vegetables and fruit. Other chemical compounds in fruit and vegetables, known as flavonoids, also act as antioxidants. Flavonoids are found in red wine too. Some minerals, such as zinc and selenium, can also act as antioxidants.

So, make sure you eat a wide range of foods to get all the vitamins and minerals you need. If in doubt, consider taking a micronutrient (vitamin/mineral) supplement.

Women planning to conceive should take an extra supplement of folic acid to reduce the risk of having a baby with a neural tube defect such as spina bifida.

Alcohol

Alcohol is a mixture of good and bad. It is a relaxant and has been acknowledged by the medical profession as having a real benefit in relieving stress. Alcohol in moderate quantities also helps to reduce the risk of heart disease. It is, nevertheless, a mild form of poison and the body works hard to get rid of it. On most of my diets, I allow a single unit of alcohol each day for women and two for men. Remember, too, that alcohol can be addictive, and we need to be mindful of the dangers. As with all things, moderation is the key.

There has been much debate and also many trials to determine the benefits and disadvantages of consuming alcohol, ranging from whether it helps your heart to whether it makes you fat. It was even suggested at one point that the calories from alcohol didn't count because the body processes calories from alcohol in a different way from other calories. But alcohol calories do count.

In its neat form, alcohol yields 7 calories per gram, but of course we never consume alcohol in its pure state. It is always diluted by water, even in the strongest spirits. The calories in your favourite tipple may not always be directly related to the alcohol content, since many drinks contain sugar, carbohydrate and sometimes even fat.

Alcohol is easily absorbed by the stomach, but the only way the body can rid itself of alcohol is by burning it in the liver and other tissues. Since alcohol is essentially a toxin and the body has no useful purpose for storing it, the body prioritises the elimination of it at the cost of processing other foods you have eaten. Consequently, other foods may be converted to fat more readily than usual, thereby increasing your fat stores.

In the many trials I have carried out for my diets I have always found that slimmers who do drink a little alcohol while following the diet do at least as well as those who don't and, in some cases, lose more weight. But rather than suggesting that alcohol has any miracle effect, I believe it's down to the fact that if you are allowed a drink you feel less restricted, can still socialise and feel as if you are leading a 'normal' life.

Iron content of foods

Food	*Serving size*	*mg*
Liver	100g cooked weight	8
Kidney	100g cooked weight	7
Venison	100g cooked weight	8
Lean beef	100g cooked weight	3
Lean lamb	100g cooked weight	2
Pork	100g cooked weight	1
Ham	100g cooked weight	1
Duck	100g cooked weight	3
Chicken/turkey	100g cooked weight	1
Egg	1	1
Chickpeas	100g cooked weight	2
Lentils	100g cooked weight	2.5
Baked beans	1 small can	2
Potatoes	100g	0.5
Spinach	50g cooked weight	2
Watercress	50g	1
Cabbage	50g cooked weight	0.5
Broccoli	50g cooked weight	0.5
Dried fruit	50g	1
White bread	1 slice	0.5
Wholemeal bread	1 slice	0.8
Branflakes	25g	7 (fortified)
Weetabix	25g	4 (fortified)

The reference nutrient intake (RNI) for the female population is 14.8mg per day and 8.7mg for the male population.

Calcium content of foods

Food	*Weight*	*mg*	
Milk	600ml	680	
Cheddar cheese	25g	225	
Cottage cheese	1 small pot	60	
Yogurt	1 small pot	360	
Egg	1	25	
Sardines	50g cooked weight	250	
Pilchards (canned)	50g	150	
Prawns	50g cooked weight	75	
Tofu	100g	500	
Ice cream	50g	70	
White bread	1 slice	30	(fortified)
Wholemeal bread	1 slice	7	
Weetabix	25g	10	
Shredded wheat	25g	12	
Spinach	50g cooked weight	300	
Watercress	50g	110	
Dried fruit	50g	30	

The reference nutrient intake (RNI) for both the female and male population is 700mg per day (800mg per day for 15- to 18-year-olds).

The key is to have a little each day, rather than drinking a lot on the occasional drinking binge. Perhaps the greatest danger from drinking alcohol when you are dieting is that it is extremely effective at diluting your willpower. Because it is a relaxant, it's so easy to think, 'Oh, what the heck, I'll diet tomorrow,' and then really overindulge on the food front!

Reading nutrition labels

Nowadays we are fortunate that most food products we buy contain lots of useful information on the nutrition label. This provides us with a breakdown of their nutritional content as well as the number of calories and amount of fat. To simplify matters, as far as weight control is concerned, the two key things to look at are energy and fat.

The figure relating to 'energy' tells you the number of calories in 100g of the product (you can ignore the kJ figure – just look at the kcal one). You then need to calculate how much of the product you will actually be eating to work out the number of calories per portion.

The fat content may be broken down into polyunsaturates and saturates but, for anyone on a weight-reducing diet, this is not significant. It is the total fat content per 100g that is relevant in our calculations. I make the general and simple rule that my dieters should only select foods where the label shows the fat content as 4g or less fat per 100g of product, i.e. 4% or less fat. I believe the actual amount of fat per portion is of lesser importance. If you follow the simple 4% fat rule and restrict your calorie intake to a number equivalent to your basal metabolic rate (see pages 19–20), the fat content of your food will look after itself. The only exceptions to this rule are your daily 150-calorie treat, lean cuts of meat such as beef, lamb and pork, which may be just over the 4% yardstick, and oily fish such as salmon and mackerel. In some recipes occasional high-fat ingredients have been used in very small quantities to introduce a special flavour or texture. As most recipes serve 4 people, the amount of fat is negligible.

NUTRITIONAL INFORMATION	
	Per 100g
ENERGY	172 kJ/40 kcal
PROTEIN	1.8g
CARBOHYDRATE	8.0g
(of which sugars)	(2.0g)
FAT	0.2g
(of which saturates)	(Trace)
FIBRE	1.5g
SODIUM	0.3g

Cooking the low-fat way

To cook the low-fat way you will need some basic non-stick kitchen essentials such as a non-stick frying pan or wok, some non-stick baking tins and the appropriate utensils to go with them. The first time you cook a stir-fry in a non-stick wok without a drop of oil is quite a revelation. The moisture that comes from the meat and vegetables prevents the food from sticking or tasting dry.

Once you have got used to low-fat cooking there will be no turning back. It really is easier than you think. In the following pages I have included advice on the kind of equipment you need and how to care for it, as well as outlining the various low-fat cooking techniques and suggestions for flavour enhancers to help your food taste delicious.

Equipment you will need

Utensils

At one time, non-stick surfaces used to have a very short lifespan before becoming scratched and worn. Fortunately, in recent years great progress been made with non-stick pans, although the old adage 'you get what you pay for' still holds firm. Buy a cheap non-stick pan, and the first time you slightly burn the pan, the surface begins to peel.

It is worth investing in a top-quality non-stick wok and a non-stick frying pan, both with lids. I use these two pans more than anything else in my kitchen. The lid is crucial, since this allows the contents of the pan to steam which adds moisture to the dish.

Non-stick saucepans are useful, too, for cooking sauces, porridge, scrambled eggs and other foods that tend to stick easily. Lids are essential for these too. Also, treat yourself to a set of non-stick baking tins and trays. Cakes, Yorkshire puddings, scones, and lots more can all be cooked the low-fat way.

To clean a non-stick pan, always soak the pan first to loosen any food that is still inside, then wash with a non-abrasive sponge or cloth. Any brush or gentle scourer used carefully will do the trick of cleaning away every particle without effort and without damage to the surface. Allowing pans to boil dry is the biggest danger for non-stick pans, so, when cooking vegetables, keep an eye on the water levels!

Non-scratch implements

Wooden spoons and spatulas, Teflon (or similar) coated tools and others marked as suitable for use with non-stick surfaces are a must. If you continue to use metal forks, spoons and spatulas, you will scratch and spoil the non-stick surface of pans. Treat the surfaces kindly, and good non-stick pans will last for years.

Other equipment

You will no doubt already have some of the items listed below, but I have made the list as comprehensive as possible, including the things I use most often.

Aluminium foil
Baking parchment
Chopping boards (1 small, 1 medium, 1 large)
Clingfilm
Colander (1 small and 1 large)
Fish kettle (stainless steel)
Flour shaker
Food processor
Garlic press
Good quality can opener
Juicer
Kitchen paper
Kitchen scales (ones that weigh small amounts accurately)
Lemon squeezer
Measuring jugs (1 × ½ litre/1 pint, 1 × 1 litre/2 pints)
Melon baller
Mixing bowls (1 × 1 litre/2 pints, 1 × 2 litres/4 pints, 1 × 4 litres/8 pints)
Multi-surface grater
Ovenproof dishes
Palette knife

Pasta spoon (non-scratch)
Pastry brush
Pepper mill
Pizza cutter
Plastic containers with lids
Potato masher (non-scratch)
Ramekin dishes
Rolling pin
Scissors
Set of sharp knives (all sizes)
Sieve (1 small and 1 large)
Slotted spoon (non-scratch)
Steamer
Vegetable peeler
Whisk (balloon type)
Wire rack
Zester

Store cupboard

There are many items that are very useful to have in stock. Build up your store cupboard over a period of time to avoid a marathon shopping trip!

Arrowroot
Cornflour
Plain flour
Self-raising flour
Gelatine
Marmite
Bovril
Dried herbs
Tomato ketchup
HP sauce
Fruity sauce
Barbecue sauce
Reduced oil salad dressing
Balsamic vinegar
White wine vinegar
Black peppercorns
Salt
White pepper
Vegetable stock cubes
Chicken stock cubes
Beef stock cubes
Lamb stock cubes
Pork stock cubes
Long-grain easy cook rice
Basmati rice
Pasta
Oats
Tabasco sauce
Soy sauce
Worcestershire sauce
Caster sugar
Brown sugar
Artificial sweetener

fresh items
Eggs
Fresh herbs
Garlic
Lemons
Oranges
Tomatoes

Low-fat cooking techniques

Dry-frying meat and poultry

The secret of dry-frying is to have your non-stick pan over the correct heat. If it's too hot, the pan will dry out the food too soon and the contents will burn. If the heat is too low, you lose the crispness recommended for a stir-fry. Practice makes perfect and a simple rule is to preheat the pan until it is quite hot (but not too hot!) before adding any of the ingredients. Test if the pan is hot enough by adding a piece of meat or poultry. The pan is at the right temperature if the meat sizzles on contact. Add the rest of the meat or poultry and toss it around. Once it is sealed on all sides (when it changes colour) you can reduce the heat a little as you add your seasonings, followed by vegetables and any other ingredients.

Cooking meat and poultry is simple, as the natural fat and juices run out almost immediately, providing plenty of moisture to prevent burning.

When cooking mince, I dry-fry it first and place it in a colander to drain away any fat that has emerged. I wipe out the pan with kitchen paper to remove any fatty residue and then return the meat to the pan to continue cooking my shepherd's pie or bolognese sauce.

Dry-frying vegetables

Vegetables contain their own juices and soon release them when they become hot, so dry-frying works just as well for vegetables as it does for meat and poultry. When dry-frying vegetables, it's important not to overcook them. They should be crisp and colourful so that they retain their flavour and most of their nutrients. Perhaps the most impressive results are with onions. When they are dry-fried, after a few minutes they go from being raw to translucent and soft and then on to become brown and caramelised. They taste superb and look for all the world like fried onions but taste so much better without all that fat.

Good results are also obtained when dry-frying large quantities of mushrooms, as they 'sweat' and make lots of liquid. Using just a few mushrooms produces a less satisfactory result unless you are stir-frying them with lots of other vegetables. If you are using a small quantity, therefore, you may find it preferable to cook them in vegetable stock.

Alternatives to frying with fat

Wine, water, soy sauce, wine vinegar, balsamic vinegar, and even fresh lemon juice all provide liquid in which food can be cooked. Some thicker types of sauces can dry out too fast if added early on in cooking, but these can be added later when there is more moisture in the pan.

When using wine or water, make sure the pan is hot before adding the other ingredients so that they sizzle in the hot pan.

Flavour enhancers

Low-fat cooking can be bland and dry, so it's important to add moisture and/or extra flavour to compensate for the lack of fat.

I have found that adding freshly ground black pepper to just about any savoury dish is a real flavour enhancer. You need a good pepper mill and you should buy your peppercorns whole and in large quantities. Ready ground black pepper is nowhere near as good. Sometimes it has other things mixed with the ground pepper, so give this one a miss.

When cooking rice, pasta and vegetables, I always add a vegetable stock cube to the cooking water. Although the stock cube does contain a little fat, the amount that is absorbed by the food is negligible and the benefit in flavour is very noticeable. I always save the water I've used to cook vegetables to make soups, gravy and sauces. Again, the fat from the stock cube that will be contained in a single serving is very small.

When making sandwiches, spread sauces such as Branston, mustard, horseradish and low-fat or fat-free dressings straight onto the bread. This helps the inside of the sandwich to stay 'put' and, because these sauces or dressings are quite highly flavoured, you won't miss the butter. Make sure you use fresh bread for maximum taste.

Here is a quick reference list of ingredients or cooking methods that can be substituted for traditional high-fat ones.

Cheese sauces Use small amounts of low-fat Cheddar, a little made-up mustard and skimmed milk with cornflour.

Custard Use custard powder and follow the instructions on the packet, using skimmed milk and artificial sweetener in place of sugar to save calories.

Cream Instead of double cream or whipping cream, use 0% fat Greek yogurt or low-fat fromage frais. Do not boil. For single cream, substitute low-fat natural or vanilla-flavoured yogurt or fromage frais.

Cream cheese Use Quark (skimmed soft cheese).

Creamed potatoes Mash the potatoes in the normal way and add fromage frais in place of butter or cream. Season well.

French dressing Use two parts apple juice to one part wine vinegar, and add a teaspoon of Dijon mustard.

Mayonnaise Use fromage frais mixed with two parts cider vinegar to one part lemon juice, plus a little turmeric and sugar.

Marie Rose dressing Use reduced oil salad dressing mixed with yogurt, tomato ketchup and a dash of Tabasco sauce and black pepper.

Porridge Cook with water and make to a sloppy consistency. Cover and leave overnight. Reheat before serving and serve with cold milk and sugar or honey.

Roux Make a low-fat roux by adding dry plain flour to a pan containing the other ingredients and 'cooking off' the flour. Then add liquid to thicken. Alternatively, use cornflour mixed with cold water or milk. Bring to the boil and cook for 2–3 minutes.

Thickening for sweet sauces Arrowroot, slaked in cold water or juice, is good because it becomes translucent when cooked.

Herbs

Herbs are fine fragrant plants that have been used to enhance and flavour food since the development of the art of cookery. As well as adding the finishing touches to a dish, many are attributed with hidden medicinal strengths that contribute to our wellbeing. Never before has there been such a wide variety of herbs introduced to our palate, from Mediterranean influences and worldwide cultures. You can buy them fresh, freeze-dried or dried, or grow your own. They all have an important role to play. Since dried herbs have a stronger flavour, they should be used more sparingly than fresh ones.

Fresh herbs fall into two categories: hard wood and soft leaf. Generally, hard wood herbs, such as rosemary, thyme and bay, are added at the beginning of a recipe in order to allow the herbs to soften and release their flavours. Soft leaf herbs, such as parsley, chervil, and basil, have more delicate flavours and are added near the end of cooking time so that they retain their flavour.

Spices

Spices were originally used to disguise ill-flavoured meat and sour foods as a result of insufficient means of chilled storage. Mainly derived from distant shores such as Sri Lanka and the East Indies, spices have over the years developed into flavour-enhancing additions. Today, they are appreciated for their aroma, colour and ability to blend together to give unique flavours.

Since spices are made from seeds, they are quite high in fat. However, because of the relatively small quantities used in recipes, their fat content is insignificant.

Spices can be kept longer than herbs, although once opened they will deteriorate. Keep out of direct sun and seal well after use.

The strongest flavours are achieved by grinding fresh seeds or whole spices as opposed to buying them already ground.

Always add spices at the beginning of a recipe, as they need to be allowed to 'cook out' to allow the flavour to develop fully. Berries such as juniper need to be crushed before cooking to release their flavours, whereas some spices such as fennel or cumin seeds benefit from being toasted in a non-stick pan.

The best way is to experiment with different spices, adding them in tiny quantities, to give a unique flavour to your cookery.

Further food tips

Rice

Rice is a nutritious, energy-giving carbohydrate food which is cheap to buy, convenient to cook and a great standby to have in your store cupboard. 25g (that's 1oz) dry weight rice gives you 100 calories. When it is cooked it will weigh 65g (2½oz). If you want to lose weight you should monitor the quantity carefully and stick to the portion sizes given. Other family members can of course eat more. Enhance the flavour of your boiled rice by adding a vegetable stock cube to the cooking water. First bring the water to the boil, then add the stock cube and then the rice. I find 'easycook' long-grain rice is the best, as it doesn't require any rinsing once it's been cooked and keeps hold of some of the flavour from the stock cube.

Pasta

Pasta is another useful high-energy carbohydrate. It is low in fat and comes in all shapes and sizes, giving great versatility to your meal planning. 25g (1oz) dry weight pasta gives you 80 calories and weighs 75g (3oz) when cooked. Watch the portion sizes while you are trying to lose weight. Family members who are not on a weight-reducing diet can of course have larger portions. As with rice and vegetables, you can enhance the flavour of pasta by adding a vegetable stock cube to the cooking water before adding the pasta. This removes the need to add butter or oil during cooking or serving.

Yogurt

Yogurt is a great low-fat protein food. It comes in so many different flavours these days and is a great aid to any menu. Although most yogurt falls within the 4% fat rule, the calorie content can vary significantly because of its sugar content. Always check the calories per pot from the nutrition label before you buy. For a thicker, creamier natural yogurt, try 0% Greek yogurt, and if you're buying natural fromage frais, look for the Normandy variety, which is creamier, smoother and more luxurious.

Milk

On the diet you can have skimmed or semi-skimmed milk. Skimmed milk is excellent if you like it because it contains less fat and fewer calories than semi-skimmed or full-fat milk. The only problem is that many people find skimmed milk too watery – I know I do – and prefer semi-skimmed milk, which is 2% fat. This is perfectly acceptable on a weight-reducing plan. Milk is our main source of calcium and we need to drink 450ml (¾ pint) milk each day in order to obtain sufficient quantities. Both skimmed and semi skimmed milk contain more calcium than the full-fat milk. If you don't like milk you will need to take a calcium supplement. Ask your pharmacist for advice. Alternatively you could eat 3 × 150g pots of low-fat yogurt, but the total calories should not exceed 200 for all three.

Spreads, sauces and dressings

I recommend that you make your sandwiches without butter on your bread, so you may like to use some of the low-fat sauces listed earlier to moisten the bread and to help hold the filling intact. If you really can't bear your bread without low-fat spread, find one that is no more than 5% fat and use sparingly. If you must use butter or polyunsaturated margarine, deduct the calories from your 150-calorie daily treat allowance.

There are lots of sauces, such as tomato ketchup, mustard, BBQ sauce, pickle, HP fruity sauce, that are really useful to spice up your food and add moisture. Any 95% fat free salad dressing is acceptable, too, and some reduced-oil salad dressings up to 9% fat can be used in moderation. Tartare and horseradish sauce can also be taken in moderation. If any of these are used in small quantities there is no need to count the calories.

Fruit and vegetables

Fruit and vegetables are very important for good health and have an important part to play with any diet plan. You should aim to eat at least five portions of fruit and/or vegetables each day. One portion means approximately 115g (4oz). If you take your fruit in juice form, 150ml or a quarter of a pint will give you an average of 50 calories per portion. So your recommended daily intake could be taken as an apple and a pear, or perhaps 115g (4oz) grapes and 115g (4oz) strawberries, plus a salad and/or vegetables at lunch or dinner.

To enhance the flavour of vegetables during cooking, place a vegetable stock cube in the cooking water. If you do this there is no need to add salt and the cooking water is great for making gravy.

Just remember to count the calories of your fruit and vegetables into your daily total of calories. If vegetables are included in the menus listed, there is no need to count the calories, as they are already included in the meal calculations.

Drinks

It is important to drink sufficient fluids to stay healthy. I recommend that you drink as much water as possible and, of course, it's calorie free. I don't believe it matters whether it's carbonated or still. Diet drinks are also allowed freely on this weight-reducing plan. You can also drink unlimited quantities of tea and coffee, using the milk from your daily allowance. If you take sugar in your drinks you need to remember to include the calories in your daily allowance.

Alcoholic drinks are also permissible, but the calories for those should be taken from your treat allowance unless you have a higher daily allowance of calories than 1400.

It's important to be aware that, while fruit juices are healthy, they are quite high in calories. However, you could drink 150ml (¼ pint) in place of a fruit portion, if you wish.

The Eat Yourself Slim diet

I hope you will find this diet the easiest healthy eating plan ever. Before you start you must calculate your personal calorie allowance as directed on pages 19–20. This allowance is based on the number of calories that you would burn up if you stayed in bed all day, doing absolutely nothing. Eating sufficient calories each day to meet this basic requirement will help your body believe it isn't dieting, which in turn helps to maintain your metabolic rate – that's the rate at which you burn food. If you stick closely to this calorie allowance, the great news is that every bit of physical activity that you do once you get out of bed in the morning is going to be fuelled from the fat stores around your body, so the more active you are, the more calories you will burn and the more weight you will lose.

All you have to do is select a breakfast, lunch, dinner and dessert of your choice from the already calorie counted meal suggestions so that the total doesn't exceed your daily allowance. Remember to include in your daily total the 200 calories for your milk allowance and your 150-calorie treat if you have it. If you eat fruit or anything else outside of meal times you must include the calories in your total. If you have plenty of calories to play with because of your age or weight, you can always select a meal and then supplement it with more bread, rice, pasta, fruit, or whatever. But remember, high-fat foods can only be taken from your treat allowance.

As I have explained earlier, there is no need to worry about the total fat grams per portion in a recipe, as most of the ingredients will be 4% fat or less. The exception to this is oily fish, which is higher than 4% but needs to be included for good health. There is also the occasional ingredient such as low-fat Cheddar cheese, which, even in small quantities, can make a tasty low-fat vegetarian dish.

This diet is wholly versatile. If you would like one of the lunches for your main evening meal you can have it. You can increase or reduce the serving size, you can add or subtract different accompaniments. The secret is to make it work for you and it will do if you keep within your calorie allowance.

I want to help you achieve real success so that you'll never look back. I want you to experience happiness, confidence and, most importantly, better health for you and your family in the future. If you adopt this way of eating long term, you will be making a very great step forward. On the next few pages I offer you a selection of meals which have been calorie counted for your convenience.

The diet

(V) = suitable for vegetarians

Daily allowance

450ml (3/4 pint) skimmed or semi-skimmed milk
1 × 150-calorie treat

BREAKFASTS

150-calorie breakfasts

1 (V) 2 slices light bread, toasted, plus 2 teaspoons honey, marmalade or preserve

2 (V) 50g (2oz) portion of any unsweetened bran cereal served with milk from allowance and 1 teaspoon sugar

3 (V) Fresh fruit platter, approximately 350g (12oz) in weight, of any fresh fruit of your choice in addition to your allowance

4 (V) 1 medium banana chopped into 1 low-fat yogurt (maximum 70 kcal)

5 (V) 1/2 grapefruit; 1 small egg, boiled or poached, served on 1 slice light bread, toasted

6 (V) 30g (1 1/4oz) portion of any chocolate-coated cereal served with milk from allowance, plus 1 piece fresh fruit of your choice excluding bananas

7 (V) 30g (1 ¼oz) portion of any sugar-coated cereal served with milk from allowance; 1 piece fresh fruit

8 (V) 2 × 100g pots of low-fat yogurt (maximum 150 kcal in total)

9 (V) 1 small banana sliced, 50g (2oz) strawberries, sliced and mixed with 1 × 100g low-fat yogurt or fromage frais (maximum 70 kcal)

10 (V) 2 slices light bread, toasted, topped with 2 heaped tablespoons baked beans

250-calorie breakfasts

1 1 × 50g (2oz) bread roll spread with mustard or pickle and filled with 75g (3oz) wafer thin ham, pastrami or chicken

2 (V) 50g (2oz) porridge oats cooked with water and served with milk from allowance, 2 teaspoons honey or brown sugar

3 1 egg, dry-fried or poached, served with 2 turkey rashers plus unlimited grilled mushrooms and tomatoes and 1 medium slice wholemeal toast

4 (V) 2 M&S pikelets, toasted and spread with 1 teaspoon preserve of your choice and topped with 2 teaspoons low-fat Greek yogurt

5 (V) 50g (2oz) portion of sweetened muesli served with milk from allowance and topped with 1 chopped apple

6 2 slices light bread, toasted, topped with 1 small can (205g) baked beans plus 1 grilled turkey rasher

7 (V) 225g (8oz) fresh cherries plus 1 × 150g pot low-fat yogurt, any flavour (maximum 150 kcal)

8 (V) 2 medium slices wholemeal toast spread with 2 teaspoons marmalade or preserve

9 (V) ½ a melon seeded and filled with 115g (4oz) fresh raspberries and topped with 1 × 150g pot of low-fat yogurt of your choice (maximum 150 kcal)

10 (V) 1 medium banana, 115g (4oz) strawberries plus 1 × 150g low-fat yogurt or fromage frais, any flavour

LUNCHES

250-calorie lunches

1 3 slices light wholemeal bread spread with low-calorie reduced-fat salad dressing and filled with unlimited salad vegetables plus 25g (1oz) wafer thin ham or chicken or beef or low-fat cottage cheese

2 50g (2oz) salmon, mackerel or trout, 1 teaspoon horseradish sauce plus large salad tossed in 2 teaspoons reduced-fat salad dressing; 1 banana

3 (V) 350g (12oz) chopped salad vegetables (e.g. peppers, onions, tomatoes, cucumber, celery, carrots, baby sweetcorn) with soy

sauce to taste plus 1 chicken drumstick (all skin removed) or 1 small can (205g) baked beans

4 (V) 1 × 115g (4oz) jacket potato topped with 50g (2oz) cottage cheese mixed with 2 garlic cloves, crushed, ½ teaspoon dried mixed herbs and 1 teaspoon low-fat natural fromage frais or yogurt, plus large salad tossed in fat free dressing

5 (V) 2 × 48g soft brown bread rolls, filled with salad and 50g (2oz) low-fat cottage cheese

6 (V) Any prepacked sandwich or snack with no more than 250 calories and 4% fat

7 1 medium wholemeal pitta slit open and filled first with shredded lettuce then topped with 50g (2oz) tuna (in brine) mixed with 25g (1oz) canned sweetcorn and 1 teaspoon reduced-fat salad dressing

8 (V) Cream of asparagus soup (page 62) served with 50g (2oz) French bread plus 1 piece fresh fruit

9 (V) Simple tomato and roast garlic soup (page 60) served with 115g (4oz) French bread, plus 1 low-fat yogurt (maximum 70 kcal)

10 Black bean and smoked bacon soup (page 61) served with 1 slice light bread

11 (V) Sweetcorn and red pepper soup (page 66) served with 50g (2oz) French bread and 1 large banana

12 (V) Spiced cauliflower soup (page 72) served with 50g (2oz) French bread, and 1 low-fat yogurt (maximum 70 kcal)

13 (V) Sundried tomato hummus with roasted summer vegetables (page 168) plus 1 medium banana

14 (V) Potato and spinach soufflé (page 124) served with a mixed salad and 1 piece fresh fruit

15 Hattie's crunchy baked chicken (page 97) served with a large mixed salad tossed in oil free dressing, plus 1 piece fresh fruit

16 (V) 2 Roasted pepper tarts (page 158) served with a large mixed salad tossed in oil-free dressing

17 (V) Spanish omelette (page 133) served with a green side salad

18 (V) 3 pieces of any fresh fruit, 1 medium banana and 1 pot low-fat yogurt (maximum 70 kcal)

300-calorie lunches

1 Lobster couscous salad (page 108) served with chopped green salad topped with cherry tomatoes

2 Red Thai beef (page 86) served with 25g (1oz) [dry weight] boiled rice and a side salad

3 Salt cod and red pepper brandade (page 168) served with 50g (2oz) crusty bread

4 Smoked mackerel and sweet mustard pâté (page 166) served with 2 slices light bread, toasted

5 Omelette made with 2 eggs whisked together with a little milk. Season well and cook in a non-stick frying pan. When half-cooked, add unlimited peas, sweetcorn, chopped peppers and 50g (2oz) diced cooked ham. Serve with salad

6 Griddled swordfish with tomato and lime salsa (page 111) served with 115g (4oz) new potatoes, plus salad; 1 kiwi fruit

7 (V) Any prepacked readymade wholemeal sandwich with up to 300 kcal or 250 kcal plus 1 apple or pear

8 1 medium jacket potato (approximately 180g) topped with one of the following:
- (V) 50g (2oz) baked beans, plus salad
- (V) 50g (2oz) low-fat cottage cheese (with flavourings if desired), plus salad
- 50g (2oz) salmon or tuna (in brine) mixed with reduced-oil salad dressing, plus salad

9 4 slices 'light' wholemeal bread spread with Waistline or similar dressing. Fill with mixed salad ingredients plus 115g (4oz) wafer thin ham, chicken, beef, turkey or 150g (5oz) low-fat cottage cheese

10 French bread margarita (page 130) served with a large salad tossed in low-fat dressing

11 Minted green pea and cucumber soup (page 168) served with 50g (2oz) crusty bread and 2 piece fresh fruit

12 Thai noodle soup (page 78) plus 1 piece fresh fruit and 1 × 150g (5oz) pot low-fat yogurt (maximum 70 kcal)

13 Celeriac and nutmeg soup (page 74) with 50g (2oz) crusty bread plus 2 pieces fresh fruit.

14 (V) Papaya, beansprout and hot banana salad (page 192), plus Lime cheesecake ice cream (page 150)

15 (V) Quick vegetable korma (page 118) served with 50g (2oz) [dry weight] boiled rice

16 (V) Honey roast corn on the cob (page 193) served with chopped salad and 25g (1oz) crusty bread

DINNERS

400-calorie dinners

1 Hot pan smoked duck with orange salad (page 106) served with 175g (6oz) new potatoes and unlimited other vegetables of your choice

2 225g (8oz) any white fish cooked without fat and served with 225g (8oz) potatoes plus unlimited other vegetables and low-fat parsley sauce

3 115g (4oz) salmon cooked without fat and served with 175g (6oz) potatoes plus unlimited other vegetables and 2 teaspoons tartare sauce

4 115g (4oz) lean lamb or pork steak (all visible fat removed) served with 115g (4oz) new potatoes plus unlimited other vegetables and low-fat gravy

5 3 low-fat sausages (max 4% fat) served with 115g (4oz) mashed potatoes plus unlimited other vegetables and low-fat gravy

6 175g (6oz) calf's or lamb's liver, braised with onions in low-fat gravy served with 115g (4oz) mashed potatoes and unlimited other vegetables of your choice

7 (V) Cherry tomato and courgette tarte tatin (page 122) served with Garlic and herb roasted new potatoes (page 195), plus a large mixed salad tossed in oil-free dressing

8 Seafood pie (page 114) served with 50g (2oz) French bread and a green salad

9 (V) Any 95% fat free readymeal (maximum 400 kcal including accompaniments)

10 (V) 1 dry-fried egg, 3 grilled turkey rashers or 1 vegetarian burger, 3 grilled tomatoes, 115g (4oz) mushrooms boiled in vegetable stock, plus 175g (6oz) 95% fat-free oven chips and 115g (4oz) peas served with sauce of your choice

11 (V) Spiced creamy vegetables with coconut milk (page 126) served with 25g (1oz) [dry weight] boiled rice, sweet mango chutney and cucumber salad

12 (V) Aubergine and spinach pasta bake (page 142) served with unlimited vegetables excluding potatoes

13 Jamaican jerk chicken (page 98) served with a small green salad

14 Pot roast lamb with celery and peppers (page 94) served with 115g (4oz) potatoes

500-calorie dinners

1 Stir-fried chicken (serves 4): chop 450g (1lb) skinned chicken breasts and season well. Dry-fry in a non-stick pan with unlimited chopped mushrooms, peppers, onion, mange tout (or any vegetables of your choice) until half-cooked. Add 1 jar of any readymade sauce (max. 4% fat) and heat thoroughly. Serve with boiled rice (50g/2oz dry weight per person)

2 1 × 175g (6oz) gammon steak grilled, served with 1 slice pineapple, pineapple sauce plus 175g (6oz) potatoes and unlimited vegetables. To make a pineapple sauce, thicken pineapple juice with cornflour or arrowroot mixed with a little cold water and cook for 2 minutes

3 Pork Provençale (page 89) served with 175g (6oz) potatoes and unlimited other vegetables

4 Preserved lemon chicken (page 100) served with 50g (2oz)[dry-weight] rice and 225g (8oz) other seasonal vegetables

5 Balsamic pork chop with tangerine (page 91) served with 175g (6oz) potatoes and 300g (10oz) other seasonal vegetables

6 Coconut roasted sea bass wrapped in banana leaves (page 180) served with unlimited vegetables excluding potatoes

7 115 (4oz) lean steak, grilled, served with 115g (4oz) jacket potato or new potatoes plus grilled tomatoes, mushrooms cooked in stock and unlimited other vegetables

8 2 lamb chops or steaks trimmed of all visible fat, grilled and served with 115g (4oz) potatoes and unlimited other vegetables, mint sauce and low-fat gravy

9 Baked trout with smoked garlic and pesto topping (page 181) served with 115g (4oz) new potatoes plus a large salad

10 Hot pan smoked salmon (page 184) served with 115g (4oz) new potatoes plus 300g (10oz) other seasonal vegetables

11 Griddled lamb's liver with tomato and bacon salsa (page 93) served with 115g (4oz) new potatoes and salad

12 (V) Lentil and roast vegetable loaf (page 132) served with 1 medium (approximately 180g) jacket potato

13 (V) Leek and sundried tomato risotto (page 140) served with 75g (3oz) French bread and a green salad

14 Chicken spaghetti (page 138) served with 75g (3oz) French bread and green salad

PUDDINGS

Here is a selection of puddings which you may or may not choose to include in your everyday eating plan. Some are as quick as just a couple of pieces of fresh fruit, or a branded readymade pudding, or you can make one of the delicious recipes included in this book. Any of these would grace a dinner party or could be offered as a treat for the family.

All these puddings are low in fat and so do not need to be included in your treat allowance unless you have no other calories to play with.

100-calorie puddings

1 (V) Fresh fruit salad verde (page 149)

2 (V) 1 meringue nest topped with 25g (1oz) any fresh fruit and 1 tablespoon low-fat yogurt

3 (V) 2 scoops fruit sorbet

4 1 × 150g pot low-fat yogurt or fromage frais (maximum 100 kcal)

5 Raspberry bavarois (page 154)

6 (V) 150g Total 0% fat Greek yogurt mixed with 1 level teaspoon runny honey

7 (V) Mango and white rum ice (page 147)

8 (V) Chestnut meringue roulade (page 148)

9 Orange Panna Cotta with fresh orange (page 153)

10 (V) Kiwi and passion fruit salad with balsamic dressing (page 156)

150-calorie puddings

1 (V) Lime cheesecake ice cream (page 150)

2 (V) Cinnamon and lemon prunes with saffron fromage frais (page 146)

3 (V) Burgundy poached peaches with strawberry salsa (page 152)

4 (V) 225g (8oz) strawberries topped with 115g (4oz) Wall's 'Too Good to be True' iced dessert

5 (V) 2 × 150g pots low-fat yogurt (maximum 150 kcal in total)

6 (V) 175g (6oz) fresh fruit salad topped with 1 × 150g low-fat yogurt (maximum 100 kcal)

7 (V) 1 meringue nest filled with 50g (2oz) fresh fruit plus 2 tablespoons low-fat yogurt or fromage frais

8 1 × 125g pot ready-to-eat raspberry flavour jelly topped with 175g (6oz) fresh raspberries

9 (V) 150ml ($\frac{1}{4}$ pint) instant custard made with semi-skimmed milk plus $\frac{1}{2}$ a small chopped banana

10 (V) 75g (3oz) dried apricots

TREATS

Here is a selection of treats from which you may choose each day, or save up for a bigger one. Some are low fat (less than 4% fat) and some are high fat. The choice is yours. Don't feel guilty if you want to select from the high-fat ones. Have your treat and enjoy it but then stop. If you find that having a taste of chocolate sets you off on a chocolate binge, then don't tempt yourself again for the moment. In time you may be able to be satisfied with small amounts and find you *can* be trusted. Only you can know when you reach this healthy balance of a relaxed attitude to those foods that once controlled you. But please be assured it can be done. I've been there. I know! My passion for ice cream is well known but now I can keep tubs of Häagen-Dazs in the freezer and only eat it on special occasions. It has no hold over me any more. And when I do have some, it is just a scoop, not the whole tub!

If you know there is a food type that you just adore, acknowledge it to yourself. The last thing you should do is pretend that it isn't tempting! Avoid keeping it in the house until you think you can be trusted and when you do, only buy one (don't stock up) to limit your likely downfall. Only eat it *with* someone so that second and third helpings are more difficult. Savour the flavour and appreciate it. Once you've had it, forget about it and move on to do something that takes your mind off food. Then give yourself a great big pat on the back if you get to the end of the day without giving into temptation.

Remember it's fear that you won't be able to control your eating of it that makes your consciousness towards the 'treat' much more acute. Try to chill out about it. Yes you can have more – another day. This is not your last chance to eat it. Tomorrow it is not going to be declared a 'banned substance'! Relax!

150 calories (4% or less fat)

50g (2oz) seedless raisins
8 sponge fingers
50g (2oz) slice malt loaf
6 Trebor barley sugars
10 Liquorice Allsorts
1 packet fruit gums
115g (4oz) oven chips
3 Matteson's turkey rashers, grilled and served on 1 medium slice wholemeal bread
1 × 150g pot low-fat custard plus ½ small chopped banana

150 calories (more than 4% fat)

30g bag potato hoops
39g Cadbury's Crème Egg
1 snack size Picnic
2 treat size bags Cadbury's Chocolate Buttons
1 Dime bar
5 chocolate orange éclair sweets
2 Wispa treat size bars
25g (1oz) Bombay Mix
4 Cadbury's Roses chocolates
25g bag ready salted crisps
10 Peardrop sweets

200 calories (more than 4% fat)

25g (1oz) butter
1 onion bhaji
1 small avocado
2 level tablespoons mayonnaise
30g (1¼oz) Bombay Mix
50g (2Oz) Parmesan cheese

250 calories (more than 4% fat)

25ml (1fl oz) oil (all varieties)
1 vegetable samosa
50ml (2fl oz) double cream
30ml (1½fl oz) clotted cream
50g (2oz) taramasalata

300 calories (more than 4% fat)

3 large chocolate Digestive biscuits
4 Ferrero Rocher chocolates
1 Bounty bar
65g size Mars bar
61g Snickers bar
6 McDonald's Chicken McNuggets
1 chip shop cod in batter
49g bar Cadbury's Dairy Milk
49g bar Cadbury's Wholenut
60g bag Skittles

450 calories (more than 4% fat)

85g bar Galaxy
100g Mars bar
1 McDonald's milk shake
115g (4oz) After Eight mints
115g (4oz) Quality Street chocolates
115g (4oz) Cheddar cheese
1 Sharwoods Pot Noodle (Chinese curry flavour)

9 McDonald's Chicken McNuggets
1 McDonald's Quarter Pounder
1 portion McDonald's Large Fries

Fat and calorie content of foods

Here are some at-a-glance calorie calculations to help you plan your meals.

	Per 100g	
	Kcal	*Fat (%)*
Meat products		
Beefburgers	265	20.5
Black pudding	305	21.9
Corned beef	217	12.1
Cornish pasty	332	20.4
Faggots	268	18.5
Haggis	310	21.7
Luncheon meat	313	26.9
Meat paste	173	11.2
Pâté	316	28.9
Pork pie	376	27.0
Salami	491	45.2
Sausage roll	477	36.4
Sausages	299	24.1
Steak and kidney pie	323	21.2
Stewed steak (canned)	176	12.5
Bolognese sauce	145	11.1
Moussaka	184	13.6
Shepherd's pie	118	6.2
White fish		
Cod	76	0.7
Haddock	73	0.6

	Per 100g	
	Kcal	*Fat (%)*
Halibut	92	2.4
Lemon sole	81	1.4
Plaice	91	2.2
Whiting	92	0.9
Fatty fish		
Anchovies	280	19.9
Herring	234	18.5
Kipper	205	11.4
Mackerel	223	16.3
Pilchards	126	5.4
Salmon	182	12.0
Sardines	177	11.6
Trout	135	4.5
Tuna in brine	99	0.6
Tuna in oil	189	9.0
Whitebait (fried)	525	47.5
Crab	127	5.2
Lobster	119	3.4
Prawns	107	1.8
Scampi	316	17.6
Shrimps	73	0.8
Cockles	48	0.3
Mussels	87	2.0
Squid	66	1.5
Fish cakes	188	10.5
Fish fingers	233	12.7
Fish paste	169	10.4
Fish pie	105	3.0
Kedgeree	166	7.9
Roe	202	11.9
Taramasalata	446	46.4

	Per 100g Kcal	Fat (%)
Fruit		
Apples	47	0.1
Apricots: fresh	31	0.1
dried	158	0.6
Avocado	190	19.5
Bananas	95	0.3
Blackberries	25	0.2
Blackcurrants	28	Tr
Cherries	48	0.1
Clementines	37	0.1
Currants	267	0.4
Damsons	34	Tr
Dates	227	0.2
Figs	209	1.5
Gooseberries	19	0.4
Grapefruit	30	0.1
Grapes	60	0.1
Kiwi	49	0.5
Lemons	19	0.3
Lychees	58	0.1
Mandarins (canned in juice)	32	Tr
Mangoes	57	0.2
Melon: cantaloupe	19	0.1
honeydew	28	0.1
watermelon	31	0.3
Mixed peel	231	0.9
Nectarines	40	0.1
Olives	103	11.0
Oranges	37	0.1
Passion fruit	36	0.4
Peaches	33	0.1
Paw paw	36	0.1
Pears	40	0.1
Pineapple	41	0.2
Plums	36	0.1
Prunes	79	0.2
Raisins	272	0.4
Raspberries	25	0.3
Rhubarb	7	0.1
Satsumas	36	0.1
Strawberries	27	0.1
Sultanas	275	0.4
Tangerines	35	0.1
Vegetables		
Asparagus	25	0.6
Aubergine	15	0.4
Baked Beans	84	0.6
Beans: green	24	0.5
broad	81	0.6
red kidney	103	0.5
butter	77	0.5
runner	22	0.4
Beetroot (raw)	36	0.1
Broccoli	33	0.9
Brussels sprouts	42	1.4
Beansprouts	31	0.5
Cabbage	26	0.4
Carrots	35	0.3
Cauliflower	34	0.9

	Per 100g Kcal	Fat (%)
Celery	7	0.2
Chicory	11	0.6
Courgettes	18	0.4
Cucumber	10	0.1
Curly kale	33	1.6
Fennel	12	0.2
Leeks	22	0.5
Lettuce	14	0.5
Marrow	12	0.2
Mushrooms	13	0.5
Okra	31	1.0
Potatoes	75	0.2
Onions	36	0.2
Parsnips	66	1.2
Peas	83	1.5
Peas: mange tout	32	0.2
Peppers	20	0.6
Pumpkin	13	0.2
Quorn	86	3.5
Radish	12	0.2
Runner beans	22	0.4
Spinach	25	0.8
Spring greens	33	1.0
Spring onions	23	0.5
Swede	24	0.3
Sweetcorn (canned)	23	0.4
Tomatoes	17	0.3
Turnips	23	0.3
Watercress	22	1.0

ALCOHOL

	Kcal
Beer 300ml (½ pint)	90
Cider 300ml (½ pint)	100
Cider vintage 300ml (½ pint)	280
Lager 300ml (½ pint)	90
Spirits: 1 pub measure	50
Wine: 150ml (5fl oz)	
Dry white	95
Sparkling	110
Rosé	100
Red	100

Non-alcoholic drinks

	Kcal
Fruit juice: 150ml (5fl oz)	
Apple	50
Grape	75
Grapefruit	50
Orange	50
Pineapple	70
Tomato	30
Squashes: 25ml (1fl oz) undiluted	30
Mixers: 120ml (4fl oz)	
Ginger ale	40
Bitter lemon	50
Dry ginger	25
Tonic water	35
Lemonade	30
Fizzy drinks: 330ml can	
Cola	130
Ginger beer	100
Lemonade	80

Motivation: finding the willpower

I am often asked how it's possible to drum up the willpower to stick to a diet and exercise regime. My experience shows that if you have a good enough reason for wanting to lose weight, you can definitely do it. Imagine if someone were to offer you £50,000 if you could lose all your excess weight by a certain date. Do you think you could do it? Yes, of course you could. Why? Because the reward would be great enough to inspire you to make the effort and put into practice all that was needed to achieve your goal. You'd pull out all the stops to ensure that nothing got in your way to make you to stray off course. Motivation and having a positive mental attitude are crucial to the success of your diet and fitness campaign, as indeed they are in any aspect of life. Those people who just drift through life tend to get nowhere. It is the ones who have the motivation to succeed who become the great achievers.

Here are my top ten tips to help you get in the right frame of mind. Take these on board, and you will be well on the way to becoming a great achiever.

Set yourself some goals

If you want to lose weight and get fit you need to have some goals. In this instance I am not talking about losing a set amount of inches or being able to get into a size 10, but a goal that provides a deadline for you to work towards and a reason for losing as much weight as possible by that date. Be realistic – don't expect to lose four stone in two months – but your goal should provide a sufficient challenge so that you have to concentrate your mind and energy to achieve it. Decide to join your local Rosemary Conley Diet and Fitness class, join a running or walking club, tennis club, dance class. Include some short-term and some long-term goals. Write them down.

As you achieve your first goal tick it off. Then you need to set another goal to *keep* you motivated. Even if you've already achieved your target weight, you still need an incentive to encourage you to stay at that weight.

Reward yourself

As you achieve each goal, it's important that you reward yourself. It may be sufficient to be able to look stunning in a new outfit at a wedding or special celebration but that is pretty short term. If you don't have a specific event to attend, then reward yourself with a day at a health spa, a meal out with your partner or friend, or treat yourself to a new outfit. You need to give yourself an enjoyable 'pat on the back' for making the effort. We deserve self-care time and we deserve reward for our efforts. And to remind yourself of what you have achieved, place tins or packets of food of an equivalent weight that you have lost in a carrier bag and keep it in your wardrobe. Pick it up often to remind yourself of your progress. Realise that you used to carry that weight around with you all the time – and now you don't.

Stop making excuses

There'll never be a week or month when there isn't a birthday, a special meal out, or a million and one other reasons why it isn't a good time to start a diet. Stop making excuses – I think I've heard them all – and get on with the job in hand. If you want to lose weight and get fit, you can. Only you can do it, but you have to want to do it badly enough.

Be realistic

Just as we cannot change our height or our genes, neither can we change our bone structure or our basic physiological shape. But there is an enormous amount we can do to improve the way we look. As well as losing weight, set yourself a goal to restyle your hair, maybe colour it. Have a 'colour analysis' so you only buy clothes in colours that suit you. Remember, too, that healthy eating and regular exercise can make us glow with health, tone us up as we slim down and give us a greater sense of wellbeing. Truly, you *can* transform yourself yet still be realistic.

Record your progress

It's so easy to forget what we looked like at our heaviest, so before you start your diet and fitness campaign, ask someone to take a couple of photographs of you – a front view and a side view. Next, find yourself a pair of tight-fitting trousers or a skirt and set this garment aside as your measuring tool. Try it on every few days so that you have tangible proof of how many inches you are actually losing. Often, we don't realise how much progress we are actually making and we need a constant reminder of our achievements.

Develop the habit of enthusiasm

Be enthusiastic and focus on the many benefits you will be enjoying within days of starting your diet and fitness campaign. Make a note in your diary of all the good things you feel about yourself. As your whole attitude towards yourself and your body changes your self-esteem will increase.

Remove temptation

It is essential that you remove temptation from your kitchen and place of work. If you must have any sort of high-fat foods in the house – chocolate, biscuits, crisps and so on – keep them stored away in a place that is difficult to reach or under lock and key. If the food isn't there, you won't miss it, but if it is staring you in the face every time you open the cupboard, you will find it very difficult to resist.

Learn to cope with the difficult times

No matter how determined and conscientious you may be, there'll be occasions when your willpower weakens and your determination begins to flag. If you do have a minor indiscretion – or even a major one – don't think you've ruined all your hard work so far. You haven't. Just get right back on track, eat normal meals for the rest of the day and try to be more physically active to compensate. Do not skip meals ever!

Keep a scrapbook of your success

Buy yourself a scrapbook and make a note in it of all the good things that happen to you from now on. Fill it with photographs of yourself as you lose each stone or each time you do something new, something that you wouldn't have done when you were overweight. Looking back at this scrapbook on the 'bad' days could provide you with just the motivation you need to continue.

Picture yourself succeeding

Picture yourself wearing that beautiful dress or suit that you have had in your wardrobe for years but haven't been able to get into. Visualise yourself standing tall and slim, full of confidence, feeling really healthy and fit with lots of energy. If you want a better body, you can have one.

Honestly you can achieve it. Start today. What have you got to lose, except those unwanted pounds and inches?

Here are ten benefits you will enjoy if you lose weight and get fitter.

1 Clothes will fit!

Your clothes size will reduce faster than you think. Very soon you will feel so good wearing smaller clothes and you'll look great in them.

2 More energy!

You will have lots more energy. At the moment as you walk around it's as if you are carrying around a shopping bag or even a suitcase. Imagine how different it will feel when you have shed some of that weight. You will feel like you're dancing on air.

3 Your body will change!

Your body shape will improve dramatically. No matter whether you are heart shaped, apple shaped or pear shaped, as you lose weight your general shape will improve and your figure will become much more balanced. You will be amazed at how a low-fat eating plan can help you to change shape and look better than you ever dreamed you could.

4 Fashionable clothes!

You will be able to wear more fashionable clothes and look terrific. Trendy outfits that you never dreamt you would be able to wear will look fabulous on you. Can you imagine how good you're going to feel when you walk into the fashion store and choose something off the smaller rail and every garment you try on looks great?

5 Your metabolic rate increases!

You can actually increase your metabolic rate through taking regular exercise, but it must be exercise that you enjoy. If you don't have fun exercising you are not going to carry on doing it, so it is crucial that you find a way of exercising that stimulates you. It can be going for a walk with the dog, playing football with the children, working out to one of my videos or going along to a fitness class. A combination of all of these is ideal as they all burn fat and all of them will make you fitter.

6 Feel fit! Feel healthy!

You will feel fitter and healthier. You will probably find that you don't have so many aches and pains. You will sleep better and will have more zest for life. It really is a win/win situation.

7 Stand by for compliments!

Be prepared to accept some compliments from your family and friends and when people comment that you've lost weight, try not to rebuff it and say: 'Well, I've still got a huge stomach or backside,' or whatever. Try to acknowledge the compliment as a generous gift and appreciate it. Say: 'I'm glad you can see the difference! I feel so much better now. Thank you!' You wouldn't like it if nobody commented, would you?

8 Confidence booster!

In a very short period of time you will find your self-confidence increasing greatly. You will find your whole attitude to life will improve and, amazingly, people won't irritate you so much! You will find you have more patience and your whole outlook on life will be a sunnier one. You may even find that you are better at doing your job. Even your relationship with your husband or partner and your children may improve. We just need to feel good about ourselves, and losing weight and getting fitter helps us achieve that.

9 Do your family a favour!

Don't feel that you have to cook special food just for you and give the family other foods. A healthy, low-fat diet is suitable for everyone, though very young children can be given additional foods that contain more fat, such as cheese, eggs and even a little butter.

10 Look ten years younger!

Without doubt, one of the things that I have noticed when we photograph the successful slimmers for my magazine is that they all look years younger than when they were overweight. Being overweight does make us look older, so if you want to look younger, lose those excesses. You'll be so glad you did. Teaching everyone healthy eating habits now will change their lives and their family's lives in the future. It is probably the best gift you could give them and, remember, *nothing* tastes as good as being slim feels!

Keeping trim for good

When you reach your goal weight you will feel on top of the world, but the big challenge is yet to come – keeping that weight off for ever.

Hopefully, on this diet, you have not found it too difficult to eat healthily yet enjoyably. The key now is to still keep to the low-fat way of cooking and eating. If you do, and you don't consciously *overeat*, then you shouldn't find maintaining your weight a problem. You will certainly find it easier if you keep up your activity levels and also refrain from nibbling between meals.

However, it is important that you eat more now than you did when you were trying to lose weight and you can be more relaxed with regard to carefully looking at the fat content of every food you buy. But beware the slippery slope of getting the taste for fat back again. Having a little butter on that bread roll in a restaurant, a little cream on your dessert, and chips more than occasionally can find you right back where you started. Just picture yourself as you felt then. Remember what you felt like, how tired you were all the time, how you never felt good in your clothes, how much older you looked, how much higher your blood pressure and/or cholesterol used to be. Don't go back there. You've done the hard work, don't throw it away now.

You know from the tables on pages 19–20 how many calories you need to eat to lose weight. When you reach your goal weight you need to gradually increase this total, initially by 200 calories daily and then a further 100 calories until you have increased your daily intake by around 600–800 calories, depending how physically active you are..

You may be thinking 'If I ate that much I know I will gain weight'. The fact is that most of us eat more calories than we think we do. So, in short, proceed with caution and you should be able to find the right level for you.

If you find you want to eat more, then just balance it with increased physical activity. Given time, your body (and your clothes) will tell you that your weight is either staying constant or increasing. I rarely weigh myself now – perhaps three or four times a year – as I know from the mirror and my clothes how I'm doing.

At our Rosemary Conley Diet and Fitness Clubs we do not pressurise the members who have reached their goal to weigh in every week. We suggest once a month is quite sufficient. What is so great about our classes is that whether you are aiming to lose weight or have reached your goal and are just maintaining your target weight, the exercise session included in the classes helps members burn fat and calories as well as keeping them fit and toned.

Some of the members in my own classes have been joining me every Monday night in Leicester for over 20 years! They have better, trimmer figures and much healthier bodies as a result. If I had been running a 'slimming only' club they would not have kept coming and would no doubt be much heavier and less healthy as a result.

So, keep up the good habits learnt within this or any of my earlier books. Keep as active as you can – any and every bit of activity will help to keep you slim.

Soups

The foundation of good soup lies in having fresh core ingredients coupled with a good flavoursome stock. These days, fresh stocks are readily available, along with bouillon stock powder, which simplifies the seasoning of soups and sauces. This instant powder can be sprinkled into the dish during cooking or at the finish, allowing total control over flavouring.

Soup has many forms, from clear crisp consommés garnished with baby vegetables or grains such as pearl barley, to others that are roux based, thickened with flour; a more substantial preparation is to purée, giving a rich, thick, velvety consistency.

Some of the recipes call for a little low-fat fromage frais stirred in just prior to serving. Low-fat Normandy fromage frais (available from most supermarkets) is preferable, as it is smoother than other brands. This adds a rich, creamy effect. Always use this as the finishing touch, as otherwise it may cause the soup to curdle if it is reboiled.

Simple tomato and roasted garlic soup

This soup requires forward thinking. The garlic needs to be roasted for approximately 45 minutes before you make the soup. Roasting the garlic gives it a much mellower flavour than usual, so it's a good idea to roast a couple of whole heads together while you have the oven on. Wrapped in foil, it will keep in the refrigerator for up to one week. It makes a good substitute for smoked garlic.

SERVES 4
PER SERVING:
62 KCAL/0.7G FAT
PREPARATION TIME:
5 MINUTES
COOKING TIME:
50 MINUTES

1 whole head garlic
3 × 400g (3 × 14oz) cans plum tomatoes
6 spring onions, finely chopped
3 teaspoons vegetable bouillon stock powder
1 tablespoon chopped fresh basil
salt and freshly ground black pepper

1. Preheat the oven to 200C, 400F, Gas Mark 6.
2. Remove the outer skin from the garlic bulb and slice the top off. Place in a square piece of foil and wrap around to form a parcel.
3. Place in the oven for 45 minutes until soft. Remove from the oven and allow to cool.
4. Pour the canned tomatoes into a liquidiser or food processor and purée until smooth.
5. Squeeze out the garlic purée from the roasted bulb and add to the food processor.
6. Push the mixture through a sieve into a saucepan to remove the tomato seeds. Add the spring onions and the vegetable stock with sufficient water to give a good consistency and bring to the boil. Stir in the basil.
7. Season to taste with salt and pepper and serve.

Black bean and smoked bacon soup

SERVES 6
PER SERVING:
182 KCAL/5G FAT
PREPARATION TIME:
20 MINUTES
COOKING TIME:
40–45 MINUTES

- 175g (6oz) black beans, soaked overnight
- 2 medium onions, finely chopped
- 2 carrots, finely diced
- 1 celery stick, finely diced
- 2 garlic cloves, crushed
- 1 teaspoon ground coriander
- 1.2 litres (2 pints) vegetable stock
- 1 tablespoon chopped fresh marjoram
- 2 bay leaves
- 115g (4oz) lean smoked bacon, finely chopped
- salt and freshly ground black pepper
- 4 tomatoes, peeled, seeded and finely chopped to garnish
- 2 tablespoons chopped fresh coriander to garnish

Serve this soup as a wholesome lunch or liquidise and serve as an evening soup flavoured with a little Madeira wine.

IMPORTANT: Black beans should always be soaked overnight and boiled rapidly for at least 10 minutes at the start of cooking. Do not eat uncooked beans.

1 After soaking overnight, rinse the black beans well in plenty of cold running water and place in a large saucepan with the onions, carrots, celery, garlic, ground coriander and stock.
2 Bring to the boil, and boil rapidly for 10 minutes, then reduce the heat to a gentle simmer, add the marjoram, bay leaves and smoked bacon. Cover and simmer gently for 40–45 minutes until the beans are soft.
3 Season to taste with salt and pepper and adjust the consistency, adding more stock if required.
4 Ladle into warmed serving bowls and garnish with the chopped tomato and fresh coriander.

Cream of asparagus soup

Asparagus can be bought in many different grades from thick jumbo stems to the thin fine spear. Choose a thick to medium thickness of stem, as the finer stems will disintegrate when cooked over this length of time.

SERVES 4
PER SERVING:
105 KCAL/1.3G FAT
PREPARATION TIME:
10 MINUTES
COOKING TIME:
30–35 MINUTES

225g (8oz) fresh asparagus
2 medium onions, finely chopped
2 garlic cloves, crushed
1 teaspoon chopped fresh thyme
450ml (3/4 pint) vegetable stock
1 tablespoon plain flour
450ml (3/4 pint) skimmed milk
2 bay leaves
salt and freshly ground black pepper
1 tablespoon chopped fresh chives to garnish

1 Prepare the asparagus by trimming away the stalk at the point where the stem breaks when snapped in half. Trim off the tips and reserve. Chop the remaining stems into small pieces.
2 In a non-stick pan dry-fry the onions until soft. Add the garlic and thyme and continue cooking for 1–2 minutes. Add 3 tablespoons of vegetable stock, then sprinkle the flour over and cook out for 1 minute, stirring well with a wooden spoon.
3 Gradually add the remaining stock along with the skimmed milk and asparagus stems. Add the bay leaves and gently simmer for 15–20 minutes until the asparagus is just cooked and the soup has slightly thickened.
4 Five minutes before serving stir in the asparagus tips and season to taste.
5 Serve piping hot garnished with chopped chives.

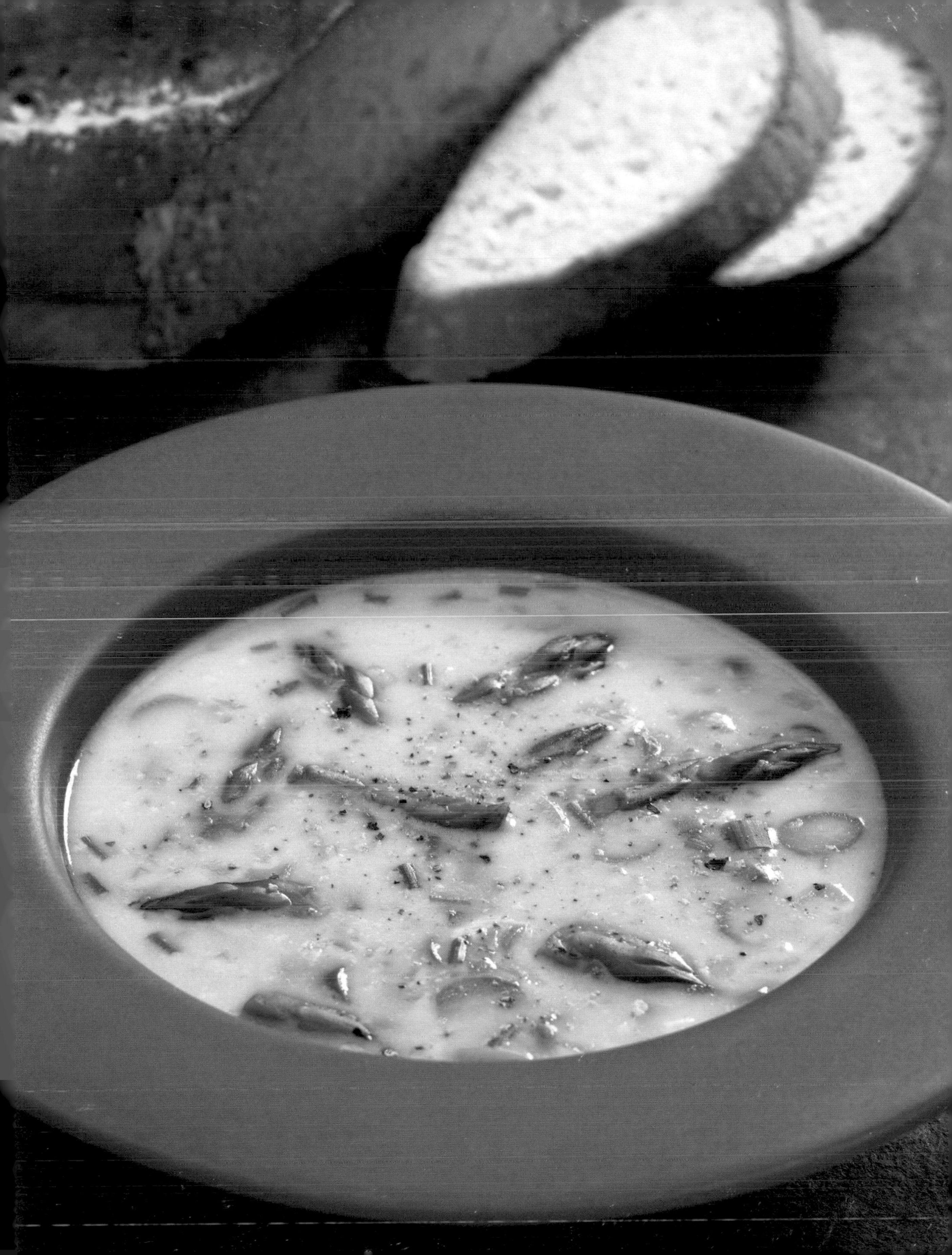

Cream of leek and wild mushroom soup

Be selective when buying dried mushrooms. Check for good-sized pieces, not broken or shrivelled dark flakes, as these can be hard and chewy when reconstituted. Adding a little lemon zest to the soup really enhances the strong mushroom flavours.

SERVES 4
PER SERVING:
91 KCAL/1.6G FAT
PREPARATION TIME:
10 MINUTES
COOKING TIME:
35–40 MINUTES

40g (1 ½oz) good quality dried wild mushrooms
2 garlic cloves, crushed
1 teaspoon chopped fresh thyme
450ml (¾ pint) vegetable stock
4–5 young leeks, finely chopped
1 teaspoon finely grated lemon zest
1 tablespoon plain flour
450ml (¾ pint) skimmed milk
2 bay leaves
1 tablespoon chopped fresh parsley
salt and freshly ground black pepper

1 Place the mushrooms, garlic, thyme and stock into a small saucepan and gently simmer for 10 minutes in order to soften the mushrooms.
2 In a separate non-stick pan dry-fry the leeks until soft. Add the lemon zest with 3 tablespoons of the mushroom stock.
3 Sprinkle the flour over and cook out for 1 minute, stirring well with a wooden spoon.
4 Gradually add the mushroom stock and the contents of the saucepan along with the skimmed milk. Add the bay leaves and gently simmer for 20–25 minutes until the mushrooms are soft and the soup has slightly thickened.
5 Just before serving, stir in the chopped parsley and season to taste.
6 Serve with crusty bread.

Courgette and basil soup

SERVES 4
PER SERVING:
102 KCAL/1.7G FAT
PREPARATION TIME:
10 MINUTES
COOKING TIME:
30 MINUTES

1kg (2lb) young courgettes
2 medium onions, chopped
2 garlic cloves, crushed
600ml (1 pint) vegetable stock
1 teaspoon fresh thyme leaves
2 bay leaves
300ml ($^1/_2$ pint) skimmed milk
salt and freshly ground black pepper
20 fresh basil leaves to garnish

Always select small young courgettes with a brightly coloured skin free from wrinkles. Aged courgettes can taste bitter and sour. Make the soup in advance and store chilled until required.

1 Top and tail the courgettes and roughly chop.
2 Place in a large saucepan with the remaining ingredients except the skimmed milk and basil. Bring to the boil, then reduce the heat and simmer gently for 15–20 minutes until the vegetables are soft.
3 Allow to cool slightly, then liquidise in batches, adding a little of the milk and basil to each batch until smooth and lump free. Return to the pan and season to taste.
4 Adjust the consistency with a little extra milk if required, garnish with finely shredded basil leaves and serve immediately.

Sweetcorn and red pepper soup

An easy colourful soup to brighten up your day. Most of the ingredients can be stored in your food cupboard, making it a quick and easy lunch for all the family.

SERVES 4
PER SERVING:
50 KCAL/1.1G FAT
PREPARATION TIME:
10 MINUTES
COOKING TIME:
20 MINUTES

4 small shallots, finely chopped
1 teaspoon paprika
2 smoked garlic cloves, crushed
2 red peppers, finely diced
1 × 175g (6oz) can sweetcorn, drained
pinch of dried chilli flakes
600ml (1 pint) vegetable stock
2 teaspoons cornflour
1 tablespoon finely chopped chives to garnish

1. In a large non-stick pan dry-fry the shallots until soft.
2. Sprinkle the paprika over, add the garlic and cook for 2–3 minutes, stirring well. Add the peppers, corn and chilli and stir in the stock. Bring to the boil, then reduce the heat to a gentle simmer.
3. Slake the cornflour with a little cold water and add to the soup, stirring well to prevent any lumps forming. Cook for 5–6 minutes until the soup thickens slightly.
4. Serve garnished with chopped chives.

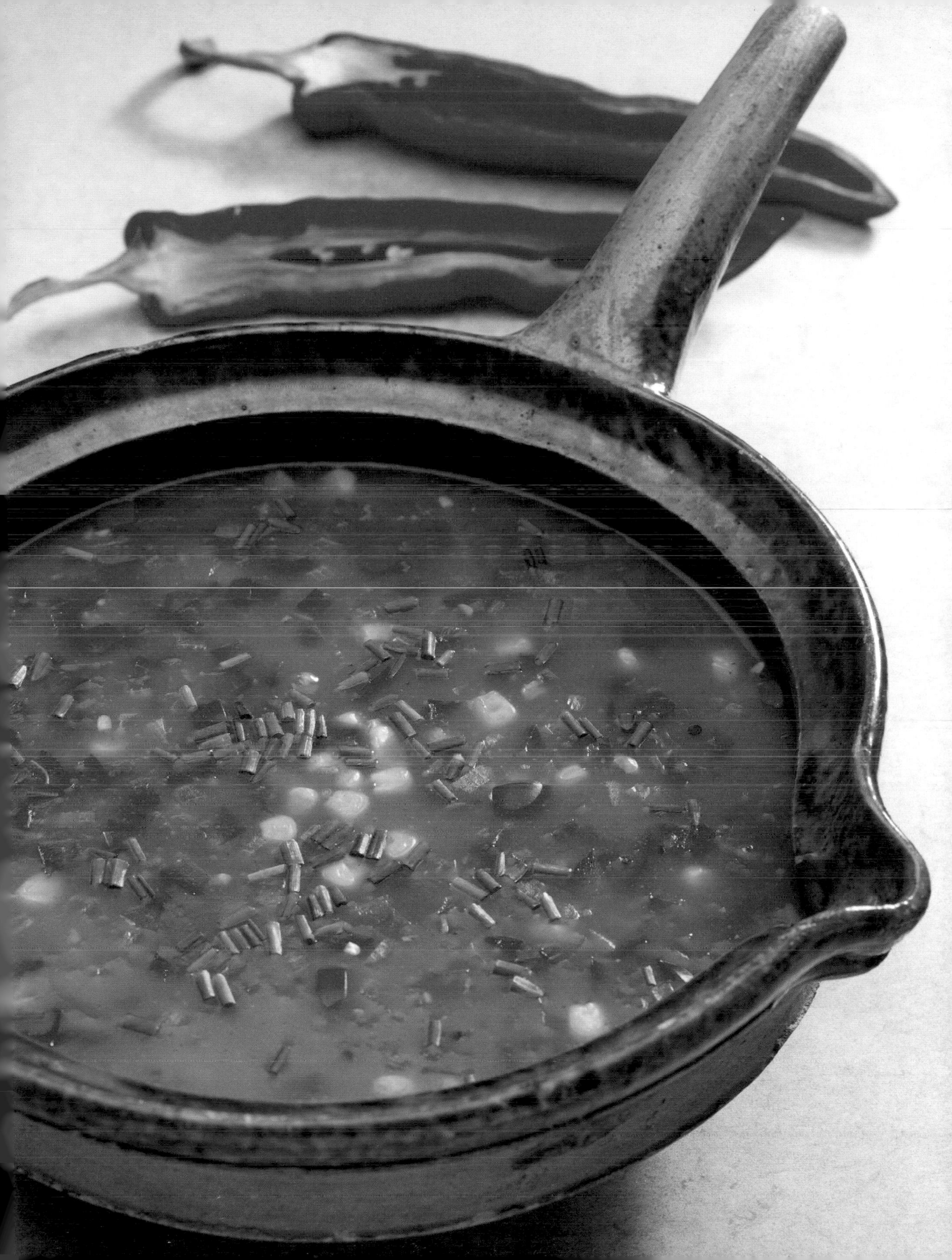

Parsnip and apple soup with Calvados

A classic combination of sweet and sour. The flaming Calvados adds a finishing touch to this delightful, comforting soup.

SERVES 4
PER SERVING:
249 KCAL/3.4G FAT
PREPARATION TIME:
20 MINUTES
COOKING TIME:
30 MINUTES

1 kg (2lb) fresh young parsnips
3 celery sticks, sliced
2 medium onions, chopped
1 garlic clove, crushed
2 large Bramley cooking apples
2 teaspoons chopped fresh thyme
1.2 litres (2 pints) vegetable stock
2 bay leaves
2 tablespoons virtually fat free fromage frais
2 tablespoons Calvados brandy
salt and freshly ground black pepper

1 Peel and slice the parsnips, place in a saucepan with the celery, onions and garlic and dry-fry over a low heat for 2–3 minutes.
2 Peel, core and slice the apples. Add them, the thyme, stock and bay leaves and simmer gently until the vegetables are soft. Remove the bay leaves and liquidise until smooth.
3 Return the soup to the pan, adjust the consistency with a little extra stock if required and season with salt and black pepper.
4 Just before serving, remove from the heat and stir in the fromage frais.
5 Divide into serving bowls. Heat the Calvados in a metal ladle over a low heat, then ignite with a long match. Pour the flaming brandy over the soup and serve.

Watercress and potato soup

SERVES 4
PER SERVING:
138 KCAL/1G FAT
PREPARATION TIME:
10 MINUTES
COOKING TIME:
20 MINUTES

4 baby leeks, finely sliced
2 garlic cloves, crushed
3 baking potatoes, peeled and diced
1.2 litres (2 pints) vegetable stock bouillon
1 tablespoon plain flour
½ teaspoon ground mace
1 tablespoon finely chopped fresh marjoram
1 bunch watercress, tops removed
salt and freshly ground black pepper
a little low-fat fromage frais to garnish

Ground mace is the outer husk of the spice nutmeg. It has a very unusual flavour, but use sparingly, as too much may result in a strong bitter aftertaste.

1 In a non-stick pan dry-fry the baby leeks and garlic for 2–3 minutes over a moderate heat, until softened but not coloured.
2 Add the potatoes and 3 tablespoons of stock and stir in the flour and the ground mace. Cook over a low heat, stirring well, for 1 minute in order to cook out the flour.
3 Gradually add the remaining stock, stirring well to prevent any lumps forming. Add the marjoram and bring to the boil, then reduce the heat and simmer for 20 minutes.
4 Just before serving, season to taste with salt and black pepper and add the watercress. Pour into a warmed serving tureen and garnish with a little low-fat fromage frais.

Spring vegetable soup

A celebration of fresh new spring vegetables. Make the soup in advance and reheat as required, adding the spring greens just at the end to prevent them overcooking.

SERVES 4
PER SERVING:
69 KCAL/1.4G FAT
PREPARATION TIME:
10 MINUTES
COOKING TIME:
20 MINUTES
SUITABLE FOR FREEZING

4 baby leeks, finely sliced
2 small carrots, cut into thin strips
2 small courgettes, diced
1.2 litres (2 pints) vegetable stock bouillon
1 × 400g (14oz) can chopped tomatoes
2 teaspoons cornflour
2–3 leaves spring greens, finely chopped
salt and freshly ground black pepper

1 In a non-stick pan dry-fry the baby leeks, carrots and courgettes for 2–3 minutes over a moderate heat, until softened but not coloured.
2 Stir in the stock and chopped tomatoes.
3 Slake the cornflour with a little water and stir into the soup, bringing the soup up to the boil. Reduce the heat and simmer gently for 10–15 minutes.
4 Five minutes before serving, add the spring greens and season to taste with salt and black pepper. Serve immediately.

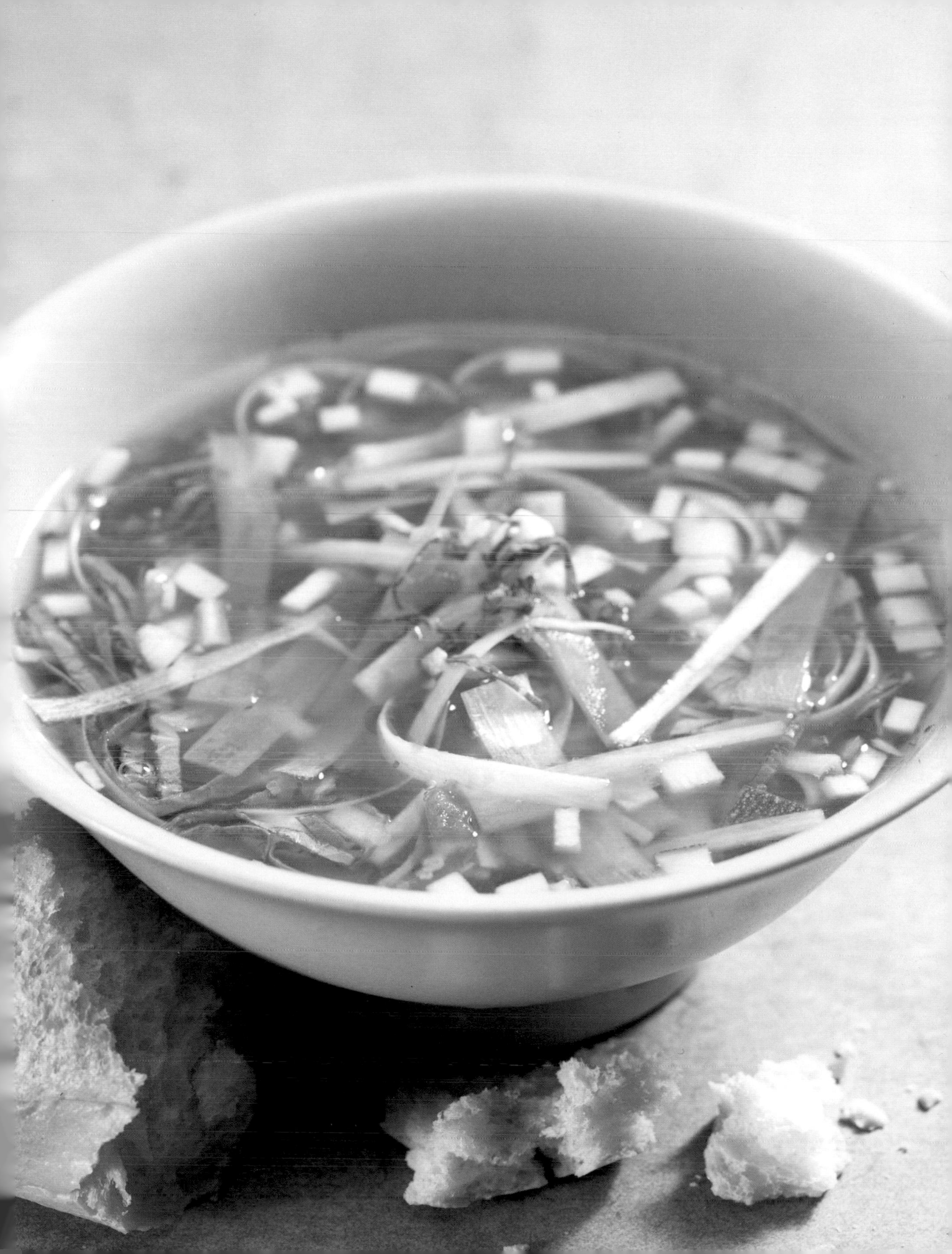

Spiced cauliflower soup

Cauliflower makes wonderful thick creamy soup. It is best to make it fresh and be sure not to re-boil the soup after it has been liquidised, as this may impair the flavour.

SERVES 4
PER SERVING:
82 KCAL/1.4G FAT
PREPARATION TIME:
10 MINUTES
COOKING TIME:
30 MINUTES

- 1 large cauliflower
- 2 medium onions, chopped
- 2 smoked garlic cloves
- 600ml (1 pint) vegetable stock
- 2 teaspoons medium curry powder
- 1 teaspoon ground coriander
- 1 red chilli, finely chopped
- 300ml (½ pint) skimmed milk
- 2 tablespoons chopped fresh coriander
- salt and freshly ground black pepper

1. Remove and discard the outer leaves from the cauliflower and coarsely chop the rest, including the stalk. Place in a large saucepan with the remaining ingredients except the skimmed milk and fresh coriander. Bring to the boil, then reduce the heat and simmer gently for 15–20 minutes until the vegetables are soft.
2. Allow to cool slightly, then liquidise in batches, adding a little of the milk and coriander to each batch until smooth and lump free. Return to the pan and season to taste.
3. Adjust the consistency with a little extra milk if required, garnish with finely chopped coriander leaves and serve immediately.

Roasted shallot and spinach soup

SERVES 4
PER SERVING:
100 KCAL/1.6G FAT
PREPARATION TIME:
10 MINUTES
COOKING TIME:
40 MINUTES

450g (1lb) long shallots, peeled
300ml ($^1/_2$ pint) skimmed milk
2 garlic cloves, peeled and chopped
2 teaspoons fresh thyme
4 teaspoons cornflour
1 tablespoon Dijon mustard
225g (8oz) young baby leaf spinach
1.2 litres (2 pints) vegetable stock
salt and freshly ground black pepper
grated fresh nutmeg to garnish

Roasting the shallots releases their sweet natural juices, adding a distinctive roasted flavour to this flavoursome soup. If you are unable to get shallots, substitute baby leeks.

1 Preheat the oven to 200C, 400F, Gas Mark 6.
2 Slice the shallots in half and place on a non-stick baking tray. Season with salt and black pepper and roast in the top of the preheated oven for 20–25 minutes until soft.
3 Heat the milk, garlic and thyme in a medium-sized saucepan. Slake the cornflour with a little water and stir into the milk. Keep stirring as the sauce thickens, then reduce the heat and simmer for 2–3 minutes.
4 Stir in the mustard and spinach – if using large leaf spinach roughly chop first. Add half the stock along with the roasted shallots. Allow to cool.
5 When the mixture is quite cool, pour into a liquidiser and blend until smooth.
6 Return the soup to the pan, add the remaining stock and reheat.
7 Serve garnished with a little grated fresh nutmeg.

Celeriac and nutmeg soup

Celeriac is an unusual root vegetable with a distinctive nutty flavour – ideal for thick wholesome winter soups. It can also be boiled with potatoes to add flavour to mashed potatoes.

SERVES 4
PER SERVING:
81 KCAL/1.3G FAT
PREPARATION TIME:
15 MINUTES
COOKING TIME:
40 MINUTES

- 2 medium onions, chopped
- 2 garlic cloves, crushed
- 450g (1 lb) celeriac, peeled and cut into chunks
- 1 tablespoon fresh thyme
- 1.2 litres (2 pints) vegetable stock
- a little fresh nutmeg
- salt and freshly ground black pepper
- 3 tablespoons low-fat fromage frais
- flat leaf parsley to garnish

1. Dry-fry the onion and garlic in a non-stick saucepan until soft. Add the celeriac, thyme and stock. Simmer gently for 25–30 minutes until tender.
2. Pour the soup into a liquidiser or food processor and blend until smooth.
3. Return to the saucepan, adjusting the consistency with a little more stock or skimmed milk if required. Grate over a little fresh nutmeg and season with salt and black pepper.
4. Before serving, remove from the heat and stir in the fromage frais. Serve garnished with a sprig of parsley and a little grated fresh nutmeg.

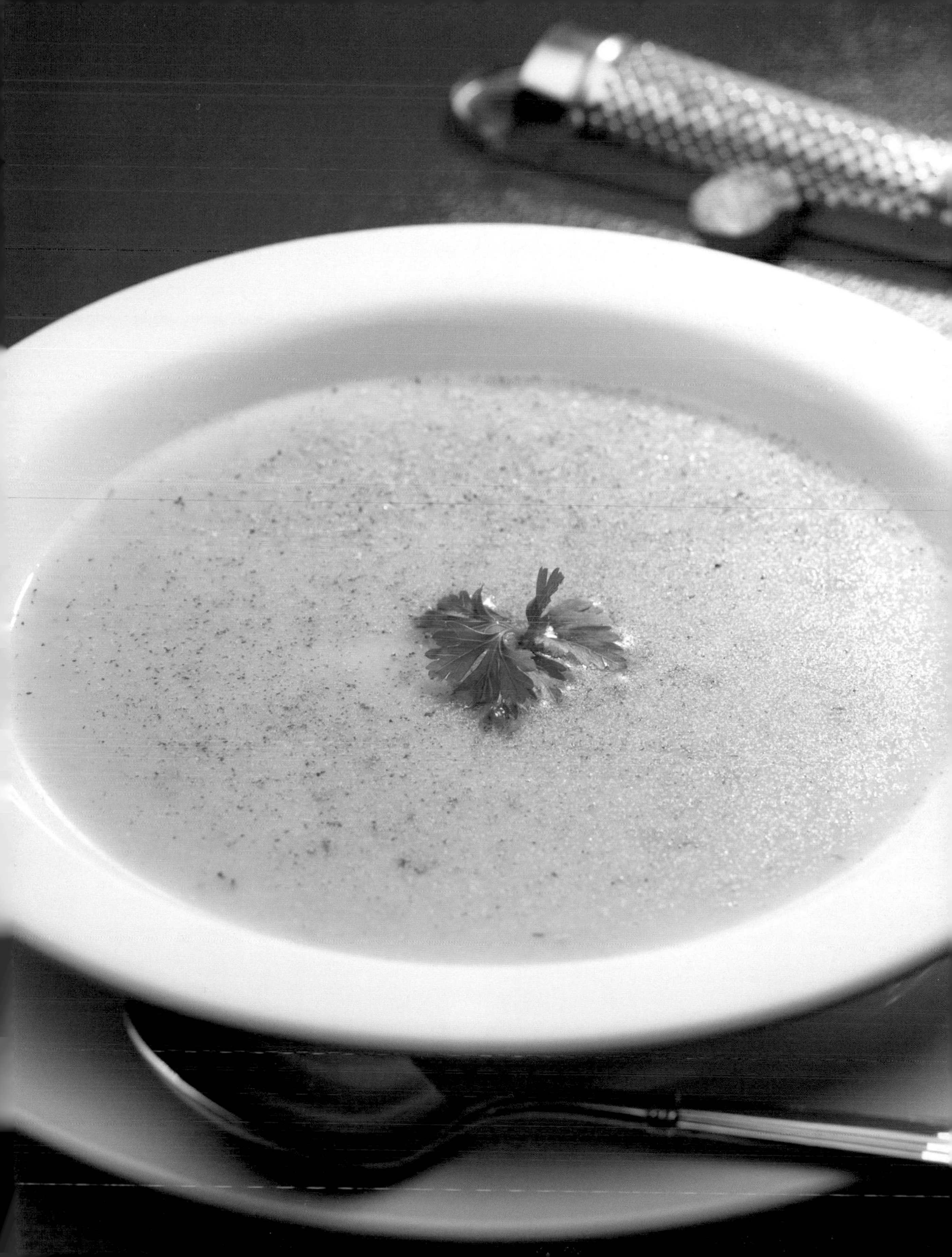

Potage paysanne

Cutting all the vegetables into similar-sized pieces adds style to a basic clear soup. Use fresh seasonal vegetables for maximum flavour.

SERVES 4
PER SERVING:
53 KCAL/1.6G FAT
PREPARATION TIME:
10 MINUTES
COOKING TIME:
20 MINUTES

- 4 baby leeks, finely sliced into small circles
- 2 small carrots
- 4 small turnips
- 2 sticks celery
- 6 spring onions
- 1.2 litres (2 pints) vegetable stock bouillon
- 50g (2oz) French green beans
- 50g (2oz) fresh peas
- 2 tablespoons chopped fresh parsley
- salt and freshly ground black pepper

1. Thinly slice all the root vegetables, and then cut them into small shapes, the size of a one-penny piece.
2. In a non-stick pan dry-fry the vegetables except the beans and peas for 2–3 minutes over a moderate heat, until softened but not coloured.
3. Stir in the stock and bring to the boil. Reduce the heat and simmer gently for 10–15 minutes.
4. Chop the beans into diagonal slices and add to the soup 10 minutes before serving, along with the peas.
5. Season to taste with salt and black pepper and stir in the chopped parsley.
6. Serve straight away with warm crusty bread.

Minted green pea and cucumber soup

SERVES 4
PER SERVING:
104 KCAL/1.7G FAT
PREPARATION TIME:
10 MINUTES
COOKING TIME:
25 MINUTES

450g (1lb) frozen petit pois
1 medium onion, finely chopped
8 fresh mint leaves
1 young cucumber, peeled and chopped
600ml (1 pint) vegetable stock
1 tablespoon virtually fat free fromage frais
salt and freshly ground black pepper

Cucumber is a vegetable we tend to limit to salads and cold dishes. When cooked, it has a very delicate flavour. Try it in soups or simply stir-fried.

1 Place the peas and onion in a large saucepan, barely cover with salted water and boil for 20 minutes. Pour into a liquidiser or food processor and purée until smooth.
2 Add the mint and cucumber, along with the vegetable stock, and blend again until smooth. Return to the saucepan and reheat.
3 Season to taste with salt and pepper.
4 Just before serving, stir in the fromage frais.

Thai noodle soup

Bring the flavours of the orient to your table with this spicy wholesome soup. If you find you have to buy fresh spices such as lemongrass or ginger in large quantities, prepare them, then place in food bags and freeze for a later time.

SERVES 1
PER SERVING:
175 KCAL/4.1G FAT
PREPARATION TIME:
20 MINUTES
COOKING TIME:
20 MINUTES

1 small shallot, finely sliced
1/4 teaspoon coriander seed
1/2 smoked garlic clove, crushed
1/2 teaspoon lemongrass, finely chopped
small piece fresh ginger, peeled and finely chopped
pinch of dried chilli flakes
pinch of ground turmeric
300ml (1/2 pint) vegetable stock
25g (1oz) [dry weight] egg noodles
25g (1oz) beansprouts
1 tablespoon virtually fat free Normandy fromage frais
mint leaves to garnish

1 In a large non-stick pan dry-fry the shallot until soft.
2 Crush the coriander seed on a chopping board with the broad side of a chopping knife and add to the pan. Add the garlic and cook for 2–3 minutes, then add the lemongrass, ginger, chilli, turmeric and stir well to combine the spices. Add the vegetable stock and bring to the boil. Reduce the heat to a gentle simmer and add the noodles.
3 Cook for 5–6 minutes until the noodles become soft, then remove from the heat and stir in the beansprouts and fromage frais.
4 Just before serving, garnish with mint leaves.

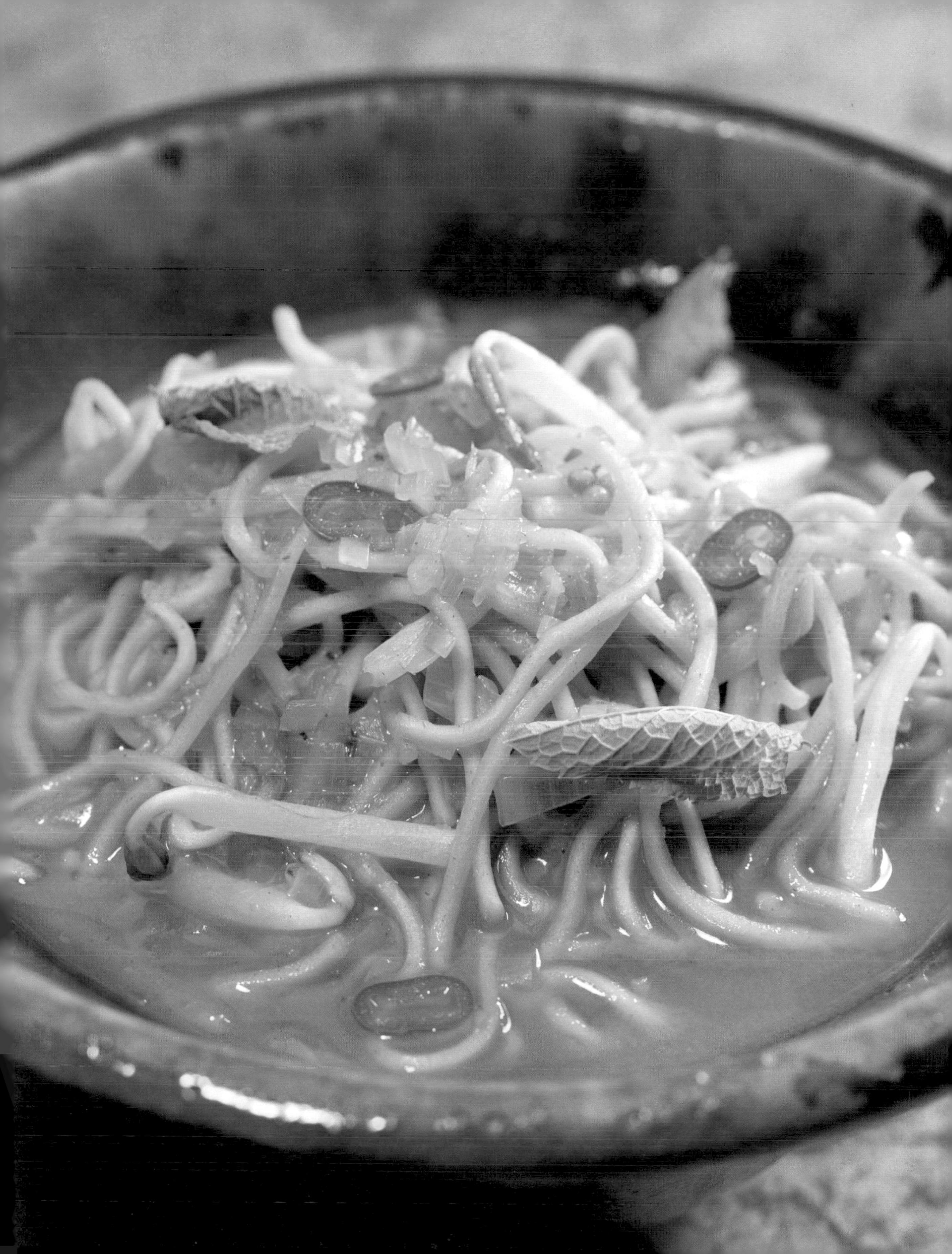

Meat and poultry

The selection of prepared meats available is endless and choosing the right cut can sometimes become quite daunting. Basic butchering can determine many factors, but the key rule is to choose clean, clear-coloured meat, not dull and grey in appearance and certainly without dried edges.

Small cuts should be evenly sliced or diced into uniform-sized pieces to ensure that they cook properly at the same time.

Organic or free range meat may seem slightly more expensive, but the compensation is well worth it in the form of both flavour and texture.

Meat should always be stored well-wrapped in the coldest part of the refrigerator. Most small cuts, including mince, are best used within 1–2 days of purchase. Generally red meat tends to keep better than white, but if in doubt – throw it out!

As with meat, the selection of poultry has expanded, offering farm-produced birds, again organically fed, or free range with a fuller flavour.

Supermarket birds are generally very lean, which can mean a compromise on flavour, so use marinades and stir-fry spices to pep them up. Proper chilled storage is imperative, as is making sure the poultry is completely cooked through.

Chilli beef enchiladas

SERVES 4
PER SERVING:
351 KCAL/13.4G FAT
(EXCLUDING TORTILLA)
PREPARATION TIME:
10 MINUTES
COOKING TIME:
35 MINUTES

450g (1lb) lean steak mince
2 medium onions, finely chopped
3 garlic cloves, crushed
2 beef stock cubes
1–2 fresh red chillies, chopped
2 red peppers, seeded and finely chopped
1 tablespoon chopped fresh oregano
1 × 400g (14oz) can chopped tomatoes
300ml ($^1/_2$ pint) tomato passata
300ml ($^1/_2$ pint) skimmed milk
3 teaspoons cornflour
4 Navajo Tortillas (see recipe, page 120)
50g (2oz) low-fat Cheddar cheese, grated
salt and freshly ground black pepper

Tortillas form the base to this Mexican feast. If you wish, replace the beef with minced chicken or pork, and a good vegetarian filling is roasted vegetables.

1 Preheat the oven to 200C, 400F, Gas Mark 6. In a preheated non-stick pan dry-fry the mince until lightly browned. Pour into a sieve to drain away the fat and wipe out the pan with kitchen paper.
2 Add the onions and garlic to the pan and dry-fry for 2–3 minutes until soft.
3 Return the meat to the pan and crumble the stock cubes over. Add the chillies, peppers, oregano and both the chopped and passata tomatoes. Simmer gently for 20–25 minutes until the sauce has thickened and the meat is tender.
4 In a separate pan heat the milk. Slake the cornflour with a little cold water and whisk into the milk. Stir as the sauce thickens, seasoning well with salt and freshly ground black pepper.
5 Take a tortilla and place a line of the beef mixture down the centre. Roll up and place in an ovenproof dish. Repeat with the remaining tortillas, placing any meat mix on top of each. Pour the sauce over and sprinkle with grated cheese.
6 Bake in the preheated oven for 20–25 minutes until golden brown. Serve with red pepper salsa and mixed green leaves.

Roast beef with Yorkshire pudding, dry-roast potatoes and parsnips

SERVES 6
PER SERVING:
BEEF: 218 KCAL/8.3G FAT
DRY–ROAST POTATOES AND PARSNIPS: 106 KCAL/0.9G FAT
YORKSHIRE PUDDING: 79 KCAL/1.3G FAT
PREPARATION TIME: 30 MINUTES
COOKING TIME: 1–1½ HOURS

1kg (2lb) joint lean beef, topside
1 onion, finely diced
1 carrot, diced
1 celery stick, diced
2 teaspoons mixed dried herbs
600ml (1 pint) beef stock
1 tablespoon cornflour
1–2 drops gravy browning

for the Yorkshire pudding batter
115g (4oz) plain flour
1 egg
pinch of salt
150ml (¼ pint) skimmed milk

for the dry-roast potatoes and parsnips
450g (1lb) potatoes, peeled and cut in half
8 medium parsnips, peeled and left whole
1 tablespoon soy sauce diluted in 2 tablespoons of water (optional)

1 Preheat the oven to 180C, 350F, Gas Mark 4.
2 Prepare the beef by removing as much fat as possible. Place the onion, carrot, celery and herbs in the bottom of a roasting tin or ovenproof dish. Sit the beef on top and pour 300ml (½ pint) water around. Place in the oven. Allow 15 minutes per 450g (lb) plus 15 minutes for rare beef, 20 minutes per 450g (1lb) plus 20 minutes over for medium rare, and 25 minutes per 450g (1lb) plus 30 minutes if you like your beef well done.
3 Cook the potatoes and parsnips separately in boiling water. Drain and place in a non-stick roasting tin. Place in the top of the oven for 35–40 minutes until golden brown. You can baste the vegetables with the diluted soy sauce if they appear to dry out, depending on your oven.
4 Forty minutes before the beef is ready, make the Yorkshire pudding batter by blending the flour with the egg and a little milk to a smooth paste. Whisk in the remaining milk until smooth. Preheat a six-hole non-stick Yorkshire pudding tin for 2 minutes in the oven. Remove and half fill each mould with batter. Return to the oven and increase the heat to 200C, 400F, Gas Mark 6 for 35–40 minutes.
5 When the beef is cooked, remove from the tin and wrap in foil to keep warm. Allow to rest for 5–10 minutes. Meanwhile, add 600ml (1 pint) of beef stock to the pan juices. Slake the cornflour with a little water and add to the pan. Stir well as the gravy thickens. Add 1–2 drops of gravy browning as required.
6 To serve, carve the beef thinly and serve with Yorkshire pudding, dry–roast potatoes and parsnips, beef gravy and seasonal vegetables.

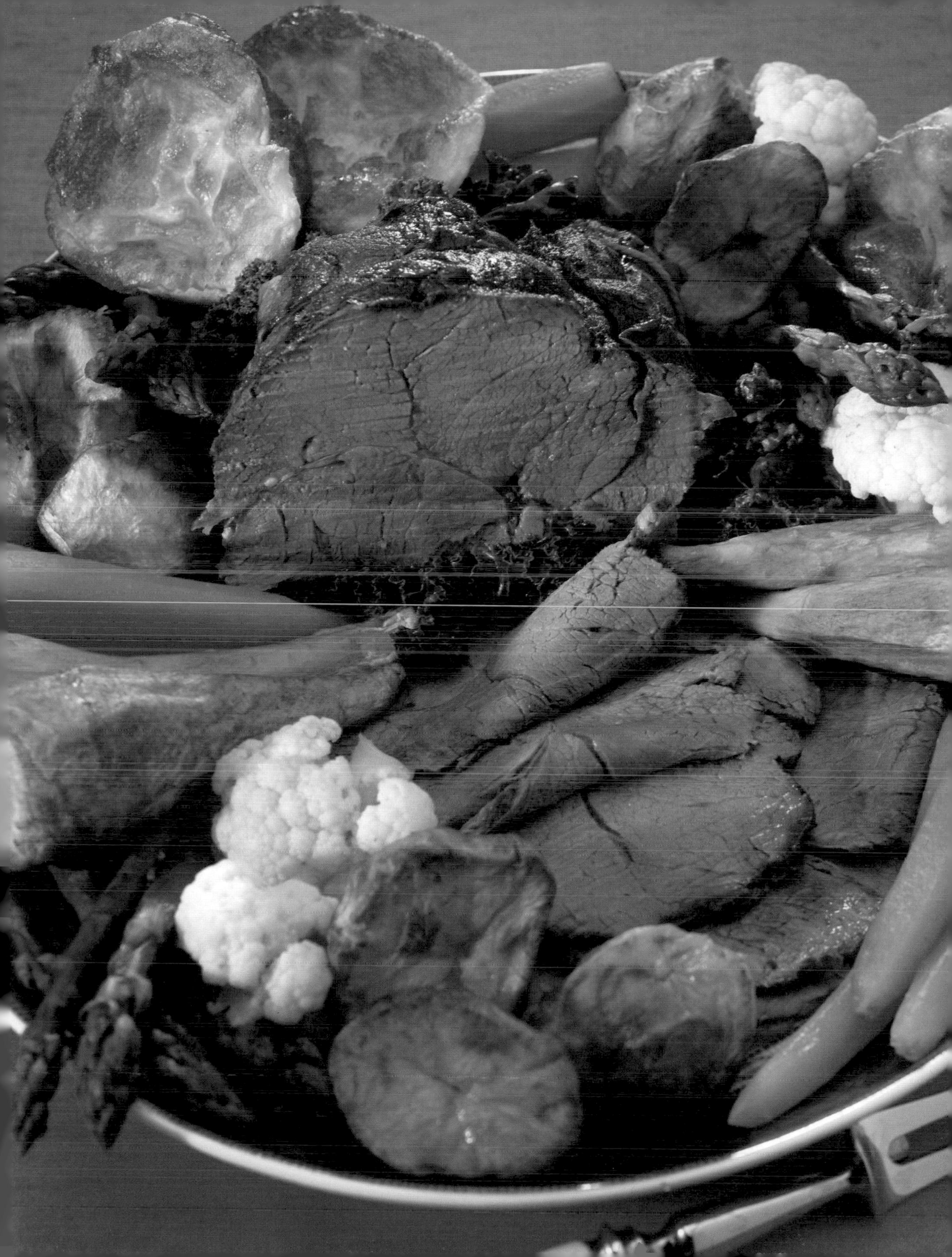

Steak and kidney pie

SERVES 4
PER SERVING:
355 KCAL/6.8G FAT
PREPARATION TIME:
20 MINUTES
COOKING TIME:
50 MINUTES

225g (8oz) lean rump or sirloin steak, cut into cubes
225g (8oz) kidneys cut into bite-sized pieces
2 medium onions, chopped
1 wine glass red wine
2 beef stock cubes
1 tablespoon gravy powder
1kg (2lb) potatoes, peeled
2 tablespoons low-fat natural yogurt
4–5 tablespoons skimmed milk
salt and freshly ground black pepper

1 Preheat the oven to 180C, 350F, Gas Mark 4.
2 Trim the steak, removing all the fat, then cut the steak into cubes.
3 Preheat a non-stick frying pan. Dry-fry the cubes of beef steak and kidneys until well browned. Place in a 12 × 8in (30 × 20cm) pie dish. Dry-fry the onions until soft and add this to the meat in the pie dish.
4 Place 300ml (½ pint) water in the pan. Add the wine and stock cubes to the pan and bring to the boil. Mix the gravy powder with a little cold water and add to the boiling stock in the pan, stirring continuously. The gravy should be quite thick. Add more gravy powder mixed with a little water as necessary. Pour the gravy over the meat in the pie dish.
5 Boil the potatoes and drain. Mash the potatoes with the yogurt and sufficient skimmed milk to make the consistency quite soft. Season to taste.
6 Using a fork or a piping bag with a star nozzle, carefully spoon (or pipe) the 'creamed' potato on top of the meat and gravy and ensure that it covers it completely. If you spoon the potato on top, spread it carefully with a fork.
7 Place in the oven for 30–40 minutes, or until crisp and brown on top.

Serrano calf's liver

SERVES 4
PER SERVING:
184 KCAL/7G FAT
PREPARATION TIME:
30 MINUTES
COOKING TIME:
10 MINUTES

4 slices calf's liver
150ml (1/4 pint) skimmed milk
1 teaspoon green peppercorns, crushed
4 thin slices Serrano ham
2 garlic cloves, crushed
300ml (1/2 pint) tomato passata
1 tablespoon mixed chopped fresh herbs (parsley, oregano, chives)
salt and freshly ground black pepper

Spain has long been a devotee of cured ham. The quality and flavour is determined by many factors, including the animal feed and curing process. Serrano ham is cured using only sea salt without the use of additives, resulting in lightly pink coloured meat with a sweet aroma and a firm texture.

1 Preheat the oven to 150C, 300F, Gas Mark 2.
2 Soak the liver in the milk for 30 minutes to clean the remove any bitter flavours.
3 Preheat a non-stick griddle pan. Add a little vegetable oil, then wipe out with kitchen paper.
4 Remove the liver from the milk and pat dry with kitchen paper. Season each piece on both sides with the green peppercorns and wrap individually with a slice of Serrano ham.
5 Cook the meat quickly in a hot pan for 2 minutes on each side. Remove and place in a warm oven while you make the sauce.
6 Add the garlic to the pan and cook quickly until soft. Pour in the passata, stirring well to pick up the pan juices. Add the herbs and season to taste with salt and freshly ground black pepper.

Red Thai beef

A quick hot and spicy beef dish that's packed full of flavour. Prepare the night before and leave covered overnight in the refrigerator for a tasty dinner accompanied with an exotic salad.

SERVES 4
PER SERVING:
169 KCAL/6G FAT
PREPARATION TIME:
10 MINUTES
COOKING TIME:
5 MINUTES

450g (1lb) lean steak (rump or sirloin)
1 beef stock cube dissolved in 150ml (¼ pint) boiling water
4 tablespoons light soy sauce
1 teaspoon ground coriander
300ml (½ pint) tomato passata
1 small red chilli, finely sliced
1 teaspoon finely chopped lemongrass
2 garlic cloves, crushed
1 tablespoon chopped fresh coriander
salt and freshly ground black pepper

1 Remove any fat from the meat and discard. Slice the meat into thin strips and place into a shallow dish. Season well with salt and freshly ground black pepper.
2 Combine the remaining ingredients except the fresh coriander and pour over the beef. Leave to marinate for at least 1 hour, mixing periodically.
3 Strain the marinade from the beef and reserve. Preheat a non-stick frying pan and stir-fry the beef quickly over a high heat for 1–2 minutes until cooked to your liking. Add the reserved marinade and heat through.
4 Stir in the fresh coriander and serve on a bed of rice.

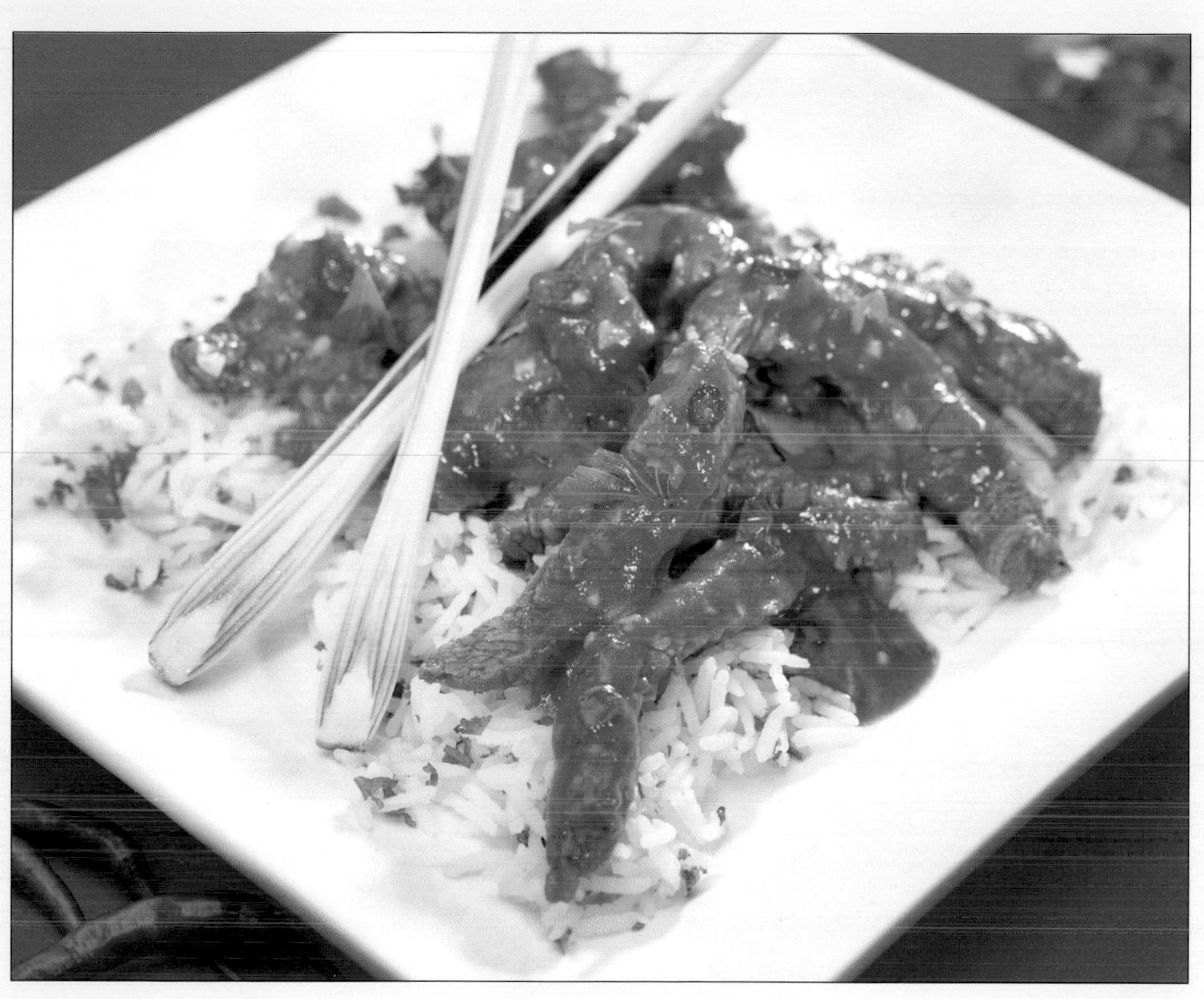

Tarragon pork

Tarragon is a primary herb with a strong distinctive flavour. It can be substituted with either sage or coriander if you prefer.

SERVES 4
PER SERVING:
298 KCAL/7G FAT
PREPARATION TIME:
20 MINUTES
COOKING TIME:
40 MINUTES

- 4 lean pork steaks
- 1 medium red onion, finely chopped
- 2 red eating apples, cored and chopped
- 1 × 2.5cm (1in) piece of fresh ginger, peeled and finely chopped
- 1 vegetable stock cube dissolved in 300ml (½ pint) water
- 1 tablespoon plain flour
- 225g (8oz) chestnut mushrooms, sliced
- 1 wine glass white wine
- 1 tablespoon chopped fresh tarragon

1. Season the pork steaks on both sides with plenty of salt and freshly ground black pepper then place in a preheated non-stick pan.
2. Dry-fry on both sides for 5–6 minutes until lightly browned, then remove from the pan and place on a plate.
3. Add the onion and apples to the pan and cook gently until lightly coloured. Add the ginger and 2 tablespoons of stock. Sprinkle the flour over and cook out for 1 minute. Gradually stir in the remaining stock with the mushrooms and wine.
4. Return the pork to the pan and add the tarragon. Simmer gently for 15–20 minutes until the sauce has reduced and the pork is cooked through.

Pork Provençale

SERVES 4
PER SERVING:
315 KCAL/10.2G FAT
PREPARATION TIME:
10 MINUTES
COOKING TIME:
20 MINUTES

4 lean pork slices
1 medium red onion, finely chopped
2 garlic cloves, crushed
1 small aubergine, finely diced
1 red pepper, seeded and finely chopped
600ml (1 pint) tomato passata
2 teaspoons vegetable stock powder
1 tablespoon chopped fresh mixed herbs
salt and freshly ground black pepper

Quick and easy, these tender pork slices make a perfect tasty meal. Cutting the vegetables into small dice allows them to cook much quicker and also adds texture to the thick tomato sauce.

1 Preheat a non-stick pan. Trim away any traces of fat from each pork slice. Using a rolling pin, beat the pork into a thin slice, then season generously with salt and freshly ground black pepper. Seal the slices in a hot pan on both sides then remove and keep warm.
2 Add the onion, garlic, aubergine and red pepper to the pan. Cook quickly over a high heat to soften. Add the tomato passata, stock powder and herbs, stir well then return the pork to the pan. Cover and simmer for 5–6 minutes to allow the pork to cook through.
3 Serve straight away with potatoes and a selection of fresh vegetables.

Chinese spiced pork fillet

Lemon marmalade forms the base to a rich sticky sauce that is perfect for the finest cut of pork. This recipe also works well with duck breast, but do remember to remove the skin before cooking.

SERVES 4
PER SERVING:
438 KCAL/10G FAT
PREPARATION TIME:
10 MINUTES
COOKING TIME:
35 MINUTES

1kg (2lb) lean pork fillet
2 garlic cloves, finely chopped
50ml (2fl oz) dry sherry
2 tablespoons lemon marmalade
50ml (2fl oz) tomato passata
1 red chilli, finely chopped
½ teaspoon Chinese five spice powder
salt and freshly ground black pepper

1 Preheat the oven to 200C, 400F, Gas Mark 6.
2 Trim away any fat from the pork and cut into 4 equal-sized pieces. Season well with salt and freshly ground black pepper and set aside.
3 Preheat a non-stick frying pan until hot. Carefully add the pork, turning quickly to seal all sides. Transfer to an ovenproof dish, place in the hot oven and continue cooking for 15–20 minutes.
4 Add the garlic to the pan and soften. Add the sherry and the remaining ingredients. Simmer gently until the pork is cooked.
5 Remove the pork from the oven and allow to rest for 4–5 minutes before slicing into medallions. Arrange on a serving plate and pour the sauce over.

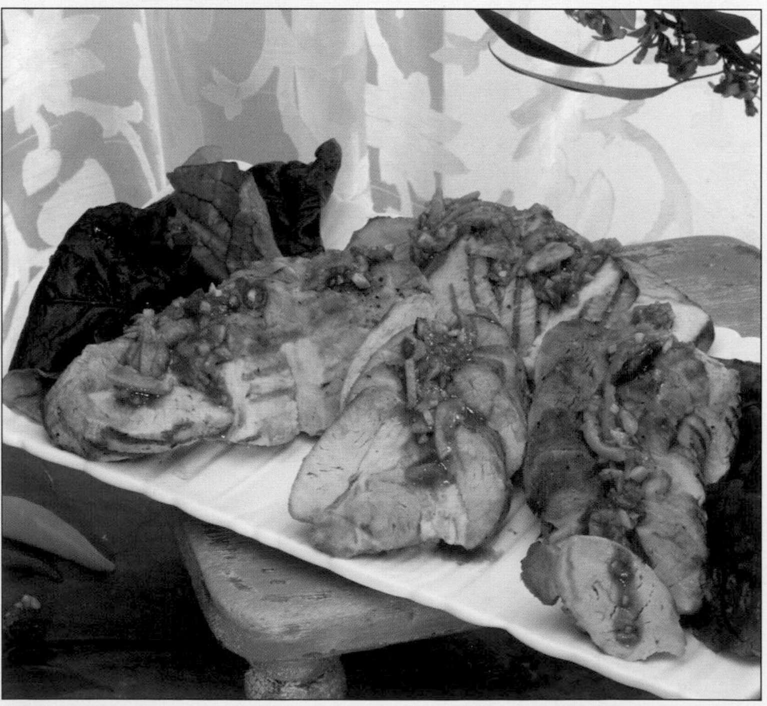

Balsamic pork chop with tangerine

SERVES 1
PER SERVING:
325 KCAL/8.2G FAT
PREPARATION TIME:
5 MINUTES
COOKING TIME:
12–15 MINUTES

1 lean pork chop or slice
1 orange
½ red pepper, seeded and finely diced
2 teaspoons good balsamic vinegar
2–3 basil leaves
1 tangerine, segmented
salt and freshly ground black pepper

This recipe requires a good balsamic vinegar, which will be thick and sweet, unlike cheaper types that are still quite sharp in flavour. The pork may be left in the marinade overnight to absorb all the flavours.

1 Remove all visible fat from the pork and place the pork in a shallow dish.
2 Using a zester, remove strands of peel from the orange and place on top of the pork. Cut the orange in half and squeeze the juice over the pork.
3 Scatter the red pepper over the pork and drizzle with balsamic vinegar.
4 Coarsely shred the basil leaves and add to the dish. Turn the pork over to coat both sides, cover and refrigerate for at least 1 hour.
5 Preheat a non-stick griddle pan until hot. Remove the pork from the marinade and season to taste.
6 Place the pork in the griddle pan and cook for 5–6 minutes on each side. Just before the end of cooking, add any marinade residue and the tangerine segments and heat through.

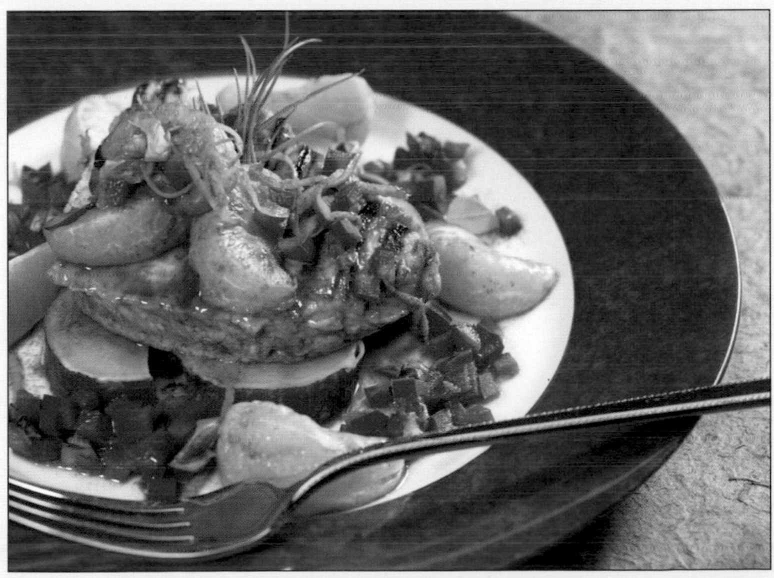

Grilled lamb steaks with cranberry and mint

Choose a lean cut of lamb such as fillet as opposed to fatty chops with very little lean meat. The meat can be marinated overnight in the refrigerator for added flavour.

SERVES 4
PER SERVING:
285 KCAL/15G FAT
PREPARATION TIME:
10 MINUTES
COOKING TIME:
40 MINUTES

450g (1lb) lean lamb filet
2 garlic cloves, crushed
a few sprigs fresh rosemary
300ml ($^1/_2$ pint) fresh orange juice
50g (2oz) fresh cranberries
1 tablespoon cranberry sauce
1 tablespoon cornflour
2 tablespoons chopped fresh mint
salt and freshly ground black pepper

1. Cut the lamb into steaks and place in a shallow dish. Sprinkle the rosemary and garlic over and season well with salt and freshly ground black pepper. Pour the orange juice over and leave to marinate for 30 minutes.
2. Remove the lamb from the marinade and place on a grill tray. Cook under a hot grill for 5–6 minutes each side.
3. Pour the marinade into a small saucepan, add the cranberries and cranberry sauce and heat gently.
4. Slake the cornflour with a little water and add to the sauce. Stir well until the sauce starts to thicken.
5. Arrange the lamb steaks on a serving dish, add the mint to the sauce and pour the sauce over. Serve with potatoes and a vegetable selection.

Griddled lamb's liver with tomato and bacon salsa

SERVES 4
PER SERVING:
405 KCAL/17G FAT
PREPARATION TIME:
25 MINUTES
COOKING TIME:
10 MINUTES

1 kg (2lb) lamb's liver, sliced
2 garlic cloves, crushed
300ml ($^1/_2$ pint) semi-skimmed milk
salt and freshly ground black pepper
2 teaspoons oil (for lining the pan and then removed)

for the salsa
4 rashers lean back bacon
6 ripe tomatoes
4 sundried tomatoes, soaked in boiling water
1 lime
1 tablespoon chopped fresh chives
1 tablespoon balsamic vinegar
1 teaspoon clear honey
salt and freshly ground black pepper

Liver, bacon and tomatoes in a different style. The milk removes any bitterness from the liver as well as having a tenderising effect.

1 Place the liver in a shallow dish. Dot with the crushed garlic and pour the milk over. Allow to sit for 30 minutes while you make the salsa.
2 Make the salsa. Skin the tomatoes by plunging them into boiling water for 10 seconds. Remove and submerge in ice-cold water. Peel away the skin, then slice each tomato in half and remove the seeds, using a teaspoon.
3 Chop the tomato flesh and place in a bowl with the reconstituted sundried tomatoes. Using a zester, remove thin strips of zest from the lime and add to the bowl along with the juice. Stir in the chives, balsamic vinegar and honey, seasoning to taste.
4 Preheat a non-stick griddle pan, lightly greasing with a little oil and removing the excess with kitchen towel.
5 When the pan is very hot add the bacon and cook quickly for 4–5 minutes on each side until crisp. Remove from the pan and drain on kitchen paper before chopping into small pieces. Add to the salsa.
6 Wipe out the griddle pan, adding a little oil if necessary. Remove the liver from the milk and drain on kitchen paper. Add to the pan and cook quickly for 3–4 minutes on each side. If overcooked, the texture will become tough and rubbery.
7 Serve with the salsa.

Pot roast lamb with celery and peppers

A delicious lamb dish full of flavour. Choose a very lean piece of meat, as lamb is naturally high in fat. Other cuts of meat are equally suited such as silverside or topside of beef.

SERVES 4
PER SERVING:
353 KCAL/13.5G FAT
PREPARATION TIME:
15 MINUTES
COOKING TIME:
2 HOURS

1kg (2lb) leg of lamb, skin removed
2 garlic cloves, sliced
3–4 sprigs fresh rosemary
2 medium red onions, chopped
1 head celery, sliced
2 red peppers, seeded and sliced
1.2 litres (2 pints) meat stock
2 tablespoons plain flour
2 tablespoons tomato purée
2 pieces lemon peel
salt and freshly ground black pepper

1 Preheat the oven to 180C, 350F, Gas Mark 4.
2 Using a small sharp knife, make incisions all over the lamb. Push slices of garlic and small sprigs of rosemary into the holes and season well with salt and pepper.
3 Preheat a non-stick frying pan until very hot. Add the lamb and quickly brown on all sides, then transfer the meat to an earthenware dish.
4 Add the onions, celery and peppers and cook until lightly coloured. Add 2–3 tablespoons of stock and sprinkle the flour over, cook briefly, then gradually mix in the remaining stock. If the pan is not sufficiently big enough to hold the total liquid transfer the mixture to the earthenware pot and add the remaining stock along with the tomato purée and lemon peel.
5 Cover the pot and place in the preheated oven for 2–2½ hours until tender.
6 Before serving, scoop off any fat from the top of the dish with a small ladle, then remove the meat from the sauce onto a serving plate. Adjust the consistency of the sauce by reducing in a saucepan over a high heat.
7 Serve with seasonal vegetables.

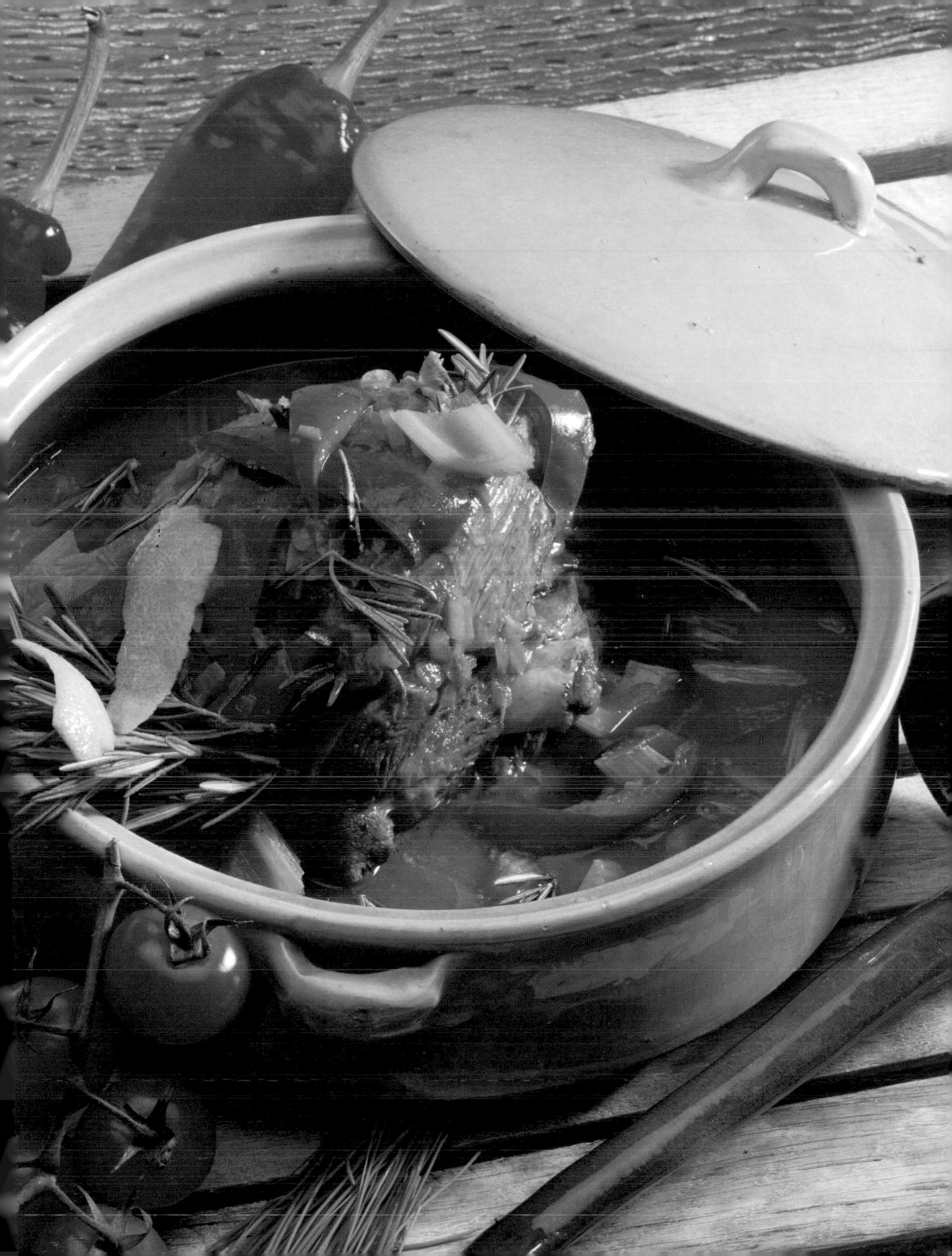

Kidneys in chilli tomato sauce

This chilli sauce is ideal to use hot or cold with grilled meat or fish. Always buy fresh kidneys for use straight away, as they are unsuitable even for short-term storage.

SERVES 4
PER SERVING:
156 KCAL/4.8G FAT
PREPARATION TIME:
20 MINUTES
COOKING TIME:
10 MINUTES

8 large kidneys
1 red onion, finely chopped
2 garlic cloves, crushed
1 red pepper, seeded and finely chopped
300ml ($^1/_2$ pint) tomato passata
1 red chilli, seeded and finely chopped
8–10 basil leaves
salt and freshly ground black pepper

1. Preheat the grill to high.
2. Wash the kidneys well and slice open through the crescent side of the meat, not cutting right the way through but sufficient to be able to open out the kidney. Cut away any white core and splay open by inserting 2 cocktail sticks across each open kidney. Season well with salt and freshly ground black pepper.
3. In a non-stick frying pan dry fry the onion for 2–3 minutes until soft, add the garlic and pepper and cook for 2–3 minutes more.
4. Add the passata and chilli, bringing the sauce to a gentle simmer. Season to taste with salt and freshly ground black pepper.
5. Grill the kidneys for 5–8 minutes, depending on their size, turning frequently.
6. Place the kidneys on a serving dish and sprinkle with shredded basil leaves. Pour the sauce over and serve.

Hattie's crunchy baked chicken

SERVES 4
PER SERVING:
106 KCAL/0.7G FAT
PREPARATION TIME:
10 MINUTES
COOKING TIME:
35 MINUTES

- 4 skinless chicken pieces
- 4 tablespoons spicy tomato chutney
- 4 handfuls cornflakes
- salt and freshly ground black pepper
- 1 tablespoon chopped fresh coriander to garnish

This is a particular favourite with children. The crunchy coating tastes absolutely delicious – just as good as Southern Fried without the fat.

1 Preheat the oven to 200C, 400F, Gas Mark 6.
2 Place the chicken pieces in an ovenproof dish and season well with salt and freshly ground black pepper. Coat each piece of chicken thoroughly with the tomato chutney and place a thick layer on the top.
3 Crush the cornflakes by placing them in a plastic food bag and roll a rolling pin over or alternatively press between two large flat plates.
4 Roll the chicken pieces in the crushed cornflakes until totally coated, sprinkling any excess on the top.
5 Bake in the preheated oven for 30–35 minutes until thoroughly cooked. Check by inserting a knife into the thickest part of the meat. The juices should run clear when fully cooked. If in any doubt return to the oven for a further 10–15 minutes.
6 Just before serving, garnish with the coriander.

Jamaican jerk chicken

There are many variations of this spicy flavoursome chicken dish. This one uses Habanero or Scotch Bonnet chillies, some of the hottest chillies available. If your palate doesn't stretch to this heat scale, then substitute with the milder bullet variety or play safe with a little chilli sauce.

SERVES 4
PER SERVING:
396 KCAL/5.8G FAT
PREPARATION TIME:
20 MINUTES
COOKING TIME:
25–30 MINUTES

8 pieces skinless chicken (drumstick, breast or thighs)
6–8 allspice berries
1 small red onion, finely chopped
2 garlic cloves, crushed
1 teaspoon finely chopped fresh ginger
½ teaspoon ground mace
1 Habanero or Scotch Bonnet chilli, finely chopped
2 tablespoons light soy sauce
zest and juice of 3 limes
2 tablespoons chopped fresh coriander
salt and freshly ground black pepper

1 Prepare the chicken by removing all traces of fat and any white strands of sinew. Slash the flesh of each piece with a sharp knife several times and place in a non-metallic bowl. Season each piece well with salt and freshly ground black pepper.
2 Prepare the jerk seasoning by crushing the allspice berries in either a pestle and mortar or use the broad edge of a large chopping knife, pressing the berries against a solid chopping board. Place in a small glass bowl and add the red onion and garlic. Add the remaining ingredients except the coriander and mix well. Spread the mixture over the chicken, turning each piece to coat. Allow to marinate for 2–3 hours.
3 Cook the chicken either under a preheated hot grill or on a barbecue for approximately 20–25 minutes. It is very important to check the chicken is fully cooked through to the centre before serving. The juices should run clear when a knife is inserted into the thickest part of the chicken.
4 Just before serving, sprinkle with chopped coriander. Serve hot or cold with rice and a selection of salads.

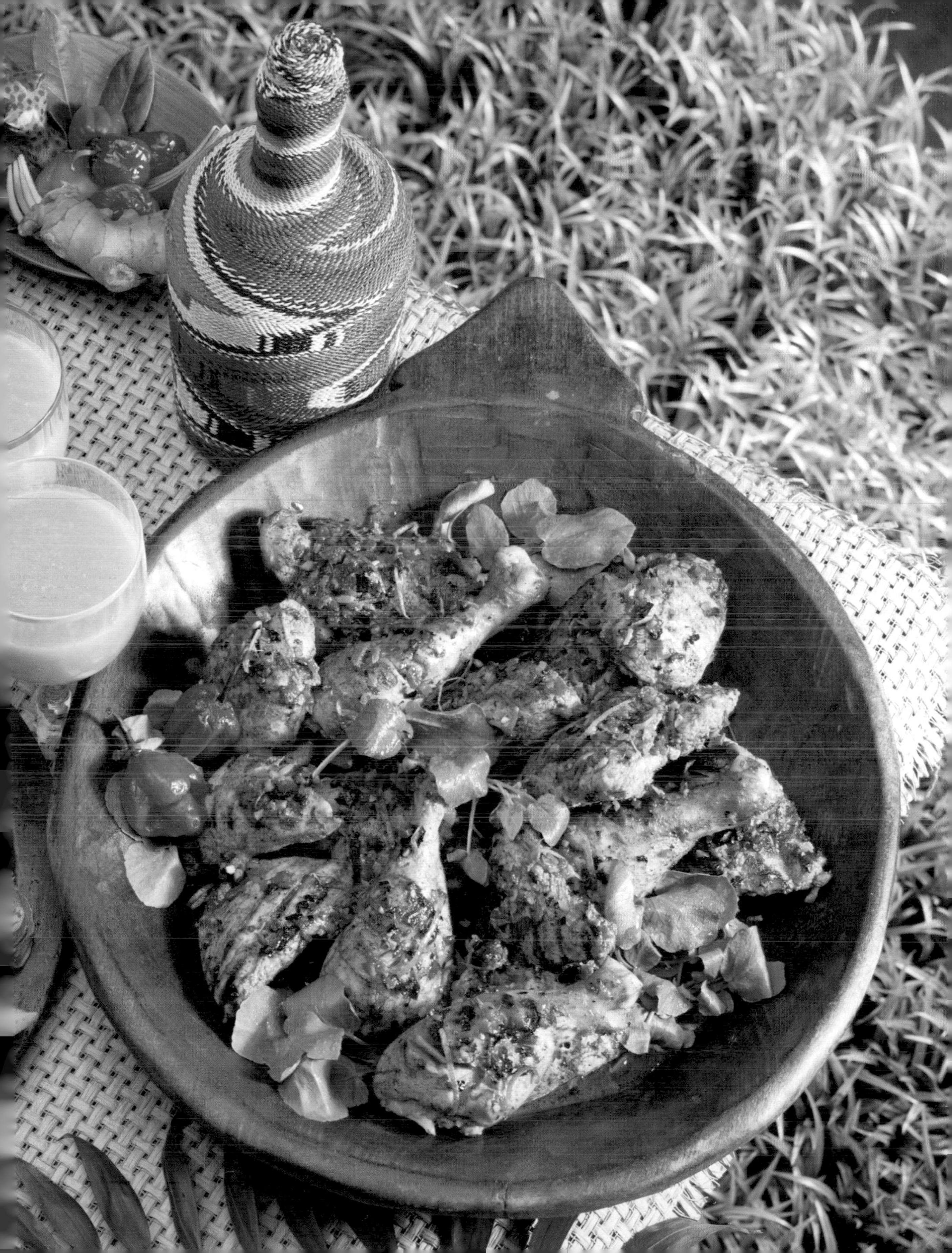

Preserved lemon chicken

Preserved lemons are a fundamental part of Moroccan cookery. The thin-skinned fruits are heavily salted and stored in a brine solution for a minimum of three weeks. The flavour is quite different to fresh lemons, as the salt draws out the bitter flavours of the lemon.

SERVES 4
PER SERVING:
265 KCAL/4.5G FAT
PREPARATION TIME:
15 MINUTES
COOKING TIME:
45 MINUTES

1 large onion, diced
450g (1 lb) skinless chicken breasts, cut into pieces
2 garlic cloves, finely chopped
450ml ($^3/_4$ pint) chicken stock
2 tablespoons plain flour
1 tablespoon chopped fresh sage
1 teaspoon fennel seeds
1 teaspoon ground cumin
6 cardamom pods, crushed
1 small red chilli, finely sliced
1 × 400g (14oz) can chopped tomatoes
1 preserved lemon, cut into quarters and core removed
salt and freshly ground black pepper

Preserving lemons

To preserve lemons, cut 2 large lemons into quarters. Place 50g (2oz) salt in a clean pint jar. Pack the lemons in and pour sufficient lemon juice over to cover. Seal the jar and shake to dissolve some of the salt. Keep in a cool place or refrigerator and shake the jar every day. It is ready to use at this point. It will keep indefinitely in a refrigerator.

1 In a non-stick pan dry-fry the onion until soft. Add the chicken and garlic and continue to cook until lightly coloured.
2 Add 2–3 tablespoons of stock to the pan, sprinkle the flour over and mix well, cooking the flour out for 1 minute. Gradually stir in the remaining stock.
3 Add the herbs and spices, tomatoes and preserved lemon. Cover and simmer gently for 20–25 minutes until the sauce thickens.
4 Season to taste and serve with either rice and sala, or potatoes and a variety of vegetables.

Hot coronation chicken

SERVES 4
PER SERVING:
312 KCAL/3.9G FAT
PREPARATION TIME:
15 MINUTES
COOKING TIME:
20 MINUTES

- 4 skinless chicken breasts, cut into chunks
- 2 medium onions, finely chopped
- 2 garlic cloves, crushed
- 1–2 tablespoons korma curry powder
- 1 vegetable stock cube, dissolved in 150ml ($\frac{1}{4}$ pint) boiling water
- 1 tablespoon plain flour
- 300ml ($\frac{1}{2}$ pint) skimmed milk
- 1 tablespoon chopped fresh flat leaf parsley
- 2 tablespoons virtually fat free Normandy fromage frais
- 1 tablespoon spicy mango chutney
- 50g (2oz) seedless white grapes
- salt and freshly ground black pepper

A hot version of this very popular family dish. For variety substitute the mango chutney with finely diced fresh mango and serve with a jacket potato or rice.

1. Season the chicken pieces with salt and pepper and dry-fry in a non-stick pan for 6–7 minutes until they start to colour. Remove from the pan and set aside.
2. Add the onions and garlic to the pan and cook gently until soft. Sprinkle the curry powder over and add 2 tablespoons of stock. Mix well, then add the flour and cook out for 1 minute. Gradually add the remaining stock and milk, stirring continuously to prevent any lumps forming.
3. Return the chicken to the pan and add the parsley. Simmer gently for 8–10 minutes to ensure the chicken is fully cooked. Remove from the heat, stir in the fromage frais, mango chutney and grapes and serve with boiled rice.

Thai chicken curry

Marinating the chicken overnight maximises the flavour of this very spicy curry. Once cooked, the finished curry can be stored chilled or frozen and reheated as required.

SERVES 4
PER SERVING:
240 KCAL/3.3G FAT
MARINATING TIME:
1 HOUR
PREPARATION TIME:
25 MINUTES
COOKING TIME:
30 MINUTES

for the paste
3 garlic cloves, peeled
1 tablespoon ground coriander
½ teaspoon ground turmeric
½ teaspoon fenugreek seeds or ground fenugreek
2–3 small whole fresh chillies
seeds removed from 4 crushed cardamom pods

1 large red onion, finely chopped
4 large skinless chicken breasts, cut into pieces
2 tablespoons tomato purée
600ml (1 pint) chicken or vegetable stock
1 tablespoon tamarind paste or hot fruit chutney
4 kaffir lime leaves
2 tablespoons chopped fresh coriander

1 Make the paste by grinding all the ingredients in either a food processor or liquidiser.
2 Scrape the paste into a bowl then rinse out the food processor bowl with a little stock. Add the chicken pieces to the paste and mix well. Allow to marinate for a minimum of 1 hour or ideally overnight.
3 In a non-stick pan dry-fry the onion until soft, then add the chicken and cook for 5–6 minutes, stirring continuously. Add the remaining ingredients except the fresh coriander and simmer gently for 15–20 minutes until the sauce thickens and the chicken is fully cooked through.
4 Just before serving, stir in the fresh coriander.

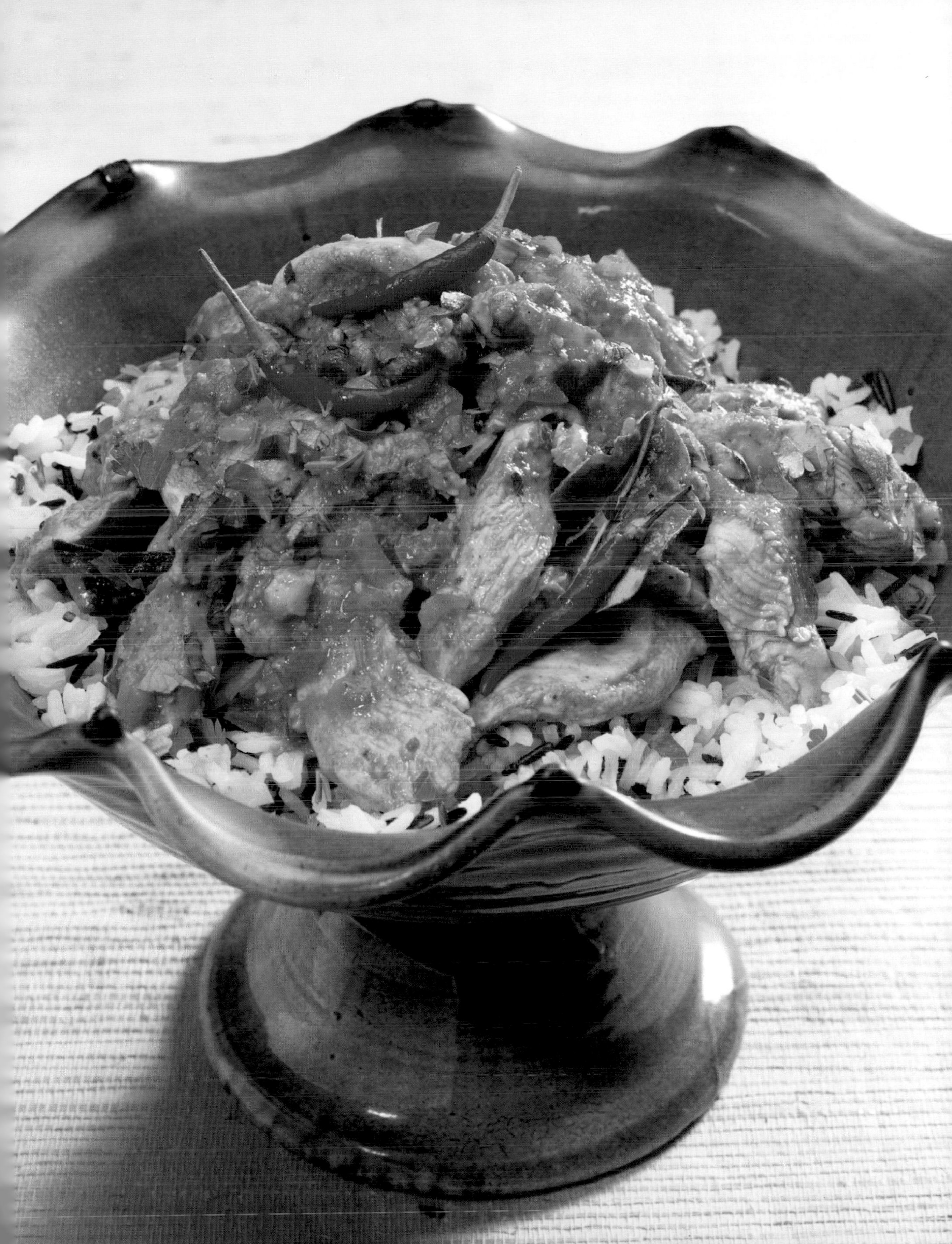

Chicken and coriander meat balls

These tasty chicken nuggets make ideal lunch box bites or picnic food. Serve hot tossed in a little tomato passata for a great pasta accompaniment.

SERVES 4
PER SERVING:
361KCAL/5.4G FAT
PREPARATION:
15 MINUTES
COOKING TIME:
20 MINUTES

1kg (2lb) lean minced chicken
1 small onion, finely chopped
1 garlic clove, crushed
2 teaspoons ground coriander
2 teaspoons ground cumin
1 tablespoon fruit chutney
2 tablespoons chopped fresh coriander
2 teaspoons vegetable bouillon stock powder
1 tablespoon tomato purée

1 Preheat the oven to 190C, 375F, Gas Mark 5.
2 Place all the ingredients in a large bowl and mix well. Mould the mixture into 16 small balls, each about the size of a golf ball, and place on a non-stick baking tray.
3 Bake in the oven for 20–25 minutes.
4 Serve hot with pasta and salad or cold with extra chutney.

Pancetta chicken with white wine

SERVES 4
PER SERVING:
321 KCAL/8.7G FAT
PREPARATION TIME:
20 MINUTES
COOKING TIME:
40 MINUTES

4 lean skinless chicken breasts
1 medium red onion, finely chopped
4 thin slices pancetta or smoked bacon
1 chicken stock cube dissolved in 300ml (½ pint) water
1 tablespoon plain flour
225g (8oz) chestnut mushrooms, sliced
1 wine glass white wine
2 tablespoons chopped fresh mixed herbs

Pancetta is a lightly smoked cured Italian bacon. It adds good flavour to stocks and sauces. If unavailable, substitute smoked streaky bacon.

1 Season the chicken breasts on both sides with plenty of salt and freshly ground black pepper, then place in a preheated non-stick pan.
2 Dry-fry on both sides for 5–6 minutes until lightly browned, then remove from the pan and place on a plate.
3 Add the onion and pancetta to the pan and cook gently until lightly coloured. Add 2 tablespoons of stock. Sprinkle the flour over and cook out for 1 minute.
4 Gradually stir in the remaining stock with the mushrooms and wine.
5 Return the chicken to the pan and add the herbs. Simmer gently for 15–20 minutes until the sauce has reduced and the chicken has cooked through.

Hot pan smoked duck with orange salad

Pan smoking is a variation of barbecuing with the food being totally encased in the cooking smoke. The food is cooked in a smoker over wood chippings, adding flavour directly to the food *(See page 184)**. Timing is essential as over-smoking can result in a dark film encasing the food, resulting in a strong bitter flavour.*

SERVES 4
PER SERVING:
195 KCAL/2.2G FAT
PREPARATION TIME:
5 MINUTES
COOKING TIME:
20 MINUTES

2 packs of 2 Gressingham skinless duck breasts (available from Sainsbury's)
salt
2 tablespoons mixed peppercorns
a few fresh sprigs thyme
4 large oranges
50g (2oz) fresh rocket leaves
1 tablespoon redcurrant jelly
a few fresh mint leaves, chopped

1. Preheat the oven to 200C, 400F, Gas Mark 6.
2. Place the peppercorns in a pestle and mortar or grind between two flat plates.
3. Prepare the duck by removing the skin with a sharp knife. Season each breast well with salt and the peppercorns.
4. Prepare the smoker and place the duck pieces onto the wire rack. Cover the whole smoker with aluminium foil and stand the smoker over a low heat.
5. Smoke for 8–10 minutes, reducing the heat if the smoke smells strong.
6. Turn off the heat and allow the smoker to stand for 2–3 minutes before removing the foil. Transfer the duck to a baking tray and cover with the thyme sprigs, place in the preheated oven for 5–6 minutes to finish cooking.
7. Remove the duck from the oven and allow to rest for 5 minutes.
8. Segment the oranges by removing the outer skin and pith with a sharp knife. Cut in between the thin membrane, separating each orange segment.
9. Place the orange segments in a serving bowl and toss through the rocket leaves. Arrange on serving plates.
10. Drain away the meat juices from the duck into a small bowl and stir in the redcurrant jelly and the mint.
11. Slice the duck into pieces, add to the salad and drizzle with the dressing.

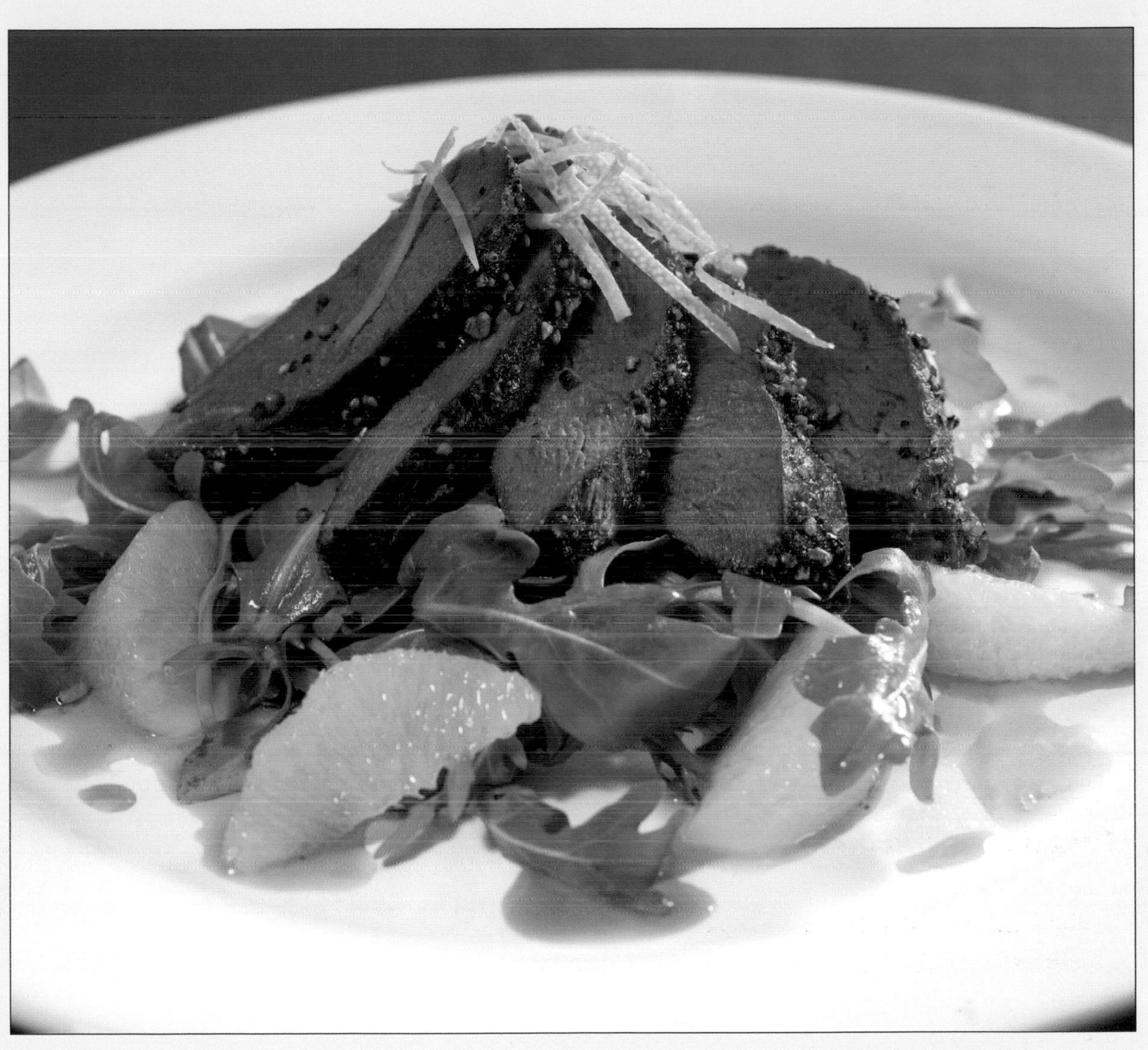

Fish and shellfish

Fresh fish is probably the easiest option on a low-fat diet. High in protein and naturally low in fat, bought prepared, it takes only minutes to cook in many versatile ways from steaming, grilling to baking and the barbecue.

Non-stick griddle pans are perfect for cooking firm, meaty fish steaks such as fresh tuna or swordfish. With the variety available, it makes sense to include fish more in our weekly menu planning.

Oily fish such as salmon and mackerel contains essential fatty acids, important for good health, and is therefore acceptable in moderation on a low-fat eating plan.

The key to maximising the flavour is to cook fish lightly, using fresh herbs and spices as a coating or sauce addition.

Lobster couscous salad

SERVES 4
PER SERVING:
270 KCAL/3.3G FAT
PREPARATION TIME:
20 MINUTES
COOKING TIME:
5 MINUTES

meat from 1 large cooked lobster
1 vegetable stock cube dissolved in 400ml (14fl oz) boiling water
1 teaspoon ground coriander
1 garlic clove, crushed
175g (6oz) couscous
1 tablespoon finely chopped chives
1 tablespoon chopped fresh coriander
4 tomatoes, skinned, seeded and diced
½ cucumber, peeled and diced
salt and freshly ground black pepper

for the dressing
150ml (¼ pint) fresh apple juice
juice of 2 limes
1 tablespoon good quality white wine vinegar
1 teaspoon Dijon mustard
fresh coriander to garnish

Lobster turns a simple salad into a luxurious seafood delight. If you are unsure about how to prepare or cook lobster, then buy it freshly cooked and use straight away. For a vegetarian option cook the couscous in the same manner and top with a selection of oven roasted vegetables or dry-fried Quorn.

1 Cut the cooked lobster meat into bite-sized pieces.
2 In a large saucepan bring the stock to the boil, adding the ground coriander and garlic. Gradually pour in the couscous, stirring well. Cover with a lid, remove from the heat and allow to stand for 1 minute.
3 Remove the lid and, using 2 forks, fluff up the couscous grains. Add the herbs, tomato and cucumber and mix well, seasoning to taste.
4 Pile the couscous mixture into a serving dish and arrange the cooked lobster on top.
5 Combine the dressing ingredients and spoon over the lobster, sprinkle with fresh coriander and serve.

See photograph on page 110.

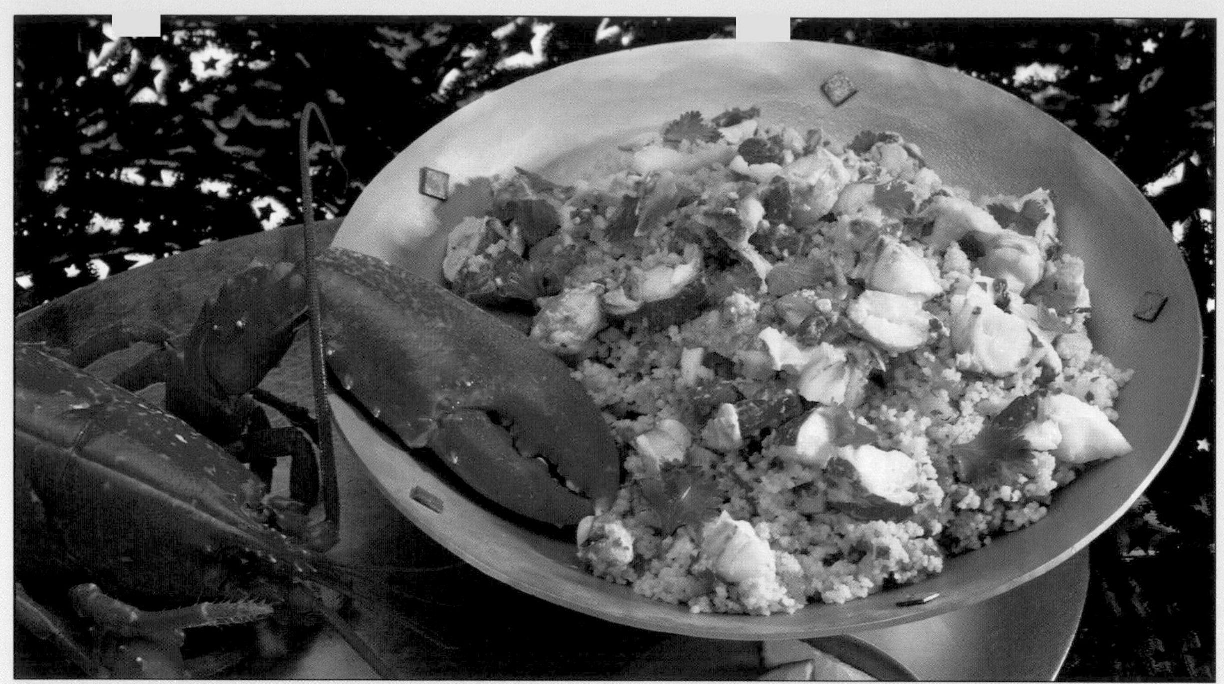

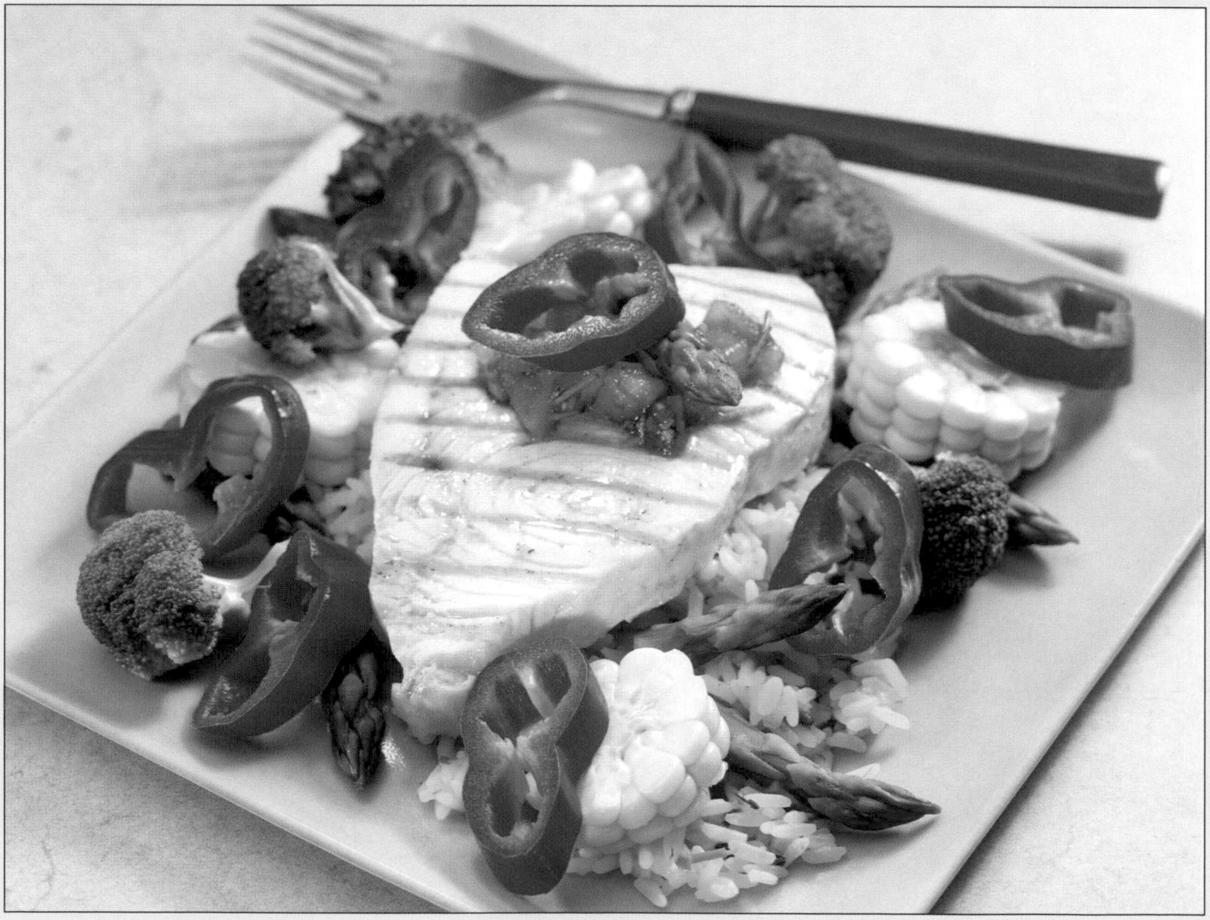

Griddled swordfish with tomato and lime salsa

SERVES 4
PER SERVING:
169 KCAL/5G FAT
PREPARATION TIME:
25 MINUTES
COOKING TIME:
10 MINUTES

4 fresh swordfish steaks

for the marinade
4 tablespoons light soy sauce
zest and juice of 2 limes
1 small red chilli, seeded and finely chopped
1 × 2.5cm (1 in) piece fresh ginger, peeled and finely chopped
salt and freshly ground black pepper
2 teaspoons oil to line pan

for the salsa
6 ripe tomatoes
1 lime
1 tablespoon chopped fresh chives
1 tablespoon balsamic vinegar
salt and freshly ground black pepper

Top left: *Lobster couscous salad*

Left: *Griddled swordfish with tomato and lime salsa*

1 Place the swordfish steaks in a shallow dish.
2 Combine all the marinade ingredients together in a small bowl and pour over the swordfish steaks. Leave to marinate for 20 minutes.
3 To make the salsa, skin the tomatoes by plunging them into boiling water for 10 seconds. Remove and submerge in ice-cold water. Peel away the skin, then slice each tomato in half and remove the seeds, using a teaspoon.
4 Chop the tomato flesh and place in a bowl. Using a zester, remove thin strips of zest from the lime and add to the bowl, along with the juice. Stir in the chives and balsamic vinegar. Season to taste.
5 Preheat a non-stick griddle pan, lightly greasing with a little oil and removing the excess with kitchen paper.
6 When the pan is very hot, carefully add the swordfish and season with salt and freshly ground black pepper. Cook it quickly for 4–5 minutes on each side. If overcooked the texture will become tough and rubbery.
7 Garnish with the salsa and serve hot.

Griddled monkfish with dill and lemon dressing

Monkfish is very dense and chunky in texture, making it ideal to griddle or barbecue. It needs very little cooking, although it does depend on the thickness of each tail. Because of its density, always make sure it is cooked through to the centre, but be careful not to overcook.

SERVES 4
PER SERVING:
184 KCAL/1.3G FAT
PREPARATION TIME:
20 MINUTES
COOKING TIME:
15 MINUTES

1kg (2lb) monkfish tail fillets, boned and skinned
300ml (1/2 pint) apple juice
juice of 1 lemon
2 teaspoons Dijon mustard
2 teaspoons finely chopped dill
1/2 teaspoon ground fenugreek
1 teaspoon green peppercorns in brine
2 tablespoons virtually fat free Normandy fromage frais
salt and freshly ground black pepper

1. Prepare the monkfish by removing the thin outer skin and cut into chunky pieces. Season well with salt and freshly ground black pepper.
2. Preheat a non-stick griddle pan until hot, and cook the fish over a high heat for 2–3 minutes on each side. Remove from the pan and cover to keep warm.
3. Add the remaining ingredients except the fromage frais to the pan, stirring continuously to combine. Bring the dressing to a low simmer and return the sealed fish to the pan. Cover with a lid for 2–3 minutes until the fish is heated through.
4. Just before serving, stir in the fromage frais.

Bouillabaisse

SERVES 4
PER SERVING:
368 KCAL/7.2G FAT
PREPARATION TIME:
20 MINUTES
COOKING TIME:
30 MINUTES

3 banana or French shallots, finely chopped
3 baby leeks, sliced
2 garlic cloves, finely chopped
good sprig of fresh thyme
$\frac{1}{2}$ teaspoon fennel seeds
2 pieces orange rind
1 small red chilli, finely chopped
good pinch of saffron
1 × 400g (14oz) can chopped tomatoes
1.2 litres (2 pints) fish stock
1kg (2lb) mixed fish (John Dory, bass, red snapper or mullet, monkfish, parrot fish)
salt and freshly ground black pepper

for the rouille
4 tablespoons fine breadcrumbs
1 tablespoon marinated red pimento peppers
1 garlic clove, crushed
2–3 tablespoons stock from the bouillabaisse

Probably the most famous fish stew, which has been adapted from a simple, peasant- style dish to a glamorous feast. It is traditionally served with either rouille, a rust orange garlic sauce, or aïoli (a garlic, olive oil and egg yolk sauce – see page 164 for a low-fat recipe). In this recipe you can use either small, whole, gutted fish or fish steaks cut from larger fish.

1 In a large shallow non-stick pan dry-fry the shallots, leeks and garlic until soft. Add the herbs and spices and continue cooking for 1–2 minutes. Pour the tomatoes and stock into the pan and bring to the boil.
2 Place the fish on top of the stock, cover with a lid and simmer gently for 15–20 minutes until the fish is cooked. Carefully lift the fish from the pan and place in warmed serving dishes.
3 Increase the heat and boil the sauce (reserve 2–3 tablespoons for the rouille) to reduce to a rich consistency. Pour the sauce over the fish.
4 To make the rouille, place all the ingredients into a food processor and blend until smooth. Season with salt and freshly ground black pepper.
5 Garnish the stew with the rouille and serve with aïoli and boiled new potatoes.

Seafood pie

As the fish is uncooked, it is essential the pie is cooked in a hot oven to get the heat through to the centre of the pie. If the pie starts to brown quickly, cover the top with foil and place lower in the oven to finish cooking.

N.B. The sauce may boil over the sides of the dish, so line the base of the oven with foil for easy cleaning.

SERVES 6
PER SERVING:
283 KCAL/3.5G FAT
PREPARATION TIME:
10 MINUTES
COOKING TIME:
40 MINUTES

675g ($1\frac{1}{2}$lb) potatoes, peeled
2 tablespoons virtually fat free fromage frais
225g (8oz) smoked haddock
225g (8oz) peeled prawns
115g (4oz) smoked or cooked mussels (optional)
225g (8oz) fresh crab meat
2 baby leeks, finely chopped
150ml ($\frac{1}{4}$ pint) fish stock
1 tablespoon plain flour
$\frac{1}{2}$ wine glass white wine or sherry
2–3 teaspoons mild Dijon mustard
600ml (1 pint) skimmed milk
1 tablespoon freshly chopped chives
salt and freshly ground black pepper
chopped fresh parsley to garnish

1 Preheat the oven to 220C, 425 F, Gas Mark 7.
2 Boil the potatoes in a saucepan of salted water until well cooked. Drain and mash well until smooth, adding the fromage frais and seasoning well.
3 Remove the skin and bones from the smoked haddock and place in the bottom of an ovenproof dish. Add the prawns and mussels, if using.
4 Check the crab meat for pieces of shell or tendons and place on top.
5 Place the leeks and the fish stock in a medium-sized saucepan and cook for 1–2 minutes. Sprinkle the flour over and mix well. Cook out for 1 minute over a low heat, then add the white wine and mustard, beating well. Gradually add the skimmed milk, stirring continuously to prevent any lumps forming. Bring to the boil, allowing the sauce to thicken.
6 Pour the sauce over the fish and allow to cool, stirring in the chives. Cover with the potatoes, either using a fork or piping through a piping bag with a large star nozzle.
7 Bake in the oven for 30–40 minutes until golden.

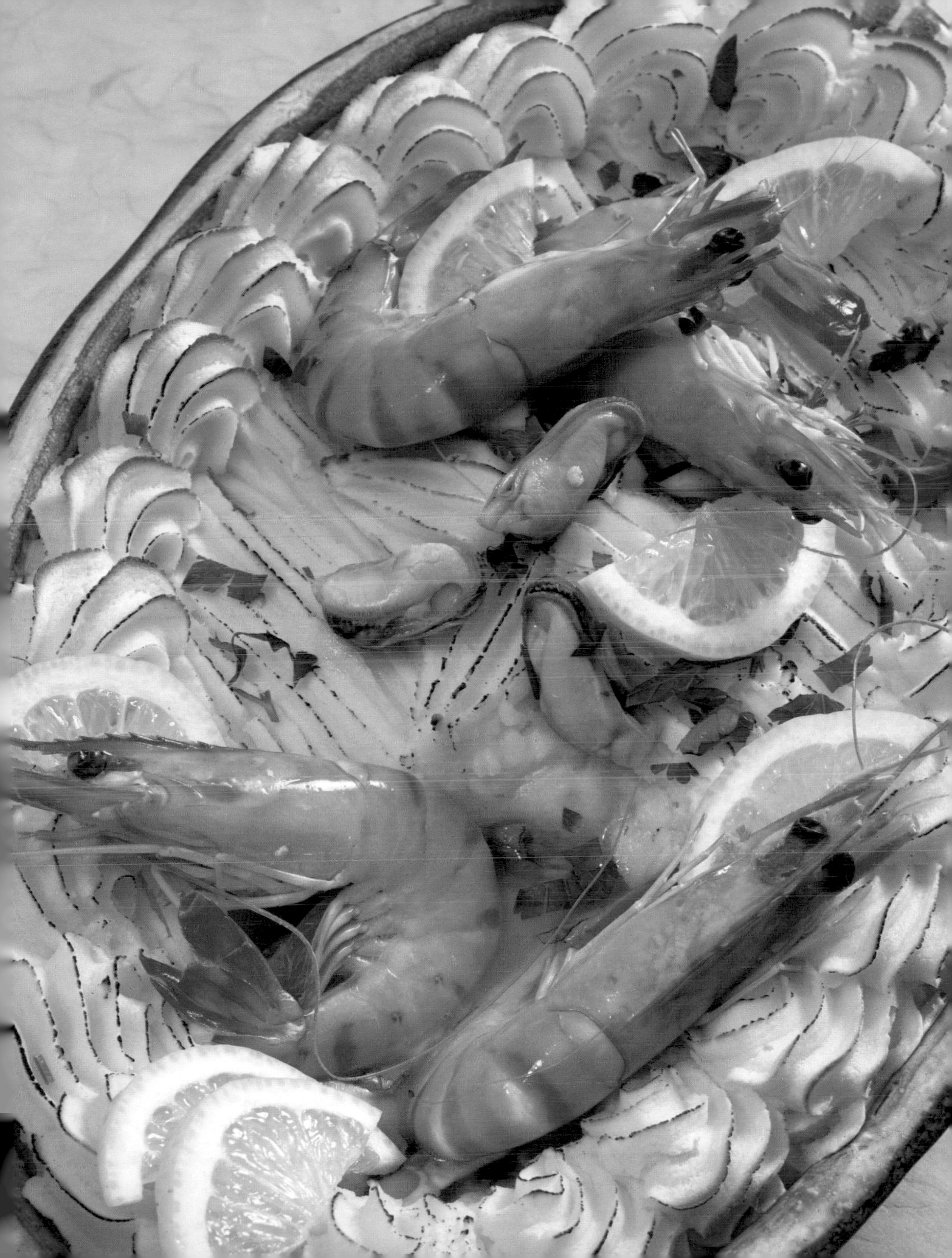

Vegetarian

We know that a good balance of nutritional meals is essential to our wellbeing. Eating some foods in excess, whether carbohydrates or protein-based foods such as meat, can have an adverse effect. With this in mind, many people now choose to incorporate vegetarian meals as part of their weekly plan.

It is essential to include foods from each of the four main food groups – proteins, milk and dairy products, cereals and grains, and fruit and vegetables.

Avoiding meat means you need to find alternative sources of protein in the form of beans and pulses. New plant-based products include TVP, tofu and Quorn, all of which can act as meat substitutes. Nuts stand alone since they are a high-fat commodity, so use sparingly.

Dairy products are essential for providing calcium. If wished, cow's milk may be substituted with soya milk and other vegetarian alternatives.

Look out for reduced-fat cheeses, particularly the mature type, which have a stronger flavour than the regular kind.

Carbohydrates such as bread, breakfast cereals, potatoes, pasta, rice and other grains should provide the bulk of food at every meal. Avoid serving these and vegetable accompaniments with additional fat. Use yogurt and low-fat cheese toppings. Serve pasta with tomato-based sauces, not cream-based, and use Parmesan shavings sparingly.

When preparing and cooking meals, you can reduce the fat by replacing oily marinades with fruit juices, soy sauce or diluted stock. Dry-frying and dry-roasting vegetables means that they cook successfully in their natural juices. Aubergine and mushrooms are a prime example, as these usually soak up oil or butter when fried.

Allow plenty of moisture in the form of well-flavoured herb stocks and tomato products such as passata or canned chopped tomatoes, which add volume as well as flavour.

If you choose not to eat fish, you may add a drop of oil to your cooking, one that is rich in essential fatty acids such as soya or rapeseed oil, but do use in moderation.

Quick vegetable korma

A quick and easy way to spice up vegetables. It is suitable for home freezing, so make up in a large batch and portion into small freezer containers. Once fully cooked, if liquidised it makes a great fresh curry sauce.

SERVES 1
PER SERVING:
114 KCAL/1.5G FAT
PREPARATION TIME:
10 MINUTES
COOKING TIME:
15 MINUTES

1 courgette, sliced
½ red pepper, diced
2–3 chestnut mushrooms, sliced
4 spring onions, finely chopped
1 garlic clove, crushed
1–2 teaspoons korma curry powder
1 teaspoon vegetable bouillon stock powder, dissolved in 4 tablespoons boiling water
1 teaspoon plain flour
4 tablespoons skimmed milk
chopped fresh flat leaf parsley
1 tablespoon virtually fat free Normandy fromage frais
salt and freshly ground black pepper

1. Preheat a non-stick pan, add the courgette, red pepper and mushrooms and dry-fry for 6–7 minutes until they start to colour.
2. Add the spring onions and garlic to the pan and cook gently until soft. Sprinkle the curry powder over and add 2 tablespoons of stock. Mix well, then add the flour and cook out for 1 minute.
3. Gradually add the remaining stock and the milk, stirring continuously to prevent any lumps from forming.
4. Add the parsley and simmer gently for 8–10 minutes. Remove from heat, stir in the fromage frais and serve with boiled rice.

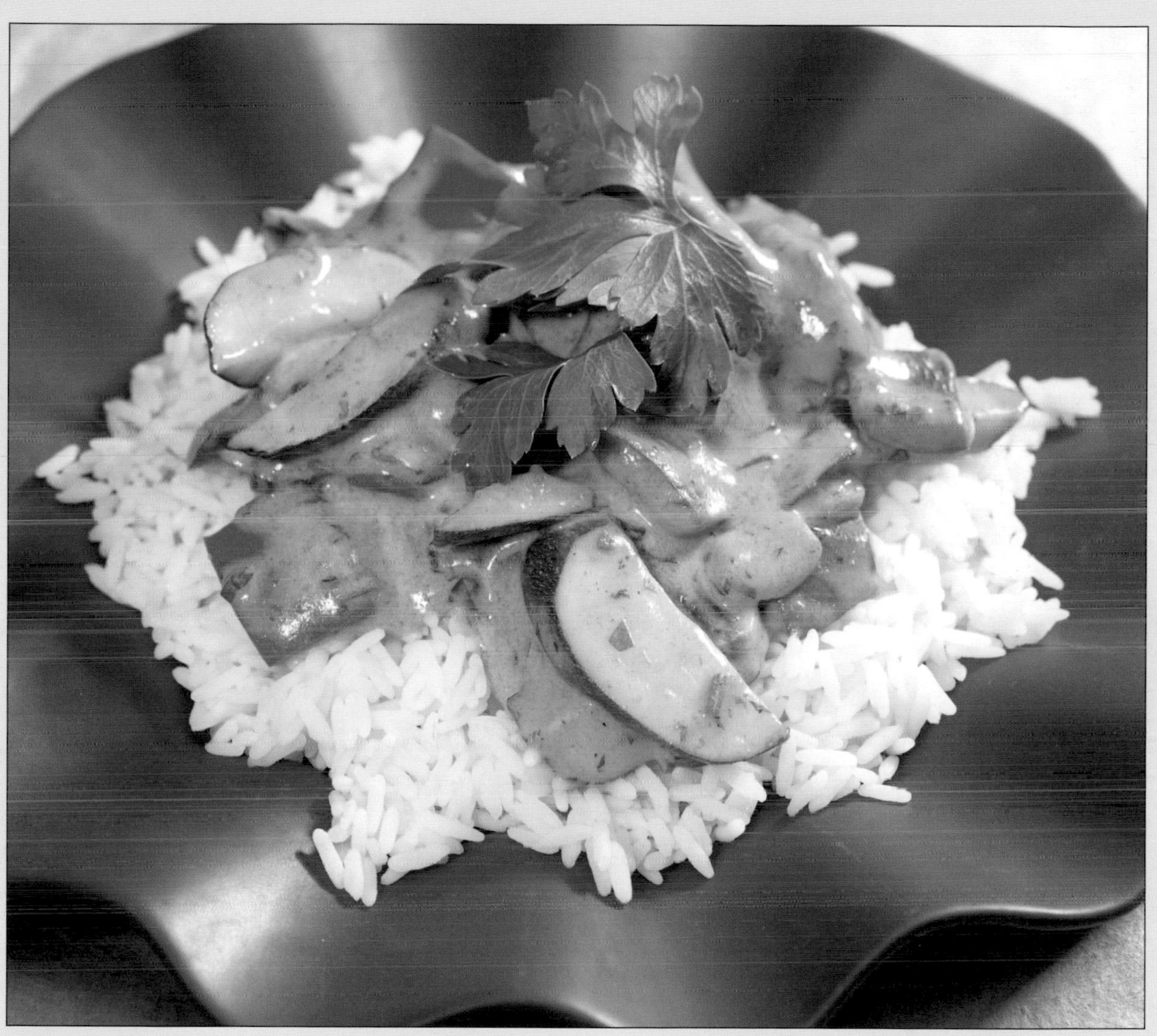

Navajo tortillas

These simple flat breads taste delicious eaten straight from the pan, but for ease cook them in advance and reheat for 4–5 minutes in a low oven. The mustard powder adds a golden colour as well as flavour.

MAKES 8
PER TORTILLA:
209 KCAL/0.9G FAT
PREPARATION TIME:
5 MINUTES
COOKING TIME:
20 MINUTES

- 450g (1lb) soft white flour
- 1 teaspoon fine salt
- 2 teaspoons baking powder
- 2 teaspoons English mustard powder
- 2 tablespoons chopped fresh coriander
- 250–300ml (8–10fl oz) skimmed milk
- a little vegetable oil

1. Sieve all the dry ingredients into a large mixing bowl. Add the coriander and mix in.
2. Using a flat edged knife, make a well in the centre of the flour and slowly add sufficient milk, bringing the mixture together with the knife to form a soft dough.
3. Divide the dough into 8 equal balls. Using a rolling pin, roll out each ball onto a floured surface into a circle, getting the dough as thin as you can.
4. Stack the breads, dusting in between with flour.
5. Preheat a large non-stick frying or griddle pan until hot. Add a small amount of vegetable oil, then wipe out with a thick pad of kitchen paper.
6. Cook the tortillas in the hot pan for approximately 1 minute each side. Don't worry if the bread has black markings, as this will add flavour.
7. Stack the breads onto a warm plate and serve or reheat as required.

Pinto bean chilli burros

SERVES 4
PER SERVING:
242 KCAL/5G FAT
PREPARATION TIME:
15 MINUTES
COOKING TIME:
40 MINUTES

2 red onions, finely chopped
2 garlic cloves, crushed
2–3 fresh green chillies, seeded and chopped
2 thin courgettes, grated
1 × 400g (14oz) can pinto beans, drained and rinsed
1 × 400g (14oz) can chopped tomatoes
300ml ($^1/_2$ pint) tomato passata
2 teaspoons chopped fresh oregano
3 teaspoons vegetable bouillon stock powder

Pinto beans are beige in colour with brown speckles. They are native to Mexico but now mostly grown in the United States.

1 Preheat a non-stick frying pan. Dry-fry the onions and garlic for 1–2 minutes until soft. Add the chillies and courgettes and continue to cook for 2 minutes.
2 Stir in the remaining ingredients and bring to the boil. Reduce the heat and cover. Simmer gently for 20–25 minutes until the sauce thickens.
3 Serve as a filling for floured tortillas with shredded lettuce and chopped spring onion.

Cherry tomato and courgette tarte Tatin

A savoury version of the famous French apple tart. This vegetarian pie makes a great alternative to high-fat quiche and also works particularly well with roasted peppers.

SERVES 4
PER SERVING:
265 KCAL/5.9G FAT
PREPARATION TIME:
10 MINUTES
COOKING TIME:
35 MINUTES

12 large cherry tomatoes
3 small courgettes, sliced
300ml (½ pint) skimmed milk
1 teaspoon vegetable bouillon stock powder
1 tablespoon Dijon mustard
1 garlic clove, crushed
1 tablespoon cornflour
2 tablespoons chopped fresh mixed herbs
50g (2oz) low-fat Cheddar cheese
1 egg
2 tablespoons skimmed milk
8 sheets filo pastry

1 Preheat the oven to 200C, 400F, Gas Mark 6.
2 Preheat a non-stick frying pan. Slice the tomatoes and arrange in the base of a 20cm (8in) ovenproof flan dish.
3 Dry-fry the courgettes quickly until coloured and add to the flan dish.
4 In a small saucepan heat the milk with the stock powder, mustard and garlic. Slake the cornflour with a little milk and add to the saucepan, whisking well. Simmer until the sauce thickens, stir in the herbs and cheese and pour onto the tomatoes and courgettes.
4 Beat together the egg and milk.
5 When the sauce is cool, place a sheet of pastry on top of the sauce, brush with beaten egg and milk, then add another layer of pastry. Continue until all the pastry is used up.
6 Brush the top and place in the oven for 20–25 minutes.
7 Allow to cool for 5 minutes, then turn out onto a tray or large serving plate.

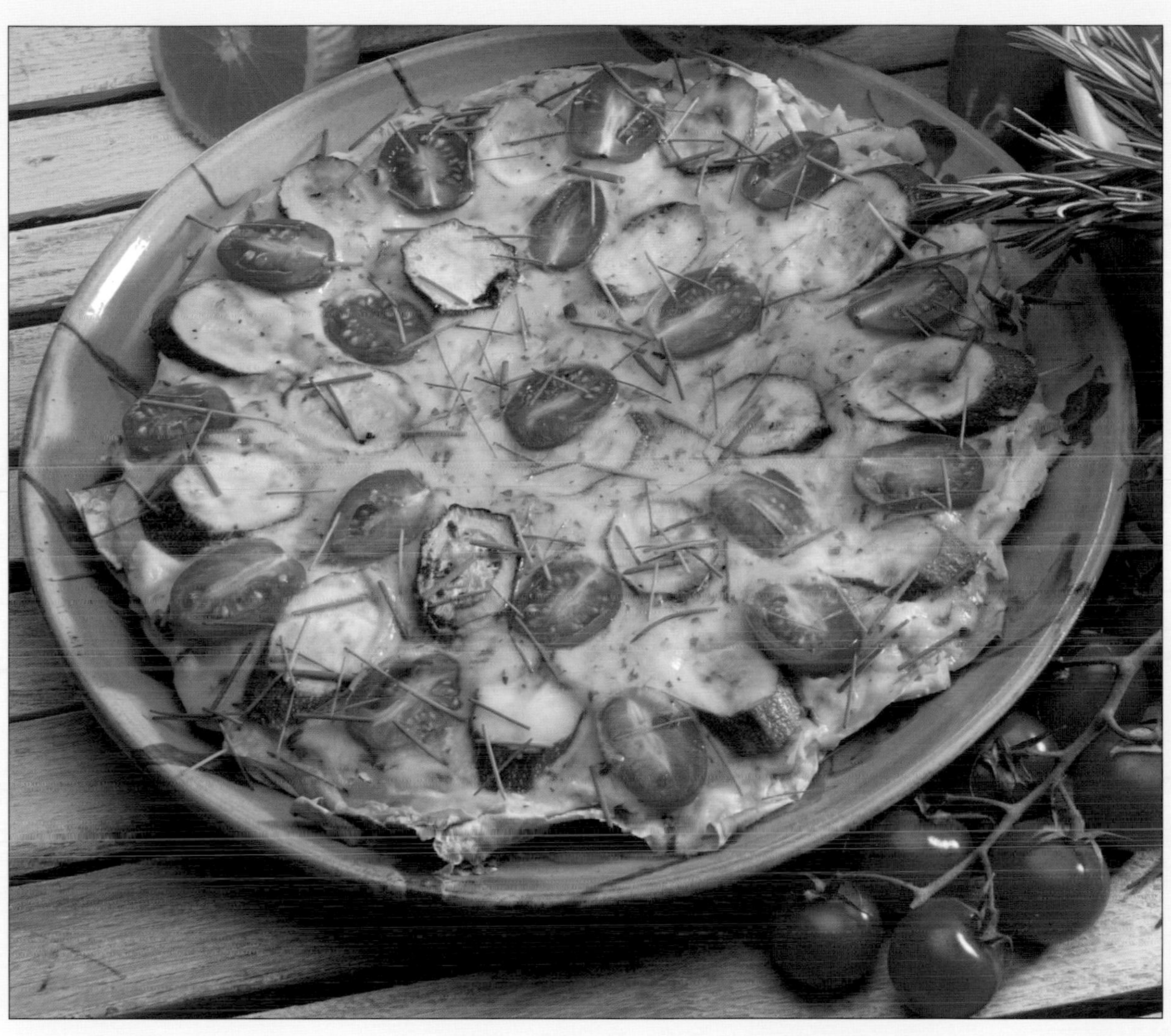

Potato and spinach soufflé

The secret of a good soufflé is to make sure the mixture is well beaten before adding the egg whites, then gently fold in the whites, retaining as much air as possible. The soufflé will start to deflate as soon as it leaves the oven, so serve straight away.

SERVES 4
PER SERVING:
147 KCAL/6.4G FAT
PREPARATION TIME:
15 MINUTES
COOKING TIME:
55 MINUTES

225g (8oz) cooked potatoes
1 tablespoon virtually fat free fromage frais
1 garlic clove, crushed
3 eggs, separated
225g (8oz) fresh leaf spinach, stalked and finely shredded
grated fresh nutmeg (optional)
25g (1oz) grated low-fat Cheddar cheese
salt and freshly ground black pepper

1 Preheat the oven to 180C, 350F, Gas Mark 4.
2 Place the potatoes in large bowl and, using a potato masher, mash well to remove any lumps. Beat in the fromage frais, garlic, egg yolks and spinach. Season well with salt and black pepper and a little nutmeg if desired. Add the grated cheese, reserving a pinch for later, and mix well.
3 In a clean bowl, whisk the egg whites until stiff. Fold into the mixture until fully combined and pour into a lightly greased 18cm (7in) soufflé dish.
4 Sprinkle the reserved cheese over the top and bake in the oven for 30–35 minutes until well risen and golden brown. Serve straight away with salad or vegetables.

Ribbon vegetable stir-fry

SERVES 4
PER SERVING:
186 KCAL/2.9G FAT
PREPARATION TIME:
20 MINUTES
COOKING TIME:
10 MINUTES

2 carrots
2 small parsnips
2 small courgettes
1 red pepper, seeded and finely sliced
4 baby leeks, sliced
2 teaspoons finely chopped fresh ginger
1 tablespoon light soy sauce
2 tablespoons chopped fresh chives
115g (4oz) fine noodles
1 vegetable stock cube
zest and juice of 1 lime
1 medium red onion, finely sliced
2 garlic cloves, crushed

This large quantity of thinly sliced vegetables soon cooks down when tossed in a hot pan. However, I find they are best cooked in batches to ensure they cook evenly. Reheat in a moderate oven, then toss with the hot noodles.

1 Prepare the vegetables by peeling if required, then, using a vegetable peeler, take thin strips from the length of the carrots, parsnips and courgettes. Place in a bowl with the other vegetables, add the ginger, soy sauce and half of the chives. Mix well.
2 Cook the noodles in a pan of water containing a vegetable stock cube. Drain and toss with the lime zest and juice.
3 Heat a non-stick wok or frying pan, add the onion and garlic and cook until soft.
4 Add the vegetables and cook quickly over a high heat until they are just cooked.
5 Add the noodles and mix together well.
6 Serve in warmed bowls and sprinkle with the remaining chopped chives.

Spiced creamy vegetables with coconut milk

The perfect light summer curry. Coconut adds sweetness to the creamy sauce as well as a thickening agent. Serve with a sweet mango chutney and cucumber salad.

SERVES 4
PER SERVING:
253 KCAL/10.9G FAT
PREPARATION TIME:
20 MINUTES
COOKING TIME:
35 MINUTES

50g (2oz) desiccated coconut
450g (1lb) young tender carrots, scraped
600ml (1 pint) skimmed milk
2 medium onions, finely chopped
2 garlic cloves, crushed
2 teaspoons fresh thyme, chopped
½ teaspoon allspice
2 teaspoons ground cumin
1 teaspoon ground turmeric
1 tablespoon chopped fresh ginger
2 red chillies, finely chopped
150ml (¼ pint) strong vegetable stock
1 tablespoon plain flour
4 baby leeks, finely chopped
225g (8oz) baby asparagus
115g (4oz) baby broad beans, shelled
115g (4oz) green beans

1. In a small saucepan boil together the coconut, carrots and milk for 10 minutes, then set aside.
2. In a preheated non-stick pan dry-fry the onions and garlic until soft, add the thyme and spices and continue cooking for a further 2 minutes.
3. Add 3 tablespoons of stock, then stir in the flour, cooking it out over a low heat.
4. Gradually stir in the remaining stock and the hot milk mixture.
5. Add the remaining vegetables and simmer gently until the vegetables are tender.

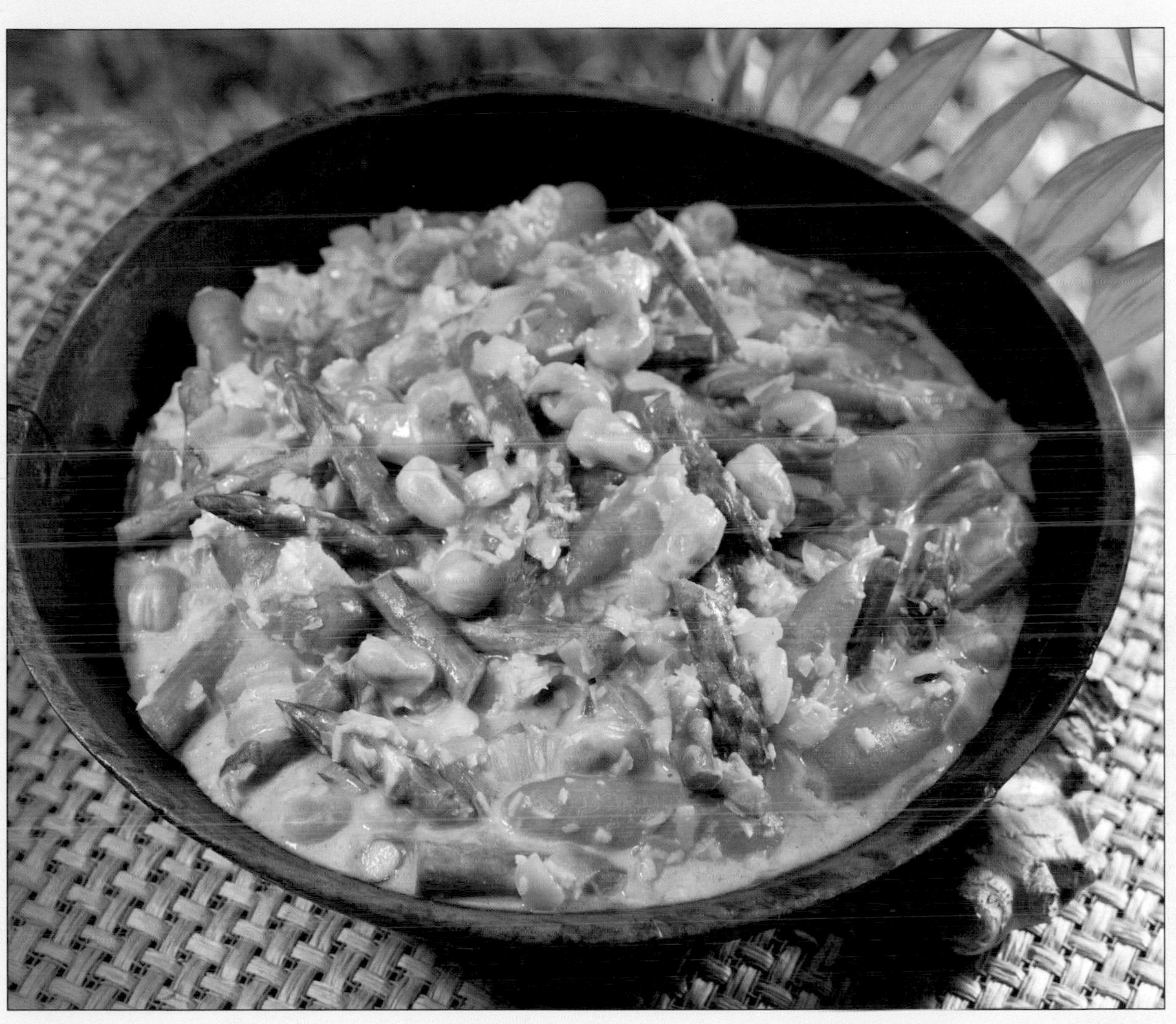

Wet polenta with Gorgonzola sauce

Polenta is made from ground corn or maize. It offers an alternative to potatoes or pasta. Although virtually all cheese is high in fat, the stronger-flavoured types can be used in small quantities when coupled with a low-fat base such as polenta or a jacket potato.

SERVES 4
PER SERVING:
340 KCAL/5G FAT
PREPARATION TIME:
10 MINUTES
COOKING TIME:
45 MINUTES

- 225g (8oz) Bramata polenta flour
- 1.2 litres (2 pints) vegetable stock
- 1 tablespoon chopped fresh mixed herbs
- 3 garlic cloves, crushed
- 2 long shallots, finely chopped
- 1 tablespoon dry sherry
- 600ml (1 pint) semi-skimmed milk
- 1 heaped tablespoon plain flour
- 1 teaspoon chopped fresh sage
- 2 tablespoons virtually fat free fromage frais
- 50g (2oz) Gorgonzola cheese, crumbled
- salt and freshly ground black pepper
- 1 tablespoon chopped fresh coriander to garnish

1 Weigh the polenta flour into a large jug so that it can be poured easily.

2 In a large saucepan bring the stock to the boil. Add the herbs and half the garlic, then slowly pour in the polenta flour in a continuous stream, stirring with a whisk to prevent lumps forming. Change the whisk for a wooden spoon and beat well until smooth. Reduce the heat to a gentle simmer and cook for 40–45 minutes, stirring occasionally.

3 Make the sauce by dry-frying the shallots and remaining garlic in a non-stick pan. Add the sherry and 2 tablespoons milk. Sprinkle the flour over and cook out for 1 minute, adding a little extra milk if it seems dry. Gradually mix in the remaining milk, add the sage and simmer to allow the sauce to thicken.

4 Just before serving, beat the fromage frais into the polenta, season well with salt and black pepper, add the crumbled Gorgonzola to the sauce and check the seasoning.

5 Arrange the polenta on a serving plate, pour the sauce over, then sprinkle with chopped coriander.

Roasted vegetable curry

SERVES 4
PER SERVING:
148 KCAL/5.6G FAT
PREPARATION TIME:
15 MINUTES
COOKING TIME:
45 MINUTES

1 small aubergine, diced
2 red peppers, seeded and diced
2 yellow peppers, seeded and diced
1 red onion, chopped
2 courgettes, sliced
12 cherry tomatoes
2 garlic cloves, crushed
1 tablespoon mild curry powder
2 tablespoons light soy sauce
600ml (1 pint) tomato passata
seeds from 8 crushed cardamom pods
salt and freshly ground black pepper
1 tablespoon chopped fresh coriander

Try this recipe with many different combinations of vegetables. For a creamy sauce stir in 2 tablespoons of virtually fat free fromage frais just before serving.

1 Preheat the oven to 200C, 400F, Gas Mark 6.
2 Place all the vegetables in a non-stick roasting tray and season well with salt and black pepper. Dot with crushed garlic and sprinkle the curry powder over. Drizzle with the soy sauce and place in the top of the preheated oven. Roast for 20–25 minutes until the vegetables start to soften.
3 In a large saucepan heat the passata with the cardamom and add the cooked vegetables. Simmer over a low heat for 15 minutes to allow the sauce to thicken.
4 Check the seasoning, add the fresh coriander and serve.

French bread margarita

An express low-fat pizza for when you have little time to spare. However, do make sure you spread the mixture right up to the edges of the bread, as they may burn slightly when the baguette is returned to the grill.

SERVES 1
PER SERVING:
214 KCAL/4G FAT
PREPARATION TIME:
5 MINUTES
COOKING TIME:
15 MINUTES

1 small French baguette, split in half lengthways
1 garlic clove, peeled and cut in half
1 × 115g (4oz) can chopped tomatoes
4–5 fresh basil leaves
1 tablespoon low-fat salad dressing
1 tablespoon grated low-fat Cheddar cheese
8 cherry tomatoes, sliced
salt and freshly ground black pepper

1. Preheat the grill to high.
2. Lightly toast the bread on both sides, then using the cut side of the garlic rub the top of the toasted bread, pressing the centre down.
3. Empty the tomatoes into a small bowl. Mix in the basil leaves and season well with salt and black pepper.
4. Spread the mixture onto both pieces of bread, making sure it goes right up to the outside edges, and top with the sliced tomato.
5. In a small bowl mix together the salad dressing and cheese and spread on the top. Return to the grill until brown and bubbling.
6. Serve straight away with a mixed salad.

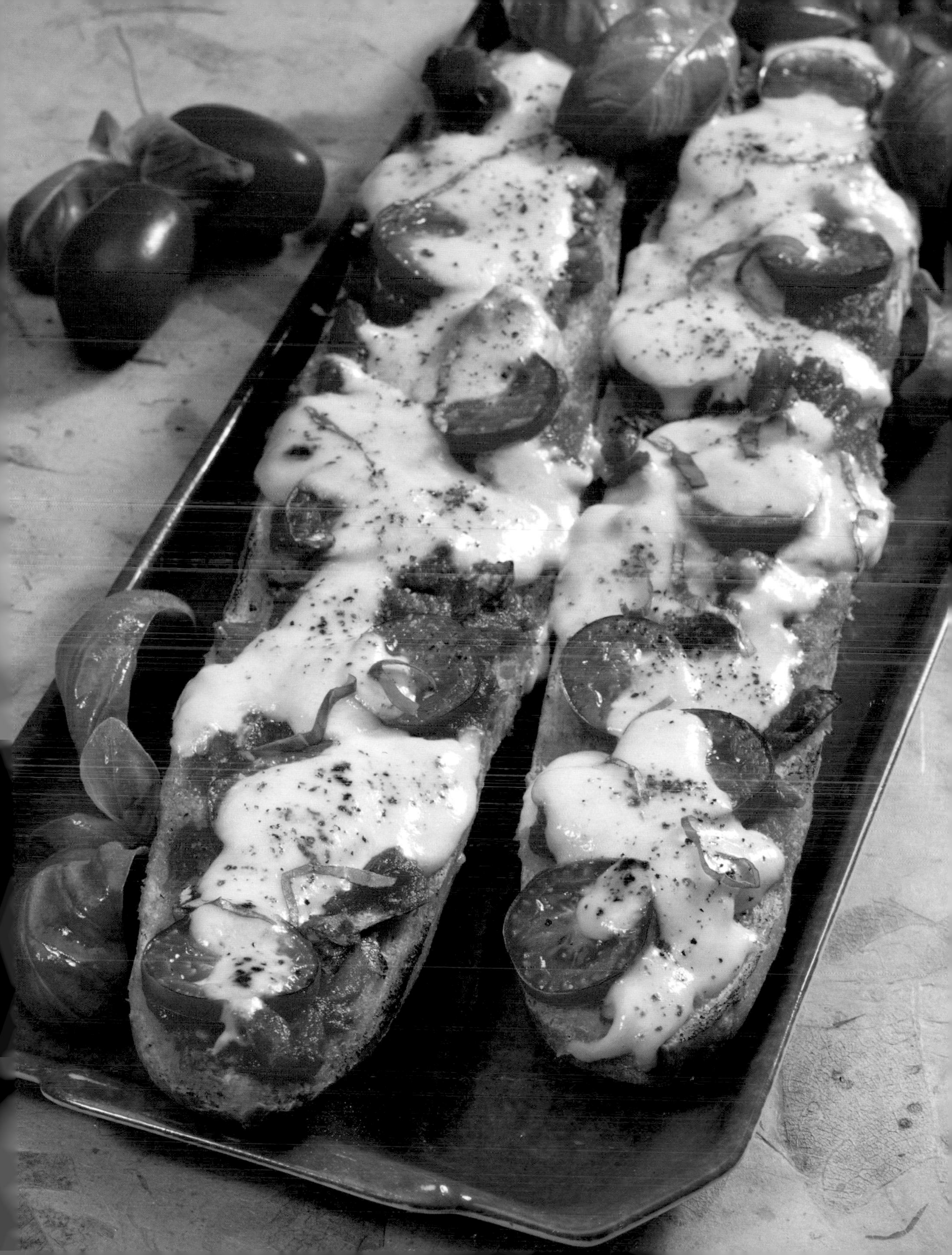

Lentil and roast vegetable loaf

Although the loaf can be served straight from the oven, it is best if allowed to cool and set completely and then reheated as required either as a whole or sliced.

SERVES 4
PER SERVING:
258 KCAL/4.8G FAT
PREPARATION TIME:
25 MINUTES
COOKING TIME:
40 MINUTES

2 medium onions, finely chopped
2 courgettes, diced
1 small aubergine, diced
1 large red pepper, seeded and diced
175g (6oz) red lentils
1 × 400g (14oz) can chopped tomatoes
150ml (¼ pint) vegetable stock
2 garlic cloves, crushed
2 teaspoons chopped fresh thyme
2 eggs, beaten
salt and freshly ground black pepper
fresh basil to garnish

1 Preheat the oven to 200C, 400F, Gas Mark 6.
2 Place the prepared vegetables into a roasting tin, season well with salt and black pepper and bake at the top of the oven for 25–30 minutes until lightly roasted.
3 In a saucepan bring to the boil the lentils, tomatoes, stock, garlic and thyme. Simmer for 15 minutes to soften the lentils and allow them to absorb the liquid. Mix the lentil mixture with the vegetables in a mixing bowl, adding the beaten egg.
4 Pour the mixture into a lightly greased 1kg (2lb) loaf tin and stand in a baking tray containing 2.5cm (1in) water. Bake in the middle of the oven for 40 minutes until risen and set. Allow to cool slightly before serving.
5 Just before serving, sprinkle with fresh basil.

Spanish omelette

SERVES 1
PER SERVING:
238 KCAL/13.5G FAT
PREPARATION TIME:
10 MINUTES
COOKING TIME:
10 MINUTES

- ½ red onion, finely sliced
- ½ red pepper seeded and diced
- 1 garlic clove, crushed
- 1 tomato, skinned, seeded and finely diced
- 2 eggs, beaten and seasoned with salt and freshly ground black pepper

As the vegetables will release liquid when they are dry-fried, there is no need to add any milk to the egg mixture, although a teaspoon or two could be added if desired.

1. Preheat a non-stick frying pan. Dry-fry the onion, pepper and garlic for 3–4 minutes until soft.
2. Add the beaten egg and cook gently, using a wooden spatula to bring the set mixture from around the outside of the pan into the centre.
3. When the omelette is almost set, add the chopped tomato and turn the omelette over, either whole or split down the centre to make it easier.

Pasta and rice

There are many different types of pasta available with varying ingredients. Some use higher quantities of egg yolk than others, so check the labels carefully when buying dried pasta, as this can increase the calorie and fat content. Shapes and styles vary from fine noodles to large shapes suitable for filling. All require cooking in a large quantity of boiling water. Adding a vegetable or herb stock cube to the water does away with the need to use olive oil, which is usually added. The same applies to cooking rice, as the stock cube adds flavour to the cooking liquor. Always rinse rice well under cold running water before cooking to remove some of the starches. This will help keep the rice fluffy and loose once cooked.

Generally pasta and rice are low in fat; it is just the additions that bump up the fat grams, so choose tomato-based sauces and add chopped herbs such as basil or coriander to your stock boiled rice.

Allow 25g (1oz) dry weight pasta per person when serving as a starter and 50g (2oz) dry weight per person when serving as a main course.

Mushroom stir-fry with lemon noodles

SERVES 4
PER SERVING:
148 KCAL/2.7G FAT
PREPARATION TIME:
10 MINUTES
COOKING TIME:
10 MINUTES

115g (4oz) fine noodles
1 vegetable stock cube
zest and juice of 1 lemon
1 medium red onion, finely sliced
2 garlic cloves, crushed
450g (1lb) assorted mushrooms, sliced
2 teaspoons fresh ginger, peeled and finely chopped
1 tablespoon light soy sauce
chopped fresh chives to garnish

1 Cook the noodles in a pan of water containing a vegetable stock cube. Drain and toss with the lemon zest and juice.
2 Heat a non-stick wok or frying pan, add the onion and garlic, cooking until soft. Add the mushrooms, ginger and soy sauce. Cook quickly over a high heat until the mushrooms are just cooked.
3 Add the noodles and mix well together.
4 Serve in warmed bowls and sprinkle with chopped chives.

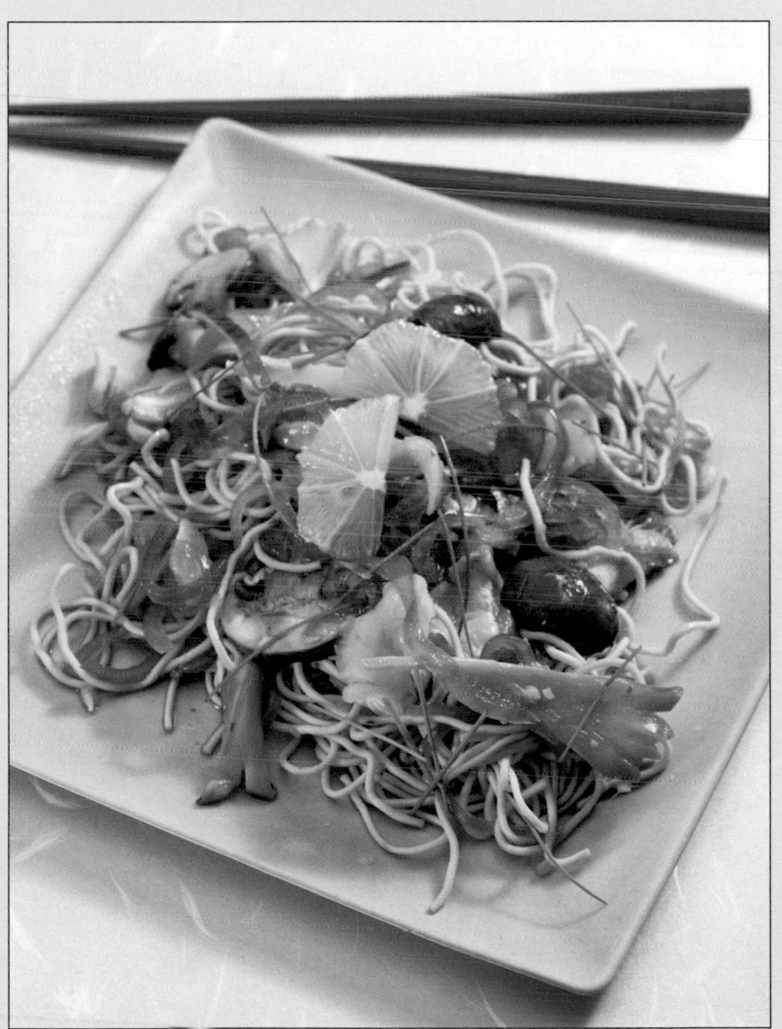

Three pepper rice

Adding just a few spices to rice really makes quite a difference. Kaffir lime leaves add a unique flavour. If you have difficulty in obtaining them, try fresh bay leaves as a substitute.

SERVES 4
PER SERVING:
199 KCAL/2G FAT
PREPARATION TIME:
15 MINUTES
COOKING TIME:
30 MINUTES

1 medium onion, finely chopped
1 garlic clove, crushed
1 teaspoon crushed coriander seed
good pinch of saffron
175g (6oz) basmati rice
450ml (3/4 pint) vegetable stock
2 Kaffir lime leaves (optional)
1 red, 1 green, 1 yellow pepper, seeded and diced
salt and freshly ground black pepper
lemon and lime to garnish

1 In a preheated non-stick pan dry-fry the onion and garlic until soft. Add the coriander seed and continue to cook for 3–4 minutes.
2 Add the saffron, rice and stir in the stock. Bring to the boil, adding the Kaffir lime leaves. Reduce the heat and cover with a lid.
3 Simmer gently for 20 minutes until all the stock has been absorbed, adding a little more stock if the mixture appears a little dry.
4 Once the rice is fully cooked add the diced peppers and stir well. Taste, adjusting the seasoning as required, and transfer to a warmed serving dish. Garnish with lemon and lime.

Szechuan noodles

SERVES 4
PER SERVING:
161 KCAL/1G FAT
PREPARATION TIME:
10 MINUTES
COOKING TIME:
10 MINUTES

115g (4oz) dried noodles
2 vegetable stock cubes
4 spring onions, finely sliced
1 green pepper, seeded and finely sliced
1 celery stick, finely chopped
1 × 2.5cm (1in) piece ginger, peeled and finely chopped
115g (4oz) peeled prawns, chopped
1 small red chilli, sliced
2 tablespoons brandy
1 tablespoon soy sauce
1 tablespoon tomato purée
4 tablespoons vegetable stock

This is a great dish for using up odds and ends of vegetables, so vary according to your taste. If you wish, you can replace the prawns with finely chopped ham or extra vegetables.

1 Cook the noodles in boiling water, adding the stock cubes for extra flavour.
2 Preheat a non-stick wok or frying pan. Dry-fry the onions, pepper, celery and ginger together until lightly coloured.
3 Add the prawns and chilli and continue cooking for 2–3 minutes. Stir in the remaining ingredients, taking the vegetable stock from the noodle pan.
4 Drain the noodles and add to the vegetables. Mix well and serve.

Chicken spaghetti

1 Cook the spaghetti in a large pan of boiling water with a stock cube added for extra flavour.
2 In a non-stick pan dry-fry the onions and garlic until soft. Add the chicken, cooking until it completely changes colour. Add 2 tablespoons of stock and stir in the flour.
3 Cook out the flour for 1 minute, then gradually stir in the passata and herbs, seasoning with salt and black pepper. Reduce the heat and simmer for 2–3 minutes until the sauce thickens.
4 Drain the spaghetti and pour into a warmed serving dish. Spoon the sauce on top and garnish with chopped chives or rocket.

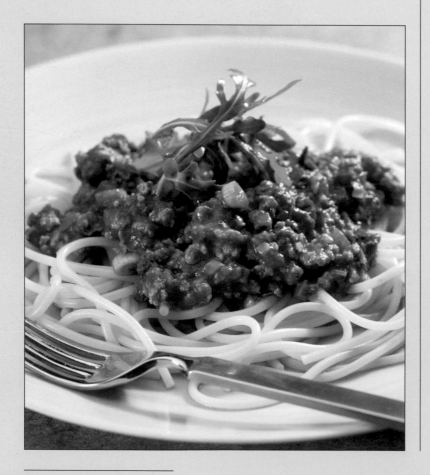

SERVES 4
PER SERVING:
312 KCAL/5.7G FAT
PREPARATION TIME:
10 MINUTES
COOKING TIME:
20 MINUTES

225g (8oz) [dry weight] spaghetti
1 vegetable stock cube
6 spring onions, finely chopped
1 garlic clove, crushed
115g (4oz) minced chicken
150ml (1/4 pint) vegetable stock
1 tablespoon plain flour
300ml (1/2 pint) tomato passata
1 tablespoon chopped fresh mixed herbs
salt and freshly ground black pepper
a few chopped fresh chives or some fresh rocket to garnish

Pasta Sombrero

SERVES 4
PER SERVING:
296 KCAL/7.5G FAT
PREPARATION TIME:
10 MINUTES
COOKING TIME:
25 MINUTES

225g (8oz) pasta shapes
1 vegetable stock cube
1 small red onion, finely chopped
2 smoked garlic cloves, crushed
$\frac{1}{4}$ teaspoon fennel seeds
1 red and 1 green pepper, finely diced
pinch of sweet paprika
1 small red chilli, finely chopped
450g (16oz) tomato passata
1 teaspoon vegetable bouillon stock
a few anchovy fillets to garnish (optional)

The taste of Spain filters through this peppery pasta dish. Try to get the Sombrero pasta shapes or alternatively use other large shapes. You can buy smoked garlic.

1 Cook the pasta in a large saucepan of boiling water containing the stock cube.
2 In a preheated non-stick pan dry-fry the onion until soft. Add the garlic and fennel seeds and continue cooking for 2–3 minutes.
3 Add the remaining ingredients and simmer gently for 5–6 minutes.
4 Drain the pasta thoroughly and arrange on warmed serving plates. Carefully fill the pasta with the sauce.
5 Garnish with thinly sliced anchovy fillets if desired.

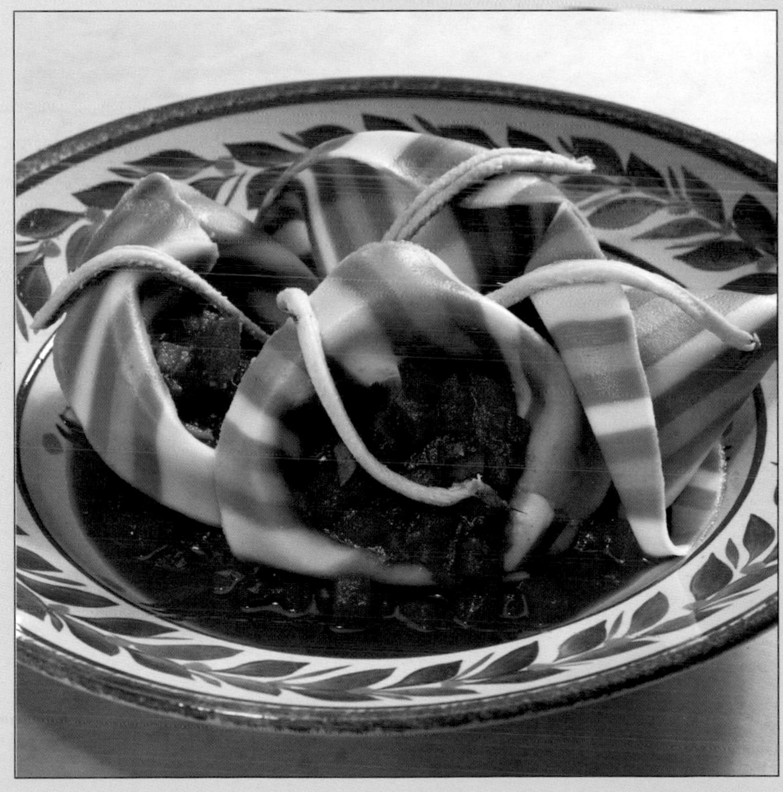

Leek and sundried tomato risotto

Sundried tomatoes can be found in most food shops. Avoid the type in oil, but if there is no alternative, then rinse well with hot water to remove as much oil as possible.

1 In a non-stick pan, dry-fry the leeks and garlic until soft.
2 Add the rice and tomatoes, then gradually stir in the stock and wine, allowing the rice to absorb it before adding more – this will take between 15 and 20 minutes.
3 Once all the liquid has been added stir in the vegetables and cover, allowing the vegetables to cook in the steam.
4 Fold in the fromage frais and remove from heat. Season with salt and black pepper. Serve hot with a little Parmesan cheese.

SERVES 4
PER SERVING:
305 KCAL/5.5G FAT
PREPARATION TIME:
10 MINUTES
COOKING TIME:
25 MINUTES

8 baby leeks, finely chopped
2 garlic cloves, crushed
225g (8oz) [dry weight] Arborio risotto rice
12 sundried tomatoes (not in oil), chopped
600ml (1 pint) vegetable stock
115g (4oz) baby asparagus
115g (4oz) frozen peas
2 tablespoons virtually fat free Normandy fromage frais
salt and freshly ground black pepper
3 tablespoons grated Parmesan cheese to serve

Smoked trout pasta bake

SERVES 4
PER SERVING:
310 KCAL/2.1G FAT
PREPARATION TIME:
10 MINUTES
COOKING TIME:
40 MINUTES

225g (8oz) pasta shapes
1 medium onion, finely chopped
2 garlic cloves, crushed
150ml ($^1/_4$ pint) vegetable stock
2 tablespoons plain flour
$^1/_2$ wine glass white wine
300ml ($^1/_2$ pint) skimmed milk
2 teaspoons Dijon mustard
1 tablespoon chopped fresh chives
225g (8oz) smoked trout fillets, flaked
3 tablespoons low-fat fromage frais
salt and freshly ground black pepper

A creamy pasta dish with wine and smoked trout to add contrasting flavours. For a vegetarian option replace the trout with roasted peppers and top with 50g (2oz) low-fat Cheddar.

1 Preheat the oven to 200C, 400F, Gas Mark 6.
2 Cook the pasta in boiling salted water until *al dente* (just tender), drain and rinse with cold water and place into a large bowl.
3 In a non-stick frying pan dry-fry the onion and garlic until soft. Add 2 tablespoons of stock, sprinkle the flour over, stir well and cook out for 1 minute before adding the remaining stock.
4 Gradually stir in the wine, milk and mustard and simmer gently for 2–3 minutes to allow the sauce to thicken.
5 Mix the sauce into the pasta, along with the chives, trout and fromage frais and season with salt and black pepper.
6 Pour into an ovenproof dish and bake in the preheated oven for 15–20 minutes until hot.

Aubergine and spinach pasta bake

This combination of vegetables works really well with the spicy tomato sauce. It can be made in advance and freezes very well.

SERVES 4
PER SERVING:
300 KCAL/6.6G FAT
PREPARATION TIME:
10 MINUTES
COOKING TIME:
30 MINUTES

175g (6oz) [dry weight] shell or rigatoni-style pasta
2 vegetable stock cubes
225g (8oz) young spinach leaves, shredded
1 red onion, finely chopped
1 aubergine, diced
2 garlic cloves, crushed
1 red pepper, seeded and finely chopped
1 × 400g (14oz) can chopped tomatoes
1 red chilli, seeded and finely chopped
8–10 basil leaves, shredded
115g (4oz) low-fat Cheddar cheese, grated
salt and freshly ground black pepper

1 Preheat the oven to 190C, 375F, Gas Mark 5.
2 Cook the pasta in boiling salted water with a vegetable stock cube. Drain well then stir in the shredded spinach.
3 Meanwhile, in a non-stick frying pan, dry-fry the onion for 2–3 minutes until soft, add the aubergine, garlic and red pepper and cook for a further 6–8 minutes until the aubergine starts to colour.
4 Add the tomatoes, chilli and remaining stock cube, bringing the sauce to a gentle simmer. Season to taste with salt and black pepper.
5 Pour the pasta into a large serving dish, cover with the sauce and sprinkle with the shredded basil leaves and grated cheese.
6 Bake in the preheated oven for 15–20 minutes until golden brown.
7 Serve with a mixed salad or fresh vegetables.

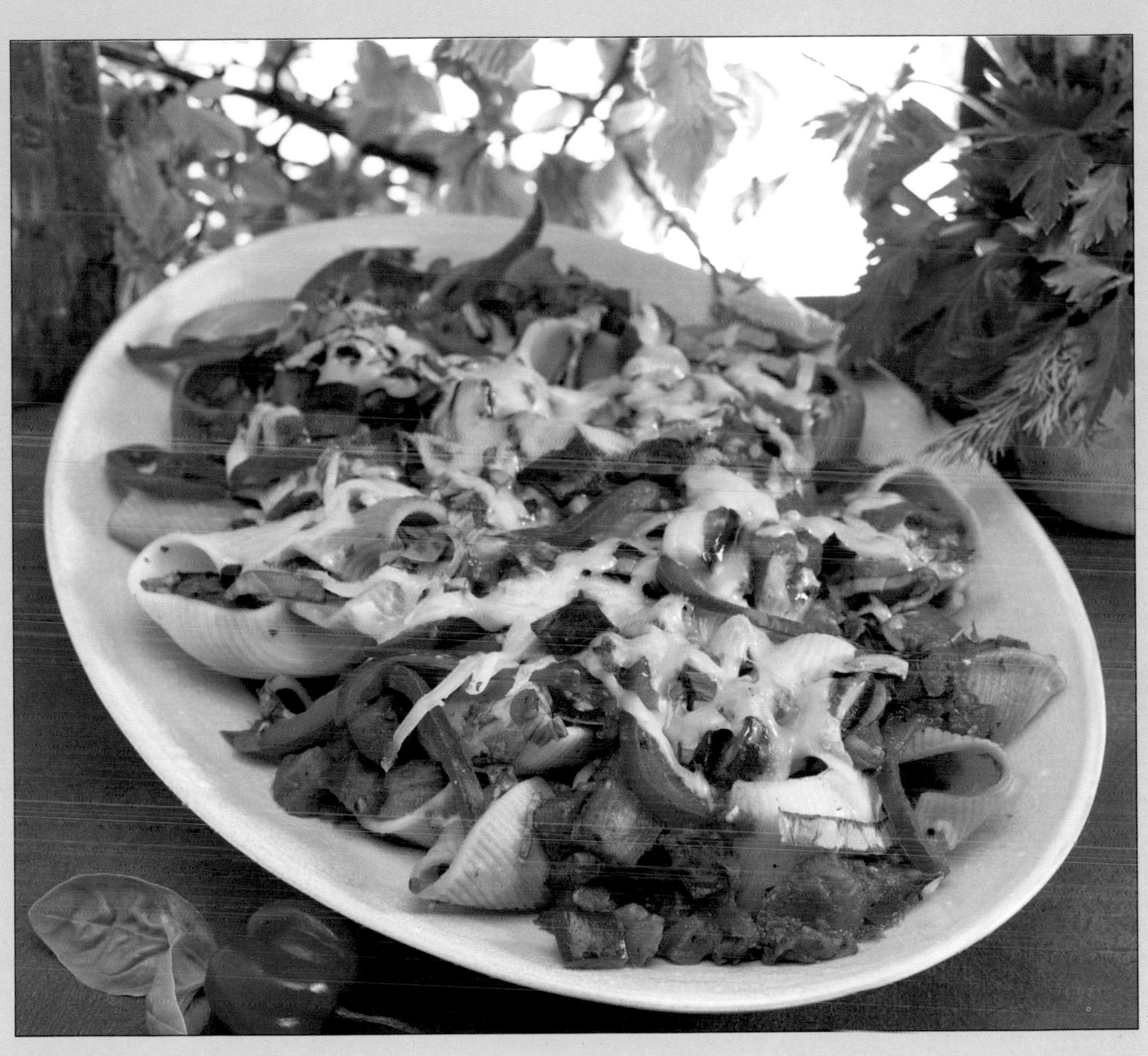

Puddings

In this chapter you'll find a great selection of traditional and some more unusual sweet offerings, both hot and cold, that keep fat to a minimum. All are easy to prepare – some need to be prepared in advance – for an instant fix. When counting the calories you need to be strict with portion sizes, dividing them into individual glasses or bowls, and top with one of the many low-fat options such as flavoured or plain yogurt, fromage frais or readymade low-fat custard, obviously taking these extras into account when totting up the calories.

Should you want a more substantial pudding, check out the recipes in the Entertaining section for further ideas.

Chocolate meringue Yule log

SERVES 8
PER SERVING (APPROXIMATELY): 168 KCAL/2.3G FAT
PREPARATION TIME: 10 MINUTES
COOKING TIME: 30 MINUTES

4 egg whites
175g (6oz) caster sugar
1 teaspoon vanilla essence
300ml ($^{1}/_{2}$ pint) Total 0% fat Greek yogurt
6 servings Valrhona Chocolate Mousse (see recipe, page 208)
or
225g (8oz) virtually fat free chocolate mousse
cocoa powder to dust

Meringue roulade makes an impressive low-fat dessert that can be made a day in advance or stored frozen. This must be the low-fat birthday cake of all time!

1 Preheat the oven to 170C, 350F, Gas Mark 3.
2 Lightly grease and line a large Swiss roll tin with baking parchment.
3 Whisk the egg whites in a dry clean bowl until stiff. Continue whisking, adding the sugar a dessertspoon at a time, allowing 10 seconds between each addition, until all of the sugar is added.
4 Add the vanilla and carefully fold into the mixture using a metal spoon. Pour the mixture into the prepared tin and level off with a palette knife. Bake in the oven for 15 minutes.
5 Reduce the oven temperature to 150C, 300F, Gas Mark 2 and bake for a further 15 minutes.
6 Turn the meringue out onto a piece of foil and peel away the parchment. Allow to cool.
7 Spread a thin layer of yogurt over the roulade, roll up like a Swiss roll and place on a serving plate.
8 Place the chocolate mousse inside a piping bag containing a star shape nozzle and pipe a lattice design across the top.
9 Just before serving, dust with cocoa powder.

Cinnamon and lemon prunes with saffron fromage frais

These prunes make a really tasty low-fat breakfast as well as a tempting dessert. Try them with muesli and low-fat yogurt – simply delicious.

SERVES 4
PER SERVING:
136 KCAL/0.2G FAT
PREPARATION TIME:
5 MINUTES
COOKING TIME:
20 MINUTES

225g (8oz) Agen or large prunes
1 lemon
1 cinnamon stick
2 tablespoons soft brown sugar
good pinch of saffron
½ wine glass white wine
300ml (½ pint) virtually fat free Normandy fromage frais
icing sugar to dust

1 Remove the stones from the prunes by squeezing them through the top of the fruit. Place the prunes in a saucepan.
2 Using a zester, zest the lemon into the saucepan, then cut the lemon in half and squeeze the juice into the pan.
3 Snap the cinnamon in half and add to the pan. Add the sugar and sufficient water to just cover, place on a low heat to simmer gently for 20 minutes.
4 Place the saffron and wine in a separate pan and simmer until the wine has almost evaporated. Scrape out and mix into the fromage frais, adding sugar to taste.
5 Serve the prunes hot or cold with a spoonful of fromage frais and a dusting of icing sugar.

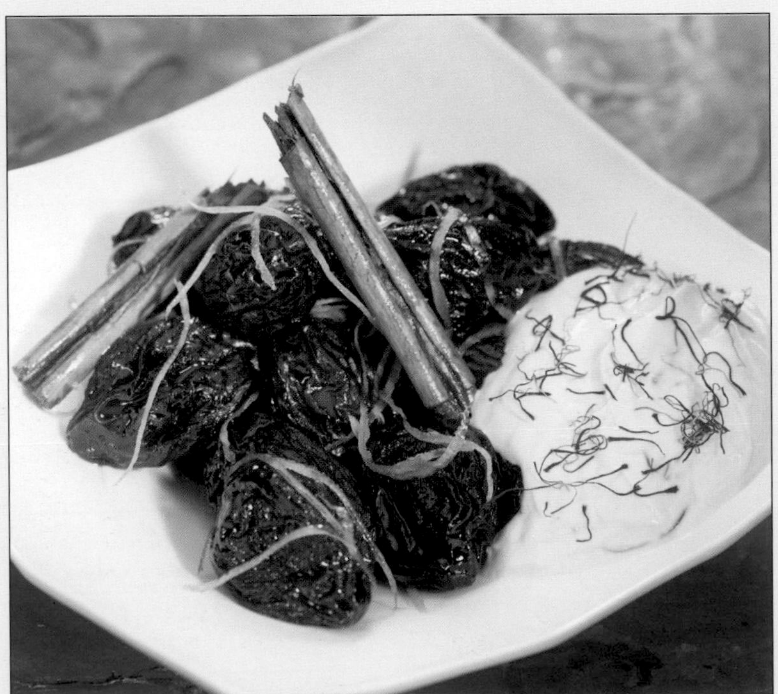

Mango and white rum ice

SERVES 4
PER SERVING:
134 KCAL/0.15G FAT
PREPARATION TIME:
15 MINUTES
COOKING TIME:
10 MINUTES
FREEZING TIME:
12 HOURS

50g (2oz) caster sugar
2 large ripe mangoes
12 pink peppercorns
grated fresh nutmeg
2 tablespoons white rum
1 egg white
fresh mint to decorate

Refreshing and tangy, this fruity iced dessert will round off any meal, especially one containing highly spiced or highly flavoured foods. If you wish, you can omit the alcohol or substitute with a cordial such as elderflower.

1 In a small saucepan dissolve the sugar in 300ml (½ pint) water and bring to the boil. Remove from the heat and allow to cool.
2 Peel the mangoes and remove the flesh from the stone. Place in a food processor, add the peppercorns and a little grated nutmeg and blend until smooth.
3 Mix the fruit purée with the cooled syrup and rum and pour into a shallow freezer container. Cover and freeze for 3 hours until mushy.
4 Remove from the freezer and break up with a fork.
5 Whisk the egg white until stiff. Fold into the loosened mixture and return to the freezer until firm, ideally overnight.
6 Twenty minutes before serving, remove from the freezer and place in the refrigerator to allow it to soften slightly.
7 Serve in a frosted glass decorated with fresh mint.

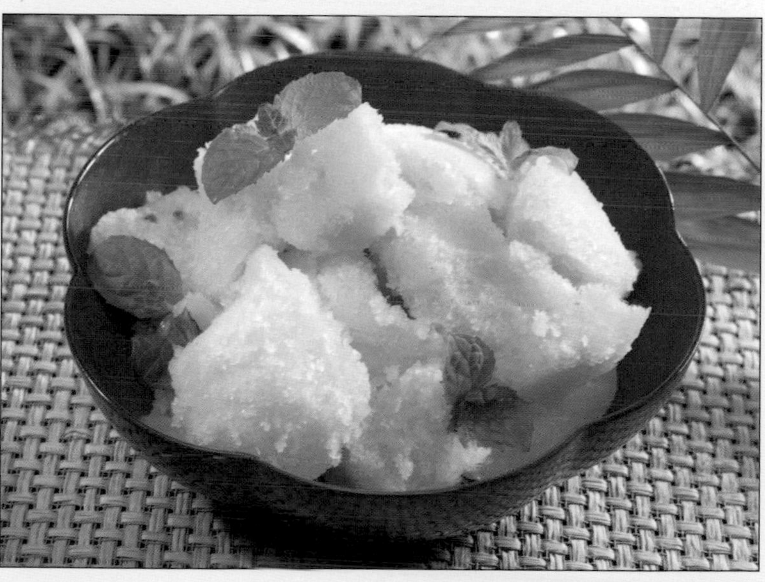

Chestnut meringue roulade

Meringue roulade makes an impressive low-fat dessert that can be made a day in advance or stored frozen. The chopped chestnuts give both added flavour and a crunchy texture. As chestnuts are the only nuts low in fat, this combination offers a tasty treat for all.

SERVES 8
PER SERVING:
112 KCAL/0.3G FAT
PREPARATION TIME:
10 MINUTES
COOKING TIME:
30 MINUTES

4 egg whites
175g (6oz) caster sugar
1 teaspoon vanilla essence
3 tablespoons chopped chestnuts
300ml (½ pint) Total 0% fat Greek yogurt
2 tablespoons chestnut purée
fresh fruit to decorate

1. Preheat the oven to 170C, 350F, Gas Mark 3. Lightly grease and line a large Swiss roll tin with baking parchment.
2. Whisk the egg whites in a dry clean bowl until stiff. Continue whisking, adding the sugar a dessertspoon at a time, allowing 10 seconds between each addition, until all of the sugar is added.
3. Add the vanilla and chestnuts and carefully fold into the mixture using a metal spoon.
4. Pour the mixture into the prepared tin and level off with a palette knife. Bake in the oven for 15 minutes.
5. Reduce the oven temperature to 150C, 300F, Gas Mark 2 and bake for a further 15 minutes.
6. Turn the meringue out onto a piece of foil and peel away the parchment. Allow to cool.
7. In a small bowl mix together the yogurt and chestnut purée, then spread a thin layer over the roulade. Roll up like a Swiss roll and place on a serving plate, decorated with fresh fruit.

Fresh fruit salad verde

SERVES 4
PER SERVING:
100 KCAL/0.4G FAT
PREPARATION TIME:
10 MINUTES

zest and juice of 2 limes
2 Granny Smith apples
3 kiwi fruit
4 ripe greengage plums, stoned and sliced
small bunch white seedless grapes, de-stalked
2 star fruit, sliced
2 teaspoons finely chopped fresh ginger
1 tablespoon crème de menthe liqueur
sugar to taste
fresh mint to decorate

Not only does this fruit salad look healthy but it also tastes equally as good. Substitute one or more of the fruits with fresh melon to suit your taste.

1. Place the lime juice and zest in a mixing bowl. Core the apples and slice directly into the bowl to prevent the apples discolouring.
2. Prepare the kiwi by removing the outer skin with a sharp knife; cut the flesh into small slices or sticks and place in the bowl with the plums and remaining fruit.
3. In a small bowl combine the ginger and liqueur then pour onto the salad. Add a little sugar if necessary and chill until required.
4. Serve in tall glasses with a little 0% fat Greek yogurt.

Lime cheesecake ice cream

Light evaporated milk forms the base to this luxurious creamy dessert. It is very important that the milk is completely chilled overnight in order to achieve the thick foam once whisked.

SERVES 6
PER SERVING:
150 KCAL/1.3G FAT
PREPARATION TIME:
15 MINUTES
COOKING TIME:
5 MINUTES
FREEZING TIME:
4–5 HOURS

4 large limes
2 × 170g cans light evaporated milk, chilled overnight
1 vanilla pod
75g (3oz) caster sugar
225g (8oz) virtually fat free fromage frais
115g (4oz) Quark (low-fat cheese)
3 × 90% fat free ginger biscuits, crushed

1 Finely grate the lime zest from all four limes into a mixing bowl and add the evaporated milk. Using an electric mixer, whisk the evaporated milk on high speed until thick and double in volume.
2 Cut the limes in half and squeeze out the juice into a small saucepan.
3 Split the vanilla pod lengthways, using a sharp knife. Scrape out the black seeds from the centre and add to the pan, along with the sugar.
4 Heat gently, stirring until the sugar has dissolved. Whisk the hot syrup into the milk until fully combined.
5 Carefully fold in the fromage frais and Quark and pour into a plastic freezer container. Cover and freeze for 4–5 hours until firm.
6 Remove from the freezer 10 minutes before serving. Serve 2–3 scoops per serving sprinkled with the crushed ginger biscuits.

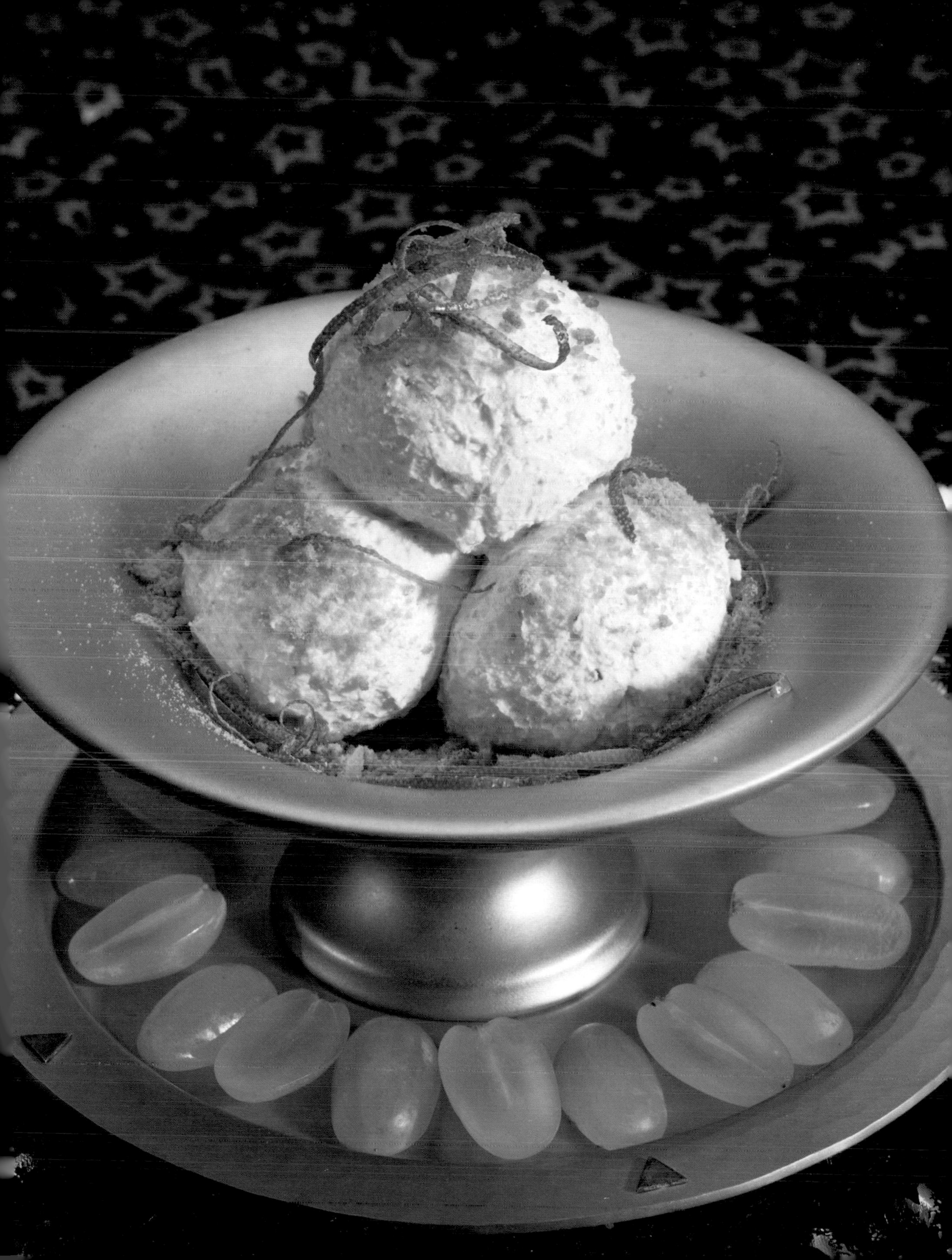

Burgundy poached peaches with strawberry salsa

Turn a simple fruit into an explosion of flavours with this classic combination of red wine and fresh fruit. White flesh peaches tend to be sweeter than the other varieties.

SERVES 4
PER SERVING:
151 KCAL/0.2G FAT
PREPARATION TIME:
10 MINUTES
COOKING TIME:
20 MINUTES

450ml (3/4 pint) Burgundy wine
zest and juice of 1 orange
8 cardamom pods, crushed seeds removed
2 tablespoons Muscovado sugar
4 large white flesh peaches
225g (8oz) fresh strawberries, hulled and chopped
fresh mint to decorate

1 In a saucepan combine the wine, orange zest and juice, cardamom seeds and sugar. Bring to the boil then reduce the heat to a gentle simmer.
2 Half-fill a separate pan with water and bring to the boil. With a slotted spoon carefully add the peaches and cook for 2–3 minutes.
3 Remove them from the pan and place immediately into cold water. Carefully peel away the outer skin and place them in the wine mixture. Cook gently for 10–12 minutes until just tender against the point of a knife.
4 Remove the peaches from the pan and place in a serving dish.
5 Place the wine back on the heat and simmer until the liquid has reduced to a thick syrup. Add the chopped strawberries and spoon over the cooked peaches.
6 Decorate with fresh mint and serve hot or cold with low-fat fromage frais.

Orange Panna Cotta with fresh orange

SERVES 4
PER SERVING:
75 KCAL/0.4G FAT
PREPARATION TIME:
5 MINUTES
COOKING TIME:
10 MINUTES

300ml (½ pint) skimmed milk
3 × 35g sachets orange Quick Jel
fine zest of 1 large orange
300ml (½ pint) low-fat natural yogurt
icing sugar to dust

Panna Cotta is an Italian dessert usually made by adding a setting agent to warmed flavoured single cream, resulting in a smooth blancmange-like texture. Our low-fat version is certainly easier to prepare and you will not believe this smooth, luxurious treat.

1. Pour the milk into a saucepan and sprinkle the Quick Jel over. Heat gently, stirring continuously, until the mixture starts to thicken. Simmer for 2–3 minutes.
2. Remove from the heat and stir in the orange zest. Allow to cool slightly, then stir in the yogurt until smooth.
3. Pour into 4 individual moulds or 1 large one and refrigerate overnight or until set.
4. Cut away the peel from the zested orange and split the orange into segments.
5. To turn out the Panna Cotta, dip the mould quickly into a bowl of boiling water, place an upturned serving plate on top and quickly flip the mould and plate over. Remove the mould and decorate with orange segments and a dusting of icing sugar.

Raspberry bavarois

There are many different types of fromage frais and low-fat yogurts available that can be used for this type of recipe. Choose good-quality varieties that tend to have a rich texture and not such sharp flavours. Make this recipe in advance and store refrigerated until ready to serve.

SERVES 4
PER SERVING:
107 KCAL/0.4G FAT
PREPARATION TIME:
5 MINUTES
COOKING TIME:
10 MINUTES

6 sheets leaf gelatine
450g (16oz) virtually fat free Normandy fromage frais
2 tablespoons Grenadine
275g (10oz) fresh raspberries
caster sugar to taste
3 egg whites
a few raspberries, blackberries and mint leaves to decorate

1 Soak the gelatine in cold water for 2–3 minutes until it becomes soft. Place it in a bowl and heat it either over a pan of boiling water or in a microwave for 1 minute until liquid.
2 Add the fromage frais and Grenadine and mix together thoroughly. Carefully fold in the raspberries with a little sugar to taste and blend again until combined.
3 Whisk the egg whites until stiff and fold into the mixture.
4 Spoon into individual glasses or place in a glass bowl and decorate with extra raspberries, blackberries and mint leaves.

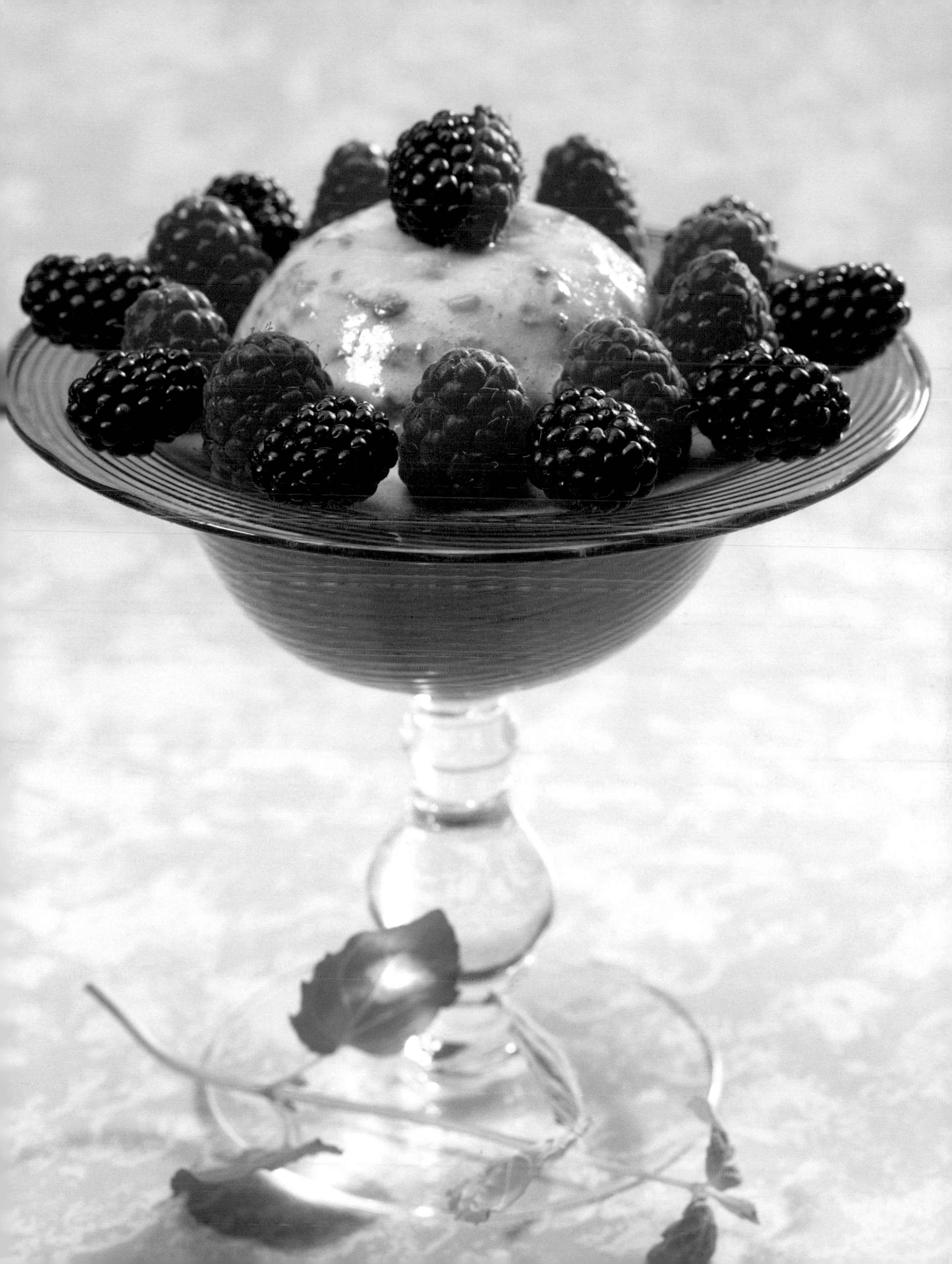

Kiwi and passion fruit salad with balsamic dressing

An unusual combination of sweet and savoury. If you find the balsamic too strong, try replacing with mild fruit vinegar such as cherry or raspberry.

SERVES 1
PER SERVING:
62 KCAL/0.4GFAT
PREPARATION TIME:
5 MINUTES

1 kiwi fruit
1 passion fruit
zest and juice of 1 lime
2–3 teaspoons balsamic vinegar
sugar to taste

1 Prepare the kiwi by removing the outer skin with a sharp knife. Cut the flesh into small slices and place in a bowl.
2 Cut the passion fruit in half, scoop out the seeds with a teaspoon and add to the kiwi.
3 In a small bowl combine the lime juice and zest with the balsamic vinegar, adding a little sugar if necessary. Arrange on a plate and chill until required.

Entertaining

Once you get into the routine of low-fat cooking you will probably find the need to expand your talents to more challenging treats or surprise guests with a low-fat creation of your own. Use this section alongside your diet recipes to add variation for all the family.

Starters

Designed as a little tasty intro, a starter can act as a useful low-calorie filler, enabling you to reduce the size of the courses to follow. Fruit, salads and fresh soups are always simple options, but sometimes we like to stretch to something a little more unusual, especially when entertaining guests.

Many of these substantial starter recipes will double up as light lunches with the addition of a salad or bread where appropriate.

Roasted pepper tarts

Simple and stylish, these attractive tarts make a great entertaining starter or buffet party food. Vary the filling, using different combinations of cooked or roasted vegetables.

MAKES 6
PER TART:
94 KCAL/1.7G FAT
PREPARATION TIME:
40 MINUTES
COOKING TIME:
20 MINUTES

3 red peppers
6 sheets filo pastry
(30 × 20cm/12 × 8in)
1 egg white, beaten
handful of fresh basil leaves
1 teaspoon vegetable bouillon stock powder
2 tablespoons tomato passata
salt and freshly ground black pepper
3 black olives to garnish

1 Preheat the oven to 190C, 375F, Gas Mark 5.
2 Cut the peppers in half, remove the seeds and place face down on a non-stick baking sheet. Roast in the top of the oven for 20–30 minutes until soft. Remove from the oven and place inside a plastic food bag. Seal the bag and leave to cool. Peel the cooled peppers and roughly chop.
2 Stack the filo pastry sheets on top of each other. Using scissors, cut the stack into 6 equal square sections, so that you end up with 36 individual squares.
3 Take 6 non-stick individual tartlet tins, 10cm (4in) in diameter. In each tin, place 6 individual pastry squares in layers, placing the squares at slight angles to each other and brushing with beaten egg white in between each layer.
4 Bake in the oven for 8–10 minutes until crisp and golden. Allow to cool.
5 To make the filling, in a mixing bowl combine the chopped peppers with the remaining ingredients except the olives and season well. Spoon the mixture into the baked shells and return to the oven to warm through.
6 Garnish each tart with half a black olive. Serve warm with a variety of freshly prepared salads.

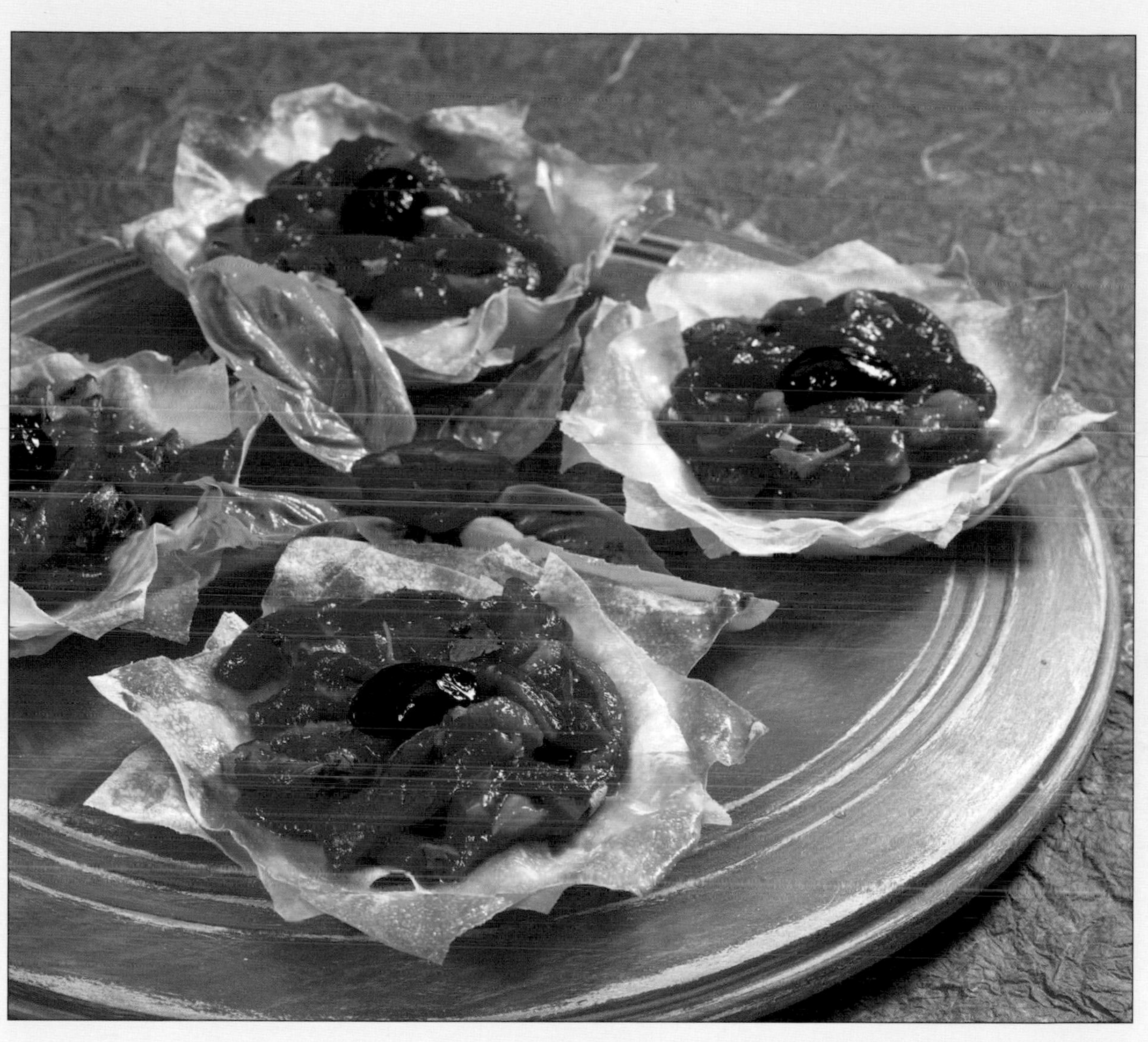

Thai cod fritters with tomato dipping sauce

This spicy fish starter can be made in advance and reheated in a warm oven. It is important to add plenty of seasoning to bring out the full flavour of the spices.

SERVES 6
PER SERVING:
75 KCAL/1.1G FAT
PREPARATION TIME:
10 MINUTES
COOKING TIME:
20 MINUTES
CHILLING TIME 1 HOUR

115g (4oz) thick cod fillet
150ml (1/4 pint) vegetable stock
150ml (1/4 pint) skimmed milk
1 red onion, finely chopped
1 small red chilli, seeded and finely chopped
2 teaspoons lemongrass, finely chopped
1 tablespoon cornflour
1 tablespoon chopped fresh coriander
salt and freshly ground black pepper

for the dipping sauce
150ml (1/4 pint) tomato passata
1 tablespoon hot mango chutney
1 tablespoon light soy sauce
1 teaspoon finely grated lime zest
salt and freshly ground black pepper

1 Poach the cod in the vegetable stock until just cooked and allow to cool.
2 In a medium saucepan combine the milk, onion, chilli and lemongrass and bring to the boil. Slake the cornflour with a little cold water and add to the pan, stirring continuously as the mixture thickens. Reduce the heat and simmer for 3–4 minutes.
3 Pour the mixture into a bowl and allow to cool. Mix in the cod and coriander, season well with salt and freshly ground black pepper, then refrigerate for 1 hour.
4 To make the dipping sauce, combine all the ingredients, season with salt and black pepper and place in a small bowl.
5 Remove the cod mixture from the refrigerator. Preheat a non-stick frying pan. Drop tablespoon-sized amounts of the mixture into the pan and dry-fry for 2–3 minutes on each side.
6 Allow 2 per person and serve with salad leaves and the dipping sauce.

Caramelised onion tarts

MAKES 6
PER TART 211 KCAL/6G FAT
PREPARATION TIME:
40 MINUTES
COOKING TIME:
20 MINUTES

6 sheets filo pastry (30cm × 20cm/12 × 8in)
1 egg white, beaten
1kg (2lb) onions, sliced
4 garlic cloves, crushed
1 teaspoon caster sugar
2 eggs
1 tablespoon fresh thyme leaves
2 teaspoons vegetable bouillon stock powder
115g (4oz) low-fat Cheddar cheese
1 tablespoon chopped fresh chives
salt and freshly ground black pepper

Caramelising onions gives a rich colour as well as a sweet nutty flavour. As the pastry is very thin, assemble at the last minute before the final cooking.

1 Preheat the oven to 190C, 375F, Gas Mark 5.
2 Stack the filo pastry sheets on top of each other. Using scissors, cut the stack into 6 equal square sections so that you end up with 36 individual squares.
3 Take 6 non-stick individual tartlet tins, 10cm (4in) in diameter. In each tin, place 6 individual pastry squares in layers, placing the squares at slight angles to each other with beaten egg white brushed in between each layer.
4 Bake in the oven for 5 minutes until dry. Allow to cool.
5 To make the filling, preheat a non-stick frying pan until hot. Add the onions, garlic and caster sugar and dry-fry for 4–5 minutes until they start to caramelise and turn brown.
6 In a mixing bowl beat the eggs, add the thyme, stock powder and cheese. Quickly mix in the onion mixture and the chopped chives, seasoning with salt and freshly ground black pepper. Spoon into the pastry cases and bake in the oven for 10–15 minutes until set.
7 Serve warm with a mixed leaf salad.

Chicken liver and bacon satés with oyster sauce

Canapés and nibbles are usually pastry based with rich creamy fillings. Try this Chinese twist on liver and bacon served hot with salad or just as simple finger food.

SERVES 4
PER SERVING:
129 KCAL/2.9G FAT
PREPARATION TIME:
15 MINUTES
COOKING TIME:
2–3 MINUTES

225g (8oz) chicken livers, soaked in milk for approx. 30 minutes
4 lean rashers smoked or plain rindless bacon
3 tablespoon Chinese oyster sauce
2 tablespoons clear honey
1 tablespoon Chinese hoisin sauce
2–3 drops Tabasco
salt and freshly ground black pepper

1 Drain the chicken livers well and cut into bite-size pieces, discarding any dark or fatty parts. Season with salt and freshly ground black pepper.
2 Cut the bacon into 8 evenly sized strips. Take 8 cocktail sticks and thread the bacon like a concertina onto the sticks, placing a piece of chicken liver in between each fold. Place in a shallow dish.
3 Combine the remaining ingredients and pour over the meat, cover and refrigerate until required.
4 Cook under a hot preheated grill for 1–2 minutes, depending on personal taste. Serve hot.

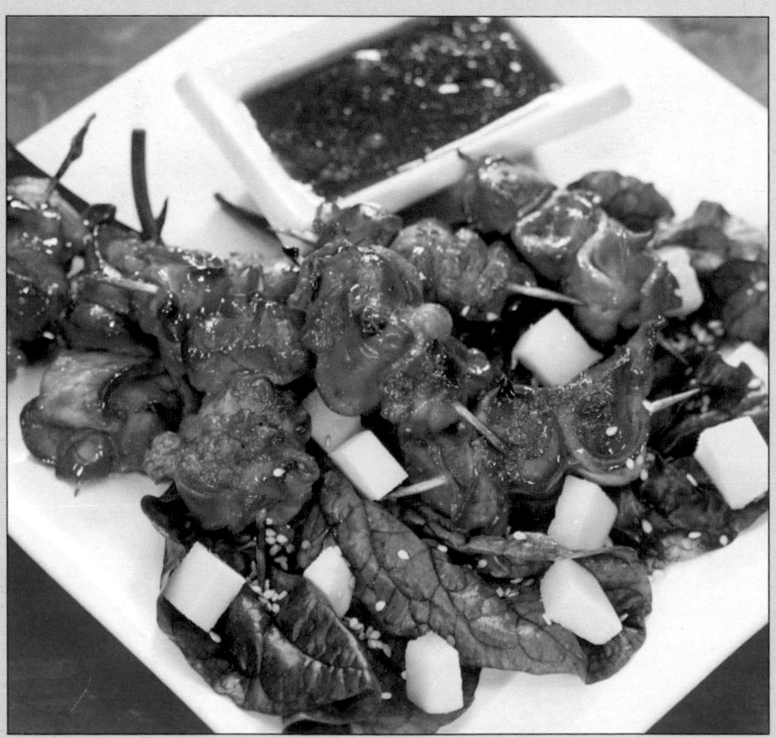

Baked aubergines

SERVES 4
PER SERVING:
91 KCAL/5.8G FAT
PREPARATION TIME:
10 MINUTES
COOKING TIME:
60 MINUTES

2 medium aubergines
4 rashers lean smoked bacon, diced
6–8 large basil leaves
2 garlic cloves, finely chopped
2 tablespoons good-quality red wine vinegar
2 tomatoes skinned, seeded and diced
salt and freshly ground black pepper
chopped fresh parsley and salad to garnish

1 Preheat the oven to 180C, 350F, Gas Mark 4.
2 Slice the aubergines in half lengthways and place in a shallow ovenproof dish. Using a sharp knife, make incisions across the cut side of each aubergine to leave a crosshatch pattern.
3 Tear the basil leaves into small pieces and mix together with the bacon and garlic in a small bowl. Press the mixture into the incisions, distributing the mixture evenly. Season with salt and pepper and drizzle with the vinegar.
4 Place in the preheated oven and bake for 1 hour or until soft.
5 Remove from the oven and cover with the diced tomato.
6 Serve hot or cold sprinkled with chopped fresh parsley on a salad garnish.

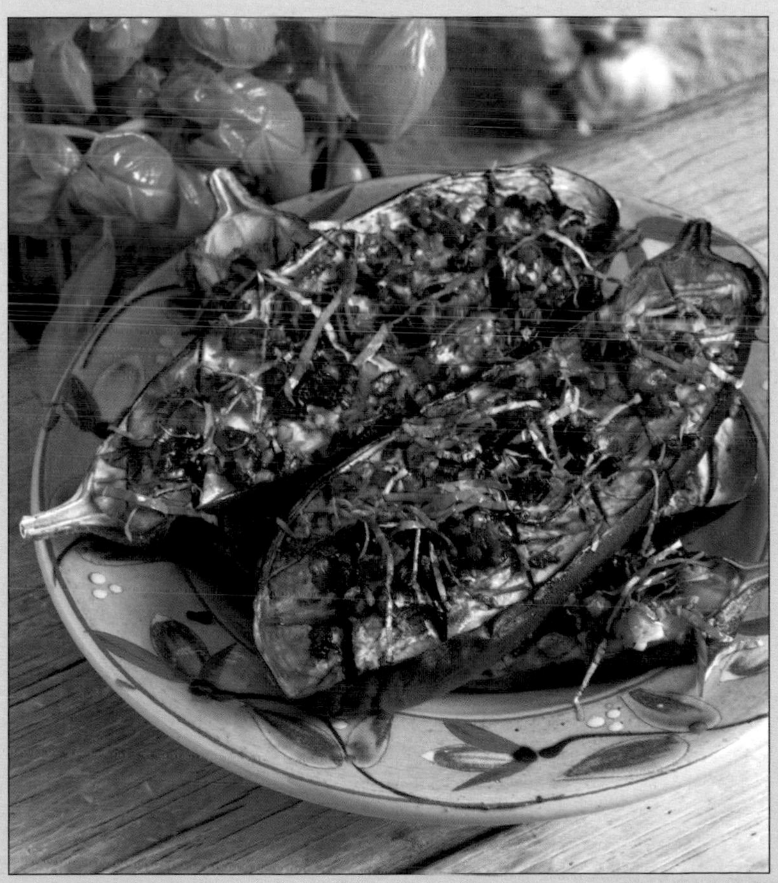

Hors d'oeuvres au aïoli

Hors d'oeuvres can vary from thin pieces of toasted bread topped with pâté or vegetable pastes to more delicate terrines and fish dishes. A selection of flavoursome vegetables lightly cooked with a garlic dipping sauce makes an ideal introduction to French cuisine. Aïoli is traditionally made using a large quantity of egg yolks and olive oil.

SERVES 4
PER SERVING:
93 KCAL/0.8G FAT
PREPARATION TIME:
10 MINUTES
COOKING TIME:
20 MINUTES

115g (4oz) French beans, trimmed
115g (4oz) small carrots
4 baby courgettes
8 cherry tomatoes
1 sweet potato, peeled and cut into wedges

for the aïoli sauce
175g (6oz) virtually fat free fromage frais
2 tablespoons cider vinegar
1 tablespoon lime juice
¼ teaspoon ground turmeric
2 teaspoons sugar
2 garlic cloves, crushed
salt and freshly ground black pepper

1 Cook the vegetables individually in a pan of boiling salted water until just tender. Drain and arrange in colourful clusters around the outside of a serving plate.
2 In a small bowl combine all the sauce ingredients, seasoning well with salt and freshly ground black pepper. Place in the centre of the plate and serve either hot or cold.

See photograph on page 166.

Mediterranean courgette boats

SERVES 4
PER SERVING:
97 KCAL/3.4G FAT
PREPARATION TIME:
15 MINUTES
COOKING TIME:
35 MINUTES

8 medium courgettes
1 small red onion, finely chopped
2 garlic cloves, crushed
1 red and 1 yellow pepper, seeded and finely diced
115g (4oz) chestnut mushrooms, finely chopped
1–2 tablespoons tomato purée
2 tablespoons chopped fresh basil
salt and freshly ground black pepper
25g (1oz) Parmesan cheese, grated

Make these cheesy vegetable boats in advance and cook when required. You may find the need to add a little water to the vegetable mixture, depending on the strength of the tomato purée.

1 Preheat the oven to 200C, 400F, Gas Mark 6.
2 Slice the courgettes down the centre and, using a teaspoon, carefully remove as much of the flesh from the centre of each half. Chop the flesh and set aside. Season the courgette shells with salt and freshly ground black pepper and place side by side in an ovenproof dish.
3 Preheat a non-stick pan. Dry-fry the onion, garlic and courgettes for 2–3 minutes until soft. Add the pepper and mushrooms, continuing to cook over a high heat. Remove from the heat and stir in the tomato purée and chopped basil.
4 Pile the mixture into the courgette shells and top with the Parmesan cheese.
5 Bake in the preheated oven for 20–25 minutes until the shells are cooked. Serve hot or cold.

See photograph on page 166.

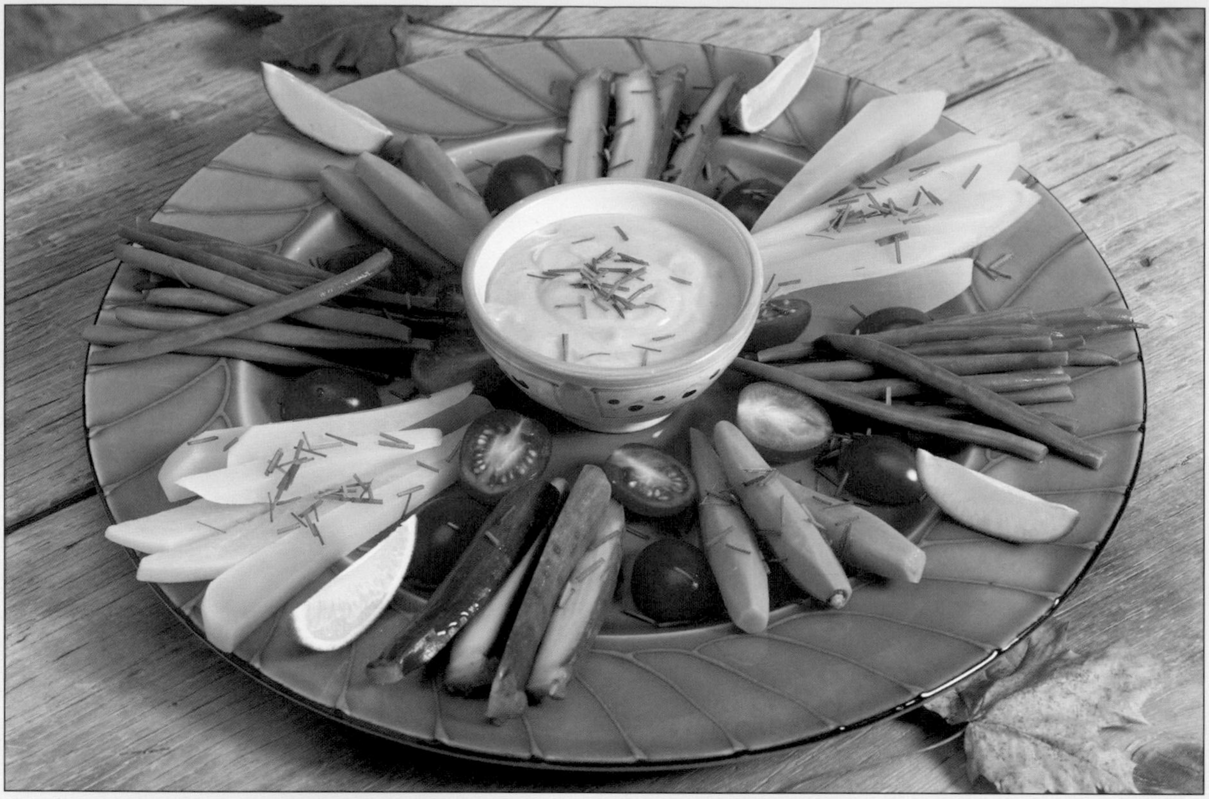

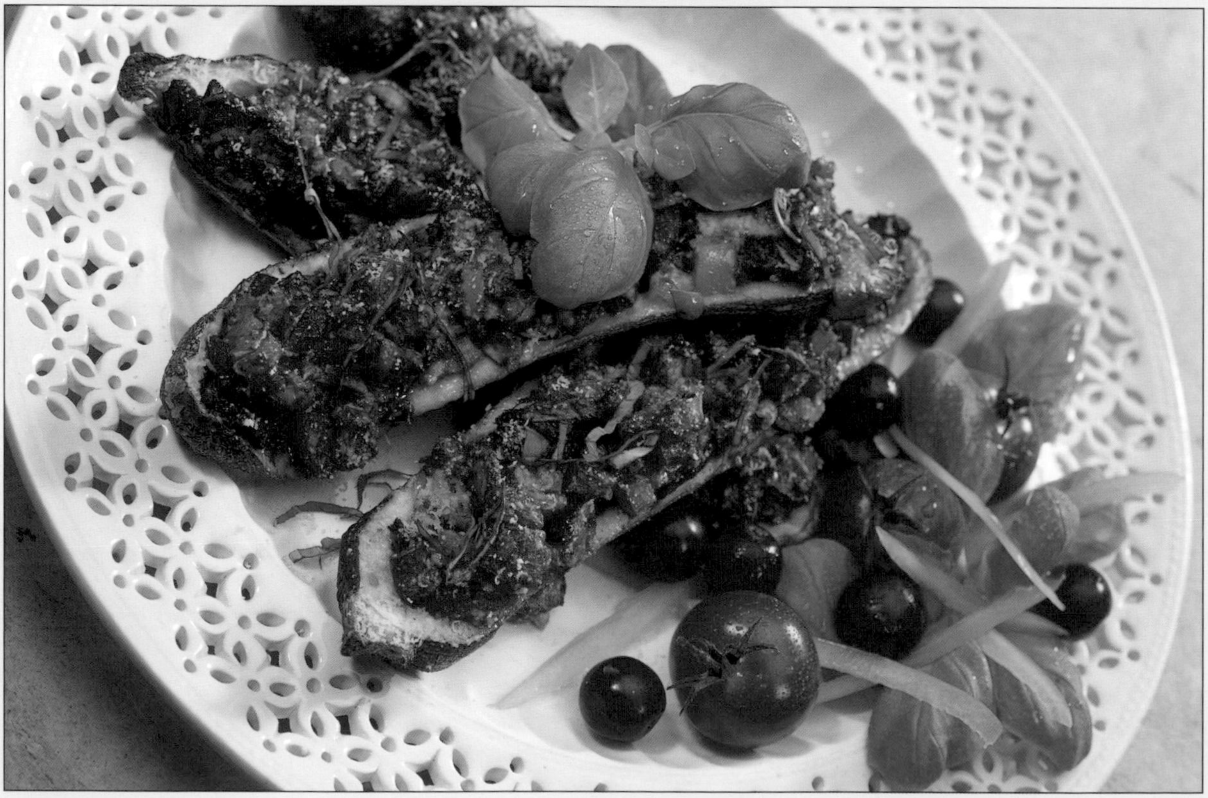

Smoked mackerel and sweet mustard pâté

SERVES 4
PER SERVING:
229 KCAL/18G FAT
PREPARATION TIME:
15 MINUTES

225g (8oz) smoked mackerel fillets
1 tablespoon coarse grain mustard
115g (4oz) Quark (low-fat cheese)
1 tablespoon chopped fresh parsley
juice of $\frac{1}{2}$ lemon
salt and freshly ground black pepper
salad to garnish

1 Using a fork, break up the mackerel fillets in a small bowl. Add the mustard, Quark, parsley and lemon juice. Mix well and season with salt and freshly ground black pepper.
2 Press the mixture into 4 ramekin dishes and smooth the tops over with a knife.
3 Refrigerate until ready to serve.

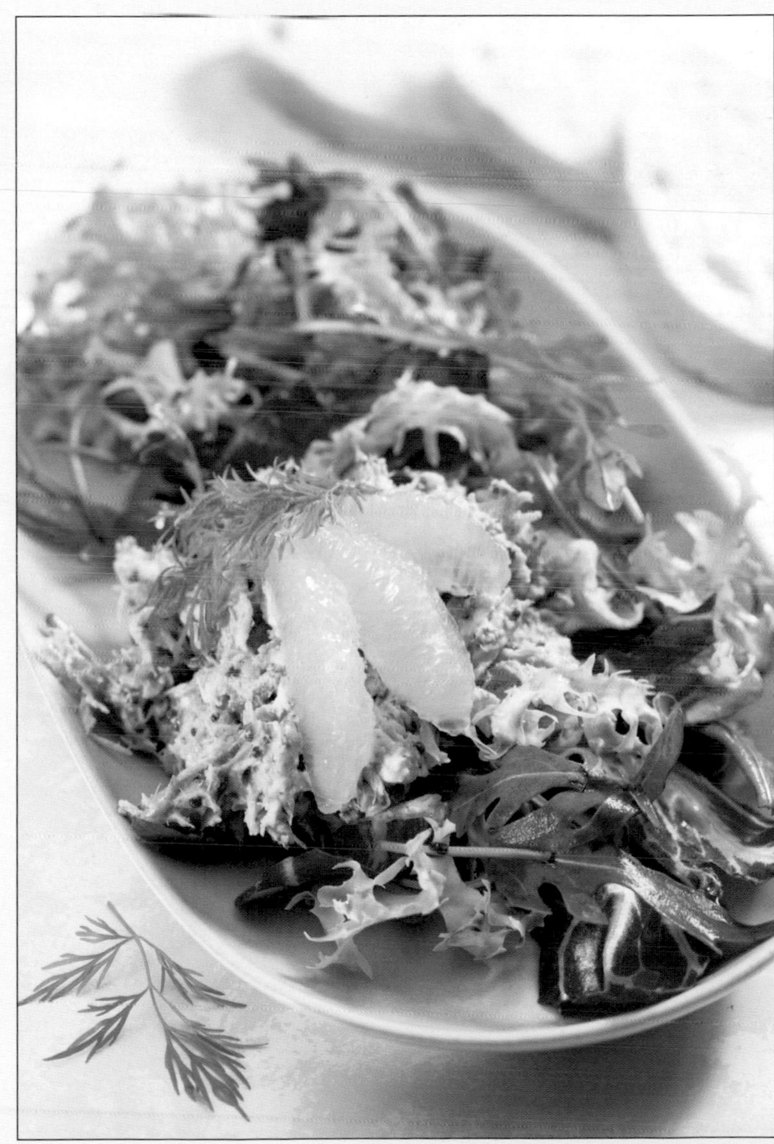

Top left: *Hors d'oeuvres au aïoli*

Left: *Mediterranean courgette boats*

Sundried tomato hummus with roasted summer vegetables

Hummus is a garlic spiked chickpea paste usually made with a large quantity of oil as well as high-fat chickpeas. The tomatoes add colour and a sweet flavour, making it much lighter to eat. Squeezing a little fresh lemon over adds that extra little touch. Stored refrigerated, it will keep for 5 days.

SERVES 4
PER SERVING:
230 KCAL/6.2G FAT
PREPARATION TIME:
20 MINUTES
COOKING TIME:
25 MINUTES

for the roasted vegetables
2 baby courgettes, sliced
2 red and 2 yellow peppers, seeded and cut into chunks
3 baby leeks, sliced
8 small vine tomatoes
1 teaspoon chopped fresh rosemary
handful of fresh basil leaves
2 tablespoons light soy sauce

for the hummus
3–4 pieces sundried tomato (non-oil type)
2 garlic cloves, crushed
300ml (½ pint) skimmed milk
1 × 425g (15oz) can chickpeas with no added salt or sugar
juice of 1 lemon
salt and freshly ground black pepper

1. Preheat the oven to 200C, 400F, Gas Mark 6.
2. Place all the vegetables into a roasting tray and drizzle with the soy sauce. Roast in the top of the oven for 20–25 minutes, turning occasionally. Allow to cool.
3. In a saucepan, heat the milk with the dried tomatoes and garlic. Reduce the heat and simmer for 8–10 minutes until the tomatoes have softened. Allow to cool.
4. Drain and rinse the chickpeas and place in a food processor. Pour in the milk mixture and process until smooth. Season with lots of salt and freshly ground black pepper, add the lemon juice, then blend again to combine. Adjust the consistency with a little extra milk if required.
5. Arrange the cooled vegetables on a serving plate, placing a spoonful of hummus in the centre.

See photograph on page 170.

Salt cod and red pepper brandade

SERVES 6
PER SERVING:
201 KCAL/1.1G FAT
(EXCLUDING FRENCH BREAD)
PREPARATION TIME:
2 DAYS' SOAKING
COOKING TIME:
35 MINUTES

700g (1lb 9oz) salt cod
600ml (1 pint) skimmed milk
1 bay leaf
3 red peppers
2 garlic cloves
juice of 1 lemon
coarsely ground black pepper
1 tablespoon chopped fresh parsley or coriander to garnish
toasted French bread to serve

1 Preheat the oven to 200C, 400F, Gas Mark 6.
2 Soak the cod in cold water for 2 days, changing the water every 12 hours.
3 Place the fish in a shallow pan containing the milk and bay leaf and poach gently until cooked. Allow to cool.
4 Cut the peppers in half, remove and discard the central core and seeds and place on a non-stick roasting tray with the garlic. Cook in the preheated oven for 25 minutes until they start to blister. Remove from the oven and place the hot peppers in a plastic food bag and seal – this will make it easier to remove the skins. Allow to cool.
5 Remove the fish from the cooking liquor and strain the liquid through a sieve into a jug. Flake the fish, removing any skin and bones, and place in a food processor with the lemon and the garlic from the roasting tray. Process on high, adding the milk gradually to create a thick paste, season with black pepper and spread onto toasted French bread.
6 Remove the peppers from the bag and carefully peel away the skins. Slice into thick strips and arrange on top of the brandade. Sprinkle with parsley or coriander and servewith toasted French bread.

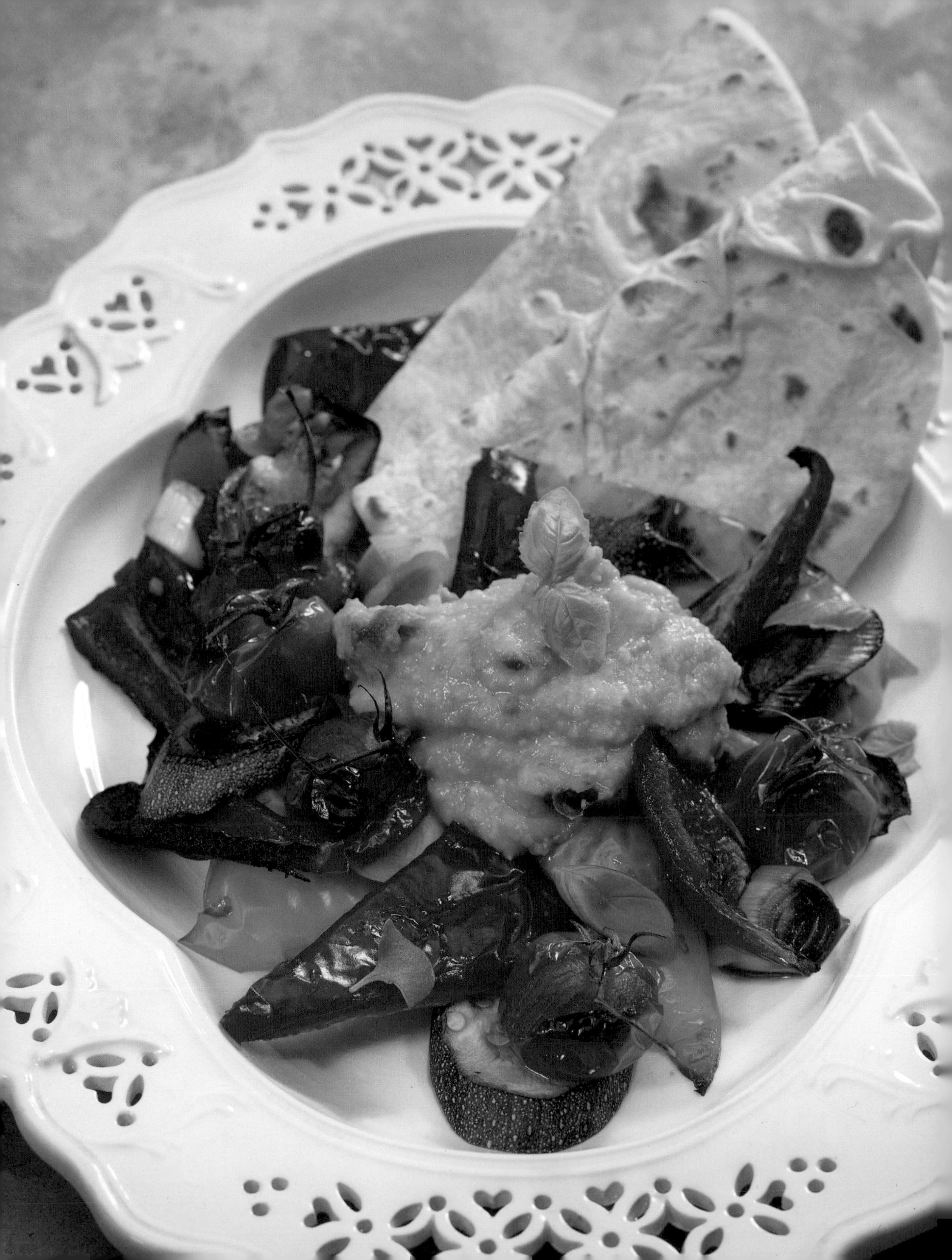

Pink grapefruit and grenadine cocktail

SERVES 4
PER SERVING:
93 KCAL/0.2G FAT
PREPARATION TIME:
10 MINUTES
COOKING TIME:
10 MINUTES

4 medium pink grapefruit
1 tablespoon soft brown sugar
zest and juice of 1 lime
2 teaspoons finely chopped fresh ginger
2 tablespoons Grenadine
mint leaves or lime zest to garnish

Left: *Sundried tomato hummus with roasted summer vegetables*

Grenadine is syrup made from the pomegranate fruit. Being red in colour it has a magical effect on fruits and salads giving them an exotic appeal.

1 Prepare the grapefruit by slicing away the skin and pith with a sharp knife to reveal the fruit. Cut in between the thin connecting membrane, separating and removing each segment into a mixing bowl. Sprinkle the sugar, lime and ginger over and spoon into serving glasses.
2 Divide the Grenadine between the 4 glasses and garnish with fresh mint or lime zest.
3 Serve chilled as a light starter or alternatively a refreshing simple dessert.

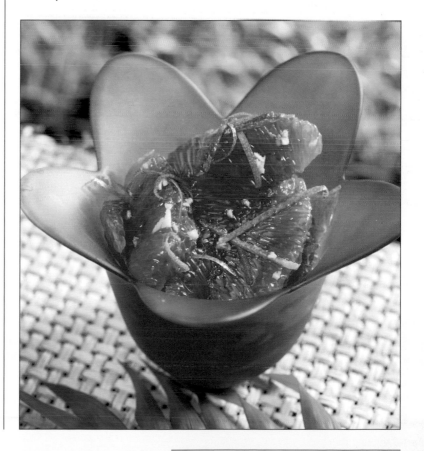

Griddled Madagascan prawns with orange and tomato glaze

Large prawns make a good starter or buffet party food. This recipe also works well with scallops or dense fish such as monkfish or fresh tuna.

SERVES 6
PER SERVING:
41 KCAL/1G FAT
PREPARATION TIME:
20 MINUTES
COOKING TIME:
2-3 MINUTES

25–30 Madagascan or jumbo prawns
4 tablespoons freshly squeezed orange juice
1 tablespoon light soy sauce
1 tablespoon chopped fresh tarragon
150ml (1/4 pint) tomato passata
2 garlic cloves, crushed

1. Peel the prawns and remove the intestinal vein by carefully making a shallow cut along the back of the prawn to reveal a dark vein. This will easily pull away from the main body of the prawn.
2. Thread the prawns onto skewers and place in the bottom of a shallow dish.
3. Combine the remaining ingredients and pour over the prawns. Allow to marinate in the refrigerator for 2–3 hours.
4. Preheat a non-stick griddle pan until hot. Place the prawns in the pan and cook for 2–3 minutes on each side, basting with the marinade during cooking.
5. Serve immediately on a bed of crisp green salad.

Melon and mango towers

SERVES 4
PER SERVING:
175 KCAL/3G FAT
PREPARATION TIME:
10 MINUTES
COOKING TIME:
10 MINUTES

selection of assorted melons (water, Ogen, Charentais, cantaloupe)
2 ripe mangoes
3 tablespoons mild mango chutney
1 × 2.5cm (1in) piece ginger, finely chopped
1 tablespoon light brown sugar

Simple, stylish appetisers are always welcome before a main meal. This recipe uses very few ingredients, yet it looks very impressive as a starter or even an alternative fruit dessert.

1 Prepare the melons by slicing down the sides of the fruit to give long thin pieces of fruit. Then, using a large pastry cutter, approximately 6cm (3in) in diameter, cut out approximately 12–16 discs of the fruit, depending on the size of the fruits. Using a smaller cutter, 2.5cm (1in) in diameter, remove the centre from each disc and reserve.
2 Peel the mangoes and again slice away the flesh in long pieces around the shape of the inner stone.
3 On a serving dish place 4 circles of melon side by side and spread lightly with the mango chutney. Add slices of mango, spread with the chutney, and then more melon. Keep building until the stacks are 3–4 melon slices deep.
4 Chop the remaining melon and mango, saving 4 inner discs for the tops. Combine the chopped fruits with the ginger and sugar, place in the centre of each tower and top with the reserved discs.
5 Chill until required.

Blinis with smoked salmon and horseradish cream

Blinis are light batter pancakes often used as a canapé or starter to serve as a base for salmon or caviar. Our low-fat version can be made in different sizes to suit. For a neat, uniform look use a round pastry cutter to trim them to equal size.

SERVES 6
PER SERVING:
226 KCAL/2.7G FAT
PREPARATION TIME:
20 MINUTES
COOKING TIME:
10 MINUTES

for the blinis

300ml (½ pint) skimmed milk
15g (½oz) fresh or dried yeast
175g (6oz) plain flour
75g (3oz) buckwheat flour
1 egg yolk
75g (3oz) virtually fat free fromage frais
4 egg whites
pinch of salt
a little vegetable oil for the pan

for the topping

115g (4oz) smoked salmon
4 tablespoons virtually fat free fromage frais
1 teaspoon horseradish sauce
salt and freshly ground black pepper
sprigs of fresh dill to garnish

1. Warm the milk to a temperature that's no more than hand hot. Add the yeast and whisk well.
2. Combine the flours in a mixing bowl, add the egg yolk and fromage frais, then, using a whisk, gradually pour in the milk, beating the mixture to a smooth, lump-free batter. Allow to stand and prove for 30 minutes.
3. Whisk the egg whites with a pinch of salt to stiff peaks, then carefully fold into the batter with a metal spoon.
4. Preheat a non-stick frying pan, then lightly oil the pan, removing the oil with kitchen paper.
5. Spoon tablespoons of the mixture separately into the pan and cook for 1 minute, flip over and cook the other side for a further 2 minutes. Allow to cool on a wire rack.
6. Place the blinis on a serving plate. Drape the smoked salmon on top.
7. Mix together the fromage frais and horseradish, seasoning well with salt and freshly ground black pepper, and spoon on top. Garnish with fresh dill.

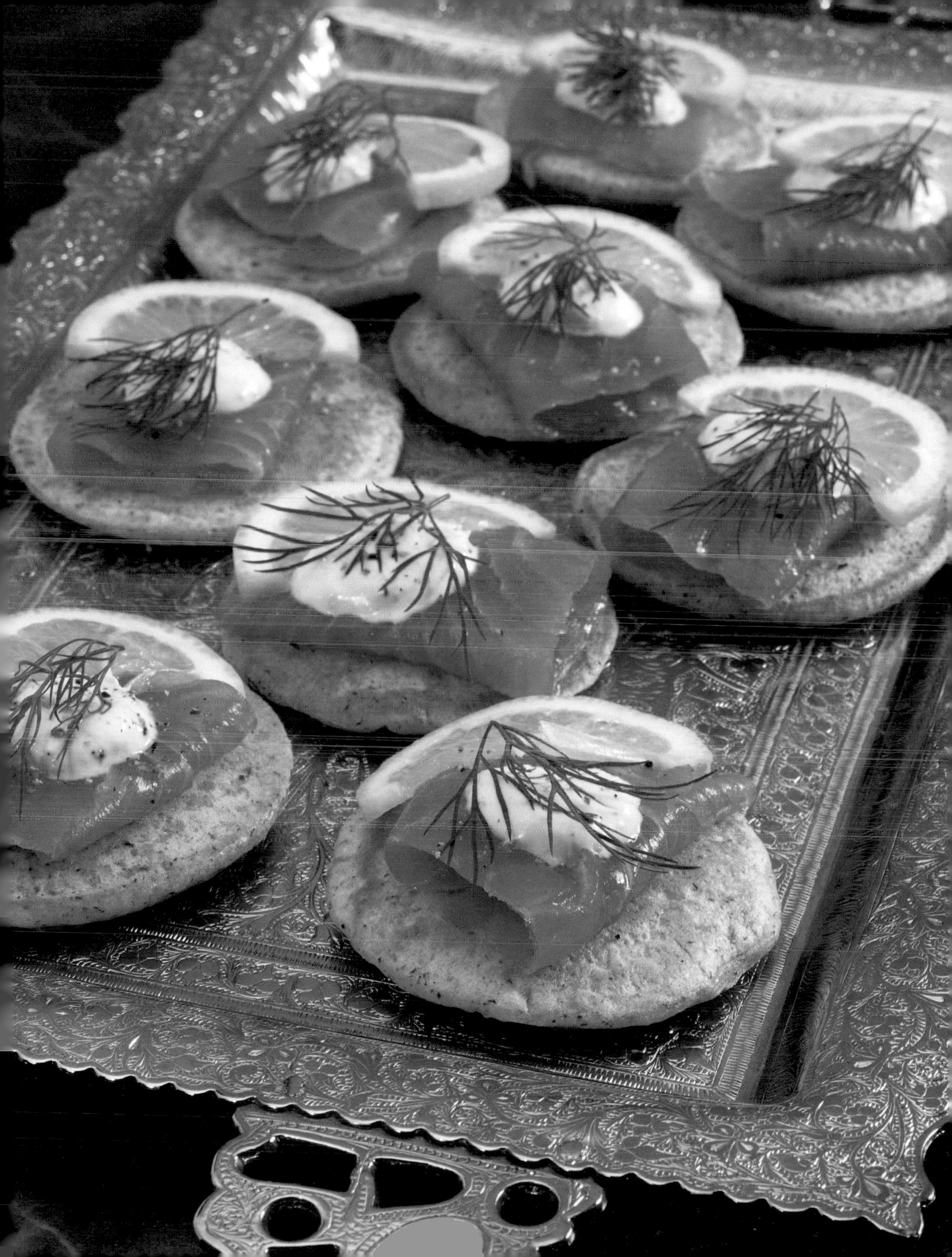

Main courses

Select from light flavoursome dishes to more elaborate creations, giving you the option to design a menu suitable for your requirements. Mix and match the accompaniments, taking into account the calorie and fat content to achieve a well-balanced meal.

Seared beef with chilli bean salad and radish salsa

SERVES 4
PER SERVING:
491 KCAL/16G FAT
PREPARATION TIME:
10 MINUTES
COOKING TIME:
10 MINUTES

4 lean fillet steaks
225g (8oz) fresh fine green beans, cut in half
1 × 450g (16oz) can red kidney beans, drained
1 × 450g (16oz) can cannellini beans, drained
1 small red onion, finely chopped
1 red bullet chilli, finely chopped
6 ripe tomatoes, skinned and finely chopped
1 tablespoon finely chopped chives
2 teaspoons horseradish sauce
salt and freshly ground black pepper

for the salsa
1 bunch of young radishes, finely chopped
1 small green pepper, finely chopped
1 tablespoon chopped fresh mint
1 tablespoon mild mango chutney

This chunky bean salad can form the base to many light lunches, not just with beef. Try it with seared lean pork or turkey slices. It also works particularly well with gammon.

1 Season the steaks with salt and freshly ground black pepper and set aside.
2 Cook the green beans in a pan of lightly salted water until tender. Drain, rinse with cold water and place in a bowl containing the drained kidney and cannellini beans. Add the remaining ingredients and season with salt and freshly ground black pepper, mixing them until fully combined.
3 Preheat a non-stick frying pan until hot. Add the steaks, cooking them for 2–3 minutes on both sides. Remove from the pan and allow to rest for 2 minutes on a chopping board.
4 Combine the salsa ingredients and place in a small serving bowl.
5 Divide the bean salad between 4 bowls, slice the beef into thick pieces and arrange on top. Garnish with the salsa.

Sage and onion roast pork

Spring onions form the centre to this traditional roast. Using fresh sage gives a much stronger flavour than using dried, adding depth and a distinctive herb flavour to the finished sauce.

SERVES 4
PER SERVING:
559 KCAL/14G FAT
PREPARATION TIME:
20 MINUTES
COOKING TIME:
2 HOURS

1.5kg (3lb) lean pork loin joint, boned
2 onions, finely chopped
1 large cooking apple, peeled and grated
2 tablespoons chopped fresh sage
12 thin spring onions
3 tablespoons clear honey
600ml (1 pint) vegetable stock
1 tablespoon cornflour
1 wine glass white wine
salt and freshly ground black pepper

1 Preheat the oven to 200C, 400F, Gas Mark 6.
2 Trim away all the fat from the pork, then weigh the joint to calculate the cooking time and lay out flat on a chopping board. Season well with salt and pepper.
3 Dry-fry the onion in a non-stick pan until soft. Add the apple and sage, stir well then remove from the heat and allow to cool.
4 Place the mixture onto the pork, then lay the spring onions across horizontally. Roll the pork up and tie with string. Place the joint in a roasting tin. Spoon the honey over the pork and pour 300ml (½ pint) stock around the meat. Cover with foil and cook in the oven, allowing 30 minutes per 450g (1lb), plus 30 minutes over.
5 Remove the pork from the tin and allow to rest, keeping it covered with foil.
6 Add the remaining stock and wine to the tin and stir well, picking up the meat juices from the bottom. Pour the mixture into a saucepan and heat.
7 Slake the cornflour with a little cold water and stir into the gravy. Simmer gently to allow the gravy to thicken.
8 Slice the pork and arrange on a serving dish with the accompanying sauce.
9 Serve with potatoes, seasonal vegetables and apple sauce.

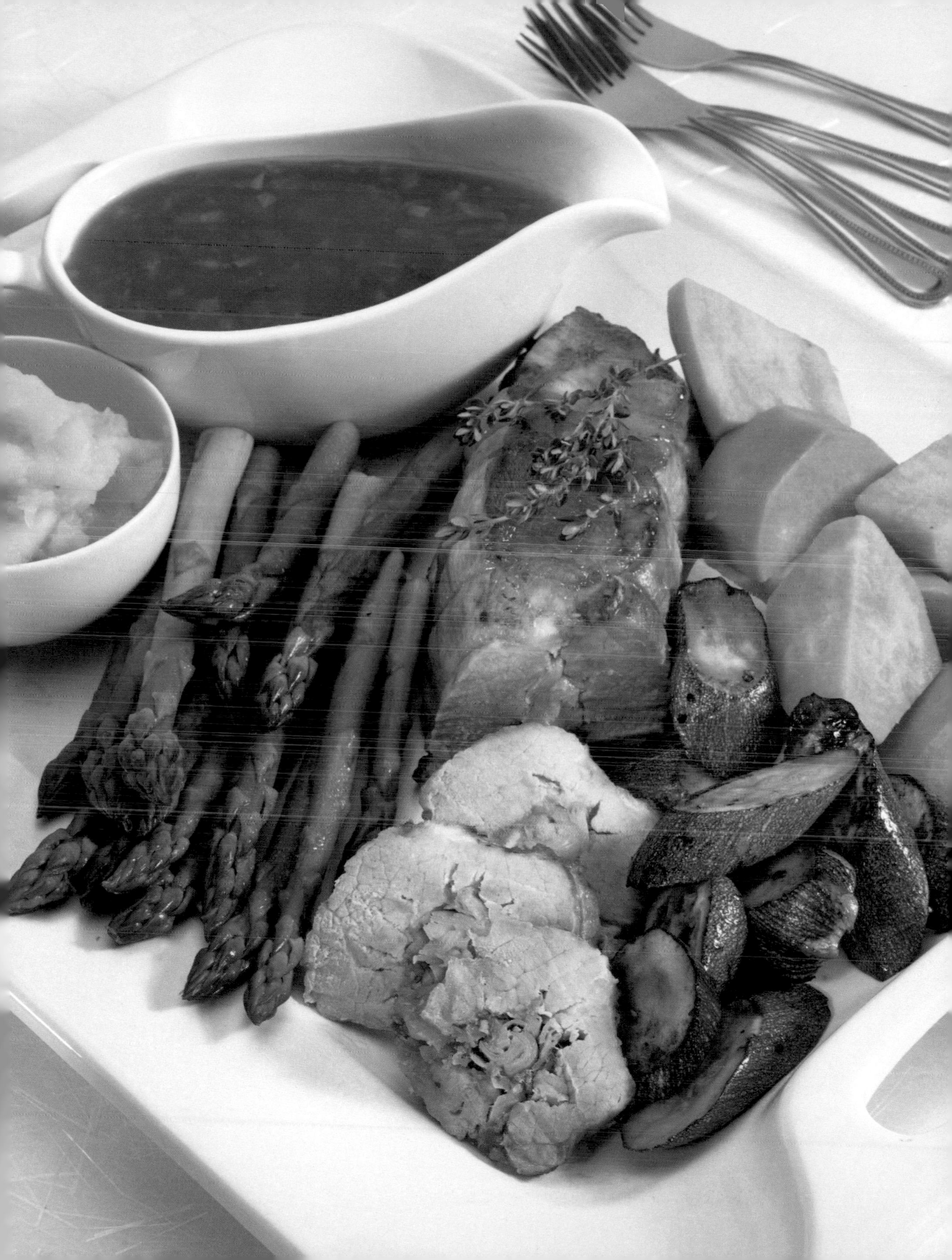

Coconut roasted sea bass wrapped in banana leaves

Toasting the coconut adds a wonderful flavour to this all-in-one fish dish. Using only a small quantity keeps the dish still fairly low in fat, bearing in mind desiccated coconut contains 62% fat. Banana leaves can be found in supermarkets alongside exotic fruit and vegetables and, more recently, in some florists. They are perfect for wrapping around foods for oven roasting since their waxy surface prevents the food from sticking. As well as being attractive, they impart a light, grassy, oriental flavour to the food.

Pre-cooked express rice, available from supermarkets, is a great time-saver and instant accompaniment. Use straight from the packet or jazz it up with herbs.

SERVES 6
PER SERVING:
424 KCAL/15G FAT
PREPARATION TIME:
20 MINUTES
COOKING TIME:
30 MINUTES

- 1.5kg (3lb) sea bass, de-scaled and gutted
- 2 limes, sliced
- 1 large or 2 small banana leaves
- 450g (16oz) [cooked weight] basmati rice
- 4–5 cardamom pods, crushed and seeds removed
- 3 tablespoons shredded, desiccated coconut
- 2–3 sprigs fresh dill
- sea salt and freshly ground black pepper

1. Preheat the oven to 180C, 350F, Gas Mark 4.
2. Wash the fish well inside and out and, using kitchen scissors, trim the fins and tail. Season the inside of the fish with plenty of salt and pepper and lay the lime slices (reserving a few for the garnish) along the length of the inside of the fish.
3. Lay the banana leaf out on a baking tray. Place the rice in a line along one edge, sprinkle with the cardamom seeds and arrange the fish on top.
4. Preheat a non-stick frying pan and dry-fry the coconut over a low heat until lightly toasted. Scatter over the top of the fish and season well with salt and freshly ground black pepper. Place the fresh dill on top, then wrap the banana leaves around the fish, covering as much of the fish as possible (you may need to wrap the head and tail in baking foil).
5. Bake in the oven for 20–25 minutes until just cooked. Remove the foil, if used, and transfer the fish to a serving dish.
6. Garnish with the reserved lime slices and extra fresh dill.

Baked trout with smoked garlic and pesto topping

SERVES 1
PER SERVING:
376 KCAL/12G FAT
PREPARATION TIME:
20 MINUTES
COOKING TIME:
25 MINUTES

1 large trout, gutted
sea salt
1 large sprig fresh rosemary
1 slice of lime
1 smoked garlic clove, finely chopped

for the pesto
1 vegetable stock cube
2 good bunches fresh basil
1 tablespoon peeled cooked chestnuts
2 teaspoons grated Parmesan cheese
salt and freshly ground black pepper

Prepare this recipe in advance to allow the flavours of the garlic and pesto to permeate the fish. You will only need 1 tablespoon of pesto for this recipe, but you can freeze the remainder or it will keep in the refrigerator for a few days.

1 Preheat the oven to 200C, 400F, Gas Mark 6.
2 Make the pesto by placing all the ingredients into a liquidiser or food processor and blending until smooth.
3 Rinse the trout well under cold running water. Scrape your finger along the inside of the backbone to remove any traces of blood. Use scissors to trim the tail and cut off all the fins.
4 Place the fish on a baking sheet and slash the top with a sharp knife, making diagonal incisions. Season the inside with sea salt and place a sprig of rosemary, a slice of lime and a little of the chopped garlic inside.
5 Using a pastry brush, spread 1 tablespoon of pesto over the fish, working it down into the incisions.
6 Bake in the oven for 20–25 minutes. Serve hot or cold.

Salmon and broccoli lasagne

This recipe can be made in advance and cooked as required. It is suitable for home freezing.

SERVES 4
PER SERVING:
658 KCAL/23G FAT
PREPARATION TIME:
5 MINUTES
COOKING TIME:
35 MINUTES

225g (8oz) broccoli, trimmed
4 × 175g (4 × 6oz) salmon fillets
600ml (1 pint) skimmed milk
2 teaspoons Dijon mustard
2 teaspoons vegetable bouillon stock powder
2 tablespoons cornflour
115g (4oz) chestnut mushrooms, sliced
50g (2oz) low-fat Cheddar cheese, grated
1 tablespoon chopped fresh dill
1 tablespoon chopped fresh parsley
225g (8oz) 'no cook' lasagne
salt and freshly ground black pepper

1 Preheat the oven to 190C, 375F, Gas Mark 5.
2 Cook the broccoli in boiling salted water, drain and set aside.
3 Place the salmon in a saucepan with the milk and cook gently over a low heat for 5–6 minutes. Allow to cool, then lift out the fish onto a plate and flake, removing all skin and bones.
4 Reheat the milk, adding the mustard and stock powder to the saucepan. Slake the cornflour with a little cold water and add to the milk, stirring well to prevent any lumps forming.
5 Add the mushrooms and cheese and mix well. Simmer gently until the sauce is of a coating consistency. Adjust if necessary with a little extra milk or diluted cornflour. Stir in the herbs.
6 Place a thin layer of sauce in the bottom of an ovenproof dish. Cover with sheets of lasagne without overlapping. Add a layer of flaked fish and broccoli then continue layering, ending with the sauce.
7 Bake in the oven for 30–35 minutes until bubbling hot.

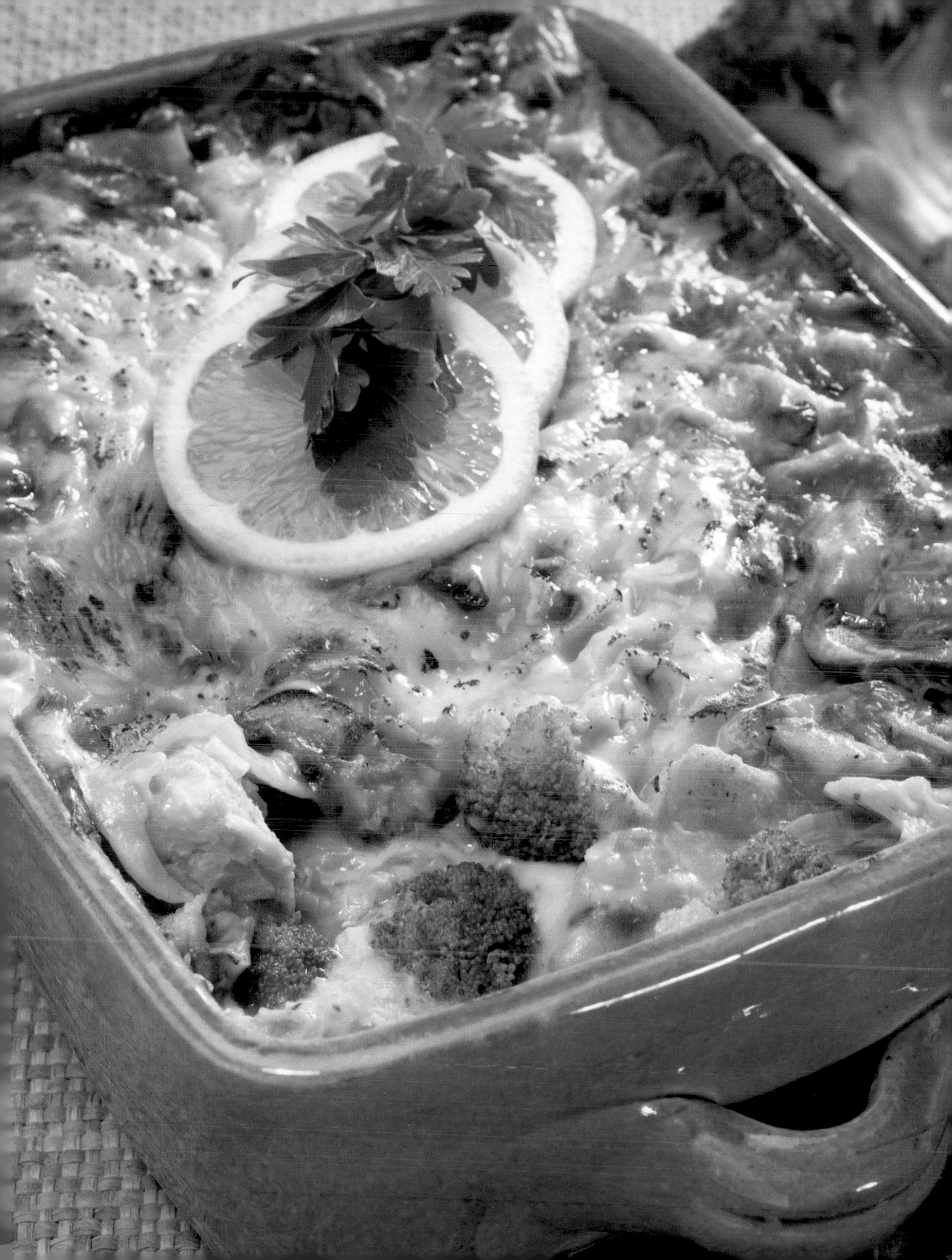

Hot pan smoked salmon

Pan smoking is a variation of barbecuing with the food being totally encased in the cooking smoke. The food is cooked in a smoker over wood chippings, which adds flavour directly to the food.

SERVES 4
PER SERVING:
358 KCAL/19.4G FAT
PREPARATION TIME:
5 MINUTES
COOKING TIME:
25 MINUTES

4 × 175g (4 × 6oz) pieces fresh salmon fillet
1 lemon
300g (10oz) virtually fat free fromage frais
2 tablespoons capers, chopped
2 teaspoons white wine vinegar
1 tablespoon chopped fresh parsley
salt and freshly ground black pepper
dill sprigs to garnish

1 Preheat the oven to 200C, 400F, Gas Mark 6.
2 Prepare the salmon by removing any bones and cut away the skin with a sharp knife. Slice each piece in half and season well with salt and freshly ground black pepper.
3 Prepare the smoker and place the salmon pieces onto the wire rack and cover the whole smoker with aluminium foil, standing the smoker over a low heat.
4 Smoke for 8–10 minutes, reducing the heat if the smoke smells strong.
5 Turn off the heat and allow the smoker to stand for 2–3 minutes before removing the foil. Transfer the salmon to a baking tray and squeeze the juice of half the lemon over. Place in the preheated oven for 5–6 minutes to finish cooking.
6 Make the sauce by combining the fromage frais with the capers, vinegar and parsley, adding lots of salt and freshly ground black pepper.
7 Check that the fish is cooked right through to the centre and serve straight from the oven with the accompanying sauce, a selection of vegetables and garnish with the remaining half lemon and fresh dill.

Hot pan smoking

This unusual method of cooking only lends itself to certain types of food such as salmon and poultry. Smokers can be purchased in good kitchen shops, but a cheaper alternative is to make your own.

All you need are 4 main items: a large turkey-style roasting tin, a small wire rack to fit inside, some hard wood oak chips (sold alongside barbecue fuel) and aluminium foil.

Simply scatter a few oak chips in the bottom of the tin. Place the rack on top, leaving a gap between the wood chips and the bottom of the rack. The food is then placed on top of the rack and the aluminium foil covers everything. Place the tin directly on the cooker hob and smoke away.

It is very important that you keep the heat as low as possible, since if too much smoke is generated it can lead to the food being ruined with a dark brown film tasting sour and bitter.

Vegetables and side dishes

Fresh vegetables are unlimited, so do make sure you offer a wide selection, taking into account flavours, colours and textures. Here we have included a few more unusual choices to serve alongside more conventional basics.

Mushrooms à la Grecque

Lemon and mushrooms make a wonderful combination and the perfect accompaniment to any fish dishes. Serve hot as a vegetable side dish or cold as a salad. Add a few fresh wild mushrooms for added flavour and colour.

SERVES 6
PER SERVING:
23 KCAL/0.7G FAT
PREPARATION TIME:
5 MINUTES
COOKING TIME:
10 MINUTES

1kg (2lb) small chestnut mushrooms
2 long shallots, finely chopped
juice of 2 lemons
2 bay leaves
12 peppercorns
1 teaspoon coriander seed
pinch of sea salt
2 tablespoons herb vinegar
1 tablespoon fresh apple juice
1 tablespoon chopped fresh parsley

1 In a non-stick pan dry-fry the shallot until soft. Wipe the mushrooms with a damp cloth, add to the pan and cook for 1–2 minutes.
2 Add the remaining ingredients except the chopped parsley and bring to the boil. Cover with a lid and remove the pan from the heat. Allow to cool.
3 Before serving, sprinkle with chopped parsley.

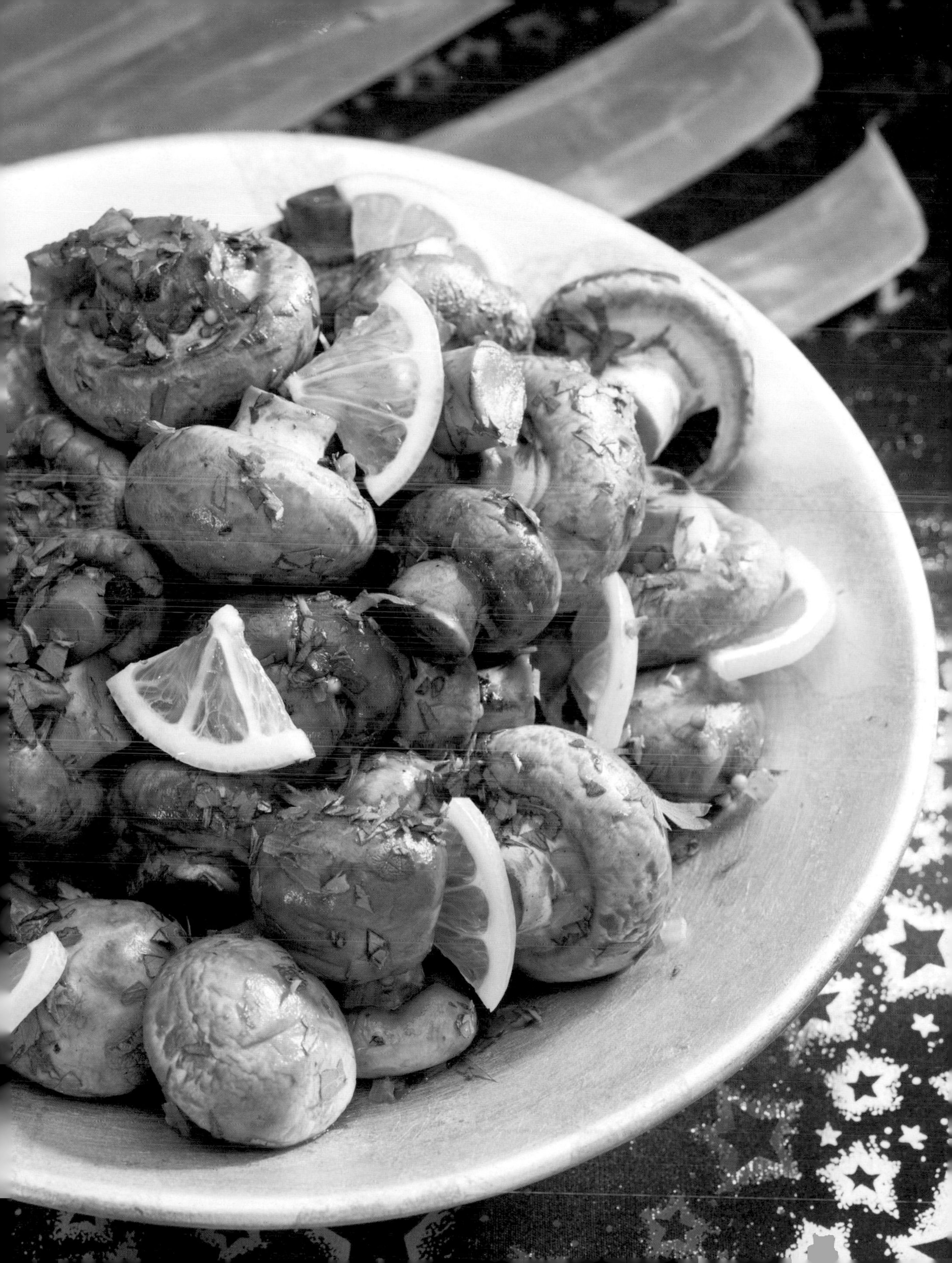

Refried beans

Refried beans are usually a no-no when it comes to low-fat eating, as the main ingredient is half a block of lard to cook everything in. Try them this way and celebrate the absence of unwanted fat.

SERVES 4
PER SERVING:
182 KCAL/6.5G FAT
PREPARATION TIME:
10 MINUTES
COOKING TIME:
25 MINUTES

2 × 400g (2 × 14oz) cans red kidney beans
2 garlic cloves, crushed
1 small red onion, finely sliced
8 spring onions, finely chopped
150ml (1/4 pint) vegetable stock
1 tablespoon chopped fresh flat leaf parsley
6 leaves Romaine lettuce, finely shredded
2 tablespoons virtually fat free fromage frais to garnish
2–3 sprigs fresh mint to garnish

1 Preheat a non-stick pan until very hot. Drain the kidney beans and rinse well under a running cold tap. Add the beans to the pan and cook over a high heat for 2–3 minutes.
2 Add the garlic and onions and continue to cook for a further 2 minutes. Add the stock and simmer until almost reduced, slightly mashing the beans with the back of a wooden spoon.
3 Fold in the parsley and lettuce and spoon into a serving dish.
4 Garnish with fromage frais and fresh mint.

Sweet red pepper salsa

SERVES 4
PER SERVING:
61 KCAL/0.6G FAT
PREPARATION TIME:
10 MINUTES
COOKING TIME:
30 MINUTES

- 2 red peppers
- 1 red onion, finely chopped
- 4 ripe tomatoes, skinned, seeded and chopped
- zest and juice of 1 lime
- 1 tablespoon chopped fresh coriander
- 1 teaspoon clear honey
- salt and freshly ground black pepper

This salsa can be used as an accompaniment to many dishes. Try it spooned over grilled fish and meat or as a sandwich filler.

1. Cut the peppers in half and remove the seeds. Place skin-side up under a preheated hot grill and leave until black and blistered. Place immediately in a plastic food bag and tie to make airtight. Leave until cold, then carefully peel away the skin under a cold running tap.
2. Dice the peppers and combine with the other ingredients. Season to taste.

Sweet and sour Chinese cabbage

Adding a little sugar to vegetables as they dry-fry helps them to caramelise much quicker, resulting in a much sweeter flavoursome dish.

SERVES 4
PER SERVING:
70 KCAL/0.4G FAT
PREPARATION TIME:
10 MINUTES
COOKING TIME:
8 MINUTES

1 Chinese cabbage
2 large carrots, coarsely grated
1 tablespoon soft brown sugar
1 × 400g (14oz) can chopped tomatoes
2 tablespoons light soy sauce
2 tablespoons white wine vinegar
salt and freshly ground black pepper

1 Preheat a non-stick deep wok.
2 Remove 2–3 outer leaves from the cabbage and reserve. Finely shred the inner part of the cabbage. Season well with salt and black pepper.
3 Dry-fry the carrots and cabbage with the sugar over a high heat for 1–2 minutes until they start to caramelise. Pour the tomatoes, soy sauce and vinegar on top and mix well until heated through.
4 Pile into a warmed serving dish, lined with the reserved outer cabbage leaves.

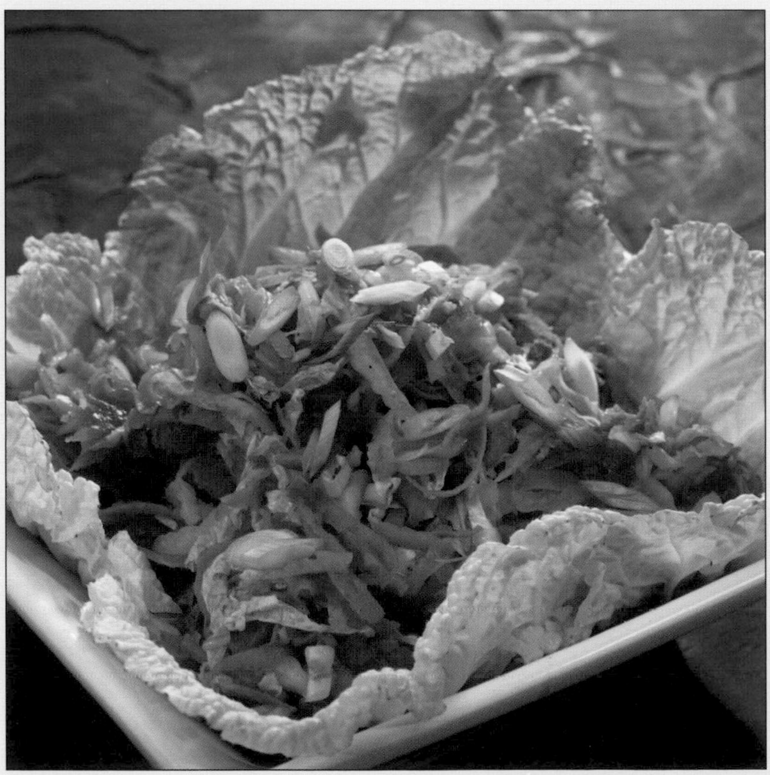

Top right: *Papaya, beansprout and hot banana salad*

Right: *Honey roast corn on the cob*

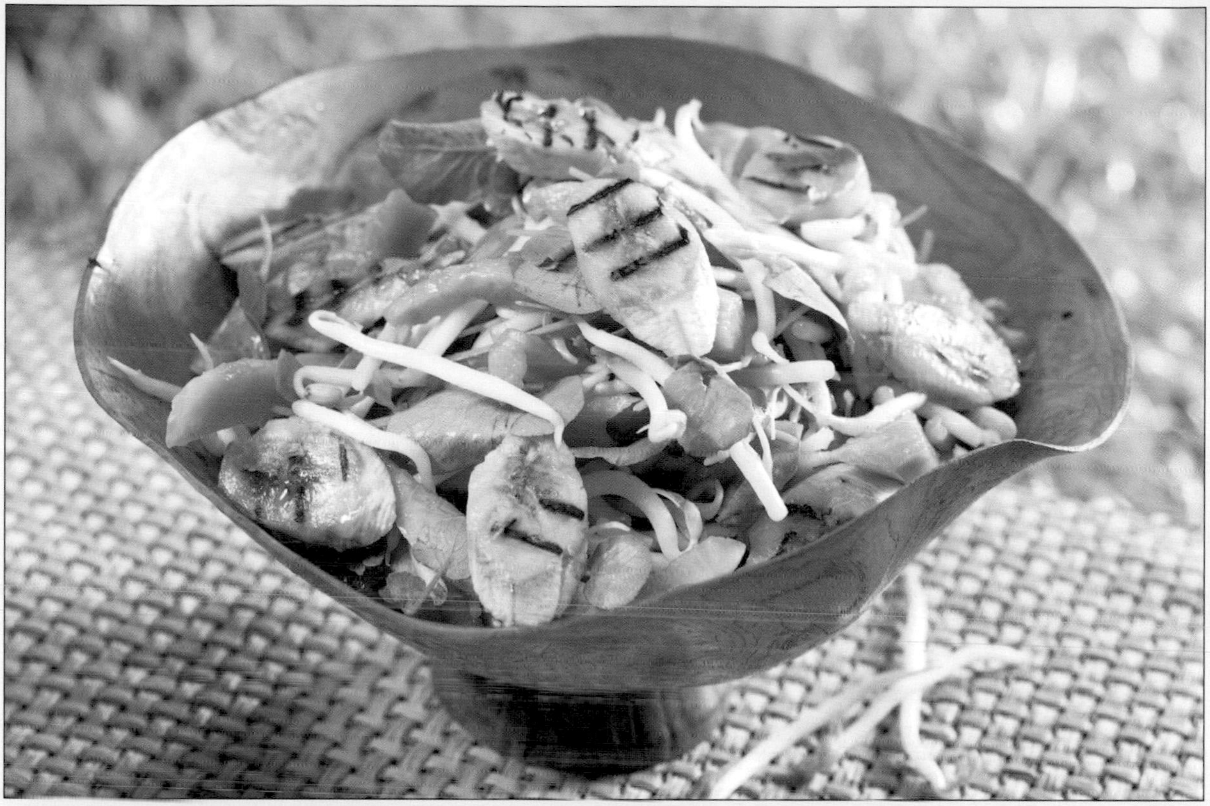

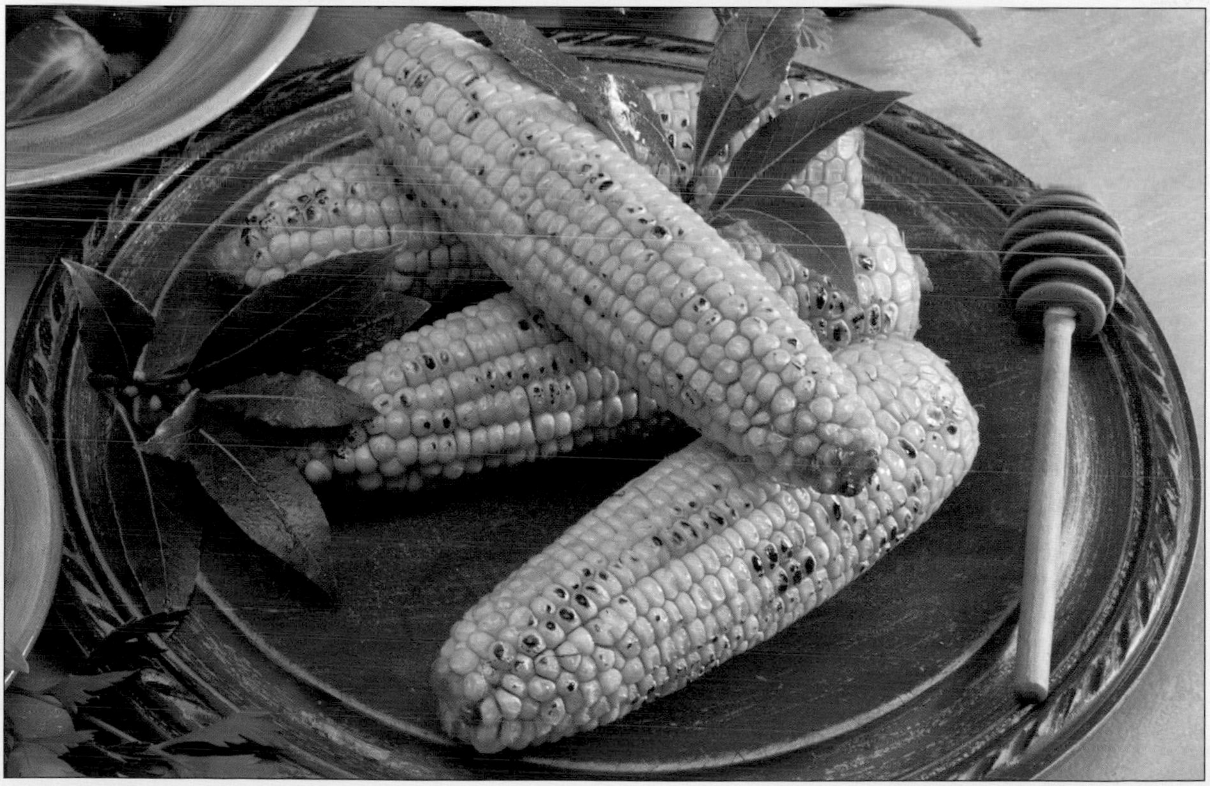

Papaya, beansprout and hot banana salad

Fresh ingredients form an essential part of this recipe. Tired beansprouts and over-ripe papaya will result in a wet, unappetising disaster. Banana takes on a different taste when cooked, so do give it a try and if you can get the cooking variety of plantain this is even better.

SERVES 4
PER SERVING:
128 KCAL/0.7G FAT
PREPARATION TIME:
15 MINUTES
COOKING TIME:
8 MINUTES

2 ripe papaya
1 small bunch watercress
225g (8oz) fresh beansprouts
6 spring onions, finely chopped
1 small red chilli, finely chopped
2 small green bananas

for the dressing
150ml (1/4 pint) orange juice
3 tablespoons blackberry or raspberry fruit vinegar
1 teaspoon mild Dijon mustard
1 teaspoon clear honey
2 tablespoons finely chopped coriander
salt and freshly ground black pepper to taste

1. Peel the papaya, then cut in half and remove the seeds and discard. Cut the flesh into thin strips and place in a large bowl.
2. Wash, drain and pick over the watercress. Add just the tender tops to the bowl, saving the stalks for soup or stock. Add the beansprouts, spring onions and chilli and toss gently to combine the ingredients.
3. Preheat a non-stick frying pan. Peel the bananas and slice on the diagonal to give long slices. Add to the pan and fry quickly for 2–3 minutes on each side so that they are lightly coloured but still firm.
4. Transfer the salad to a serving bowl and arrange the cooked banana on top.
5. Place all the dressing ingredients in a container with a tight-fitting lid – a jam jar is ideal. Shake well until combined, then drizzle over the finished salad. Serve straight away.

See photograph on page 191.

Honey roast corn on the cob

SERVES 4
PER SERVING:
172 KCAL/2.15G FAT
PREPARATION TIME:
10 MINUTES
COOKING TIME:
35 MINUTES

4 large corn on the cob
1 vegetable stock cube
1 teaspoon ground cumin
2 tablespoons runny honey
salt and freshly ground black pepper
a few chopped fresh chives to garnish

Corn on the cob tends to go hand in hand with lashings of high-fat butter. Enjoy them just as much with a sticky coating of sweet honey.

1 Preheat the oven to 200C, 400F, Gas Mark 6.
2 Remove the outer husk and silky threads from the cobs of corn and trim the ends with a sharp knife.
3 In a large saucepan dissolve the stock cube in approximately 1.2 litres (2 pints) water. Add the cumin and bring to the boil.
4 Carefully add the corn to the pan and top up with boiling water from a kettle so that the corn is completely covered. Simmer gently for 10–12 minutes until the kernels are tender when teased out with the point of a knife. Drain through a colander and place in a roasting tray. Drizzle with honey and season with salt and black pepper.
5 Place in the preheated oven for 15–20 minutes until lightly roasted.
6 Serve hot or cold with a sprinkling of chopped fresh chives.

See photograph on page 191.

Baby carrots and broad beans in a lemon sauce

Broad beans can dry out very quickly. Try adding a rich creamy lemon sauce – it can really make all the difference. This sauce can also be used alongside other vegetables as well as fish and meat dishes.

SERVES 4
PER SERVING:
110 KCAL/1.6G FAT
PREPARATION TIME:
20 MINUTES
COOKING TIME:
20 MINUTES

225g (8oz) young baby carrots, scraped
225g (8oz) shelled baby broad beans
300ml ($^1/_2$ pint) skimmed milk
2 bay leaves
1 vegetable stock cube
4 teaspoons cornflour
2 teaspoons Dijon mustard
zest and juice of 1 lemon
salt and freshly ground black pepper
1 tablespoon chopped fresh parsley to garnish

1. Top and tail the carrots and place in a large saucepan. Cover with water and boil with a pinch of salt for 10–12 minutes.
2. Add the broad beans, bring back to the boil and simmer gently until the beans are cooked.
3. In a separate pan heat the milk with the bay leaves and stock cube to near boiling. Slake the cornflour with a little cold water and whisk into the hot milk. Keep stirring as the sauce thickens. Add the mustard and lemon zest and juice and season well with salt and black pepper.
4. Drain the vegetables into a serving dish, spoon the sauce over and sprinkle with chopped fresh parsley.

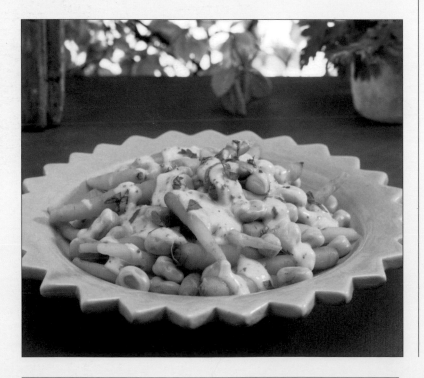

Garlic and herb roasted new potatoes

SERVES 4
PER SERVING:
85 KCAL/0.4G FAT
PREPARATION TIME:
15 MINUTES
COOKING TIME:
45 MINUTES

450g (1lb) new potatoes
2 garlic cloves, finely chopped
2–3 sprigs fresh rosemary
2–3 sprigs fresh thyme
2 tablespoons light soy sauce
chopped fresh thyme or coriander to garnish

This is a great way of dressing up leftover cooked potatoes. A good tip is to roast off a large quantity and portion them for the freezer. Cook straight from frozen in a hot oven.

1 Preheat the oven to 200C, 400F, Gas Mark 6.
2 Cook the potatoes in boiling salted water. Drain and place in a non-stick roasting tin.
3 Sprinkle with the garlic and herbs, pulling the leaves away from the stems.
4 Drizzle with soy sauce and toss the potatoes, coating them with the mixture.
5 Place in the preheated oven and roast for 35–45 minutes, shaking the pan occasionally to prevent sticking.
6 Transfer to a serving bowl and garnish with chopped fresh thyme or coriander.

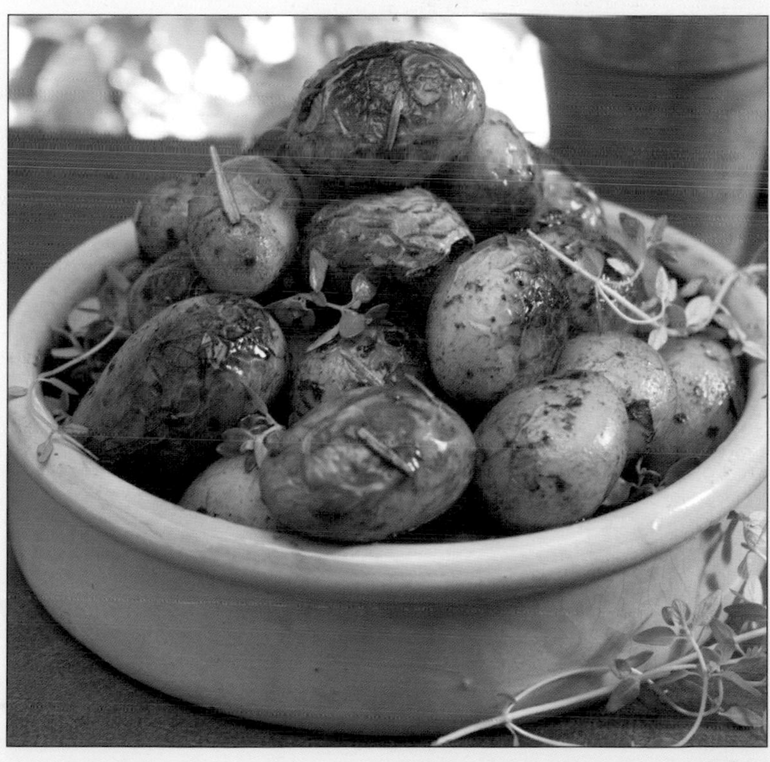

Vegetable brunoise

A colourful combination of vegetables. Cutting them small reduces the cooking time considerably. Leftover vegetables can be mixed with a little low-fat fromage frais for a creamy vegetable salad, the perfect accompaniment to cold meats.

SERVES 4
PER SERVING:
70 KCAL/0.7G FAT
PREPARATION TIME:
15 MINUTES
COOKING TIME:
10 MINUTES

4 medium sized carrots, peeled
½ butternut squash, peeled
1 small swede, peeled
1 vegetable stock cube
2 small sweet potatoes, peeled
2 small courgettes
2–3 spring onions, chopped
fresh mint to garnish

1 Prepare all the vegetables by cutting each one into regular small dice.
2 Place the carrots, squash and swede into a saucepan and cover with water, add the stock cube and bring to the boil. Simmer for 2–3 minutes, then add the remaining vegetables. Simmer until tender, then drain.
3 Just before serving, garnish with sprigs of fresh mint.

Potatoes marquise

SERVES 4
PER SERVING:
169 KCAL/0.8G FAT
PREPARATION TIME:
30 MINUTES
COOKING TIME:
25 MINUTES

675g (1½lb) potatoes, peeled and chopped
2 tablespoons skimmed milk
1 tablespoon virtually fat free fromage frais
1 medium onion, finely chopped
1 garlic clove, crushed
6 tomatoes, skinned, seeded and chopped
salt and freshly ground black pepper
2 tablespoons chopped fresh chives to garnish

1 Preheat the oven to 200C, 400F, Gas Mark 6.
2 Boil the potatoes in salted water until cooked, drain well and mash with a potato masher, adding the skimmed milk and fromage frais until lump free.
3 Dry-fry the onion and garlic in a preheated non-stick pan until it starts to colour. Add the tomatoes and remove from the heat.
4 Take a large piping bag with a star nozzle and fill with the potato mixture. On a non-stick baking tray pipe round discs of potato, 8cm (4in) in diameter, then pipe a second layer on top of each disc but only around the perimeter, leaving a void in the centre. Spoon the tomato mixture into the centre.
5 Bake in the preheated oven for 20–25 minutes until brown and crispy.
6 Serve hot, sprinkled with chives.

See photograph on page 198.

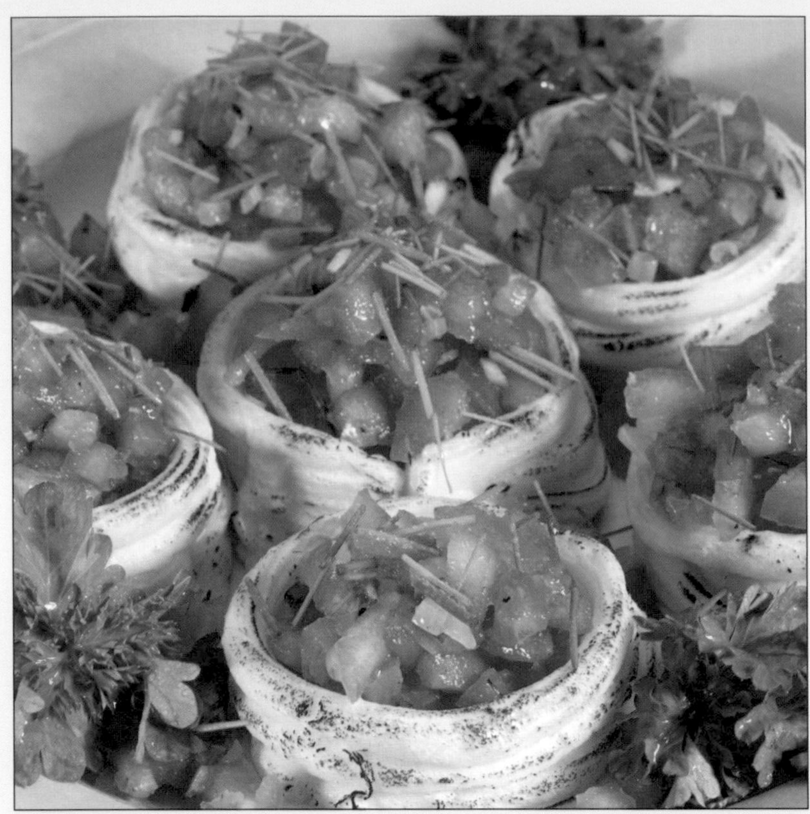

Left: *Potatoes marquise*

Below: *Baked creamed cauliflower*

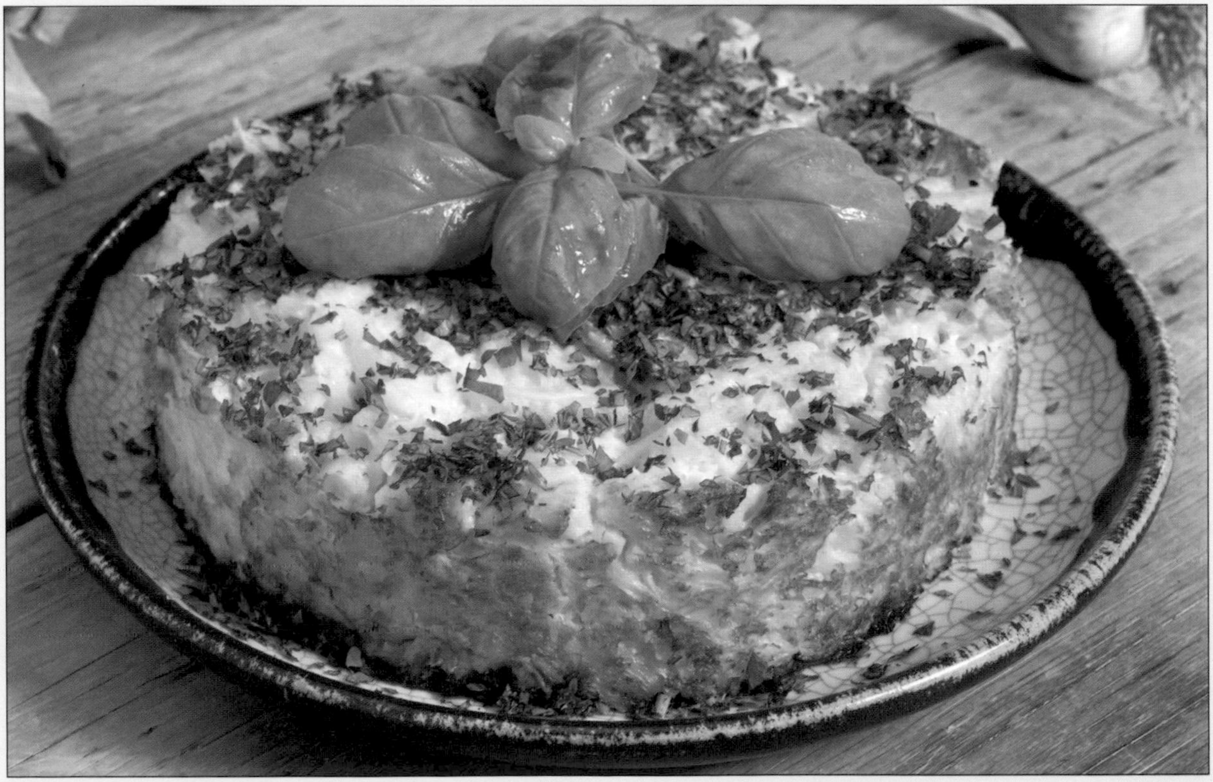

Braised fennel

SERVES 4
PER SERVING:
21 KCAL/0.3G FAT
PREPARATION TIME:
10 MINUTES
COOKING TIME:
50 MINUTES

8 small heads fennel
2 garlic cloves, crushed
1 teaspoon chopped fresh thyme
3–4 juniper berries, crushed
2 teaspoons vegetable bouillon stock powder
salt and freshly ground black pepper
4 ripe tomatoes, skinned, seeded and diced to garnish
chopped fresh chives to garnish

Fennel is an interesting vegetable with a strong anise flavour. Florence fennel is small and sweet and can be eaten both raw in salads and cooked as a vegetable. It is also a great addition to vegetable soups.

1 Trim away the root from the bottom of the fennel bulbs. Split each bulb down the centre with a sharp knife, then cut into small wedges.
2 Preheat a non-stick frying pan until hot, add the fennel and cook quickly over a high heat for 5–6 minutes until they start to colour. Add the garlic and continue cooking for 1–2 minutes.
3 Sprinkle the thyme, juniper and stock powder over the fennel, then pour 300ml (½ pint) boiling water into the pan. Season with black pepper, cover with a lid and braise gently for 10–15 minutes until tender.
4 Pour into a serving dish and sprinkle with the diced tomato and chopped fresh chives.

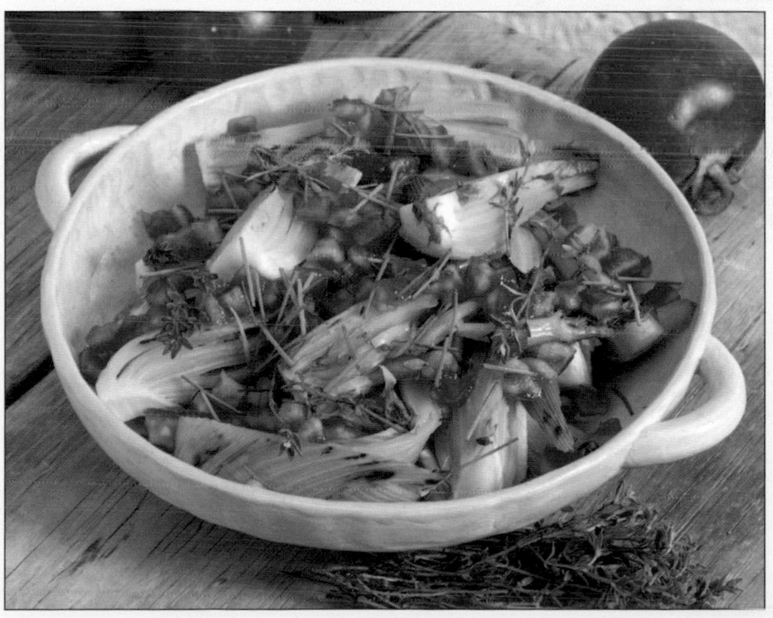

Baked creamed cauliflower

The mustard in this recipe gives the cauliflower a real lift. This vegetable accompaniment will be quite safe left in a low oven until ready to serve. Try adding fresh basil or even a little blue cheese to the mixture.

SERVES 4
PER SERVING:
117 KCAL/3.2G FAT
PREPARATION TIME:
10 MINUTES
COOKING TIME:
50 MINUTES

1 medium cauliflower
300ml ($^1/_2$ pint) skimmed milk
1 teaspoon vegetable bouillon stock powder
1 garlic clove, crushed
1 tablespoon cornflour
1 tablespoon Dijon mustard
1 egg, beaten
salt and freshly ground black pepper
2 tablespoons chopped fresh parsley to garnish

1 Preheat the oven to 200C, 400F, Gas Mark 6.
2 Remove the outer leaves from the cauliflower and break the vegetable into florets. Cook in a pan of boiling salted water until tender, then drain well.
3 In a small saucepan heat the milk with the stock and garlic until boiling. Slake the cornflour with a little cold milk and whisk into the hot milk. Simmer gently for 1–2 minutes, stirring well as the sauce thickens.
4 Remove the sauce from the heat and beat in the mustard and egg, seasoning well with salt and black pepper.
5 Place the drained cauliflower into a large bowl and break up slightly with a fork. Add the sauce and mix well. Pour into a small, round, non-stick cake tin and smooth the top with the back of a fork.
6 Place in the oven and bake for 30 minutes.
7 To serve, run a knife around the inside edge of the tin, place a serving plate on top, invert and turn out on to the plate. Sprinkle with parsley and serve.

See photograph on page 198.

Puddings

For chocolate lovers and the rest of us, here are some more tempting recipes that, without doubt, taste delicious and luxurious, even though the fat and calories have been reduced.

Some of the more substantial recipes are designed to follow a light meal, so calculate accordingly and indulge without guilt.

Banana split with hot chocolate sauce

A dessert to die for! Although low in fat, this dessert makes up for it in calories so make sure you compensate your main meals accordingly.

SERVES 4
PER SERVING:
199 KCAL/4.4G FAT
PREPARATION TIME:
10 MINUTES
COOKING TIME:
20 MINUTES

1 tablespoon Valrhona cocoa powder
300ml (1/2 pint) semi–skimmed milk
2 teaspoons cornflour
1 tablespoon caster sugar
4 small ripe bananas
2 tablespoons lemon juice
225g (8oz) fresh raspberries
8 scoops Wall's 'Too Good To Be True' iced dessert

1. In a small saucepan heat the cocoa powder with the milk, whisking continuously.
2. Slake the cornflour with a little cold milk and whisk into the milk. Simmer for 1 minute as the sauce thickens, then add sugar to taste. Keep warm over a low heat.
3. Peel the bananas, slice in half lengthways and place in a serving dish. Sprinkle with the lemon juice to prevent them turning brown.
4. Divide the raspberries between the 4 dishes. Place 2 scoops of iced dessert on top of the raspberries then pour the chocolate sauce over.
5. Serve straight away.

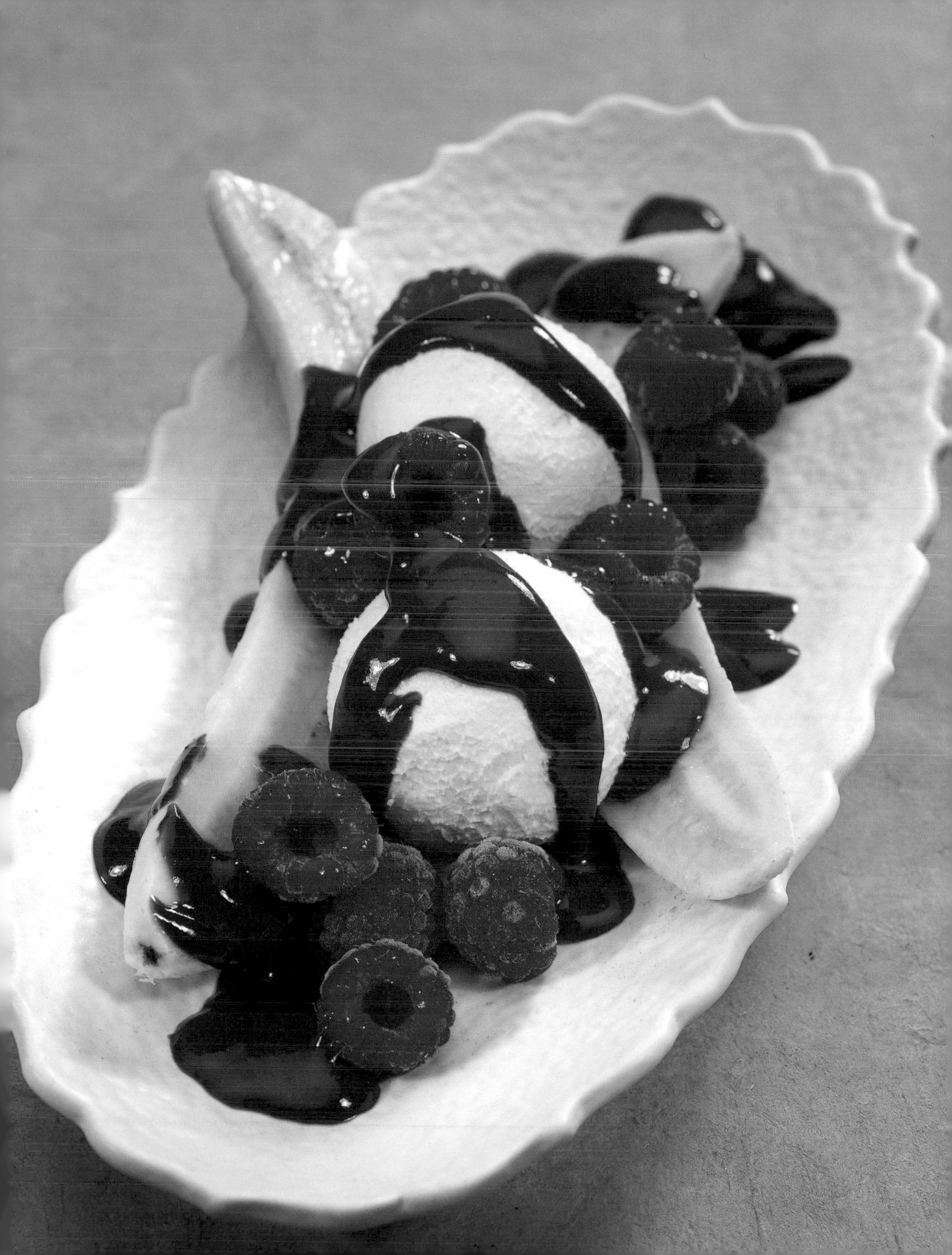

Summer berry gratin

Any combination of fruit may be used in this recipe. Firm fruits such as blueberries or peaches are cooked in a little wine for added flavour. The egg white adds bulk and a lighter texture.

SERVES 4
PER SERVING:
225 KCAL/1.1G FAT
PREPARATION TIME:
10 MINUTES
COOKING TIME:
15 MINUTES

175g (6oz) blueberries
½ wine glass white wine
2 tablespoons caster sugar
175g (6oz) raspberries
175g (6oz) strawberries, hulled and sliced
2 egg whites
600g (1lb 5oz) Total 0% fat Greek yogurt
4 tablespoons demerara sugar

1 Place the blueberries in a small saucepan and add the wine and sugar. Cook gently over a low heat until the fruit starts to pop.
2 Turn off the heat, add the raspberries and strawberries and mix well. Spoon into 4 gratin or shallow dishes and chill.
3 When the fruit is chilled, preheat the grill until it is very hot.
4 Just before you are ready to serve, whisk the egg whites to stiff peaks and fold into the yogurt. Spread the yogurt over the fruit, covering the fruit completely. Sprinkle with demerara sugar and immediately place under the grill until the sugar caramelises.
5 Serve immediately.

Pineapple crush

SERVES 6
PER SERVING:
180 KCAL/2.6G FAT
PREPARATION TIME:
20 MINUTES
COOKING TIME:
5 MINUTES

1 large pineapple
225g (8oz) low-fat sponge fingers
2 tablespoons dry sherry
2 egg whites
300ml (½ pint) Total 0% Greek yogurt
icing sugar

1 Prepare the pineapple by slicing off the top and bottom with a sharp knife. Remove the outer skin, slicing down the fruit. Cut the fruit lengthways into quarters and remove the central core.
2 Place the sponge fingers into a food processor and reduce to fine crumbs, pour into a bowl, sprinkle with the sherry and set aside.
3 Roughly chop the pineapple and add to the food processor. Using the pulse motion, reduce the flesh to a chunky purée.
4 Whisk the egg whites until stiff, then gradually fold in the yogurt and icing sugar.
5 Assemble the dessert in a glass dish or in individual sundae glasses in layers, first with sponge finger crumbs sprinkled with sherry, then pineapple and finally the yogurt mixture. Repeat, dusting the top with crumbs.
6 Refrigerate until ready to serve.

See photograph on page 206.

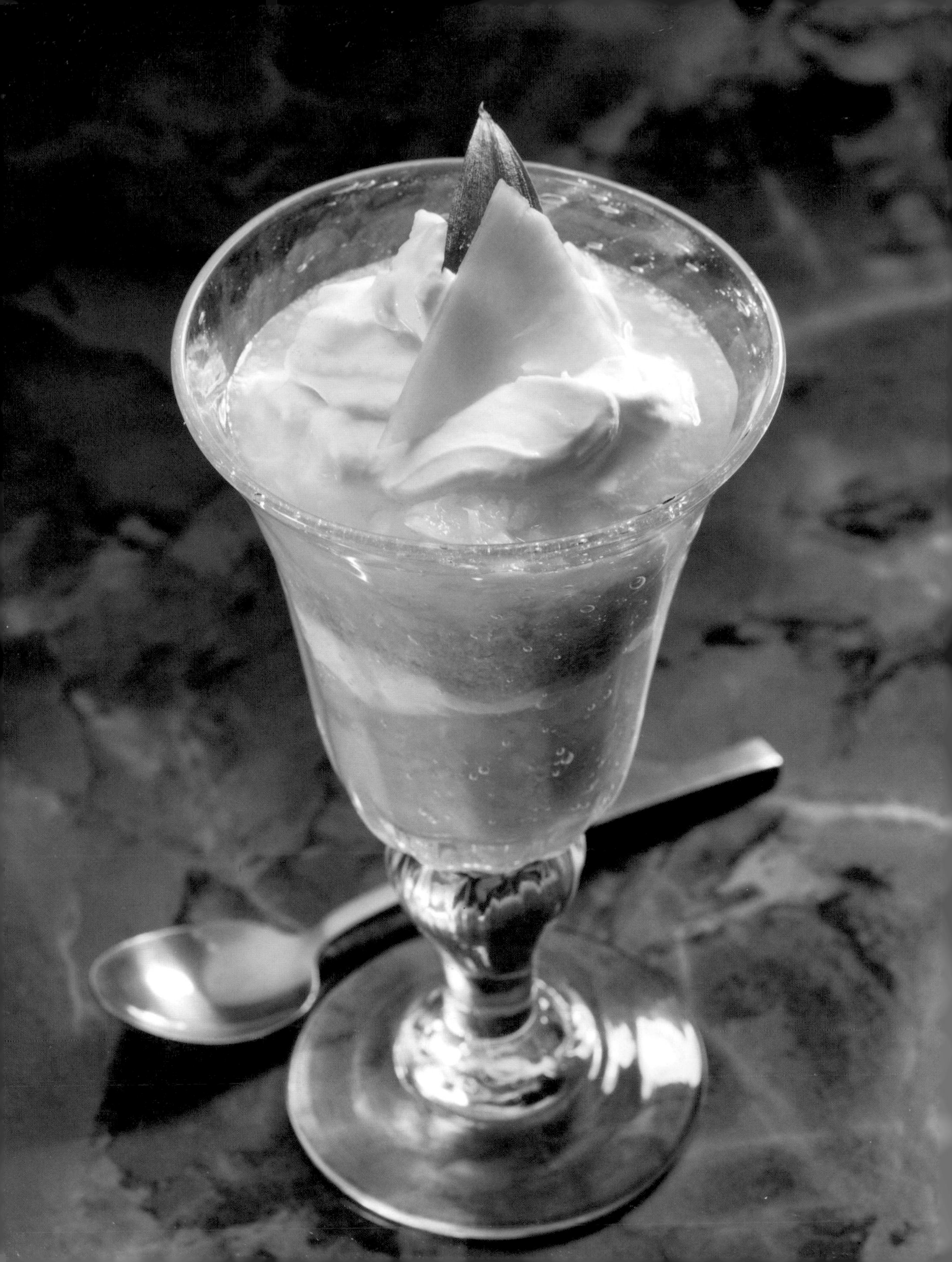

Apricot and almond syllabub

SERVES 1
PER SERVING:
174 KCAL/1.4G FAT
PREPARATION TIME:
10 MINUTES
COOKING TIME:
15 MINUTES

25g (1oz) dried apricots
zest and juice of 1 lime
4–5 tablespoons low fat Greek yogurt
2 teaspoons Amaretto liqueur
1 egg white

1 Place the apricots and lime into a small saucepan and cover with water. Bring to the boil and simmer until soft and virtually all the water has evaporated. Using a fork, mash the apricots until smooth.
2 Beat the yogurt into the apricot mixture, add the liqueur and sweeten to taste with a little sugar. Whisk the egg white to stiff peaks and gently fold into the mixture.
3 Spoon into a glass and chill until required.

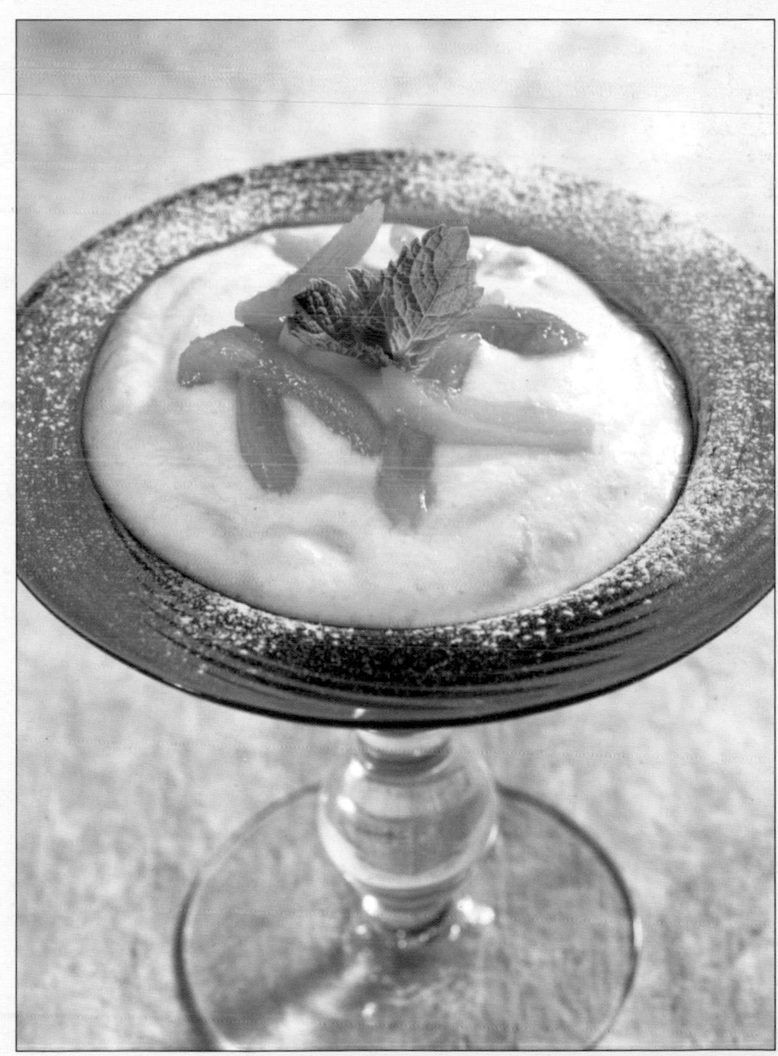

Left: *Pineapple crush*

Valrhona chocolate mousse

Valrhona cocoa powder is made using a high quantity of cocoa solids, thus giving a much stronger fuller chocolate flavour. To create a completely decadent dessert, grate a little white chocolate from a 10g Nestle's Milky Bar to give a touch of luxury on top.

SERVES 6
PER SERVING:
188 KCAL/1.4G FAT
PREPARATION TIME:
5 MINUTES
COOKING TIME:
15 MINUTES

300ml ($^1/_2$ pint) semi-skimmed milk
2 tablespoons Valrhona cocoa powder
2 tablespoons cornflour
115g (4oz) caster sugar
6 sheets leaf gelatine
450g (16oz) virtually fat free Normandy fromage frais
3 egg whites
1 × 10g Milky Bar
a few redcurrants to decorate
a few mint leaves to decorate

1 Heat the milk and cocoa powder in a small saucepan. Slake the cornflour with a little cold water and whisk into the hot milk, along with the sugar. Simmer until the sauce thickens, remove from the heat, pour into a mixing bowl and allow to cool.
2 Soak the gelatine in cold water for 2–3 minutes until it becomes soft. Place it in a bowl and heat it either over a pan of boiling water or in a microwave for 1 minute until liquid. Add to the chocolate sauce, mixing in well, along with the fromage frais.
3 Whisk the egg whites until stiff and fold into the mixture. Spoon into individual glasses or place in a glass bowl.
4 Decorate with grated white chocolate, redcurrants and mint leaves.

Chocolate marble puddings

SERVES 4
PER SERVING:
302 KCAL/2.8G FAT
PREPARATION TIME:
5 MINUTES
COOKING TIME:
30 MINUTES

- 115g (4oz) Quark (low-fat cheese)
- 115g (4oz) caster sugar
- 1 egg yolk
- 2 egg whites
- 150g (5oz) plain flour
- 2 teaspoons baking powder
- 3 tablespoons orange juice
- 1 tablespoon Valrhona cocoa powder

Create a stir with these stunning chocolate puddings. For a fruitier pudding add 2–3 teaspoons of marmalade to the bottom of each ramekin.

1. Preheat the oven to 180C, 350F, Gas Mark 4. Lightly grease 4 × 115g (4 × 4oz) ramekin dishes.
2. In a mixing bowl beat together the Quark, sugar and egg yolk until smooth. Beat in the flour and baking powder.
3. In a clean bowl whisk the egg whites until stiff and fold into the mixture.
4. In a small bowl gradually mix the orange juice into the cocoa powder to form a smooth paste. Pour the cocoa over the sponge mixture and stir to create a marbled effect.
5. Spoon into prepared dishes and bake in the centre of the preheated oven for 15–20 minutes until well risen and firm to the touch.
6. Serve hot with low-fat yogurt or fromage frais.

Caramel coffee pears with vanilla sauce

Choose firm pears without bruising, as the discoloration caused by bruising will show once peeled. The vanilla sauce can be made in advance and stored with a disc of parchment paper on the top to avoid a skin forming.

SERVES 4
PER SERVING:
255 KCAL/1.4G FAT
PREPARATION TIME:
5 MINUTES
COOKING TIME:
20 MINUTES

4 large firm pears
2 tablespoons lemon juice
115g (4oz) caster sugar
50ml (2fl oz) coffee
300ml (½ pint) semi-skimmed milk
1 vanilla pod
2 teaspoons cornflour
sugar to taste

1 Peel the pears and cut in half lengthways. Scoop out the core with a spoon and rub the surface of the pears with the lemon juice. Place the pears in a large bowl and sprinkle the sugar over to coat.
2 Preheat a non-stick saucepan. Add the pears, placing them face down in the pan. Cook gently until the sugar starts to caramelise, then add the coffee and continue cooking until the pears soften.
3 In the meantime, make the sauce by heating the milk in a saucepan. Split the vanilla pod lengthways and scrape the blade of the knife along the inside edges of the pod to remove the seeds. Add these to the milk along with the pod.
4 Slake the cornflour with a little cold water and whisk into the hot milk. Simmer gently to allow the sauce to thicken.
5 Arrange the pears in a serving dish and pour the sauce around.

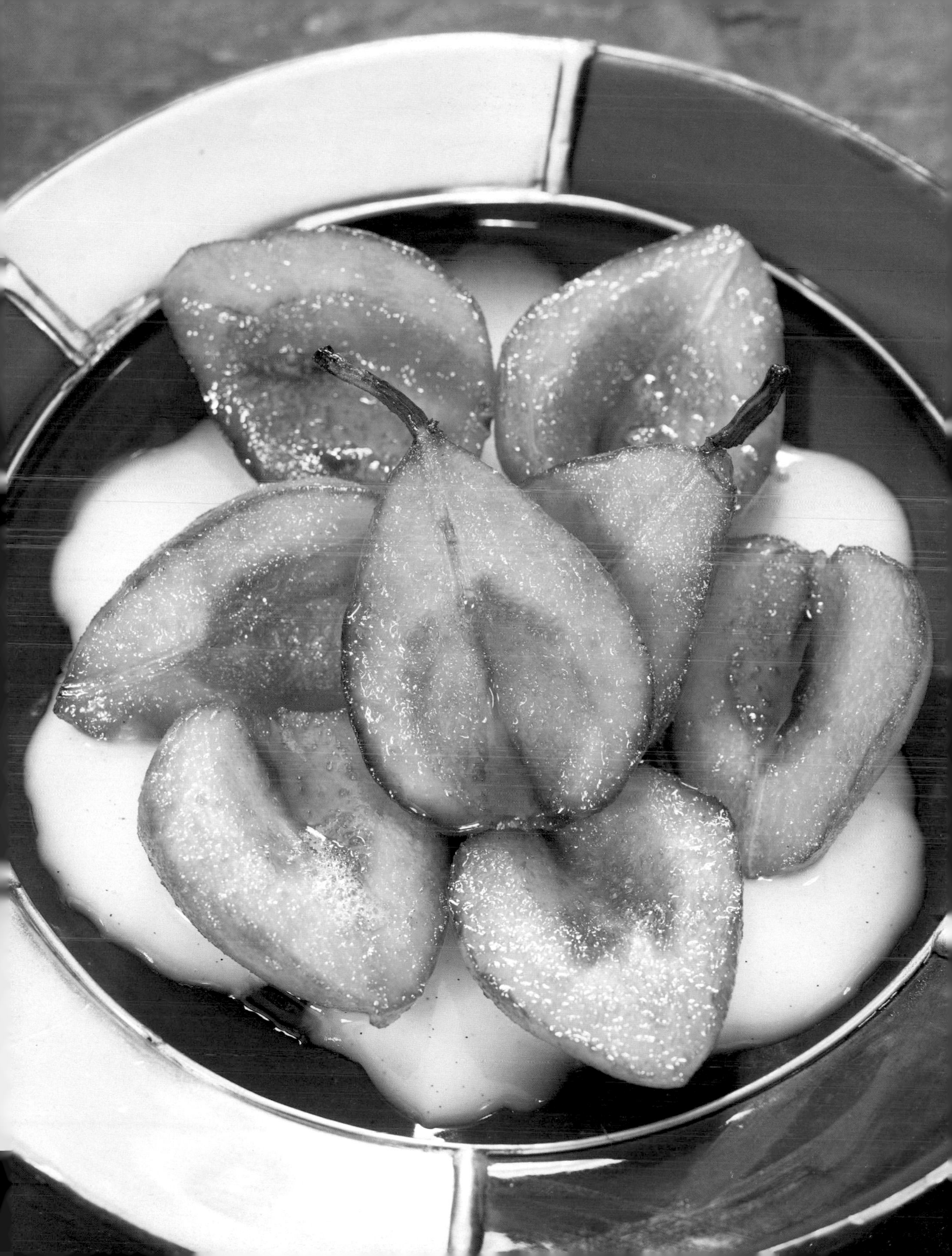

Mexican candy

Indulge in this crisp, orange-flavoured candy. Delicious dipped in hot strong coffee.

MAKES 8 PIECES
PER PIECE 188 KCAL/0.03G FAT
PREPARATION TIME: 5 MINUTES
COOKING TIME: 30 MINUTES

1 tablespoon raisins
350g (12oz) caster sugar
4 tablespoons water
fine zest of 1 orange

1 Lightly grease a 20cm (8in) square non-stick tin.
2 Scatter the raisins over the base of the prepared tin.
3 Heat the sugar with the water over a low heat in a heavy bottom saucepan until it starts to melt into a liquid. Using a wooden spoon, draw the mixture from the outside into the middle of the pan. When the sugar has caramelised, turned a golden brown colour and has completely dissolved, carefully pour over the raisins, standing well back in case the caramel spits.
4 Using a fine grater, grate the orange zest over. Allow to cool and set.
5 Cut or break into pieces and serve.

Orange velvet cream

SERVES 4
PER SERVING:
188 KCAL/0.9G FAT
PREPARATION TIME:
20 MINUTES
COOKING TIME:
15 MINUTES

4 oranges
1 tablespoon caster sugar
2 heaped tablespoons custard powder
250ml (8fl oz) skimmed milk
300g (11oz) low-fat Greek yogurt
2 egg whites
orange segments and mint leaves to decorate

1 Zest the oranges on a fine grater into a small bowl. Squeeze the juice from 2 of the oranges into the bowl.
2 In a separate bowl mix together the sugar and custard powder with a little cold milk to form a smooth paste.
3 Heat the remaining milk in a saucepan until boiling, pour onto the custard powder and whisk well. Return to the pan and cook until the mixture starts to thicken, then stir in the orange zest and juice. Remove from the heat, cover with food wrap and allow to cool.
4 Once cold, beat the yogurt into the custard mixture and sweeten to taste with a little sugar.
5 Whisk the egg whites to stiff peaks and gently fold into the mixture. Spoon into individual glasses or a large serving bowl and decorate with orange segments and mint.

Black cherry clafoutis

Clafoutis is a batter pudding baked with fruit. The original, from the Limousin province of France, was made with freshly gathered black cherries. If you find them too fiddly to stone, substitute with drained canned cherries.

SERVES 4
PER SERVING:
192 KCAL/3.2G FAT
PREPARATION TIME:
20 MINUTES
COOKING TIME:
40 MINUTES

450g (1lb) black cherries
2 tablespoons cherry liqueur
2 eggs
3½ tablespoons caster sugar
1 level tablespoon plain flour
300ml (½ pint) skimmed milk
1 teaspoon vanilla extract

1 Preheat the oven to 200C, 400F, Gas Mark 6.
2 De-stalk and stone the cherries and place in the bottom of a lightly greased shallow ovenproof dish. Drizzle with the cherry liqueur.
3 In a mixing bowl beat together the eggs and sugar until thick and creamy. Gradually blend in the flour to a smooth paste, adding a little milk if necessary.
4 Heat the milk with the vanilla in a small saucepan until near boiling. Slowly pour the milk onto the batter, stirring continuously. Pour the batter over the cherries.
5 Bake in the preheated oven for 25–30 minutes until set.
6 Serve warm with low-fat fromage frais.

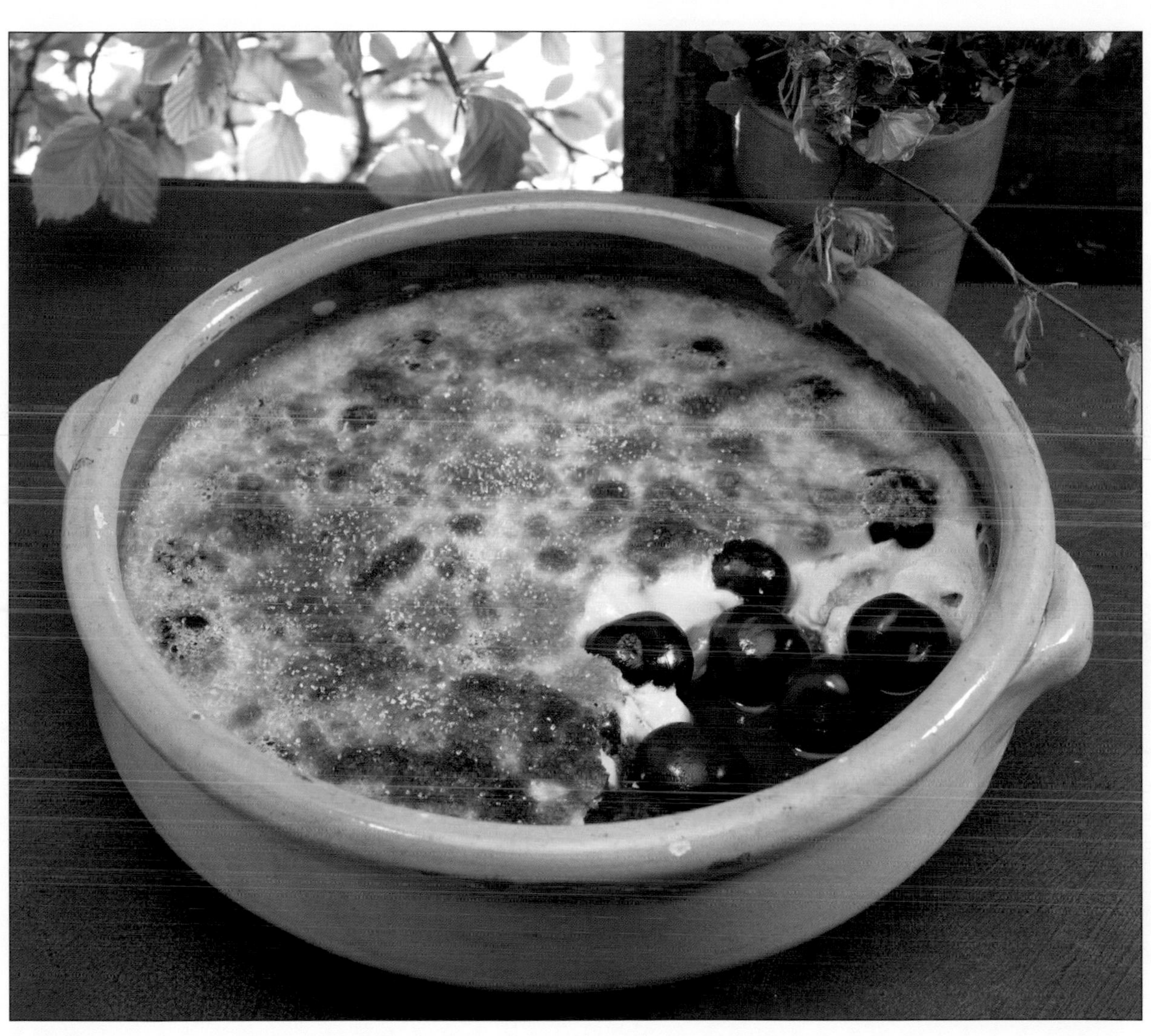

Blackberry and apple crisp

This is a lighter version of a traditional high-fat fruit crumble. While high in calories, this is a great low-fat dessert treat to have after a low-calorie main course. Vary the filling by using different combinations of seasonal fruits. Slicing apples into salted water prevents them from discolouring. Remember to rinse them well in fresh water before using to remove the salt.

SERVES 6
PER SERVING:
264 KCAL/0.8G FAT
PREPARATION TIME:
10 MINUTES
COOKING TIME:
30 MINUTES

225g (8oz) fresh brown breadcrumbs
115g (4oz) soft brown sugar
450g (1lb) cooking apples
1 tablespoon salt
225g (8oz) blackberries
2 tablespoons caster sugar
zest and juice of 1 orange
1 teaspoon ground cinnamon

1. Preheat the oven to 200C, 400F, Gas Mark 6.
2. Spread the breadcrumbs on a baking sheet and sprinkle with the brown sugar. Bake in the oven for 20 minutes, stirring occasionally until the sugar caramelises and the crumbs are toasted. Cool and break down with a fork or food processor and place in a mixing bowl.
3. Peel, core and slice the apples into a bowl of water containing the salt. Rinse well and place in the bottom of an ovenproof dish. Scatter the blackberries over the top and sprinkle with the caster sugar. Pour the orange juice over.
4. Mix the orange zest and cinnamon into the breadcrumbs and scatter evenly over the fruit.
5. Bake in the oven for 25–30 minutes until the fruit is cooked through and the topping browned.
6. Serve warm with low-fat fromage frais.

Apple tart

SERVES 6
PER SERVING:
249 KCAL/2.5G FAT
PREPARATION TIME:
20 MINUTES
COOKING TIME:
60 MINUTES

2 eggs
75g (3oz) golden caster sugar
75g (3oz) self-raising flour, sifted
1 teaspoon vanilla essence
1kg (2lb) cooking apples
1–2 tablespoons golden caster sugar
2 red eating apples
1 tablespoon lemon juice
1 tablespoon Calvados brandy
salt
apricot jam to glaze

A cheat's tart using fat-free sponge as a base to this fruity dessert. The apples need to be sliced into either salted water or lemon juice to prevent them turning brown. Add a little spice if you wish in the form of ground cinnamon or ground cloves.

1 Preheat the oven to 180C, 350F, Gas Mark 4. Grease a 20cm (8in) non-stick flan case with a little vegetable oil, then dust with caster sugar.
2 To make the sponge base, whisk together the eggs and sugar for several minutes until thick and pale in consistency. Using a metal spoon, fold in the sifted flour then the vanilla. Pour into the prepared tin and level off with a knife. Bake in the oven for 20 minutes until golden brown.
3 Allow the sponge to cool, then, using a serrated knife, cut away a 1cm (½in) layer of sponge from the centre of the flan case. Using a metal spoon, scrape away the crumbs to leave a smooth surface.
4 Peel, core and slice the cooking apples into a bowl of salted water. Rinse the apples well in fresh water then cook in a non-stick pan over a low heat for 15–20 minutes until soft.
5 Stir in the sugar to sweeten to taste, drain the apples through a metal sieve to remove any excess liquid then spoon into the sponge case.
6 Core the eating apples and cut in half. Thinly slice into a bowl containing the lemon juice. Cook the apple slices in the bottom of a non-stick frying pan until soft then arrange on the top of the flan.
7 Heat the Calvados with a little apricot jam in a small saucepan and brush over the top to glaze the apples.
8 Serve cold with virtually fat free fromage frais or Total 0% fat Greek yogurt.

See photograph on page 218.

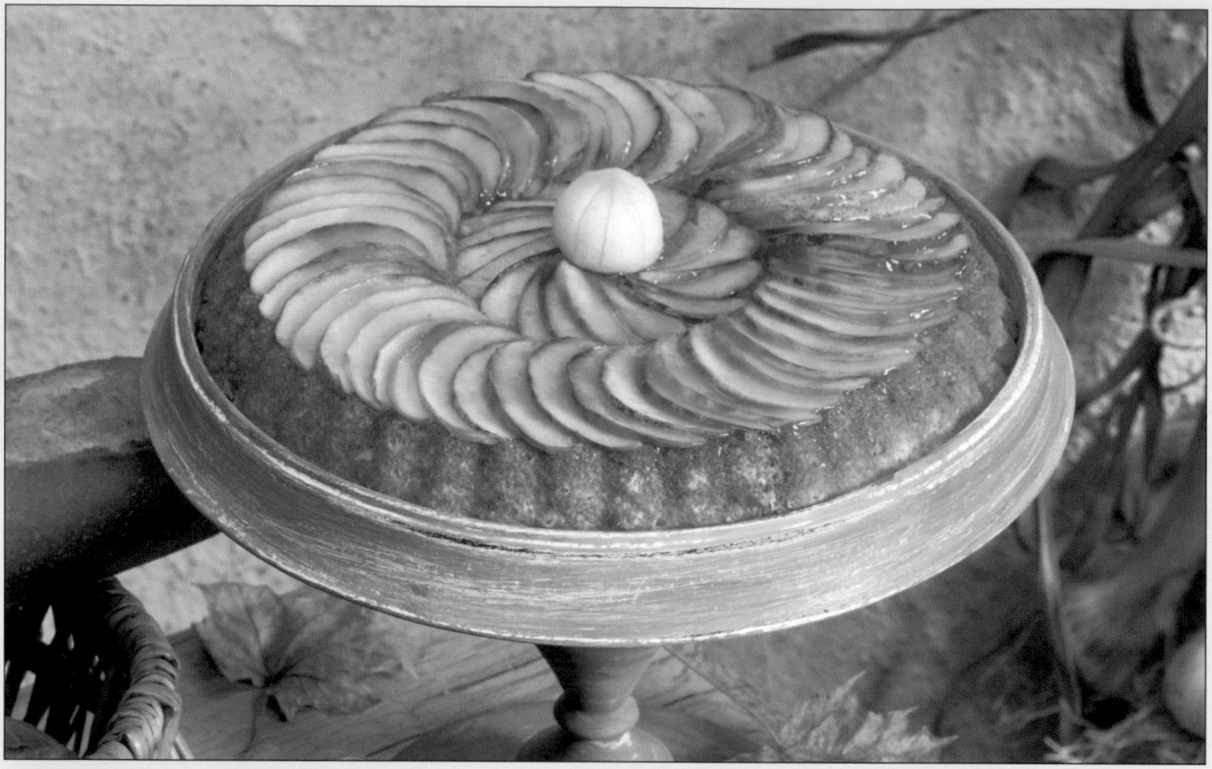

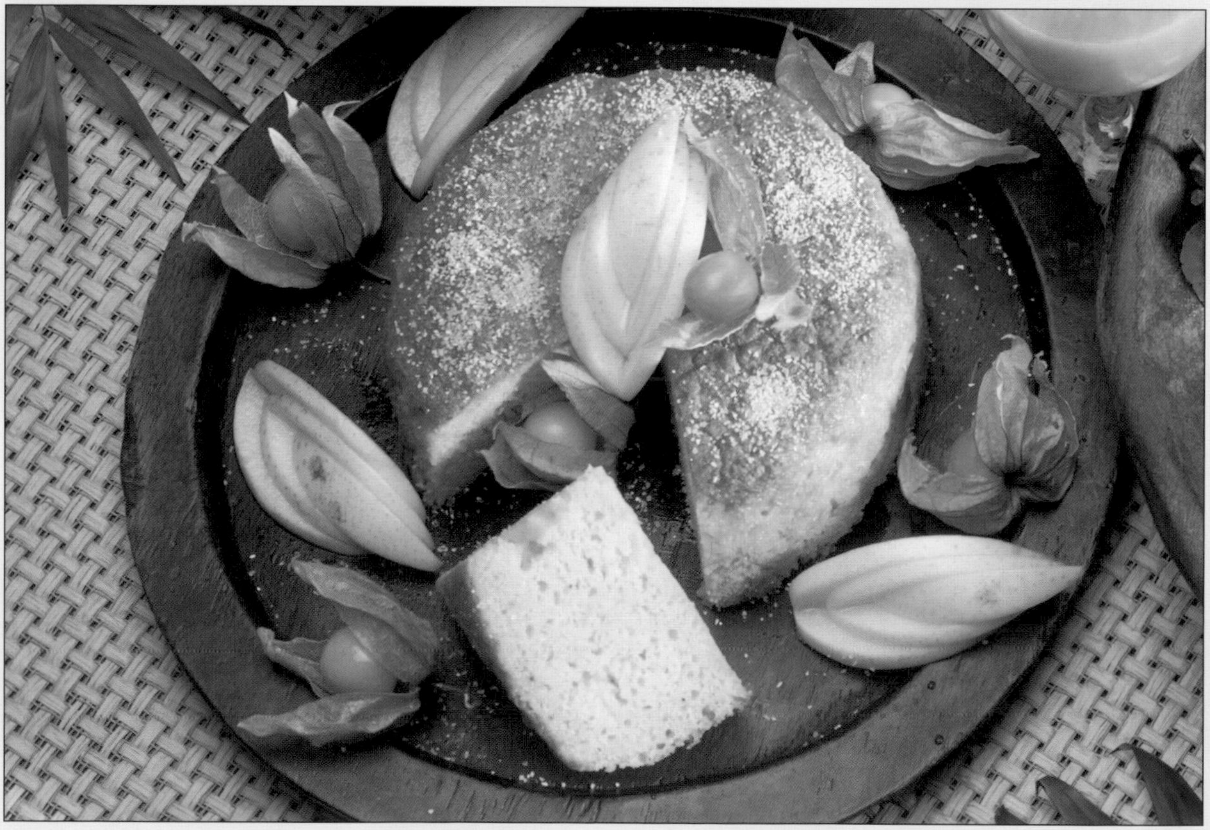

Pear and lemon polenta cake

SERVES 4
PER SERVING:
316 KCAL/5.2G FAT
PREPARATION TIME:
10 MINUTES
COOKING TIME:
40 MINUTES

175g (6oz) canned pears in natural juice, drained
115g (4oz) caster sugar
75g (3oz) plain flour
50g (2oz) fine polenta
3 eggs, beaten
2 lemons
1 teaspoon baking powder

Polenta is a versatile flour produced from ground maize or corn, hence the rich golden colour of this nutty flavoured cake.

1 Preheat the oven to 180C, 350F, Gas Mark 4. Prepare a 15cm (6in) round cake tin by lightly greasing with a little margarine, then line with greaseproof paper.
2 Drain the pears well, place in a large mixing bowl and mash down to a pulp with a large fork.
3 Beat in the sugar, using a wooden spoon, then add the flour, polenta and eggs a little at a time
4 Using a fine grater, add the zest of both lemons plus the juice of one.
5 Finally, beat in the baking powder and pour into the prepared tin.
6 Bake in the oven for 40 minutes until a skewer inserted comes out clean.
7 Allow to cool then drizzle with the lemon juice from the remaining lemon.
8 Slice and serve with low-fat fromage frais and additional pears.

Top left: *Apple tart*

Left: *Pear and lemon polenta cake*

Sauces and dressings

Low-fat sauces are very easy to make. Adding fresh herbs or other ingredients can change a sauce completely, which can make all the difference to a meal. Included in this section are basil pesto and other, more common, high-fat accompaniments – all made the low-fat way.

Fat-free mayonnaise

MAKES 220ML (7½FL OZ)
PER TABLESPOON:
9 KCAL/0.02G FAT

175g (6oz) virtually fat free fromage frais
2 tablespoons cider vinegar
1 tablespoon lemon juice
¼ teaspoon ground turmeric
2 teaspoons sugar
salt and freshly ground black pepper

Real mayonnaise contains egg yolks and oil, two very high-fat ingredients. We have managed to develop a low-fat dressing that can be substituted in recipes containing mayonnaise. The turmeric adds a rich golden colour to the finished dressing.

1 Combine all the ingredients in a small bowl.
2 Whisk until smooth. Store in the refrigerator and use within 3 days.

Fresh basil yogurt dressing

SERVES 6
PER SERVING:
22 KCAL/0.3G FAT

175g (6oz) low-fat natural yogurt
1 tablespoon lemon juice
2 tablespoons chopped fresh basil
1 garlic clove, crushed
1 teaspoon clear honey
salt and freshly ground black pepper

Basil has a strong and perfumed flavour. Its affinity with tomatoes is longstanding. Spoon this dressing over a simple tomato and red onion salad and leave to marinate for 20 minutes.

1 Combine all the ingredients in a small bowl.
2 Whisk until smooth, season well with salt and pepper. Store in the refrigerator and use within 4 days.

Fresh basil pesto

Basil pesto can be bought in many forms from jars to sachets, however the majority are made with a high percentage of fat. The chestnuts add a little body, but if you prefer they may be left out.

SERVES 4
PER SERVING:
11 KCAL/0.7G FAT

1 vegetable stock cube
2 good bunches fresh basil
1 garlic clove, crushed
1 tablespoon finely chopped peeled cooked chestnuts
2 teaspoons grated fresh Parmesan cheese
salt and freshly ground black pepper

1 Dissolve the stock cube in 150ml (¼ pint) boiling water.
2 Pluck the basil leaves from the main plant stem and place in a food processor or liquidiser.
3 Add the remaining ingredients and blend until smooth. Season to taste with salt and freshly ground black pepper and scrape out into a bowl.

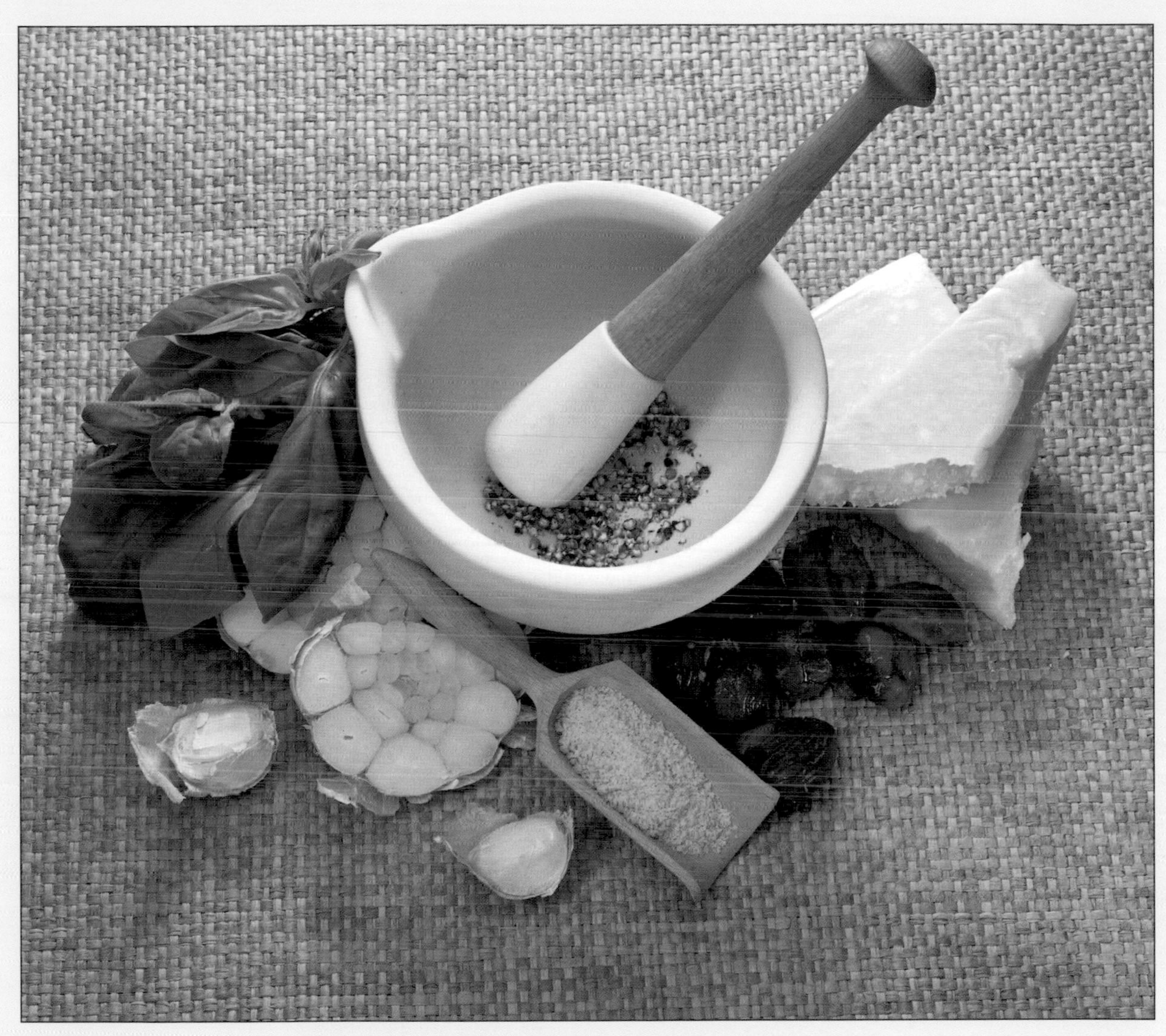

Honey and orange dressing

This dressing can be stored in the refrigerator for one week.

1 Place the orange juice, honey and vinegar in a pan. Add the Dijon mustard and orange rind.
2 Bring to the boil, allow to cool and add the chopped chives and parsley. Season to taste with salt and freshly ground black pepper.

SERVES 6
PER SERVING:
18 KCAL/0G FAT

6 tablespoons orange juice
4 teaspoons thin honey
1 tablespoon white wine vinegar
½ teaspoon Dijon wholegrain mustard
1 teaspoon grated orange rind
2 teaspoons chopped fresh chives and parsley, mixed
salt and freshly ground black pepper to taste

Prawn cocktail sauce

1 Mix all the ingredients together.
2 Store in a screw-top jar in the refrigerator until required.

SERVES 1
PER SERVING:
50 KCAL/0.5G FAT

1 tablespoon tomato ketchup
½ tablespoon reduced-oil salad dressing
1 tablespoon low-fat natural yogurt
black pepper to taste
dash of Tabasco sauce

Yogurt and mint dressing

SERVES 4
PER SERVING:
28 KCAL/0.4G FAT

175g (6oz) low-fat natural yogurt
1–2 teaspoons mint sauce
1 tablespoon finely chopped fresh parsley
salt and freshly ground black pepper to taste

1 Mix all the ingredients together in a container.
2 Store in the refrigerator and use within 2 days.

Balsamic dressing

SERVES 6
PER SERVING:
17 KCAL/0.4G FAT

300ml ($^1/_2$ pint) apple juice
2 tablespoons balsamic vinegar
1 tablespoon mild Dijon mustard
pinch of sugar
salt and freshly ground black pepper

Balsamic vinegar is a dark sweet vinegar from Modena in Italy. Its rich syrupy consistency makes a delicious fruity dressing.

1 Combine all the ingredients in a small bowl and whisk until smooth.
2 Place in a sealed jar or bottle and use as required. Use within 5 days.

Caesar salad dressing

Sometimes salad dressing can become repetitive, so pep it up with a few extra ingredients.

SERVES 4
PER SERVING:
25 KCAL/0.9G FAT

4 tablespoons low-fat salad dressing
1 tablespoon fat-free fromage frais
1 garlic clove, crushed
2–3 teaspoons fresh lemon juice
2 teaspoons grated fresh Parmesan cheese
salt and freshly ground black pepper

1 Combine all the ingredients in a bowl, cover and refrigerate for 1 hour to allow the flavours to develop.
2 Serve with grilled fish, meat or roasted vegetables.

White sauce

SERVES 4
PER SERVING:
55 KCAL/0.2G FAT

300ml (½pint) skimmed milk
1 onion, peeled and sliced
6 peppercorns
1 bay leaf
2 teaspoons cornflour
salt and freshly ground black pepper

1 Heat all but 50ml (2fl oz) of the milk in a non-stick saucepan, adding the onion, peppercorns, bay leaf and seasoning.
2 Heat gently and cover the pan. Simmer for 5 minutes. Turn off the heat and leave the milk mixture to stand with the lid on for a further 30 minutes or until you are ready to thicken and serve the sauce.
3 Mix the remaining milk with the cornflour and when it's almost time to serve it, strain the milk, add the cornflour mixture and reheat slowly, stirring continuously until it comes to the boil. If it begins to thicken too quickly, remove from the heat and stir very fast to mix well.
4 Cook for 3–4 minutes and serve immediately.

Chilli barbecue sauce

SERVES 4
PER SERVING:
48 KCAL/0.2G FAT

1 onion
1 garlic clove
150ml (1/4 pint) tomato juice
2 tablespoons Worcestershire sauce
1 teaspoon medium hot chilli powder or to taste
4 tablespoons white wine vinegar
2 tablespoons clear honey
2 tablespoons soy sauce
1 teaspoon French mustard
salt and freshly ground black pepper

1 Peel the onion and garlic. Finely chop the onion and crush the garlic. Place in a small pan.
2 Add the remaining ingredients and mix well.
3 Bring slowly to the boil and simmer for 15 minutes or until the onions are soft. Add a little water if necessary to prevent the sauce becoming too thick. Taste and check the seasoning and adjust the consistency with more water at the end of the cooking time. Serve hot.

Mustard sauce

A delicious sauce served with gammon or a good base sauce for lasagne or a pasta bake.

SERVES 4
PER SERVING:
59 KCAL/1.2G FAT

300ml ($^1/_2$ pint) skimmed milk
1 vegetable stock cube
2 teaspoons cornflour
1 $^1/_2$ tablespoons Dijon mustard
1 tablespoon chopped fresh parsley (optional)
salt and freshly ground black pepper

1 Heat the milk and stock cube in a non-stick saucepan until stock cube has dissolved.
2 Mix the cornflour with a little water to a paste, add slowly to the milk, stirring well until it comes to the boil. Cook for 2–3 minutes.
3 Stir in the mustard and parsley. Adjust the consistency with a little water if required. Season to taste.

Parsley sauce

SERVES 4
PER SERVING:
56 KCAL/0.2G FAT

300ml ($^1/_2$ pint) skimmed milk
1 onion, sliced
6 peppercorns
1 bay leaf
2 teaspoons cornflour
chopped fresh parsley or dried parsley to taste
salt and freshly ground black pepper

1 Heat all but 50ml (2fl oz) of the milk in a non-stick saucepan, adding the onion, peppercorns, bay leaf and seasoning.
2 Heat gently and cover the pan. Simmer for 5 minutes. Turn off the heat and leave the milk mixture to stand with the lid on for a further 30 minutes or until you are ready to thicken and serve.
3 Mix the remaining milk with the cornflour and when almost ready to serve, strain the milk mixture, add the cornflour mixture and reheat slowly, stirring continuously until it comes to the boil. If it thickens too quickly, remove from the heat and stir very fast to mix well.
4 Add the chopped or dried parsley to taste, cook for 3–4 minutes and serve immediately.

Spicy tomato and basil sauce

SERVES 4
PER SERVING:
16 KCAL/0.06G FAT

50g (2oz) onions, chopped
$^1/_2$ teaspoon chilli powder
1 × 115g (4oz) can plum tomatoes
2 teaspoons tomato purée
1 teaspoon caster sugar
$^1/_4$ teaspoon oregano
1 tablespoon chopped fresh basil
salt and freshly ground black pepper

1. Dry-fry the chopped onions in a non-stick pan, using a little water if necessary to prevent burning.
2. When cooked, stir in the remaining ingredients and bring slowly to the boil, stirring continuously.
3. Simmer uncovered for 10–15 minutes so that the mixture reduces and becomes thicker. Taste for seasoning. This sauce may be frozen and stored for up to 2 months.

Red pepper sauce

SERVES 4
PER SERVING:
76 KCAL/1.9G FAT

3 red peppers
1 large onion, chopped
3 garlic cloves, finely chopped
300ml ($^1/_2$ pint) tomato passata
dash of Tabasco sauce
salt and freshly ground black pepper

This thick pepper sauce is ideal served with fish or meat and accompanies braised vegetables well. It can be thinned down with a little vegetable stock if required.

1. Preheat the oven to 200C, 400F, Gas Mark 6.
2. Prepare the peppers by slicing in half lengthways, remove the seeds and discard.
3. Place the peppers, onion and garlic in a non-stick roasting tin and season well with salt and pepper. Place in the oven for 30 minutes until the vegetables soften.
4. Remove from the oven and spoon into a food processor or liquidiser, add the passata and purée until smooth. Pass through a fine sieve to remove any stray seeds or skin. Reheat as required. Add Tabasco to taste.

Mushroom sauce

SERVES 4
PER SERVING:
63 KCAL/0.6G FAT

300ml ($^1/_2$ pint) skimmed milk
1 onion, peeled and diced
6 peppercorns
1 bay leaf
$^1/_2$ teaspoon dried thyme
$^1/_2$ teaspoon dried marjoram
1 chicken stock cube
2 teaspoons cornflour
115g (4oz) button mushrooms, thinly sliced
salt and freshly ground black pepper

1 Heat all but 50ml (2fl oz) of the milk in a non-stick saucepan, adding the onion, peppercorns, bay leaf and salt and pepper.
2 Heat gently and cover the pan. Simmer for 5 minutes. Turn off the heat and leave the milk mixture to stand with the lid on for a further 30 minutes. Strain the milk through a fine sieve into a jug.
3 Rinse out the saucepan and then return the milk to it. Add the thyme, marjoram and chicken stock cube. Reheat to almost boiling.
4 Mix the cornflour and the remaining milk into a paste and slowly add this to the hot milk mixture.
5 Add the sliced mushrooms and gently heat until boiling, stirring continuously.
6 Continue stirring and cooking for a further 2 minutes. Taste to make sure there is sufficient seasoning and adjust as necessary.

Creole sauce

SERVES 4
PER SERVING:
53 KCAL/0.5G FAT

1 large onion
1–2 garlic cloves or 1 teaspoon garlic paste
1 small green pepper
1 small red pepper
1–2 tablespoons lemon juice
1 teaspoon sugar
250g (10oz) tomato passata or canned tomatoes puréed
1 teaspoon French mustard
150ml ($\frac{1}{4}$ pint) chicken stock if needed
1 tablespoon chopped parsley
salt and freshly ground black pepper

This sauce is good served with barbecued meats and fish.

1 Peel the onion and fresh garlic. Finely chop the onion and crush the garlic.
2 Remove the stalk, core, seeds and pith from the peppers and cut the flesh into small dice.
3 Place the onion, garlic, peppers, 1 tablespoon of lemon juice, sugar and the tomato passata or puréed tomatoes in a pan. Stir in the French mustard and season with salt and pepper.
4 Bring to the boil and simmer gently for 25–30 minutes until the onions and pepper are tender. If the sauce thickens too much during the cooking, add a little chicken stock while it is cooking and adjust the consistency and seasoning when the sauce is cooked.
5 Just before serving, add the parsley.

Bread sauce

1. Slowly bring the milk to the boil and add the chopped onion, cloves and bay leaf. Remove from the heat, cover the pan and leave to one side for 15–20 minutes to allow the flavours to infuse.
2. Remove the cloves and bay leaf, add the breadcrumbs and black pepper. Return to the heat, stir gently until boiling and season with salt and freshly ground black pepper.
3. Remove from the heat and place in a small covered serving dish (a small bowl covered with tin foil would work just as well). Keep warm until ready to serve.

SERVES 6
PER SERVING:
41 KCAL/0.19G FAT

300ml (½ pint) skimmed milk
1 small onion, chopped
3 cloves
1 bay leaf
6–8 tablespoons fresh breadcrumbs
salt and freshly ground black pepper

Brandy sauce

1. Heat all but 4 tablespoons of the milk with the almond essence until almost boiling and remove from the heat.
2. Mix the cornflour and remaining cold milk thoroughly and slowly pour it into the hot milk, stirring continuously until the mixture begins to thicken.
3. Return to the heat and bring to the boil. Continue to cook, stirring continuously. If it is too thin, mix some more cornflour with cold milk and add it slowly until you achieve the consistency of custard. Sweeten to taste.
4. Add the brandy a few drops at a time and stir well. Cover the serving jug and keep warm until ready to serve.

MAKES 600ML (1 PINT)
PER 600ML (1 PINT) OF SAUCE:
386 KCAL/0.8G FAT

600ml (1 pint) skimmed milk
3 drops almond essence
2 tablespoons cornflour
liquid artificial sweetener
3 tablespoons brandy

Minted fromage frais

SERVES 4
PER SERVING:
19 KCAL/0.1G FAT

fine zest and juice of 1 lemon
150ml (1/4 pint) virtually fat free fromage frais
1 tablespoon chopped fresh mint
artificial sweetener to taste

This is delicious served with stewed apple or baked fruit.

1 Using the fine section of your grater, gently grate the outside zest from the lemon, taking care not to remove any of the white pith which may make the sauce bitter.
2 Mix with the remaining ingredients and pour into a sauce boat.

Orange or lemon sauce

SERVES 4
PER SERVING:
72 KCAL/0.1G FAT

300ml (1/2pint) skimmed milk
zest and juice from 2 oranges or 2 lemons
3 teaspoons arrowroot
artificial sweetener to taste
2 teaspoons orange liqueur (optional)

1 In a non-stick saucepan heat the milk with the zest and juice from the 2 oranges or lemons to near boiling.
2 Mix the arrowroot with a little water to form a paste. Slowly stir into the hot milk and continue stirring to form a smooth sauce.
3 Sweeten to taste and add the liqueur if using.
4 Serve hot with pancakes or a baked apple.

Hot chilli sauce

Red chillies are the very hot ones, so do take care when using them. Start with just one chilli and add an extra one if necessary. When preparing them, make sure you do not touch your eyes, mouth or any tender skin with your hands. The seeds are also hot, so remove them if you want a much milder sauce. This is meant to be a thick sauce but you can dilute it with vegetable stock if you wish, although this will dilute the taste of the chillies. The sauce can be deep frozen.

SERVES 6
PER SERVING:
38 KCAL/1.6G FAT

1–2 red chillies
2–3 spring onions or 1 small onion
1–2 tablespoons lemon juice
1 × 200g (7oz) can chopped tomatoes
2 tablespoons tomato purée
salt
1–2 teaspoons caster sugar or artificial sweetener to taste

1. Trim the chillies and remove the seeds if you wish. Chop the chillies finely.
2. Trim the spring onions and slice finely, or peel the onion if using and chop it finely.
3. Heat a non-stick pan, add the onions and some or all of the chopped chillies, according to preference. Cook gently until the onions are just soft but without colour.
4. Add 1 tablespoon of the lemon juice and the remainder of the ingredients. Season to taste with salt, sugar or artificial sweetener and extra lemon juice if required. At this stage you may also wish to add more chopped chilli.
5. Bring to the boil and simmer for 6–7 minutes. Taste again and adjust the seasoning if required.

Honey and orange sauce

SERVES 6
PER SERVING:
75 KCAL/0.5G FAT

1 large onion
1 garlic clove
150ml (1/4 pint) orange juice
2 tablespoons clear honey
3 tablespoons white wine vinegar
4–5 drops (a scant 1/2 teaspoon) Tabasco sauce
2 teaspoons French mustard
1 sprig fresh rosemary
2–3 sprigs fresh thyme or 1/2 teaspoon dried thyme
salt and white pepper

This sauce is particularly good with poultry as well as lamb.

1 Peel the onion and garlic. Finely chop the onion and crush the garlic.
2 Mix all the ingredients together in a small pan and bring to the boil.
3 Simmer gently for 10 minutes or until the onion is tender. Serve hot.

Cranberry and port sauce

SERVES 6
PER SERVING:
33 KCAL/0G FAT

225g (8oz) cranberries
300ml (1/2 pint) cranberry juice drink
2 tablespoons port
artificial sweetener to taste (optional)

1 Place the cranberries in a saucepan. Add the cranberry juice drink. Bring to the boil, then simmer gently for about 5 minutes until soft. Push the mixture through a sieve to pureé it and return to the pan.
2 Stir in the port and heat through. Add a little artificial sweetener if desired.

Christmas the low-fat way

We tend to use this time of year as a celebration of food and festivity with the temptation to cast aside our regular eating pattern. Low-fat eating certainly does not mean we deny ourselves of some great traditional delights.

Making just a few minor adjustments such as reducing the fat content will make the food much lighter, allowing a little scope for that extra treat. Included are recipes for light starters, turkey and duck main courses with accompanying side dishes, wonderful vegetarian options and low-fat desserts suitable for all the family and guests alike.

Christmas would not be complete without a delicious Christmas pudding and a few mince pies for slim Santa and helpers.

Smoked salmon and lime pâté

SERVES 4
PER SERVING:
79 KCAL/1.8G FAT
PREPARATION TIME:
10 MINUTES

150g (5oz) fine sliced smoked salmon
juice of 2 limes
115g (4oz) virtually fat free fromage frais
50g (2oz) Quark (low-fat soft cheese)
1 teaspoon mixed peppercorns, crushed

This is deliciously light and tangy, making an ideal starter or simple lunch. Once refrigerated the pâté will keep for 5 days.

1 Flake the salmon into pieces and place into a food processor. Add the lime juice, fromage frais and Quark. Sprinkle a little pepper over and blend until smooth to form a soft pâté. Taste, adding a little more pepper if required, and blend again to combine.
2 Scrape the mixture out into a serving bowl or individual ramekins and refrigerate for 2 hours.
3 Serve with crusty bread and a few salad leaves as a starter or light lunch.

Seared scallops with carrot and pink ginger pickle

Scallops make an ideal starter, as they are quite fleshy in appearance yet light and delicate in both volume and flavour. Make the carrot salad in advance and store refrigerated until ready to serve.

SERVES 4
PER SERVING:
102 KCAL/1.3G FAT
PREPARATION TIME:
20 MINUTES
SITTING TIME:
30 MINUTES
COOKING TIME:
10 MINUTES

12–16 large fresh scallops
225g (8oz) young carrots, peeled
½ teaspoon coriander seed, crushed
¼ teaspoon pink peppercorns
2 teaspoons Chinese pink ginger, finely sliced
1 tablespoon white wine or fruit vinegar
1 tablespoon chopped fresh coriander
salt and freshly ground black pepper
a little vegetable oil
1 lime, sliced in half

1 Prepare the scallops by cleaning well under a cold running tap to remove any sand or grit. Pull away the small membrane attached to the side, being careful to keep the orange coral intact. Pat dry with kitchen towel and season well with salt and black pepper.
2 Using the coarse side of a grater, grate the carrot into a bowl and add the crushed coriander seed, peppercorns, ginger and vinegar. Season well, mixing the ingredients together. Mix in the fresh coriander and allow to sit for a minimum of 30 minutes.
3 Preheat a non-stick griddle pan with a little vegetable oil, then wipe out, using a good pad of kitchen paper.
4 Add the scallops to the pan and cook quickly for 1 minute on each side.
5 Arrange the carrot salad on a serving plate. Squeeze the lime over the scallops and remove from the heat. Place on top of the carrot, pouring the pan juices over.
6 Serve straight away with crusty bread.

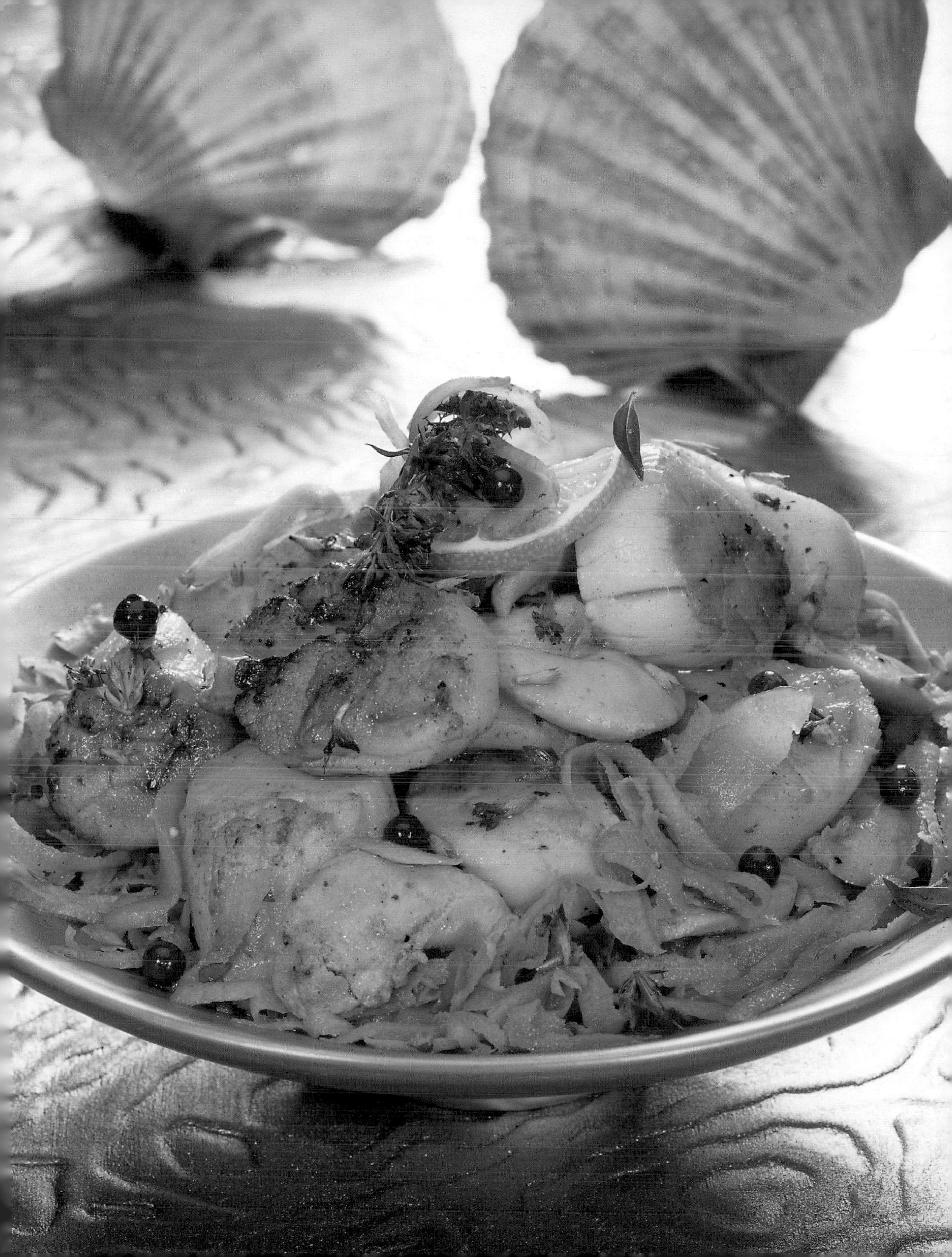

Roast turkey with chestnut stuffing and giblet gravy

SERVES 10
PER SERVING:
APPROXIMATELY
200 KCAL/4G FAT
PREPARATION TIME:
40 MINUTES
COOKING TIME:
$3\frac{1}{2}$ HOURS

1 × 5.4kg (12lb) fresh turkey
1 large onion, diced
3 bay leaves
4–5 sprigs fresh thyme
pinch of sea salt
2–3 teaspoons arrowroot
a few drops gravy browning
freshly ground black pepper

for the stuffing
1 medium onion, finely chopped
1 garlic clove, crushed
115g (4oz) fresh breadcrumbs
1 tablespoon finely chopped fresh thyme
1 tablespoon chopped fresh parsley
300ml ($\frac{1}{2}$ pint) hot chicken stock
115g (4oz) peeled chestnuts, finely chopped
1 teaspoon finely grated lemon zest
black pepper to taste

1. Preheat the oven to 180C, 350F, Gas Mark 5.
2. Calculate the cooking time, allowing 15 minutes per 450g (1lb) plus an extra 20 minutes. Wash the turkey well in cold water and remove the giblets and any excess fat. Place the giblets, onion, bay leaves, and 2 sprigs of thyme in the centre of a large roasting tin and sit the turkey on top, preferably on its side.
3. Place the remaining thyme inside the turkey and season the outside generously with salt and black pepper. Pour 600ml (1 pint) of water around the outside of the turkey to prevent the base from burning, cover with foil and place in the oven.
4. Split the total cooking time into three, turning the bird onto its other side after one third of the cooking time and placing it breast side up for the final third. This will ensure even cooking.
5. While the turkey is cooking make the stuffing. Dry-fry the onion and garlic until the onion is soft. Add the breadcrumbs and herbs with a little black pepper. Mix in the stock, chestnuts and lemon and allow to stand for 10 minutes. Mould into golf ball-sized shapes and place on a non-stick baking tray.
6. Bake the stuffing in the oven for 20–25 minutes until brown and crisp.
7. Once the turkey is cooked, remove from the roasting tin and place on a serving dish. Keep it covered with foil and allow 30 minutes standing time for easier carving.
8. Drain the contents of the roasting tin into a saucepan. Remove the giblets and bay leaves and discard.
9. Use a ladle to skim off any fat from the top of the pan. Bring to the boil, adding more liquid if required, either chicken stock or water.
10. Slake the arrowroot with a little water and gradually stir into the gravy. Add a few drops of gravy browning if desired to colour the gravy. Adjust the consistency with more liquid or arrowroot.
11. Carve the turkey and serve with the chestnut stuffing, a selection of vegetables and the giblet gravy.

Turkey pilaff

SERVES 4
PER SERVING:
355 KCAL/3.4G FAT
PREPARATION TIME:
15 MINUTES
COOKING TIME:
30 MINUTES

1 medium onion, finely chopped
2 garlic cloves, crushed
275g (10oz) [dry weight] basmati rice
750ml (1 ¼ pints) chicken stock
225g (8oz) cooked turkey
115g (4oz) chestnut mushrooms, sliced
4–5 sage leaves, finely chopped
3 bay leaves
salt and freshly ground black pepper
1 tablespoon finely chopped flat leaf parsley

Probably the simplest way of cooking rice and a great way to use up leftover turkey. For a vegetarian variation substitute the turkey with a few sundried tomatoes or canned artichoke hearts.

1 Preheat the oven to 190C, 375F, Gas Mark 5.
2 In a non-stick pan dry-fry the onion and garlic until soft. Add the rice and stock. Stir in the turkey, mushrooms, sage and bay leaves and season well with plenty of freshly ground black pepper.
3 Transfer to an ovenproof dish or casserole. Cover and place in the bottom of the oven for 25–30 minutes until the rice has absorbed all the stock.
4 Remove from the oven and serve sprinkled with chopped fresh parsley.

Braised duck with tangerine and cinnamon

This delicious duck recipe is perfect for Christmas entertaining, as all the preparation is done the day before. As it cooks it creates its own rich sauce full of aromatic flavours.

SERVES 4
PER SERVING:
282 KCAL/11.4G FAT
PREPARATION TIME:
40 MINUTES
MARINATING TIME:
OVERNIGHT
COOKING TIME:
2 HOURS

1 × 2kg (4lb) duck
4 tangerines
300ml (1/2 pint) fresh apple juice
2 garlic cloves, crushed
2 cinnamon sticks
1 tablespoon fresh thyme
1 tablespoon Teriyaki sauce
150ml (1/4 pint) chicken stock
2 tablespoons tomato purée
sea salt and freshly ground black pepper

1. Prepare the duck by dividing into 4 portions. Using a sharp knife or heavy duty scissors, cut through the breastbone along the length of the bird then the backbone. Cut each piece in half again, cutting at an angle just under where the leg joint meets the carcass. Trim away the backbone and remove all of the skin, then place the duck in a large bowl.
2. Cut the tangerines in half and squeeze the juice over, adding the shells to the bowl. Season the duck well with sea salt and black pepper. Mix together the remaining ingredients and pour over the meat. Combine well, cover and refrigerate overnight.
3. Preheat the oven to 170C, 325F, Gas Mark 3.
4. Place the duck in a large casserole dish or non-stick pan, cover with foil and cook in the middle of the oven for 1 1/2–2 hours until tender.
5. Remove from the oven and place the duck pieces on a serving plate. Pour the juices into a saucepan and adjust the consistency by adding a little more stock, or thicken by using 1 teaspoon of cornflour diluted with water.
6. Pour the sauce over the duck and serve garnished with the cooked tangerine shells.

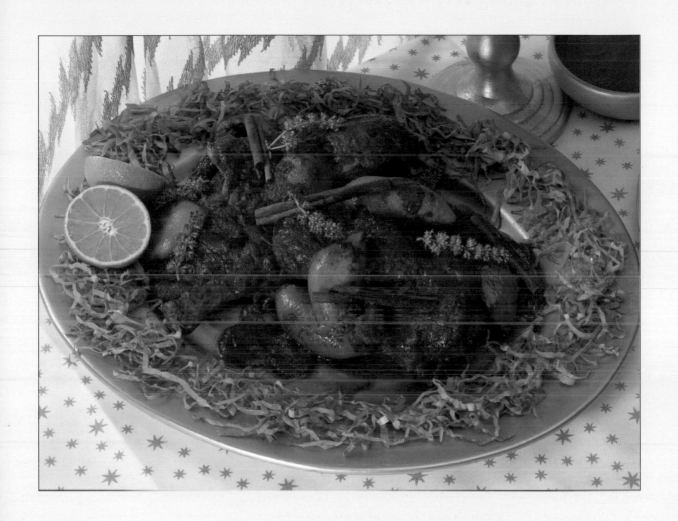

Marmalade basted gammon

A truly delicious way to prepare and serve Christmas ham. Star anise, its name deriving from its star-like shape, is popular in Asian cookery adding a sweet aniseed flavour throughout the dish. Use in moderation, as it can be bitter if used in excess.

SERVES 8
PER SERVING:
420 KCAL/12G FAT
PREPARATION TIME:
20 MINUTES
COOKING TIME:
1 HOUR 35 MINUTES

2kg (4¾lb) piece lean boiling bacon or gammon
3 oranges, sliced
2 star anise
6 whole cloves
2 cinnamon sticks
4 bay leaves
3 tablespoons Traditional thick-cut orange marmalade
2 teaspoons demerara sugar
1 orange to garnish
12 whole cloves to garnish

1 Preheat the oven to 180C, 350F, Gas Mark 5.
2 Prepare the gammon by removing all the outer skin and fat with a sharp knife. Place in a large saucepan and cover with cold water.
3 Add the orange slices, anise, cloves, cinnamon and bay. Bring the pan to the boil, cover and simmer gently for 1 hour.
4 Transfer the gammon to an ovenproof dish, pouring some of the stock around to prevent it from sticking to the bottom of the dish. Coat the meat with the marmalade and bake in the oven, uncovered, for 20–25 minutes until golden brown. Sprinkle with sugar and return to the oven for 5–10 minutes until caramelised.
5 Allow to cool, then garnish with orange slices and whole cloves. Serve sliced cold with fruit chutney.

Lentil loaf with chestnut and herb stuffing

SERVES 6
PER SERVING:
256 KCAL/6.4G FAT
PREPARATION TIME:
45 MINUTES
COOKING TIME:
40 MINUTES

225g (8oz) green lentils
1 vegetable stock cube
1 teaspoon sunflower oil
1 large onion, chopped
2 carrots, finely diced
115g (4oz) mushrooms, finely chopped
25g (1oz) chopped mixed nuts
75g (3oz) fresh white breadcrumbs
2 tablespoons chopped fresh parsley
2 tablespoons soy sauce
2 eggs, beaten
50g (2oz) herb stuffing mix
115g (4oz) canned chestnuts (drained weight)

This delicious vegetarian loaf can be served in place of the traditional turkey at the Christmas table.

1 Preheat the oven to 190C, 375F, Gas Mark 5.
2 Place the lentils in a large saucepan and cover with plenty of cold water. Add the stock cube and bring slowly to the boil, then boil rapidly for 10 minutes. Reduce the heat and simmer for 20–25 minutes until the lentils are tender. Drain.
3 Heat the oil in a large frying pan and fry the onion and carrots gently for 10 minutes until softened.
4 Add the mushrooms and cook for a further 3–4 minutes. Transfer to a large bowl and add the lentils, mixed nuts, breadcrumbs, parsley and soy sauce. Mix well. Add the beaten egg and mix again.
5 Very lightly grease the sides of a 1kg (2lb) loaf tin and line the base with baking parchment. Pile half the lentil mixture into the tin and press down well.
6 Mix the stuffing mix with 150ml (¼ pint) cold water and allow to stand for a few moments. Chop the chestnuts and add to the stuffing.
7 Spoon a layer of stuffing on top of the lentil mixture in the tin. Cover with the remaining lentils and press down well. Cover with foil and bake in the oven for 40 minutes.
8 Allow to cool in the tin for 5 minutes before turning out onto a serving dish. Serve with cranberry sauce.

Roasted pepper and leek strudel

A great vegetarian dish packed full of flavour. It can be frozen cooked or uncooked. Vary the filling by using different combinations of cooked or roasted vegetables and serve with a simple spicy tomato sauce.

SERVES 4
PER SERVING:
239 KCAL/7.3G FAT
PREPARATION TIME:
40 MINUTES
COOKING TIME:
20 MINUTES

4 red peppers
4 baby leeks, sliced
a few sprigs fresh thyme
2 garlic cloves, sliced
handful of fresh basil leaves
1 teaspoon vegetable bouillon stock powder
2 tablespoons tomato passata
6 sheets filo pastry (30 × 20cm/12 × 8in)
1 egg, beaten

for the sauce
300ml ($^1/_2$ pint) tomato passata
1 teaspoon ground cumin
1 teaspoon ground coriander
1 tablespoon chopped fresh coriander
1–2 teaspoons vegetable bouillon stock powder
salt and freshly ground black pepper

1 Preheat the oven to 200C, 400F, Gas Mark 6.
2 Cut the peppers in half, remove the seeds, and place face down in a non-stick baking tin. Roast in the top of the oven for 20–30 minutes until soft. Remove from the oven and place inside a plastic food bag. Seal the bag and leave to cool.
3 Preheat a non-stick frying pan and dry-fry the leeks with the thyme and garlic until soft, remove from the heat and stir in the basil, stock and passata.
4 Peel the cooled peppers, roughly chop and add to the leeks.
5 Separate the filo pastry sheets. Place one onto a non-stick baking tray and brush with the beaten egg. Continue adding the remaining sheets, brushing each layer with egg.
6 Spread the leek and pepper filling over the pastry, leaving a 2.5cm (1in) border around the edge. Fold in the 2 short sides and roll up like a Swiss roll. Brush the top with egg and bake in the oven for 8–10 minutes, until crisp and golden.
7 Make the sauce by heating all the ingredients in a small saucepan. Season with salt and pepper and serve piping hot.

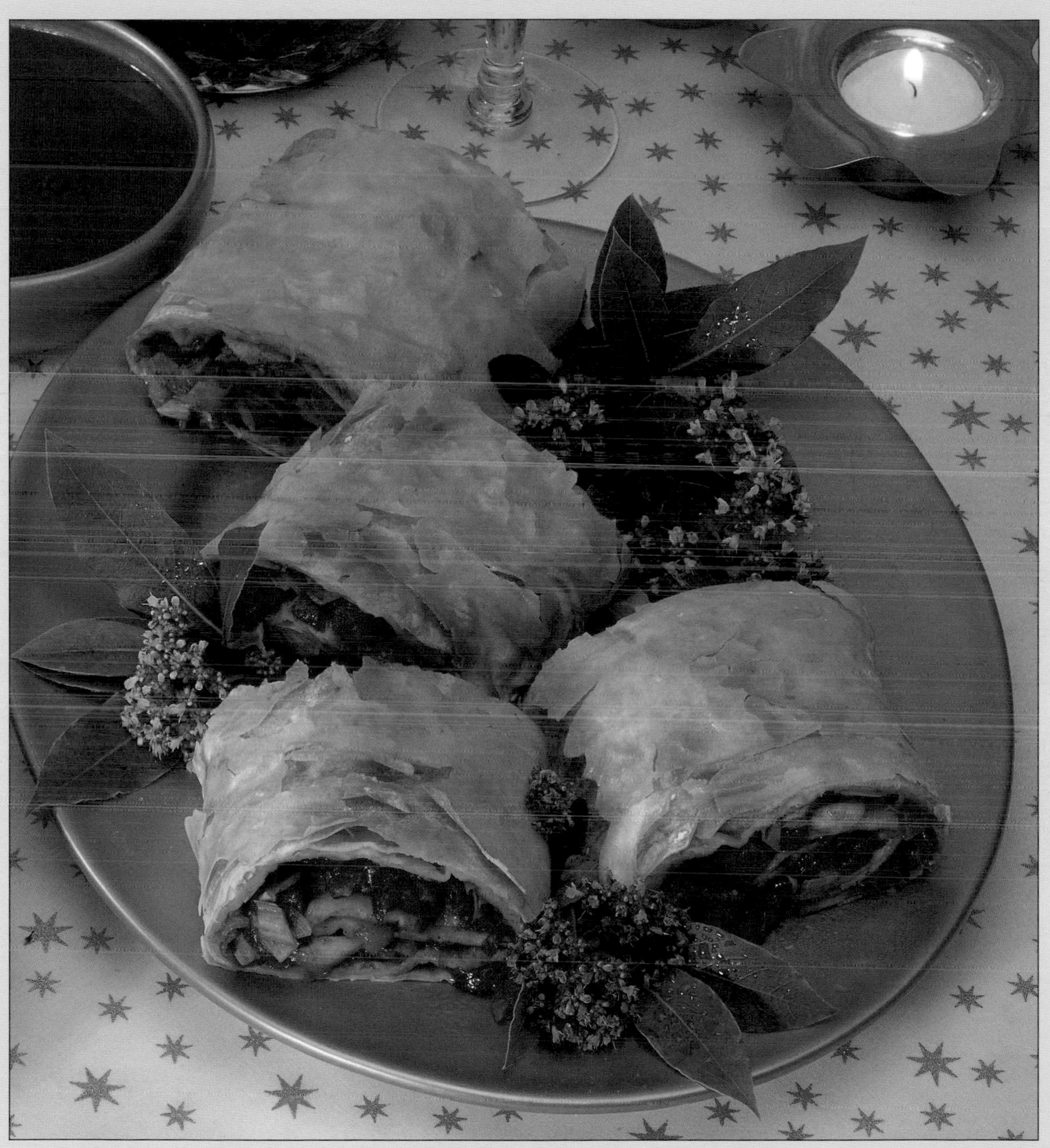

Caramelised onion bread sauce

Caramelising the onions adds a sweet concentrated flavour to this traditional sauce. The cloves add a little spice, but if you prefer, substitute with a little grated nutmeg.

SERVES 10
PER SERVING:
118 KCAL/0.7G FAT
PREPARATION TIME:
10 MINUTES
COOKING TIME:
30 MINUTES

- 4 medium onions, finely chopped
- 2 garlic cloves, crushed
- 300ml (½ pint) semi-skimmed milk
- 6–8 tablespoons fresh breadcrumbs
- 2 bay leaves
- 3 whole cloves
- 2 teaspoons vegetable bouillon stock powder
- salt and freshly ground black pepper

1. In a non-stick frying pan, dry-fry the onions and garlic for 10–12 minutes until they start to colour and caramelise. Add the milk and remaining ingredients, stirring well to combine. Bring the sauce up to a gentle simmer and cook for 10 minutes to allow the flavours to develop.
2. Season well with salt and black pepper. Remove the cloves and bay leaves and pour the sauce into a serving dish.

Cranberry and orange relish

SERVES 10
PER SERVING:
66 KCAL/0.03G FAT
PREPARATION TIME:
10 MINUTES
COOKING TIME:
20 MINUTES

225g (8oz) fresh cranberries
115g (4oz) golden caster sugar
zest and juice of 2 oranges
½ teaspoon ground cinnamon
1 tablespoon ginger preserve
salt and freshly ground black pepper

A very useful relish to serve alongside hot or cold meats. Refrigerated it will keep for up to 2 weeks.

1 Place the cranberries and sugar in a saucepan with 150ml (¼ pint) water. Add the orange zest and juice, cinnamon and ginger preserve. Bring to the boil, reduce the heat and simmer gently for 15–20 minutes until the cranberries have split and the relish has reduced to a thick paste.

2 Season to taste with salt and black pepper, then allow to cool. Refrigerate until ready to use.

Brussels sprouts with pancetta and chestnuts

Adding a few extras to vegetables transforms them, providing texture and a contrast of flavours. For a vegetarian option substitute the pancetta with veggie bacon slices and cook in the same way.

SERVES 4
PER SERVING:
124 KCAL/7.3G FAT
PREPARATION TIME:
20 MINUTES
COOKING TIME:
20 MINUTES

450g (1lb) Brussels sprouts
1 tablespoon vegetable stock bouillon or 1 stock cube
4 slices pancetta or smoked streaky bacon, finely chopped
115g (4oz) peeled and cooked chestnuts, chopped
grated fresh nutmeg
salt and freshly ground black pepper

1. Remove the loose outer leaves from the sprouts and make a small nick in the stalks. Cook in boiling water with the stock until just tender.
2. Meanwhile preheat a non-stick pan. Add the pancetta and cook quickly until it starts to crisp. Add the chestnuts and Brussels sprouts to the pan and continue cooking, mixing well.
3. Season well with salt, pepper and grated fresh nutmeg. Pile into a warm serving dish and serve.

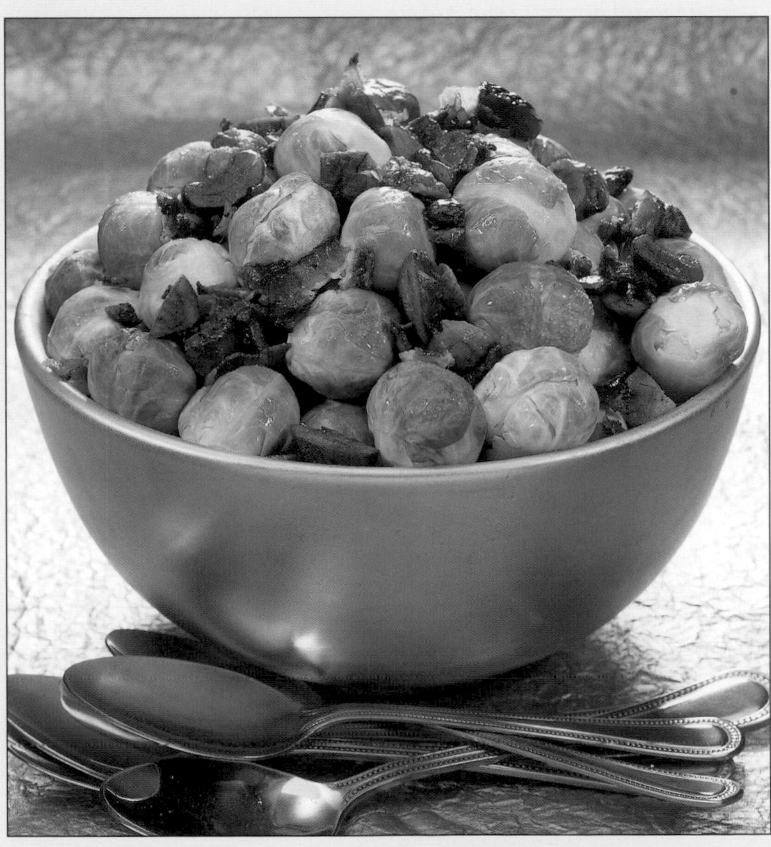

Roasted sweet potatoes with chilli glaze

SERVES 4
PER SERVING:
124 KCAL/0.5G FAT
PREPARATION TIME:
20 MINUTES
COOKING TIME:
55 MINUTES

450g (1lb) sweet potatoes
1 medium red onion, finely diced
2 tablespoons light soy sauce
1 teaspoon sea salt
1 red bullet chilli, seeded and finely chopped
1 garlic clove, crushed
2 tablespoons apple sauce
1 tablespoon chopped fresh parsley

Sweet potatoes make a good change from the regular, more common type. Naturally sweet, they complement strong meats such as duck or game. Delicious mashed with a little yogurt or fromage frais.

1 Preheat the oven to 200C, 400F, Gas Mark 6.
2 Wash, peel then rewash the potatoes and cut into 2.5cm (1in) pieces.
3 Boil in a pan of water for 5 minutes, then drain well. Place in the bottom of a non-stick baking tin with the red onion. Drizzle the soy sauce over and sprinkle with salt. Bake in the preheated oven for 20–25 minutes.
4 Remove from the oven. Combine the chilli, garlic and apple sauce and dot over the potatoes. Shake the pan well to coat, then return to the oven for 5 minutes. Sprinkle with parsley before serving.

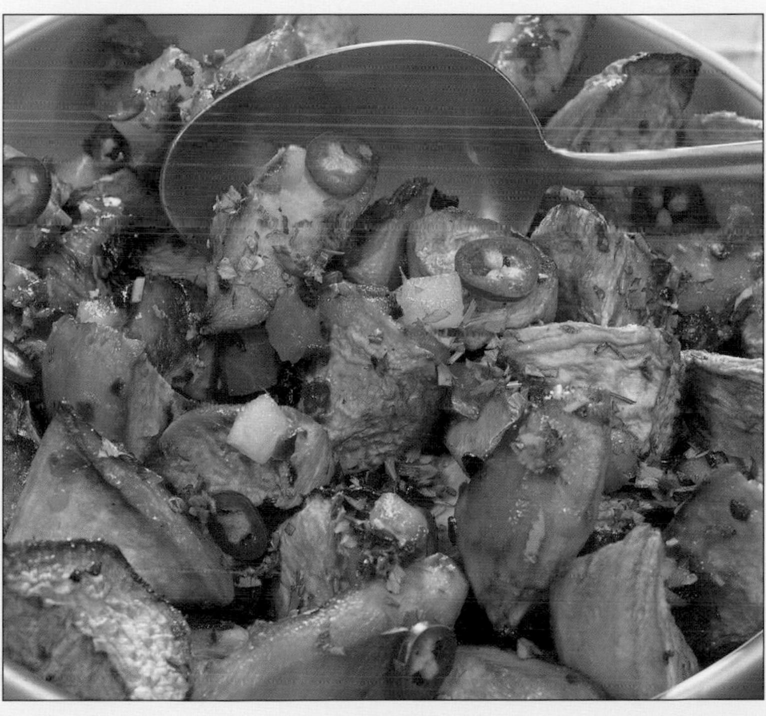

Creamed butternut squash

Butternut squash and carrot mashed together make a wonderful contrast of colours. This dish can be made in advance and reheated in the bottom of a moderate oven. Allow approximately 30 minutes.

SERVES 4
PER SERVING:
120 KCAL/0.7G FAT
PREPARATION TIME:
15 MINUTES
COOKING TIME:
20 MINUTES

1 large butternut squash or 2 small
225g (8oz) carrots, chopped
1 vegetable stock cube
2–3 sprigs fresh mint
2 tablespoons virtually fat free fromage frais
sea salt
freshly ground black pepper

1 Prepare the butternut squash by cutting in half with a large chopping knife. Scoop out the centre seeds and carefully peel away the outside skin. Chop the squash into bite-size pieces and place in a saucepan with the carrots. Cover with water.
2 Add the vegetable stock cube and mint and bring to the boil. Simmer gently for 15–20 minutes until the vegetables are tender.
3 Drain the vegetables well and return to the saucepan. Using a potato masher, mash until smooth. Stir in the fromage frais and season well with sea salt and black pepper. Pile into a serving dish and serve.

Braised spicy red cabbage

SERVES 8
PER SERVING:
62 KCAL/0.4G FAT
PREPARATION TIME:
20 MINUTES
COOKING TIME:
1 ½ HOURS

1 medium red cabbage
1 red onion, finely sliced
2 cooking apples, grated
5 juniper berries, crushed
pinch of red chilli flakes
75g (3oz) soft brown sugar
300ml (½ pint) red wine vinegar
150ml (¼ pint) vegetable stock
salt and freshly ground black pepper

This flavoursome side dish can be made in advance and reheated in a low oven. It is especially good served cold alongside meats, fish and other buffet foods.

1 Preheat the oven to 150C, 300F, Gas Mark 2.
2 Cut the cabbage into quarters lengthways and remove the stalk. Finely shred the cabbage and place in a large mixing bowl.
3 Add the onion, apples, juniper and chilli, mixing all the ingredients together thoroughly and seasoning well with salt and black pepper.
4 Pile the mixture into a large ovenproof dish and sprinkle with brown sugar. Pour the vinegar and stock over and cover with greaseproof paper.
5 Bake in the bottom of the oven for 1–1 ½ hours until soft.
6 Serve hot or cold as a vegetable accompaniment

Banoffi whip

Treat yourself to a delicious creamy dessert that combines toffee custard and bananas. Don't make it too far in advance, as it may separate when stood for a while.

SERVES 4
PER SERVING:
169 KCAL/0.8G FAT
PREPARATION TIME:
20 MINUTES
COOKING TIME:
15 MINUTES

2 bananas
1 tablespoon Muscovado sugar
1 tablespoon custard powder
250ml (8fl oz) skimmed milk
1 tablespoon rum (optional)
300g (11oz) low-fat Greek yogurt
2 egg whites
cocoa powder to dust

1 Using a fork, mash the bananas in a small bowl.
2 In a separate bowl mix together the sugar and custard powder with a little cold milk to form a smooth paste.
3 Heat the remaining milk in a saucepan with the rum, if using, until boiling, pour onto the custard powder and whisk well. Return to the pan and cook until the mixture starts to thicken. Remove from the heat, cover with food wrap and allow to cool.
4 Once cold, beat the yogurt into the custard mixture and sweeten to taste with a little sugar. Whisk the egg whites to stiff peaks and gently fold into the mixture. Spoon into individual glasses or 1 large bowl, dust with a little cocoa powder and decorate with fresh fruit.

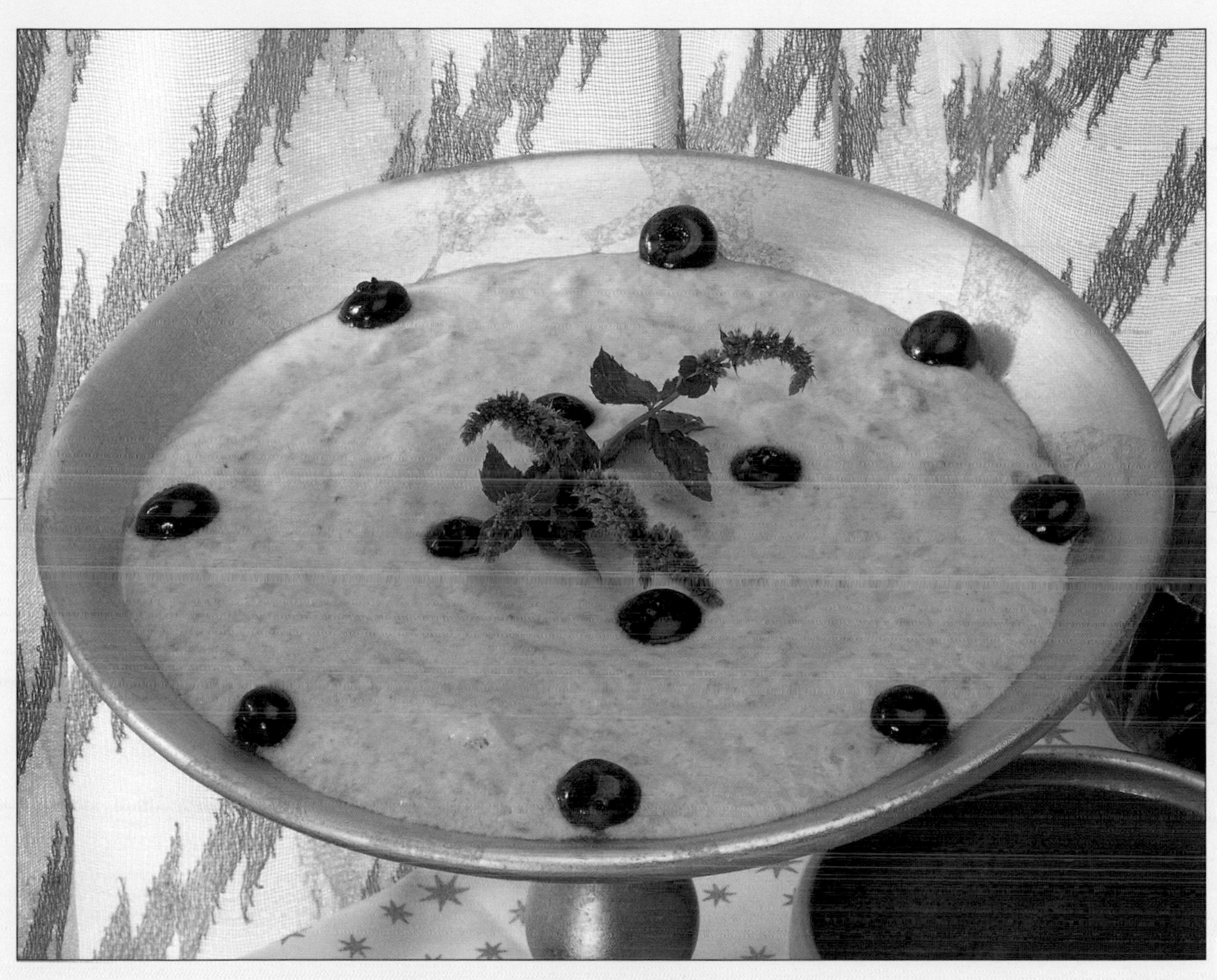

Fresh fruit flan

For a chocolate-flavoured base, substitute 25g (1oz) of flour with cocoa powder and add $^1/_2$ teaspoon of baking powder. Choose fruits that will complement such as fresh orange or pears.

SERVES 6
PER SERVING:
146 KCAL/2.5G FAT
PREPARATION TIME:
20 MINUTES
COOKING TIME:
1 HOUR

- 2 eggs
- 75g (3oz) golden caster sugar
- 75g (3oz) self-raising flour, sifted
- 1 teaspoon vanilla essence
- selection of fresh soft fruit approximately 225g (8oz) in weight, e.g. peaches, raspberries, apricots, kiwi
- 3 tablespoons Total 0% fat Greek yogurt
- apricot jam to glaze

1. Preheat the oven to 180C, 350F, Gas Mark 4. Grease a 20cm (8in) non-stick flan case with a little vegetable oil then dust with caster sugar.
2. To make the sponge base, whisk together the eggs and sugar for several minutes until thick and pale in consistency. Using a metal spoon, fold in the sifted flour and then the vanilla. Pour into the prepared tin and level off with a knife. Bake in the oven for 20 minutes until golden brown.
3. Allow the sponge to cool, then using a serrated knife cut away a 1cm ($^1/_2$in) layer of sponge from the centre of the flan case. Using a metal spoon, scrape away the crumbs to leave a smooth surface.
4. Chop half the fruit into small dice and combine with the yogurt in a small bowl. Spoon the mixture into the centre of the sponge case and level, using a knife. Slice the remaining fruit and arrange on the top.
5. Heat the apricot jam in a small saucepan until liquid, then brush lightly over the fruit to glaze. Refrigerate until ready to serve.
6. Serve cold with virtually fat free fromage frais or 0% fat Greek yogurt.

Compote of spiced fruits

SERVES 4
PER SERVING:
143 KCAL/0.3G FAT
PREPARATION TIME:
10 MINUTES
COOKING TIME:
15 MINUTES

225g (8oz) fresh dark plums
225g (8oz) fresh peaches
115g (4oz) soft dark sugar
150ml (1/4 pint) cider vinegar
2 teaspoons coriander seeds
1/2 teaspoon allspice
zest and juice of 1 lemon
pinch of sea salt

Spiced fruits make an ideal accompaniment to cereals at breakfast or can be served warm as a dessert.

1 Cut the plums and peaches in half and remove the centre stones.
2 In a large saucepan dissolve the sugar in the cider vinegar over a low heat. Add the spices, lemon zest and juice and salt.
3 Add the fruits to the pan, cover and simmer gently for 15 minutes. Remove from the heat and allow to cool, still covered. Pour into a container and refrigerate until ready to use.
4 Serve cold or warmed with low-fat yogurt or low fat fromage frais.

Christmas pudding soufflés

This is a much lighter version of this traditional celebratory pudding. Make sure the egg whites are whisked in a scrupulously clean bowl in order to achieve the maximum amount of volume.

SERVES 4
PER SERVING:
260 KCAL/0.2G FAT
PREPARATION TIME:
20 MINUTES
COOKING TIME:
10 MINUTES

a little margarine
caster sugar to dust
1 small eating apple, cored, peeled and grated
50g (2oz) dried mixed fruit
25g (1oz) black cherries, pitted
¼ teaspoon ground mixed spice
½ teaspoon grated orange zest
300ml (½ pint) fresh apple juice
1 tablespoon brandy

for the meringue
3 egg whites
175g (6oz) caster sugar
fresh fruit to decorate

1 Preheat the oven to 200C, 400F, Gas Mark 6.
2 Lightly grease 4 small ramekins with a little margarine, then dust lightly with caster sugar and set aside.
3 Place the fruit and other ingredients, except the brandy, in a small saucepan and simmer gently for 10–15 minutes until the fruit has reduced to a thick paste. Pour into a bowl, stir in the brandy and allow to cool.
4 In a clean bowl whisk the egg whites on full speed, adding only a pinch of sugar initially. Once the whites start to peak, gradually add the remaining sugar 1 dessertspoon at a time, allowing 10 seconds between each addition.
5 Place a teaspoon of fruit into the bottom of each ramekin, then gently fold the egg whites into the remaining fruit mixture. Pile into the ramekins, smoothing the top and sides with a palette knife. The mixture should stand about 5cm (2in) above the dishes.
6 Bake in the preheated oven for 5–6 minutes.
7 Serve immediately, as they will start to collapse as soon as they come out of the oven.

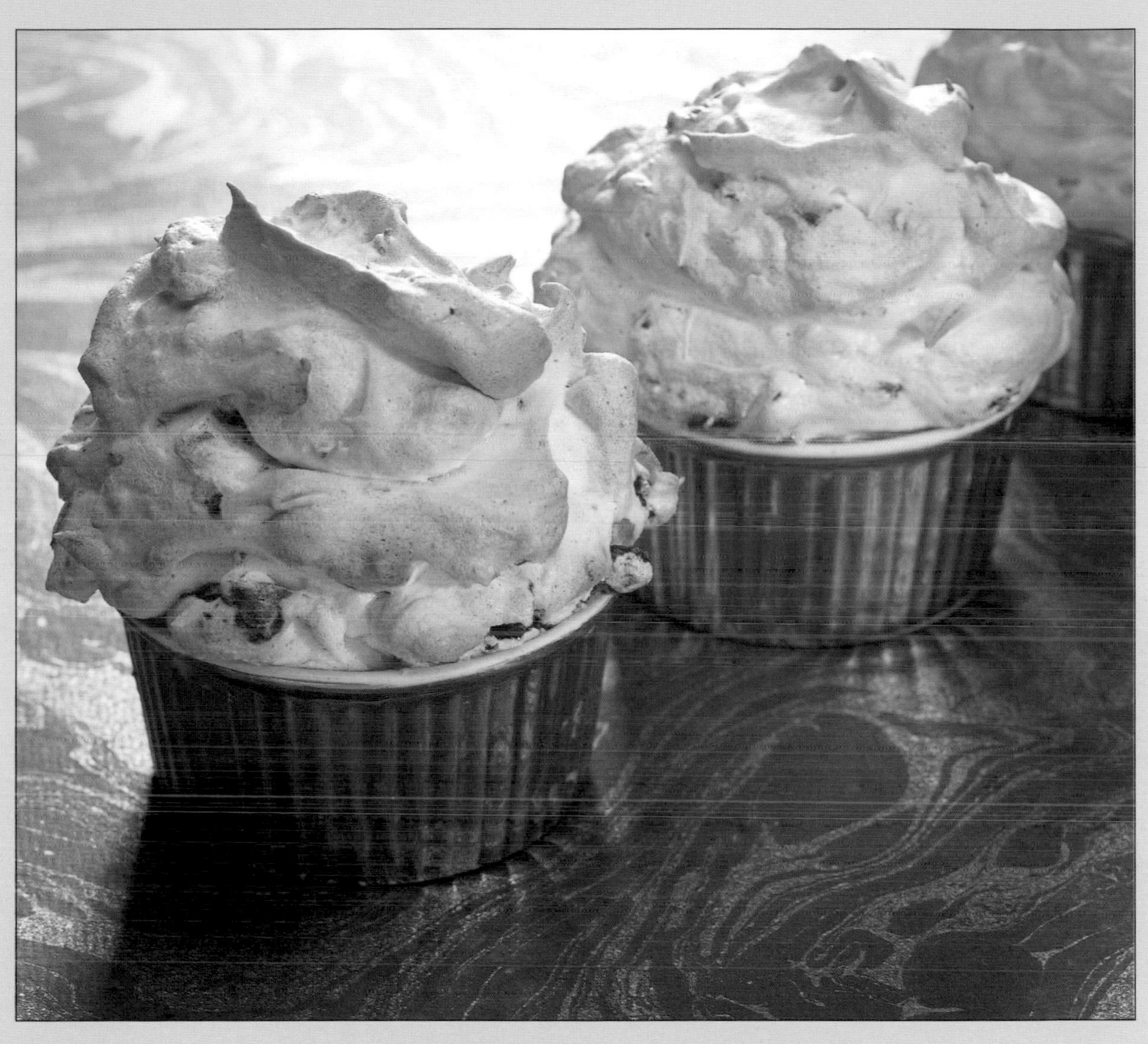

Spicy fat-free mincemeat

MAKES 1.5KG (3LB)
PER 1.5KG (3LB):
775 KCAL/1.1G FAT
PREPARATION TIME:
5 MINUTES
COOKING TIME:
20 MINUTES

225g (8oz) mixed dried fruit
150g (5oz) cooking apples, peeled and grated
$^{1}/_{2}$ teaspoon mixed spice
150ml ($^{1}/_{4}$ pint) sweet cider
2 teaspoons rum

1 Place the dried fruit in a saucepan. Add the grated apple, mixed spice and cider.
2 Simmer for 20 minutes or until the mixture has formed a pulp and most of the liquid has evaporated.
3 Stir in the rum. Pack in sterilised jars and store in the refrigerator until required.

Raspberry layer dessert

SERVES 4
PER SERVING:
240 KCAL/3G FAT
PREPARATION TIME :
20 MINUTES
COOKING TIME:
15 MINUTES

225g (8oz) low-fat sponge fingers
225g (8oz) fresh or frozen raspberries
2 egg whites
300ml ($1/2$ pint) Total 0% fat Greek yogurt
2 tablespoons icing sugar
2 tablespoons dry sherry
sprig of mint to decorate

A delicious refreshing dessert that is so simple to prepare. Try adding a little fruit liqueur in place of the sherry for a more luxurious flavour.

1 Place the sponge fingers in a food processor and reduce to fine crumbs or place in a plastic food bag and crush with a rolling pin.
2 Gently heat the raspberries, reserving a few for decoration, in a small saucepan over a low heat for 2–3 minutes until soft.
3 Whisk the egg whites until stiff then gradually fold in the yogurt and icing sugar.
4 Assemble the dessert in a glass dish in layers, first with the sponge finger crumbs sprinkled with sherry, then the raspberries and finally the yogurt mixture. Repeat, dusting the top with crumbs then place in the refrigerator until ready to serve.
5 Decorate with the reserved raspberries and a sprig of mint and serve chilled.

Filo pastry mince pies

MAKES 6 MINCE PIES
PER MINCE PIE:
144 KCAL/1.5G FAT
PREPARATION TIME:
20 MINUTES
COOKING TIME:
10 MINUTES

6 sheets filo pastry (12in × 8in/30cm × 20 cm)
1 egg white, beaten
3 tablespoons spicy fat-free mincemeat (see recipe, page 260)
icing sugar to dust (optional)

1 Preheat the oven to 190C, 375F, Gas Mark 5.
2 Stack the filo pastry sheets on top of each other on the work surface. Using scissors, cut the stack into 6 square-shaped sections, so that you end up with 36 individual squares.
3 Take 6 non-stick patty tins. In each patty tin, place 4 individual pastry squares at slight angles to each other, brushing with beaten egg white in between each layer. Place a half tablespoonful of mincemeat in the centre of each pastry case.
4 Brush the remaining 12 pastry squares with egg white and scrunch them up to make crinkly toppings for the pies. Place 2 scrunched-up squares on top of each portion of mincemeat.
5 Bake in the oven for 10 minutes until the pastry is crisp and golden.
6 Just before serving, dust with a little icing sugar, if using.

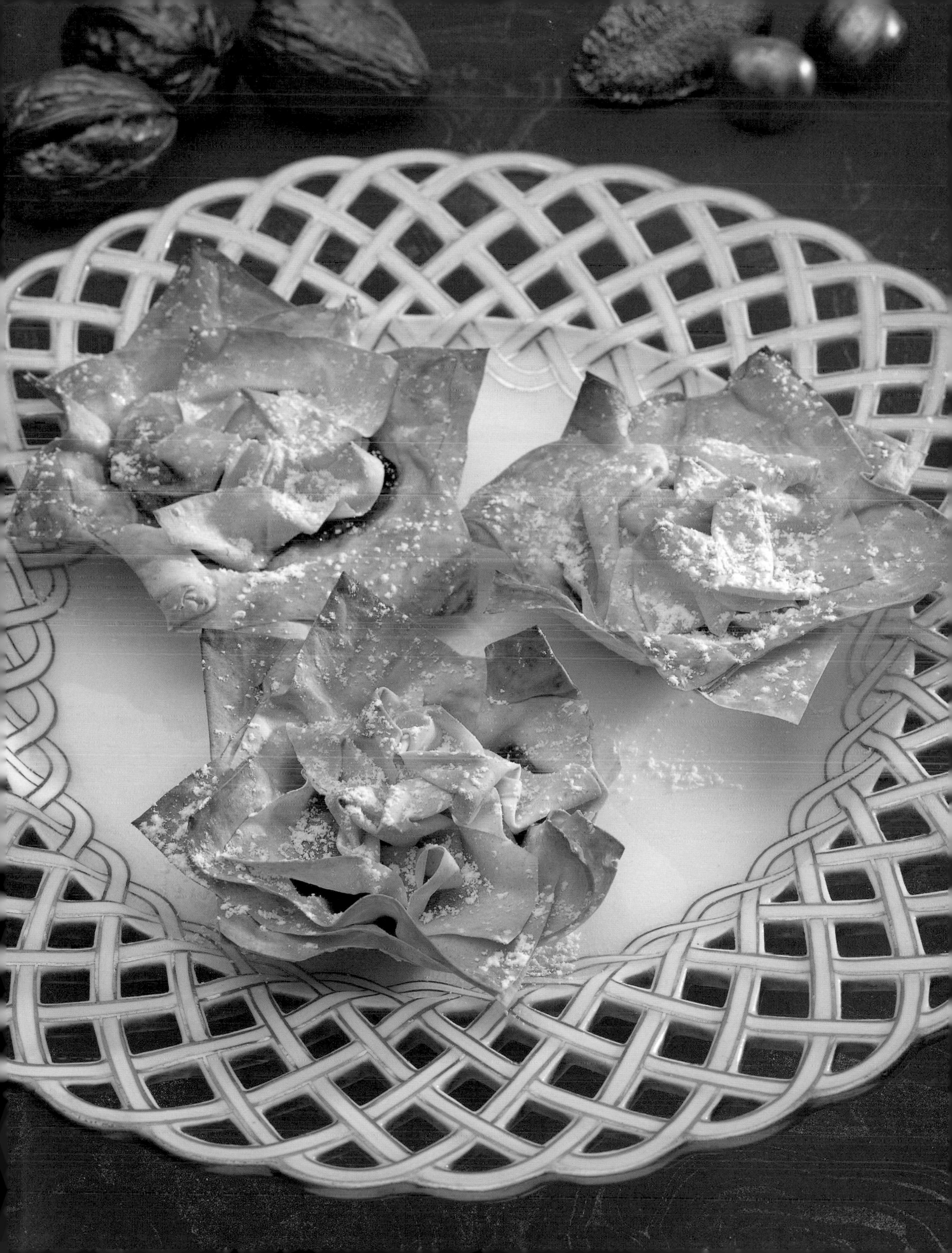

Tropical trifle

An alternative fruity dessert that makes use of unusual flavoursome fruits.

SERVES 4
PER SERVING:
290 KCAL/0.5G FAT
PREPARATION TIME:
10 MINUTES
COOKING TIME:
10 MINUTES

1 packet sugar-free jelly
2 sherry glasses sweet sherry
1 small mango, diced
1 small pineapple, cut into small pieces
4 passion fruit
1 × 425g (15oz) carton low-fat custard
1 vanilla pod
300g (10oz) virtually fat free fromage frais

1 Make up the jelly according to the packet instructions, substituting 120ml (4fl oz) of the water with 2 glasses of sweet sherry.
2 Arrange the mango and pineapple in the bottom of a glass bowl. Cut 3 of the passion fruit in half and scoop out the seeds into the bowl. Pour the jelly over and refrigerate until set, preferably overnight.
3 When set, cover with the low-fat custard.
4 Place the vanilla pod onto a chopping board. Using the point of a sharp knife, split the pod down the centre lengthways. Run the blade of the knife along the pod, scraping out the vanilla seeds.
5 Add the seeds to the fromage frais and mix well. Spoon the fromage frais over the top of the custard and smooth with a knife. Decorate with seeds from the remaining passion fruit.

Low-fat Christmas cake

MAKES APPROXIMATELY 20 SLICES
PER SLICE: 228 KCAL/2.8G FAT
PREPARATION TIME: 30 MINUTES
COOKING TIME: 2–2½ HOURS

225g (8oz) no pre-soak prunes, pitted
115g (4oz) cooking apple, grated
175g (6oz) dark Muscovado sugar
4 eggs, beaten,
zest of 1 lemon
zest of 1 orange
175g (6oz) self-raising flour, sifted
1 tablespoon mixed spice
50g (2oz) sunflower seeds
225g (8oz) currants
225g (8oz) sultanas
225g (8oz) raisins
115g (4oz) glacé cherries
120ml (4fl oz) brandy
2 tablespoons sieved apricot jam to glaze
12 glacé cherries to decorate

Cakes made without butter or margarine have a very different texture, probably best described as slightly chewy. They do, however, taste less greasy and more fruity. This cake benefits from being made at least one week in advance.

1 Preheat the oven to 170C, 325F, Gas Mark 3. Lightly grease and line a 20cm (8in), 7.5cm (3in) deep round tin with greaseproof paper.
2 In a large mixing bowl mash together the prunes and apple until smooth. Add the sugar then beat in the eggs a little at a time.
3 Mix in the zests, then carefully fold in the flour, mixed spice, sunflower seeds and dried fruit.
4 Gradually stir in the brandy and pour into the prepared tin. Arrange the cherries on the top and bake in the oven for 2–2½ hours or until a metal skewer comes out clean once inserted in to the centre of the cake.
5 Allow to cool on a wire rack, then glaze by brushing with warmed apricot jam. Decorate with the glacé cherries.
6 Once cool, store in an airtight container.

Low-fat Christmas pudding

This is an old faithful recipe that tastes even better than the full-fat traditional pudding. No one will guess this is low fat – not even the greatest sceptic! You can deep-freeze the pudding, but do take care to thaw it thoroughly before reheating.

SERVES 10
PER SERVING:
280 KCAL/2.5G FAT
SOAKING TIME:
12 HOURS
PREPARATION TIME:
20 MINUTES
COOKING TIME:
MICROWAVING: 15–20 MINUTES
STEAMING: 5 HOURS

75g (3oz) currants
75g (3oz) sultanas
115g (4oz) raisins
4 tablespoons brandy, rum or beer
75g (3oz) glacé cherries, halved
75g (3oz) plain or self-raising flour
1 teaspoon mixed spice
½ teaspoon ground cinnamon
50g (2oz) fresh breadcrumbs
50g (2oz) Muscovado or caster sugar
2 teaspoons gravy browning
grated zest of ½ lemon
grated zest of ½ orange
115g (4oz) grated apple
115g (4oz) finely grated carrot
1 tablespoon lemon juice
2 eggs
4 tablespoons skimmed milk
2 tablespoons molasses or cane sugar syrup
4 tablespoons rum or brandy for reheating

1 Soak the dried fruit in the brandy, rum or beer and leave overnight.
2 When ready to make the pudding, shake the cherries gently in the flour and then add the mixed spice, cinnamon, breadcrumbs, sugar and gravy browning.
3 Mix in the grated zest, apple and carrot, together with the lemon juice. Add the soaked fruit.
4 Beat the eggs with the milk and molasses and slowly add to the mixture, stirring well. Mix together gently and thoroughly.
5 Place in a 1.2 litre (2 pint) ovenproof basin. If you are going to microwave the pudding, place an upturned plate over the basin and microwave on high for 5 minutes. Leave to stand for 5 minutes, then microwave for a further 5 minutes. If steaming the pudding, cover with foil or a pudding cloth, and then steam gently for 3 hours (this makes a moister pudding).
6 After cooking, allow the pudding to cool and then wrap in aluminium foil and leave in a cool, dry place until required.
7 Before reheating, pierce the pudding several times with a fork and pour some more rum or brandy over the top. Steam for 1–2 hours or microwave on high for 10 minutes.
8 Serve with brandy sauce (see page 232).

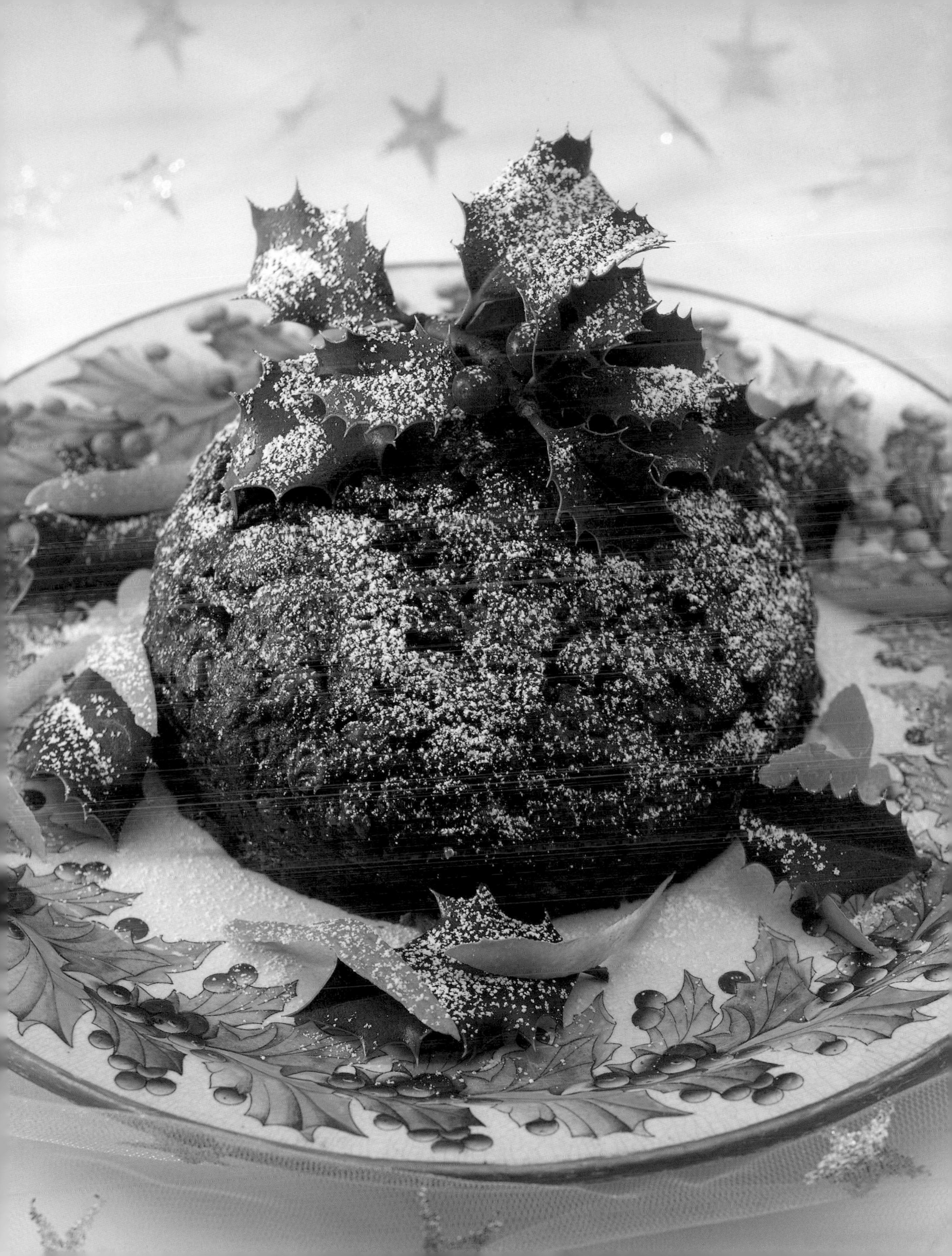

Index

SURVEY OF LONDON

VOLUME XXXIX

PREVIOUS VOLUMES
OF THE SURVEY OF LONDON

I Bromley-by-Bow.*
II Chelsea. Part I.*
III St. Giles-in-the-Fields. Part I (Lincoln's Inn Fields).†
IV Chelsea. Part II.†
V St. Giles-in-the-Fields. Part II.†
VI Hammersmith.
VII Chelsea. Part III (The Old Church).
VIII St. Leonard, Shoreditch.†
IX St. Helen, Bishopsgate. Part I.†
X St. Margaret, Westminster. Part I.*
XI Chelsea. Part IV (The Royal Hospital).†
XII All Hallows, Barking-by-the-Tower. Part I (The Parish Church).*
XIII St. Margaret, Westminster. Part II (Neighbourhood of Whitehall, vol. I).†
XIV St. Margaret, Westminster. Part III (Neighbourhood of Whitehall, vol. II).
XV All Hallows, Barking-by-the-Tower. Part II.
XVI St. Martin-in-the-Fields. Part I (Charing Cross).†
XVII St. Pancras. Part I (Village of Highgate).*
XVIII St. Martin-in-the-Fields. Part II (The Strand).*
XIX St. Pancras. Part II (Old St. Pancras and Kentish Town).*
XX St. Martin-in-the-Fields. Part III (Trafalgar Square and neighbourhood).†
XXI St. Pancras. Part III (Tottenham Court Road and neighbourhood).†
XXII St. Saviour and Christ Church, Southwark (Bankside).*
XXIII St. Mary, Lambeth. Part I (South Bank and Vauxhall).†
XXIV St. Pancras. Part IV (King's Cross neighbourhood).†
XXV St. George the Martyr and St. Mary Newington, Southwark (St. George's Fields).
XXVI St. Mary, Lambeth. Part II (Southern area).†
XXVII Christ Church and All Saints (Spitalfields and Mile End New Town).†
XXVIII Hackney. Part I (Brooke House).
XXIX, XXX St. James, Westminster. Part I (South of Piccadilly).†
XXXI, XXXII St. James, Westminster. Part II (North of Piccadilly).
XXXIII, XXXIV St. Anne, Soho.
XXXV The Theatre Royal, Drury Lane, and The Royal Opera House, Covent Garden.
XXXVI St. Paul, Covent Garden.
XXXVII Northern Kensington.
XXXVIII The Museums Area of South Kensington and Westminster.

* *Original edition out of print. Photographic facsimile available from the Greater London Council Bookshop, County Hall, London,* SE1 7PB, *or from A.M.S. Press Inc.,* 56 *East* 13*th Street, New York.*

† *Out of print.*

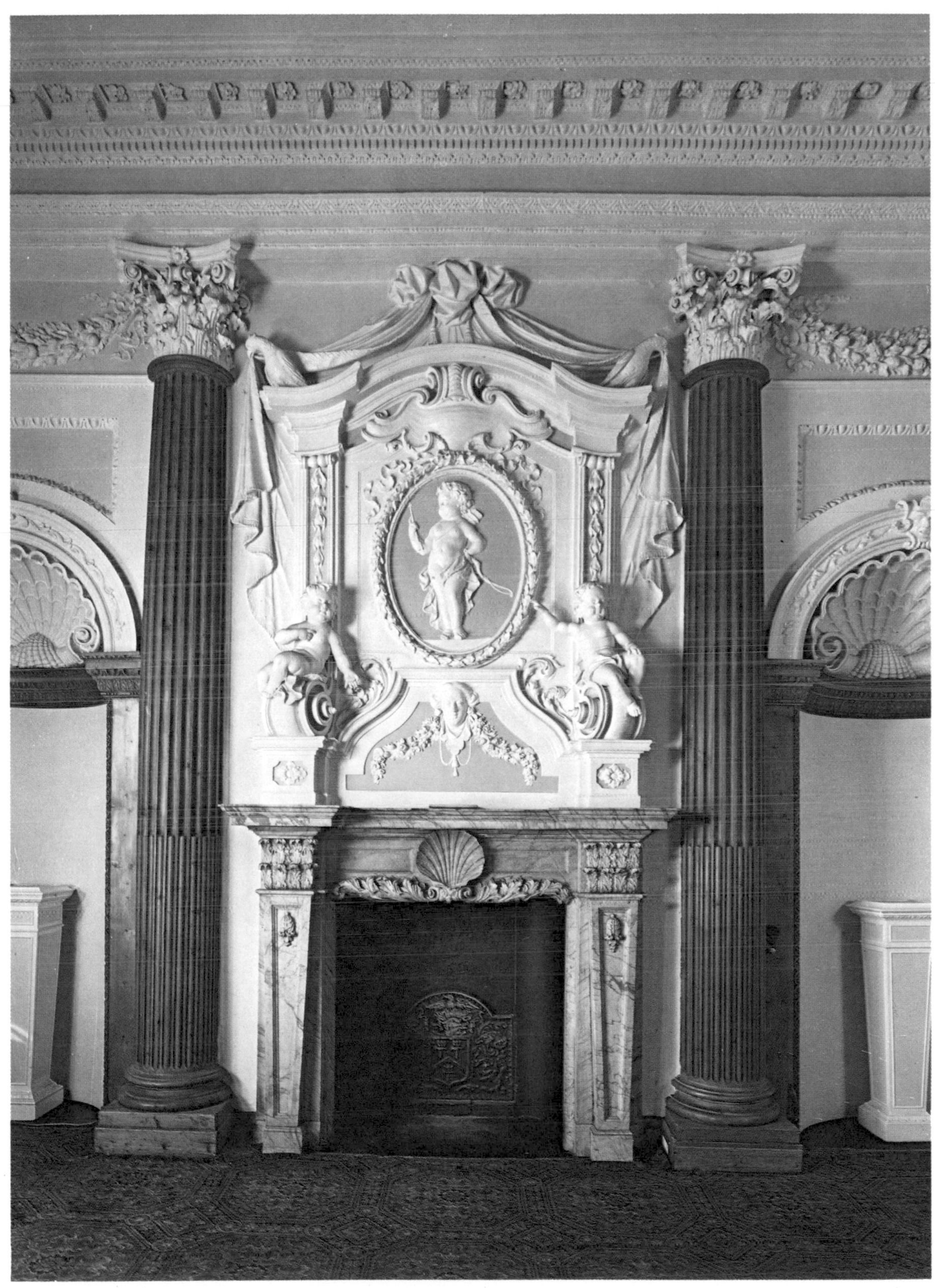

No. 66 Brook Street, now the Grosvenor Office: chimneypiece in first-floor front room in 1976. Edward Shepherd lessee, 1725

SURVEY OF LONDON

GENERAL EDITOR: F. H. W. SHEPPARD

VOLUME XXXIX

The Grosvenor Estate in Mayfair

PART I

General History

THE ATHLONE PRESS
UNIVERSITY OF LONDON
Published for the Greater London Council
1977

Published by
THE ATHLONE PRESS
UNIVERSITY OF LONDON
at 4 *Gower Street, London* WC1

Distributed by
Tiptree Book Services Ltd, Tiptree, Essex

U.S.A. and Canada
Humanities Press Inc, New Jersey

PUBLICATION NUMBER 71680859/5

ISBN 0 485 48239 8

Printed in Great Britain
at the University Press, Oxford
by Vivian Ridler
Printer to the University

Preface

The publication of this volume of the *Survey of London* coincides with the tercentenary of the establishment of the Grosvenor Estate in London. In advancing the printing of this volume by a year, the Greater London Council is giving special prominence to one of the most extraordinary and successful developments in our city. The increasingly tight control exercised by the Estate in modern times not only over the architecture but also over the use of newly erected buildings, has contributed to making Mayfair a harmonious and to a large extent visually united whole. Georgian, Victorian and Edwardian elements blend into a cohesive and dignified entity. Only occasionally, some later buildings may be felt to be unwelcome intruders.

Situated in the very heart of London, alongside Oxford Street, the capital's largest shopping thoroughfare, the area described in this volume has Grosvenor Square as its focal point, famous for its connection with the United States of America. Their mighty new embassy building dominates the western end of the large square, while the statue of Franklin Delano Roosevelt constitutes the main feature of its open space. Other embassies, including those of Italy and Japan, are sited close by. It is no accident that so many foreign missions have sought out this part of London where they exist side by side with a prosperous business community, fine residences, and some of the capital's most prestigious hotels and restaurants. The very name of Mayfair has become a byword for quality, not least because of the prevalence of strong and characteristic architecture and the total absence of mean or derelict streets.

This is the first part of the *Survey of London*'s study of the Grosvenor Estate in Mayfair. It contains a general account of the history and architecture of the estate, and will be followed by a detailed description of individual buildings which is now in course of preparation.

The Grosvenor family's estates in what are now Mayfair and Belgravia were acquired by Sir Thomas Grosvenor through his marriage on 10 October 1677 with Mary Davies, the daughter and heiress of a scrivener in the City of London. In Mayfair, development for building began in the 1720's, and within a few years Daniel Defoe was describing the 'amazing Scene of new Foundations, not of Houses only, but as I might say of new Cities' which were then springing up on the western outskirts of London. Many of the leading architects and builders of the day, notably Colen Campbell, Roger Morris and Edward Shepherd, worked on the Grosvenor Estate. Despite widespread rebuilding during the last hundred years, several splendid examples of the original Georgian work still survive, and many of the Victorian and Edwardian buildings are equally notable.

Hitherto only a few of these buildings have been studied in any detail, and the history of the estate itself—of its first development and of its subsequent management down to the present day—has remained largely unknown. The production of this volume has been made possible by the decision of the Grosvenor Estate Trustees to allow the Council's *Survey of London* staff access to their historical records kept at the Grosvenor Office in Mayfair and at Eaton Hall in Cheshire. The Council is most grateful to them and their staff at the Grosvenor Office, and in particular to Mr. Guy Acloque, for this essential assistance in the study of London's historic fabric.

On behalf of the Council I should also like to thank all those people who have given help in the preparation of this study. Many of their names are recorded in the List of Acknowledgments in this volume, and much of the research for it could not have been done without their generous assistance. I am particularly grateful to my colleagues, the advisory members of the Historic Buildings Board—Sir John Betjeman, Sir Hugh Casson, Sir Osbert Lancaster, Mr. Ian Phillips, Sir Paul Reilly and Sir John Summerson—who have given their valuable time and profound knowledge at numerous meetings of the Board. I would also like to express my great appreciation to the elected members of the Board for their devotion to the task of preserving the architectural heritage of our great city.

This volume has been prepared under the General Editorship of Mr. F. H. W. Sheppard. On the basis of research started in 1973, he and the Assistant Editors, Mr. J. Greenacombe and Mr. V. R. Belcher (all of the Director-General's Department) wrote the historical portions of the text and edited all the material. Latterly they were assisted in research and editing by the Deputy Editor, Mr. P. A. Bezodis. The typing was done by Mrs. K. Hill, who prior to her retirement in 1976 had typed the whole of the texts of seven volumes of the *Survey*, and by Mrs. B. Crawford, who also assisted with proof reading. All the contributions made by the staff of the Historic Buildings Division of the Department of Architecture and Civic Design were produced under the aegis of Mr. Ashley Barker, Surveyor of Historic Buildings. These contributions comprise portions of the text written by Mr. Andrew Saint, the Architectural Editor, who in 1974 took over from Dr. Malcolm Airs the organisation of the photographic and drawing programmes. The principal photographers were Mr. Alan Turner, Mr. Graham Slough and Mr. Stephen Tozer of the Council's Photographic Unit. The drawings were made in the Historic Buildings Division under the general guidance of Mr. F. A. Evans, M.B.E., and after his retirement in 1975, of Mr. John Sambrook. The authorship of each individual drawing is acknowledged in the List of Figures. I should like here to add a word of special appreciation for the outstanding contribution made by Mr. Evans, whose drawings appear in all eighteen of the volumes of the *Survey* published since 1949.

LOUIS BONDY
Chairman, Historic Buildings Board
Greater London Council
County Hall
March 1977

Acknowledgments

The principal acknowledgment of assistance received by the Council in preparing this volume must be to the Trustees of the Grosvenor Estate for their great courtesy in making available the records of the Mayfair estate, without which this study would have been impossible. It is a pleasure to acknowledge at the same time the ready assistance given to the Council's officers in their work by the members of the staff of the Grosvenor Office, and of the Trustees' solicitors, Boodle, Hatfield and Company.

For the work of Fernand Billerey on the estate his widow, Madame V. H. Billerey, and his son Mr. L. V. A. Billerey gave both encouragement and much valuable information. Mr. Jonathan Blow hospitably provided an opportunity to discuss the work of his father, Detmar Blow, and to examine the numerous architectural drawings in his possession. Mr. Geoffrey Singer, formerly Chief Surveyor to the Grosvenor Estates, very kindly read parts of the text at successive stages of their production.

Particular acknowledgment should also be made to Mr. Edward Hubbard and to Dr. J. M. Robinson for their generosity in allowing use to be made of their post-graduate theses on John Douglas and Samuel Wyatt respectively.

The Council tenders its grateful thanks to the following individuals, institutions and corporate bodies who have helped to make the work on this volume possible by providing or giving access to information or by allowing the inspection of buildings in their ownership or occupation:

Mr. Guy Acloque; Mr. Bengt Åkerrén; Mrs. Jill Allibone; H.E. the American Ambassador; Margaret, Duchess of Argyll; Miss Catherine Armet; Miss Rosemary Ashbee; Viscountess Astor; Mr. E. H. Aucott; Miss A. S. Bagshawe; Mr. Eustace Balfour; Mr. Nicolas Barker; the Duke of Beaufort; Mrs. Denis Berry; Mrs. E. K. Berry; Mr. G. C. Berry; Mr. T. S. Blakeney; H.E. the Brazilian Ambassador; Mrs. W. Broekema; Mr. O. Bateman Brown; Mr. S. Bywater; Mrs. Ann Campbell; Lady Iris Capell; the Earl of Carnarvon; Mr. Wayne Carter; Mrs. Carvalho; Mrs. Bridget Cherry; Miss Sarah D. Coffin; Mr. S. R. Coggan; Mr. H. M. Colvin; Mr. John Cornforth; Dr. Maurice Craig; Mr. Alan Crawford; the Earl of Crawford and Balcarres; Mr. Stephen Croad; the late Miss Jacqueline Cromie; Miss Helen Cundy; Mrs. Joan Cundy; Mr. J. Cutileiro; Mrs. Monica Dance; the Countess of Denbigh; Lady D'Erlanger; Mr. E. V. Dommett; Mr. Ian Doolittle; Mrs. M. P. G. Draper; Mr. William Drummond; Mr. Peter Dunne; Mrs. C. Dutnall; Rev. Fr. F. Edwards, S.J.; H.E. the Egyptian Ambassador; Frances, Lady Fergusson; Mr. R. B. Fisher; Rev. John Gaskell; Mr. A. Stuart Gray; Mr. B. Lund Hansen; Mr. John Hardy; Mrs. T. H. Harker; the Earl of Harrowby; Mr. M. D. Heber-Percy; Mr. J. B. Henderson; Mr. Nicholas Hill; Bishop A. Hornyk; Lady Hulse; H.E. the Indonesian Ambassador; Mr. R. Irving; H.E. the Italian Ambassador; H.E. the Japanese Ambassador; Mr. Edward Joy; Miss A. M. Kennett; Mrs. Geraldine Kunstadter; Mrs. Nancy Lancaster; Mr. Michael Levey; Mrs. Christine Loeb; the Hon. Christopher McLaren; Mr. Byron Maile; Mr. C. E. Mansfield; Miss Betty R. Masters; Mr. R. Mellin; Lord Methuen; Mr. E. Croft Murray; Mrs. Virginia Murray; Mr. R. G. Must; Mr. David Nickerson; Mrs. Y. Nothman; Prof. D. P. O'Brien; Miss Susan Orde; Sgr. L. Orsi; Count Guy de Pelet; Sir Nikolaus Pevsner; H.E. the Portuguese Ambassador; the Earl of Radnor; Mr. A. Ramsey; Mr. P. M. Rayner; Mrs. Margaret Richardson; Mr. Michael Robbins; Miss Mary L. Robertson; Mr. Michael Ross-Wills; the Marquess of Salisbury; Mr. A. W. Saxton; Mr. I. B. Scott; Mr. T. Shearing; Mrs. Smallpeice; Mr. F. T. Smallwood; Mr. R. A. H. Smith; the Duke of Somerset; Mr. H. D. Steiner; Miss Dorothy Stroud; Miss E. A. Stuart; Sir John Summerson; Miss M. Swarbrick; H.E. the Swedish Ambassador; Dr. Eric Till; Mrs. M. Travis; Mrs. P. A. Tritton; Miss Elmira Wade; Mr. Clive Wainwright; Mr. B. Weinreb; Mrs. H. J. Whetton; Mr. J. W. Wilcox; Mr. R. H. Harcourt Williams; Mrs. Dorothy Wimperis; Dr. E. J. Wimperis; Mr. R. McD. Winder; Sir Hugh Wontner; Mr. A. C. Wood.

Alpine Club; American Church in London; Ashmolean Museum; Messrs. Barrington Laurance; Barrow Hepburn Group; Bedfordshire Record Office; Bell Faultless Partnership; Berkshire Record Office; Biddle Holdings; Bodleian Library; John Bolding and Sons; British Library; British Optical Association; British Standards Institute; Buckinghamshire Record Office; Carmarthenshire Record Office; Casanova Club; Cheshire Record Office; Chester City Record Office; Church Commissioners; Claridge's Hotel; Sibyl Colefax and John Fowler; Brian Colquhoun and Partners; Commonwealth Secretariat; Connaught Hotel; Conservatoire National Des Arts et Métiers; Cornwall Record Office; Corporation of London, Guildhall

Library, and Record Office; *Country Life*; County and District Properties; Cumbria Record Office; Derbyshire Record Office; Devon Record Office, Exeter; Drummond's Branch, Royal Bank of Scotland; Duchy of Cornwall Office; Dudley Public Library; Durham Record Office; East Sussex Record Office; Essex Record Office; John Garlick Ltd.; Glamorgan Record Office; Gloucestershire Record Office; Thos. Goode and Co.; Green and Abbott Ltd.; Guildford Muniment Room; Gwent County Record Office; Gwynedd Archives Service, Caernarvon; Hammerson Group of Companies; Hampshire Record Office; Harkness House; Harrowby MSS Trust; Haslemere Estates; C. E. Heath and Co.; Hereford Record Office; Hertfordshire Record Office; Hoare's Bank; House of Lords Record Office; Huntingdon (Cambridgeshire) Record Office; Henry E. Huntington Library; The Honourable Society of the Inner Temple; Kent Archives Office; King's College, Cambridge; Lambeth Palace Library; Lancashire Record Office; Leeds Archives Dept.; Leicestershire Record Office; Lenygon and Morant Ltd.; Lincolnshire Archives Office; London Library; Lucas Industries Ltd.; Mallett at Bourdon House; Merchant Taylors' Company; Metropolitan Museum of Art; Messrs. Millar and Harris; Museum of London; National Library of Ireland; National Library of Wales; National Monuments Record; National Register of Archives; National Register of Archives (Scotland); National Trust (Hughenden Manor); W. H. Newson and Sons; Niedersächsische Staats- und Universitätsbibliothek, Göttingen; North Humberside Record Office; North Yorkshire Record Office; Northamptonshire Record Office; Nottinghamshire Record Office; Oxfordshire Record Office; Peabody Trust; Public Record Office; Public Record Office of Northern Ireland; Rank Organization; Royal Institute of British Architects; Royal Photographic Society; The John Rylands University Library of Manchester; Savile Club; Scottish Record Office; Sesame Club; Sheffield City Libraries; Shropshire Record Office; Sir John Soane's Museum; Somerset Record Office; Sotheby's Belgravia; Staffordshire Record Office; Robert Stigwood Organization; Suffolk Record Office; Surrey Record Office; Thames Water Authority; Trollope and Colls (City) Ltd.; Tupperware Company; Ukrainian Catholic Cathedral; University College of North Wales, Library; University of Hull, Brynmor Jones Library; University of Nottingham, Library; Victoria and Albert Museum; Voice and Vision Ltd.; Warwickshire Record Office; West Sussex Record Office; Westmoreland Properties; Williams and Glyn's Bank; Wiltshire Record Office; Worcestershire Record Office; Yorkshire Archaeological Society; Zinc and Lead Development Associations.

Contents

List of Plates

List of Figures

Note. Many of the following drawings show the buildings conjecturally restored to their presumed original state, and should in no case be taken as a precise record of present appearance.

TABLES

END POCKET

CHAPTER I

The Acquisition of the Estate

For three hundred years the Grosvenor family has owned large estates in what are now some of the most valuable parts of Westminster. These estates were acquired in 1677 through the marriage of Sir Thomas Grosvenor with Mary Davies, the infant daughter and heiress of a scrivener in the City of London. In the process of time Mary Davies's inheritance was developed for building, and the Grosvenors became the richest urban landlords in the country, the lustre of their name—for long synonymous with wealth and fashion—being gilded by successive advancements in the peerage, culminating in the dukedom of Westminster in 1874. Today the bulk of that inheritance is still, despite the sale of some of the less select parts, enjoyed by her descendants, and is now administered by the Grosvenor Estate Trustees.

The marriage portion which the guardians of the twelve-year-old Mary Davies were able to offer the young Cheshire baronet Sir Thomas Grosvenor in 1677 consisted of some five hundred acres of land, mostly meadow and pasture, a short distance from the western fringes of built-up London. Not all of this was to be available in immediate possession and the income from the land was at that time relatively small, but its potential for future wealth was realized even then. The area with which this volume is particularly concerned was only a part of that vast holding, approximately one hundred acres in extent and sometimes called in early deeds The Hundred Acres,[1] lying south of Oxford Street and east of Park Lane. With only minor exceptions this part of Mary Davies's heritage has remained virtually intact to the present day and forms the Grosvenor estate in Mayfair. The history of the ownership of this land before it came into the possession of the Grosvenor family is, however, best told as part of the history of the larger holding which the third baronet acquired on his marriage. To a considerable extent this story, and that of the personalities involved in it, have been recounted in the two volumes by Charles Gatty entitled *Mary Davies and the Manor of Ebury* and only a brief outline will be attempted here.

The Manor of Ebury

Most of the London estates which now belong or have belonged to the Grosvenor family—and all of that with which this volume is concerned—once formed part of the manor called Eia in the Domesday survey but later known as Eye, from which Eybury or Ebury derives. Although the manor's original bounds have not been determined with certainty it probably occupied the territory between the Roman road along the present course of Bayswater Road and Oxford Street on the north, the Thames on the south, the Westbourne river on the west, and the Tyburn, which was also known as Eye or Ay(e) Brook, on the east.[2] Even these relatively straightforward bounds are difficult to define because these tributaries tended both to change course and to have more than one outlet to the Thames. In the case of the Tyburn the westernmost of several channels, perhaps originally little more than a drainage ditch, seems to have formed the eastern boundary of the manor in its southern part.

After the Norman Conquest Geoffrey de Mandeville obtained possession of the manor, one of many which he took in reward for his services in the Conqueror's cause. Before the end of William's reign de Mandeville had given the manor to the Abbey of Westminster and it remained in the Abbey's ownership until 1536 when it was acquired by Henry VIII.[3] During this long period two areas came to be distinguished from the main manor, but although sometimes termed manors it is doubtful whether they had entirely separate jurisdictions.[4] The areas were Hyde in the north-west corner, now incorporated into Hyde Park, and Neyte or Neat(e) in the heart of the district later known as Pimlico. The so-called manor or bailiwick of Neat presents particular problems. In seventeenth- and eighteenth-century title deeds the estate belonging to the Grosvenors is described as the site of the manor of Ebury and parcel of the bailiwick of Neat,[5] but the use of these terms appears merely to have followed that in early leases in which they were probably employed loosely to describe farms. In fact the Neyte was formerly a manor house or grange of the Abbots of Westminster situated between the modern Warwick Way and Sutherland Row,[6] and its site, together with some thirty-six acres to the south and east, were not included in Mary Davies's inheritance, having been granted away separately by the Crown after 1536, and thus did not pass into the ownership of the Grosvenor family.

Surrounded by other lands belonging to Westminster Abbey the manor had lost its identity as a unit of landholding before the end of the Middle Ages, and the process of disintegration continued after its acquisition by the Crown. The many documents and maps which survive show that the subsequent history of its descent is extremely complex, but as few of these complexities affect the history of The Hundred Acres in Mayfair no attempt will be made here to unravel all of them. The 'Manor of Hyde' was enclosed into Hyde Park by

Henry VIII, and he or his successors also added some land on the east to his new park, for fifteen acres called Tyburn Close and forty acres near Stonehill (apparently the north-eastern and south-eastern extremities of the park) were specifically excluded from subsequent leases and grants of Ebury manor. Other stated exceptions in such transactions were the lands around the 'Manor of Neate'.[7]

Although not specified other lands which appear originally to have been within the manor became detached when it was in the hands of the Crown, including a substantial part of Mayfair south of The Hundred Acres. Among these was a large close or series of fields called Brick Close which was later to form part of the Berkeley estate,[8] and other fields which were incorporated into the manor or bailiwick of St. James. Some six or seven acres to the north of the modern Brick Street were, however, retained; they were included in a schedule of property to be sold to pay the debts of Alexander Davies, Mary Davies's father, by Act of Parliament in 1675,[9] and therefore did not pass to the Grosvenors.

Of the areas in Mayfair which apparently became separated from the manor, that which presents the most puzzling aspects is a plot with a frontage to Park Lane, about three acres in extent, immediately to the south of the Grosvenor estate, now occupied by the Dorchester Hotel and parts of Deanery and Tilney Streets. When first leased for building in the 1730's this was described as waste ground belonging to the manor of Knightsbridge in the ownership of the Dean and Chapter of Westminster.[10] The Dean and Chapter had acquired the manor (the full title of which was the manor of Knightsbridge with Westbourne Green) from Henry VIII in 1542[11] although it had belonged to Westminster Abbey in the Middle Ages. How that manor came to include a parcel of waste ground in the middle of the manor of Ebury is unclear. In Grosvenor estate documents of the eighteenth century the area is defined as 'a common or waste... called Ossulton Common'.[12] The name Osolstone is also used to describe this spot in a deed of 1614 and in the same document Park Lane is described as 'the highwaye from Osolstone to Tiburne'.[13] The name is also marked on an early manuscript map among the Grosvenor archives which relates to this deed. In the records of Westminster Abbey there are references to a farm 'at Osolueston' which belonged to the manor of Eye, and other references to Ossulston, always as part of this same manor.[14] The evaluation of this evidence in determining the location of the assemblies or courts of the Hundred of Ossulston, the ancient area of jurisdiction which included London, is not within the scope of this volume, and the apparent conflict of evidence about the manorial history of this small area remains unresolved.

Most of the remainder of Ebury manor was let by the Crown in two leasehold entities, the fields of one intermingling with those of the other. Reversionary leases were also granted, apparently as a way of rewarding faithful service, well before the current leases expired, and to complicate matters further each reversionary lease came to be held by more than one person so that partitions of the land had to take place when the previous leases fell in early in the seventeenth century.[15]

In 1618 a moiety of one lease was bought for £4,760 by trustees acting for Sir Lionel Cranfield, the ambitious merchant who held several offices of state under James I and was later impeached for corruption.[16] By this purchase Cranfield became the direct leaseholder of a large part of the manor including The Hundred Acres. He also contemplated purchasing the other moiety, which he estimated would cost about £5,000 or £6,000, but was evidently unable to complete the transaction before his fall, for this leasehold interest remained outstanding until its expiry in 1675.[17] In 1623, however, James I sold the freehold reversion* of the manor to two 'gentlemen' of London, John Traylman and Thomas Pearson, for £1,151 15*s*. By a conveyance dated the day following they in turn disposed of it for the same amount to two representatives of Cranfield, by then Earl of Middlesex and Lord High Treasurer of England.[19] The price was equivalent to thirty years' purchase of the nominal Crown rents obtained under leases granted by the Tudors, and by buying the manor in fee farm Cranfield could no doubt claim that he was preserving the King's rent, low as it was. Not only did the grant convey all of the manor with the exception of those parts already detached from it and a royal mulberry garden (now part of the site of Buckingham Palace and its grounds), but additionally some land elsewhere was included. Particularly important for the later history of the Grosvenor estate were some twenty acres at Millbank on the south side of Horseferry Road, for it was here that the first speculative building on the estate took place.

In 1626, when his personal and financial fortunes were at a low point, Cranfield sold his interests in the manor and the additional lands for £9,400 to Hugh Audley (also spelt Awdley or Awdeley), a clerk of the Court of Wards and Liveries who amassed a considerable fortune by lending money.[20] Although Cranfield had thus made a handsome profit on the two sums he had laid out, he felt that Audley had driven a hard bargain.[21] Audley held the property until his death at an advanced age in 1662. During this long period he sold some small parcels of land and bought others which had probably once belonged to the manor,[22] but when he died the estate he had purchased in 1626 was still virtually intact. By a settlement made shortly before his death he left the bulk of the land

* In strict terms the manor was sold in fee farm, for a perpetual annual rent of £38 7*s*. 10*d*. (equal to the total rent due under the existing leases) was payable to the Crown. In 1663 this rent was granted by Charles II to the Earl of Sandwich[18] and was thereafter paid to the Earl and his descendants.

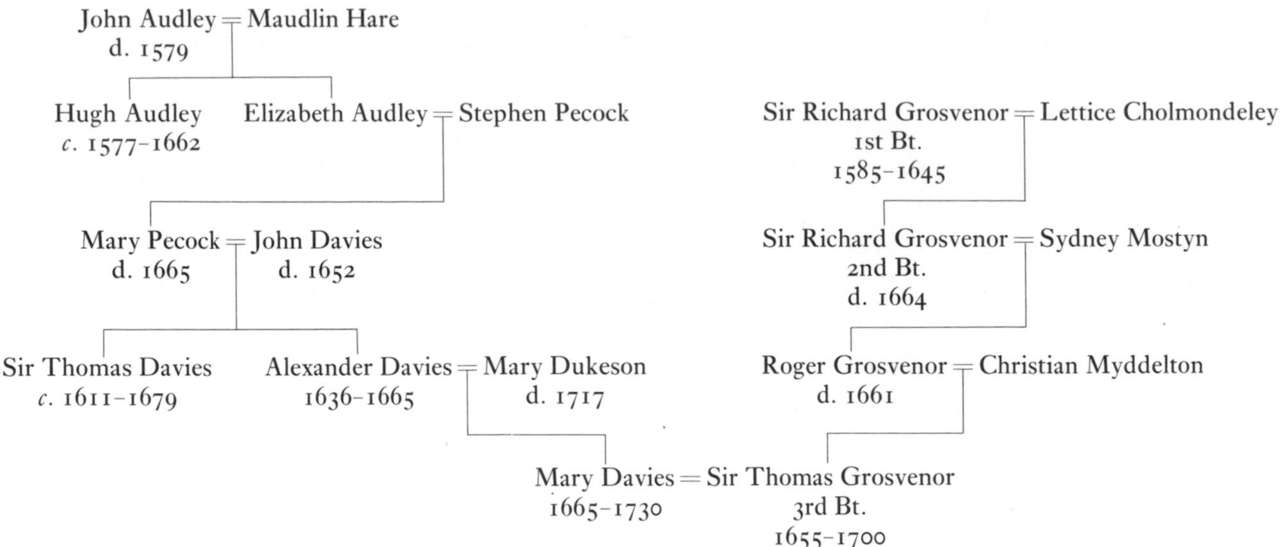

Abridged pedigree of Audley, Davies and Grosvenor families

to his great-nephew Alexander Davies and the detached part at Millbank (known as Market Meadows) to the latter's brother Thomas Davies, later Sir Thomas Davies, who was Lord Mayor of London in 1676–7.[23] After Audley's death Thomas Davies sold his holding for £2,000 to his brother[24] so that Alexander Davies possessed all of Audley's former estate in the area.

Alexander Davies was a scrivener by profession and had worked for Audley.[25] Although scriveners were technically the draftsmen of deeds they also undertook many of the functions later associated with lawyers, particularly the management of investments for clients, and Davies probably had access to ready supplies of capital. He decided to embark on speculative building on his new property and as the site chose Market Meadows at Millbank, which he had purchased from his brother. He let the land along the river front for building, reserving a large plot at the southern end as the site of a mansion for his own occupation. This was later called Peterborough House and then Grosvenor House when it became the principal London residence of the Grosvenor family in the first half of the eighteenth century. In 1665, however, 'in the time of the ... greate Sicknesse' Alexander Davies died at the age of twenty-nine, leaving the speculation unfinished, his mansion half built, and an infant daughter less than six months old as his heir.[26] This was the Mary Davies who was to marry Sir Thomas Grosvenor in 1677.

Alexander Davies had settled the estate on trustees for the benefit of his heirs with provision for an annuity of £100 to be paid to his widow.[27] The settlement did not extinguish her right of dower, however, and so his widow, also named Mary, could claim a life interest in a third of the property. She quickly remarried, her second husband being John Tregonwell, a Dorset squire, and was hereafter, of course, known as Mrs. Tregonwell. Despite the potential wealth of the estate the immediate problem facing the Tregonwells was the settlement of Alexander Davies's debts. He had not paid the £2,000 purchase money for the land at Millbank and had borrowed heavily to finance his building programme. Nearly £2,000 more had to be spent on the unfinished mansion to make it habitable and there were annuities and interest charges on the estate. A substantial part of the land yielded no income as it was still subject to the leasehold interest granted by the Crown (previously referred to) which was not due to fall in until 1675. John Tregonwell later claimed to have advanced a considerable amount of his own money in settling Alexander Davies's affairs,[28] and in 1675 an Act of Parliament was passed enabling some property to be sold to pay the debts.[9] Specified in the Act were Goring House (on the site of Buckingham Palace) and some twenty acres adjoining, five acres which now lie in the north-western corner of Green Park, the seven acres in Mayfair to the north of the line of Brick Street referred to above, and twenty-two acres in Knightsbridge. The land in Knightsbridge was repurchased by the Grosvenor family in 1763.[29] The Act also provided that several fields in the Mayfair portion of the estate should be held in dower by Mrs. Tregonwell. About fifty-six acres were involved, constituting the western part of The Hundred Acres. This had some effect on the building history of the area as the dower lands were exempted from subsequent settlements and were held under a different tenure when building leases came to be granted.

Despite these temporary difficulties, however, there was no doubt about the eligibility of the infant Mary Davies as a future wife for some aspiring young nobleman. In 1672 an agreement was drawn up whereby she was to

be married to the Hon. Charles Berkeley, the eldest son of John, first Baron Berkeley of Stratton, as soon as she reached her twelfth birthday, when she would be of age to consent to the match. As part of the contract Lord Berkeley paid £5,000 immediately to John Tregonwell, partly in recompense for money spent in finishing Alexander Davies's mansion and in the upbringing of Mary; he also agreed to settle land of a considerable annual value either on, or in trust for, the couple by the time of the ceremony.[30] The marriage, however, never took place. According to an account preserved in the Grosvenor archives and probably drawn up by Mrs. Tregonwell[31] the reason was that Lord Berkeley was unable to provide the land. Although he was a rich man he had recently built an expensive mansion, Berkeley House in Piccadilly, and at about this time he purchased Brick Close in Mayfair, immediately to the south of the fields belonging to Mary Davies.[32] The breakdown of these plans mattered little for within a few months of her twelfth birthday a husband had been found for her in the twenty-one-year-old baronet, Sir Thomas Grosvenor.

The Grosvenor Marriage

The marriage between Mary Davies and Sir Thomas Grosvenor took place on 10 October 1677 in the church of St. Clement Danes, where the bride's grandfather, Dr. Richard Dukeson, was rector.[33] The Grosvenors were an ancient Cheshire family claiming a somewhat tenuous descent from Hugh Lupus, first Earl of Chester, one of William the Conqueror's foremost knights and possibly his nephew. By the seventeenth century they owned land in Chester, Cheshire, Denbighshire and Flintshire and also valuable lead mines in the last two counties. In 1622 Sir Richard Grosvenor was created a baronet by James I, and Sir Thomas, his great-grandson, was the third baronet. The family seat was at Eaton Hall, near Chester.

All Sir Thomas Grosvenor's prospects from the marriage were in the future. In deference to her tender years his bride remained for at least two years in the care of a guardian aunt, and as part of the marriage bargain he had to expend a considerable sum of money. Lord Berkeley's £5,000 had to be repaid with interest, and among other sums required to be disbursed John Tregonwell received £1,000 for a reversionary interest in the estate which would arise in the event of the death of Mary Davies before reaching the age of twenty-one, and which he had prudently acquired by assignment.[34] While a settlement of the estates in Cheshire and North Wales for the benefit of any male heirs of the marriage in order of primogeniture was made shortly after the ceremony,[35] a similar settlement of that part of Mary Davies's lands which was free from dower had to await her twenty-first birthday and was finally made in 1694.[36] The total annual rental value of the London estates in 1677 was £2,170, but one third of this was payable to Mrs. Tregonwell in dower, and after annuities and other payments the clear income from the rest amounted to £824.[37] Besides this income, some £3,400 were obtained in 1681 when thirty-five acres were sold, apparently by royal wish, to the Earl of Arlington.[38] The land involved now constitutes parts of the grounds of Buckingham Palace, Green Park and Hyde Park Corner. A further two and a half acres in Chelsea, now or formerly part of the grounds of the Royal Hospital, were also sold.[39]

Sir Thomas Grosvenor died in 1700 leaving three sons under the age of twelve; a daughter also was born a month after his death. All three sons eventually succeeded to the baronetcy. Sir Richard, the eldest, died in 1732. His brother, Thomas, succeeded him for only seven months before his death in Naples early in 1733. The youngest son, Robert, then became the sixth baronet until his death in 1755; he was the only one of the three brothers to leave any issue.

The effect of the settlement of 1694 was that on her husband's death Dame Mary Grosvenor, as Mary Davies was now styled, was left a life interest in the London estate, with the exception of those parts held in dower by her mother. She had already shown signs of mental instability during her husband's lifetime and her illness was no doubt accelerated by his death. In 1701 while in Paris she married, or was inveigled into a bogus marriage by, Edward Fenwick, the brother of a Roman Catholic chaplain she had taken into her household. Four years of legal disputes ensued until the supposed marriage was annulled by the Court of Delegates in 1705.[40] In the same year a commission of lunacy was appointed to enquire into her mental state. She was adjudged insane and committed to the care of Francis Cholmondeley of Vale Royal in Cheshire, who had been appointed one of the guardians of her children by Sir Thomas Grosvenor's will.[41] As a result the revenues from her estate were paid into the Court of Chancery to be invested for her benefit, and any change in the use or disposition of the land could only be made by leave of the Court. Dame Mary lived on without regaining her faculties until 1730.

In 1708 Sir Richard Grosvenor married Jane Wyndham, daughter of Sir Edward Wyndham of Orchard Wyndham in Somerset. In return for a marriage portion of £12,000 he agreed to make a new settlement of the estates in his possession and of those in which his mother had a life interest, in part to secure a jointure for his wife.[42] In view of his mother's lunacy, however, it was only possible to do this with the authority of an Act of Parliament which was duly obtained in 1711 when he had reached the age of twenty-one.[43] The effect of the settlement was to preserve the descent of the estates in the male line, firstly to his male heirs if any and then to his brothers and their male heirs. Jane Grosvenor died in 1719 without issue and Sir Richard married again. His second wife was Diana Warburton, daughter of Sir George Warburton of Arley in Cheshire. This time a dowry of £8,000 was provided and a new settlement was

drawn up, but its effect was to preserve the same contingent remainders as earlier ones.[44] Diana Grosvenor died in 1730, also without issue.

A clause was inserted in the Act of 1711 to enable Sir Richard Grosvenor to grant building leases for any term up to sixty years of the land in London in which his mother held a life interest (but excluding the land held in dower by Mrs. Tregonwell). The Act referred to some old and ruinous buildings which might be rebuilt, but otherwise there is no indication that any specific development was then planned.

In 1717 Mrs. Tregonwell died[45] and the third of the estate which she had held in dower passed in fee simple to Dame Mary Grosvenor. The income from this land was also henceforth administered on her behalf by the officials of the Court of Chancery.

CHAPTER II

The Development of the Estate 1720–1785

'I passed an amazing Scene of new Foundations, not of Houses only, but as I might say of new Cities. New Towns, new Squares, and fine Buildings, the like of which no City, no Town, nay, no Place in the World can shew; nor is it possible to judge where or when, they will make an end or stop of Building.... All the Way through this new Scene I saw the World full of Bricklayers and Labourers; who seem to have little else to do, but like Gardeners, to dig a Hole, put in a few Bricks, and presently there goes up a House.' So wrote Daniel Defoe in *Applebee's Weekly Journal* in 1725.[1] He was describing the amount of building work then going on in west London. Periodic bursts of activity in house building had been common in the western suburbs of London since the Restoration, but Defoe described the latest phase which followed the Hanoverian succession as 'a kind of Prodigy'.[2] Within a dozen years builders had moved from Hanover Square through the City of London's Conduit Mead estate well into the Grosvenor estate and even north of Oxford Street, in the vicinity of Cavendish Square. More deeds were registered in the Middlesex Land Register in 1725 than in any other year until 1765—an indication of the feverish level reached by building speculation at that time. On the Grosvenor estate, where development began in 1720, only a handful of houses were occupied before 1725, but in that year the parish ratebooks show many more houses filling up and the new streets on the estate were formally named, an occasion marked by a 'very splendid Entertainment' given by Sir Richard Grosvenor.[3]

The relative stability which followed the Peace of Utrecht and the crushing of the Jacobite rebellion provided a favourable climate in which building developments could be undertaken, and there seems to have been plenty of capital available for mortgages even during the years of the South Sea Bubble, but it is difficult to find adequate demographic reasons why there should have been so many houses built in the decade after 1715. As far as we know the population of London was not rising substantially at this time,[4] but the inexorable movement of fashion westwards, partly out of the fear of disease in the more crowded parts of the capital, may have provided much of the impetus. Defoe remarked on the contrast between the depopulation of the older parts of the metropolis and the creation of new *faubourgs* in the west. 'The City does not increase, but only the Situation of it is a going to be removed, and the Inhabitants are quitting the old Noble Streets and Squares where they used to live, and are removing into the Fields for fear of Infection; so that, as the People are run away into the Country, the Houses seem to be running away too.'[5]

Against this background the decision of the Grosvenor family in 1720 to lay out The Hundred Acres in Mayfair for building is not a particularly remarkable one. The extent of the building scheme—stretching as far west as Park Lane—may have been a bold gesture, but the timing of the enterprise must have been largely dictated by the fact that builders had already reached the eastern boundary of the estate in their development of the adjoining Conduit Mead property in the vicinity of New Bond Street, and the men who initially carried through the operation on the Grosvenor lands were almost without exception those who were still working on the neighbouring estate.[6]

The Ground Landlord and his Role

A certain circumspection on the part of the ground landlord was to be expected on the Grosvenor estate during the first half of the eighteenth century, for Sir Richard Grosvenor and his brothers were country gentlemen rather than metropolitan entrepreneurs. Worthy, honest and perhaps a trifle dull, they appear to have made little mark on the national scene. They represented Chester at Westminster on the family interest as Tories, and in 1722 Sir Richard's name was included in a secret list drawn up by the Jacobites of those members of the nobility and gentry who, they thought, 'may be inclinable to join' a rebellion.[7] The Grosvenors were, however, Protestants, and there is no overt evidence that they were disloyal to the Hanoverian dynasty. The decision to erect a statue of George I as the centrepiece of the grand square which was to dominate the estate layout was probably prompted not merely by considerations of expediency, and architects and speculators more generally associated with Whig patrons apparently found little difficulty in co-operating with them. Of the three brothers who succeeded in turn to the baronetcy, Richard, the eldest, and Robert, the youngest, appear to have been most concerned with events in Mayfair. Indeed a dispute which occurred when Thomas Grosvenor became fifth baronet in 1732 suggests some degree of estrangement from his younger brother. He replaced the agents who managed the Middlesex estates, Richard and Robert Andrews, by a man of his own choice, but was apparently unable to persuade them to hand over the documents in their custody, and eventually brought a case against them in the Court of Exchequer.[8] They were supported in their

resistance by Robert Grosvenor, ostensibly on the grounds that they were also acting for him as one of the executors of Sir Richard Grosvenor's will. A consideration in the minds of Sir Thomas Grosvenor's opponents was that he was a sick man (he died in Naples in February 1733) and that it might in turn prove difficult for them to obtain the papers necessary for running the estate from his executors on his death.[9] Robert Grosvenor was actively involved in the development of Mayfair even before he became sixth baronet in 1733. He often looked after the family's interest in London while Sir Richard Grosvenor was at Eaton and lived in a new house on the site of the present No. 10 Upper Grosvenor Street from 1730 to 1733,[10] probably while Grosvenor House, Millbank, was being reconstructed. He was also a lessee (from his brother) of parts of the estate, particularly on the south side of Grosvenor Square,[11] and this property, which was largely developed by speculative builders under sub-leases in the normal manner, was referred to as his trust estate.

Robert Grosvenor's son Richard, who succeeded his father as seventh baronet in 1755 and was created Baron Grosvenor in 1761 and Viscount Belgrave and Earl Grosvenor in 1784, appears to have been a different type of person from his father and uncles. With a disastrous marital life which led to a notorious scandal when he brought an action for adultery against George III's brother, the Duke of Cumberland,[12] and with a fondness for the turf which brought him to near ruin, he represents a transition between the country gentry and the sophisticated aristocracy of the Grosvenor family in the nineteenth and twentieth centuries. A series of sycophantic letters written to him by William Pitt the elder[13] suggests that he was also fully aware of the advantages to be gained by bestowing his political favours shrewdly and it was through Pitt's influence that he was raised to the peerage. He once described Pitt as 'the shining light or rather the blazing star of this country'.[14] The hectoring tone of some of the letters written to him by his London agent, however, suggests an exasperation at delays in obtaining crucial decisions affecting his affairs, and indicates that he was less than decisive in matters of estate policy.[15]

Until 1730 the position of the Grosvenor family as landlords was complicated by the mental derangement of Dame Mary Grosvenor and the different tenures under which the land in Mayfair was held. By the Act of 1711 Sir Richard Grosvenor had power to grant leases for up to sixty years of those parts of the estate in which his mother held a life interest, but not of the land which was then held in dower by his grandmother, Mrs. Tregonwell, and which his mother was to inherit in fee simple in 1717. The lands in which Dame Mary Grosvenor had only a life interest were in the eastern part of The Hundred Acres, and as this was the quarter from which development would naturally proceed, the problem of the fee-simple land was not an immediate one. The first difficulty was that the Grosvenors thought a term of sixty years would not be a sufficient inducement to builders, even though sixty-one- and sixty-two-year leases were accepted during the contemporary development of the Burlington estate, and even shorter terms were granted in Conduit Mead. From the beginning a longer term was evidently intended for parts of the Grosvenor estate for in the very first building agreement, concluded with the estate surveyor, Thomas Barlow, in August 1720, it was specified that leases were to be granted for sixty years and 'a further term of years...as shall be agreed to be granted for building the new intended Square'.[16] Other agreements made in 1720 were either for sixty years (although the leases granted under them were for longer periods), or for ninety-nine years even though no power existed as yet to grant such a term.[17] The first lease (dated 15 July 1721) was for sixty years from Midsummer 1721, but this term was extended by a subsequent deed.[18]

This unsatisfactory situation was resolved in 1721 by a deed dated 2 June in which forty-three acres were conveyed in trust for the use of Sir Richard Grosvenor and his heirs with a proviso that leases could be granted for any term not exceeding ninety-nine years.[19] This deed explains the peculiar terminology of the early estate leases which were granted for sixty years under the Act of 1711 and a further term under the deed of 2 June 1721. This further period was generally thirty-nine years making ninety-nine in all, but for the area to the east of Davies Street an eighty-year term overall was more usual, the ninety-nine-year lease to Thomas Barlow of a large plot on the south side of Grosvenor Street to which he was entitled under the building agreement referred to above being the one notable exception.[20] Barlow, himself, granted only one sub-lease for a longer term than eighty years and several, chiefly of plots for stables, were for sixty or less,[21] the reversionary term under his direct Grosvenor lease eventually considerably enhancing the value of his estate (see page 19).

Although no leases of the western part of The Hundred Acres, which was held by Dame Mary Grosvenor in fee simple, were granted until 1727, builders were interested in staking a claim in this territory as soon as the development of the estate got under way.[22] Accordingly a petition was presented to Chancery in 1721 asking that Robert Myddelton of Chirk Castle in Denbighshire, who was then the legal guardian of Dame Mary Grosvenor, should be empowered to grant leases of this land for up to ninety-nine years. The necessity for such a term was explained by 'the intended buildings being very large'. The request was granted, subject, however, to the approval of each lease by the Master in Chancery who administered the revenues from Dame Mary's estates—a costly and time-consuming procedure.[23] The laying out of Grosvenor Square, the site of which included part of Dame Mary's lands, made the matter urgent, and after more abortive approaches to Chancery another Act of Parliament was obtained in 1726 by which Myddelton (or any subsequent guardian) acquired power to grant ninety-nine-year leases,

the consent only of Dame Mary's heir apparent being required.[24]

Myddelton was a party to all the agreements and leases concluded while Dame Mary Grosvenor was still alive. In leases of the land in which she held only a life interest Sir Richard Grosvenor was the grantor or first party and Myddelton the second, the latter nominally consenting to the transaction on behalf of Dame Mary; but in leases of the fee-simple land, Myddelton was the first party with Sir Richard Grosvenor as consenting party. The precise niceties of the correct order were not always followed in agreements, which did not have the same long-term legal force as leases.

Dame Mary Grosvenor died in January 1730 and within a few months Sir Richard Grosvenor had taken steps to simplify the whole tenure of the estate by means of the legal device of a common recovery which abolished the entail imposed in the settlement of 1694.[25] He now held all the London estates in fee simple, but in his will he established a new entail by bequeathing his property to his next brother Thomas and his male heirs in order of birth, and failing issue in that line, to his youngest brother Robert and his male heirs likewise.[26] It was not until 1755 that Sir Richard (later first Earl) Grosvenor, who had recently succeeded to the estate, abolished this entail by similar legal means.[27] For the rest of the eighteenth century encumbrances on the title to the estate did not arise through complexities of tenure but were monetary, eventually leading to the establishment of a trust whereby the control of the estate was taken out of Lord Grosvenor's sole charge (see page 37).

The peculiar circumstances that over several years the revenues from Dame Mary Grosvenor's estates, after expenses and allowances, had been 'frozen' in the Court of Chancery enabled the Grosvenors to aid the development of their Mayfair lands in a practical manner. By 1721 £8,490 was held in Chancery besides any interest which might have accrued on this sum.[28] Although they had some difficulty in freeing this money, as several Chancery petitions testify, the Grosvenors were eventually able to use it (and a good deal more) in a series of measures designed to assist the builders who took land on their estate.

Until Sir Richard Grosvenor's death the sewers which were laid under most of the new streets were built at his initial cost, the money being recovered from lessees on the granting of their leases, usually at the rate of six shillings per foot frontage for those plots which fronted on to the streets under which the sewers lay.[29] The sewers drained into 'the Great Sewer called Aybrooke' and were at first constructed without the leave of the Westminster Commission of Sewers. It was not until 1726 that the Commissioners discovered this, but they then gave permission for the work to be continued on payment of a lump sum of £204 (computed at £2 per acre on 102 acres) to the Commission.[30] Cash books among the Grosvenor records contain a day by day account of income and expenditure on the London estates beginning in 1729; these include several payments 'for sewering' to building tradesmen who also worked on the houses being erected. George Barlow, John Barnes and Thomas Hipsley, bricklayers, Lawrence Neale, carpenter, and Stephen Whitaker, brickmaker, 'on account of digging work', were paid some £300 between them for such work in 1729.[31] In the later years of the development, however, the building agreements suggest that the construction of sewers was often undertaken by the developers rather than the ground landlord.[32]

Although under the terms of agreements and leases road-making was the responsibility of undertakers and their lessees, some stable yards which formed the boundary between blocks of land taken under building agreements were laid out at the Grosvenors' expense, the money being recovered, as in the case of sewers, from lessees according to the footage of their plots abutting on the yard.[33] John Mist, paviour, was paid for 'paving the stable yard between Grosvenor Street and Brook Street with the horsepond and way leading thereto'.[31] The majority of mews, however, lay completely within large areas developed under one agreement and were not, therefore, made at the Grosvenors' cost.

Apart from the expense of the sewers, the principal capital cost met by the Grosvenor family and retrieved later, where possible, from builders, was in the laying out of Grosvenor Square. By an agreement of June 1725[34] between Sir Richard Grosvenor and the various building tradesmen and others who were already in possession of the land fronting on to the square under building agreements, Sir Richard undertook to lay out the square garden* and surround it with a brick wall topped by a wooden fence, access being provided through four iron gates. In the centre of the enclosure was to be a gilded equestrian statue of George I (by John Nost). The cost of the garden (£350) and the statue (£262 10*s.*) was specified and rates for the other work set out. The signatories agreed to repay Sir Richard's costs within one month of the work being completed, the sum due from each being determined by the extent of his frontage to the square. An initial rate of 20*s.* per foot frontage was assessed, but later Sir Richard also met the cost of paving the square around the oval enclosure and a final payment of 40*s.* 9*d.* per foot frontage was eventually sought, not always successfully, from the building lessees of the houses in the square.[36]

The sums laid out by the Grosvenors in these ways were in effect interest-free loans (not always repaid) which were designed to advance the progress of development. Another and more important method of achieving

*The work was to be done by one of his own tenants, John Alston, a gardener from Pimlico, who also provided the design for the garden layout.[35]

this object was by the granting of mortgages. An Order in Chancery of October 1722 required the Master to whom the administration of Dame Mary Grosvenor's finances had been entrusted, John Borrett, to provide mortgages at 5 per cent interest to builders approved by Sir Richard Grosvenor, his brothers and sister and Robert Myddelton. The first such loans were made in December 1722 for various amounts, generally between £400 and £600.[37] Borrett died shortly afterwards and some difficulties being encountered in securing the co-operation of his successor as Master in Chancery, permission was granted for Richard Andrews, the Grosvenors' London agent, to execute mortgages in his own name.[38] Between 1726 and 1729 Andrews lent £11,800, mostly to builders working in and around Grosvenor Square, in a series of transactions which have been preserved among the estate records.[39] Although he appears also to have been lending money on his own account, the survival of these records suggests that he was here acting as trustee for the Grosvenors. When Dame Mary Grosvenor died in 1730 an account was drawn up of her personal estate in which were itemized the various sums owing to her on mortgages to builders. Several correspond with the amounts advanced in Andrews' name and they totalled in all £9,450 (some of the principal no doubt having been repaid).[40]

The Grosvenors took a particularly direct concern in the building of Grosvenor Square, no doubt regarding its successful prosecution as the key to the progress of the whole enterprise. As already indicated, Robert Grosvenor was the head lessee for most of the south side and several of the mortgages referred to above were granted to builders who had sub-leases from him. He also apparently had one house built directly (No. 42), which he sold to the master builder Benjamin Timbrell in 1731.[41] He also assisted in the building of the important east side, which was developed uniformly by another master builder, John Simmons, by purchasing improved ground rents from Simmons while the building operations were still in progress. Between 1731 and 1733 he provided over £2,000 in this manner towards the completion of four houses, including the large centre house with a seventy-foot frontage.[42] Robert Grosvenor was also prepared to intervene elsewhere to bail out builders who found themselves in difficulties,[43] and after he succeeded to the baronetcy in 1733 he continued the policy of providing mortgages; at his death in 1755 he was owed £7,700 by builders (including £1,700 by Elizabeth Simmons, the widow of John Simmons).[44]

A less direct but probably equally valuable way of assisting builders was by allowing arrears of ground rent to accumulate. Sometimes quite substantial sums were involved. At Christmas 1731 £3,600 was owing, but Lady Day appears to have been the quarter day on which most accounts were settled, and the arrears at the end of that quarter are therefore probably more significant, the highest such total—£2,595—being at Lady Day 1732. At Sir Richard Grosvenor's death shortly afterwards the debt amounted to £2,988 and some attempt was made to clear this, but £1,239 remained outstanding and was probably never recovered.[45] In 1733 (on the succession of Sir Robert Grosvenor) a new account was begun, but arrears continued to mount up and by Lady Day 1744 totalled £2,060.[46] This was reduced in succeeding years, and on the succession of Sir Richard (later first Earl) Grosvenor in 1755 the practice of allowing rent to stand uncollected for long periods was discontinued.[47] Although evidence about the administration of the estate in these years is scanty, there is no indication that builders were hounded for back rent, and a willingness on the part of the Grosvenors to condone such casualness in the payment of rent must have helped builders to maintain an essential cash flow, particularly in the early years.

A measure of the extent to which the development of its estate was fostered by the Grosvenor family is shown in the previously cited account of Dame Mary Grosvenor's personal estate drawn up after her death in January 1730. Besides the £9,450 due on mortgages granted to builders, £12,000 was owed on a mortgage by Sir Richard Grosvenor (not necessarily, of course, used to promote the development) and £2,000 similarly by Robert Grosvenor. A further item was a debt of £4,747 due from Sir Richard Grosvenor 'to make good to the Personal Estate all such Sums of Money as have been disburst thereout to Carry on the new buildings, more than has been received from those buildings'.[40]

The Estate Agent

Little is known about the background of Richard Andrews, who was variously described as the agent, steward or 'receiver of the rents' for the Grosvenors' London estates when building began in Mayfair in 1720. He was then living 'next door to the blew Boar' in Great Russell Street, St. Giles-in-the-Fields,[48] and had first been employed as steward by Dame Mary Grosvenor in 1700, when he was some thirty-five years old.[49] In 1706 he was dismissed for alleged malpractice but was reinstated again in 1716 largely as the result of entreaties by Anne Grosvenor, Sir Richard's sister.[50] By 1730 his salary was £80 per annum and he also had an assistant, his second son Robert, at £50 per annum.[51] Robert Andrews was a member of the Inner Temple, being admitted in January 1725 when he was about twenty years old,[52] and he practised as a solicitor. He not only acted as London agent for the Grosvenors but also conducted the family's legal business in the capital.[53] No doubt partly because of his professional position Robert Andrews took a more considerable role in the management of the estate than his father, even before the latter's death in 1734 or 1735. He lived in a house in Grosvenor Street (No. 10, now demolished) from 1730,[54] and was also involved in parish affairs. He acted as attorney for the Vestry of St. George's, Hanover Square, between 1736 and 1744 and was a Vestryman

from 1741.[55] In 1763, the year of his death, he was still acting as London agent for the first Baron (later first Earl) Grosvenor.

A brief hiatus occurred, however, in the long stewardship of the Andrews family on the death of Sir Richard Grosvenor, the fourth baronet, in July 1732, when, as indicated earlier, his successor Sir Thomas Grosvenor wished to put his own man in charge. His agent was Robert Barbor, a contemporary of Robert Andrews at the Inner Temple, but the Andrewses refused to give Barbor the books and papers necessary to run the estate. Sir Thomas brought an action in the Court of Exchequer to force them to hand over the documents, but he died in Naples in February 1733, probably before the case had come to a decision. The Andrewses always had the confidence of Robert Grosvenor, now sixth baronet, and Barbor dropped out of the picture. He submitted a bill for services rendered to the late Sir Thomas, but he was probably little involved in the affairs of the estate.[56]

Both Richard and Robert Andrews were more directly involved in the development of the estate than their positions as agent would seem to warrant. Both took areas of the estate under building agreements and leases and proceeded to develop them as independent speculators by granting sub-leases to builders.[57] Robert Andrews, in particular, secured some handsome profits in improved ground rents;* for instance he obtained over £130 per annum from one large plot which he held under a direct Grosvenor lease, and £120 from another.[58] He was also concerned with others in the building of the Grosvenor Chapel in South Audley Street, eventually becoming its sole proprietor.[59] Both he and his father lent money to builders on mortgage,[60] but it is not always possible to distinguish those occasions in which they were advancing their own capital from those in which they were acting for the Grosvenors. The possible conflict between the Andrewses' role as agents (and trustees) negotiating with other developers and builders, especially after 1730 when there was no estate surveyor, and their activities as speculators profiting from the development themselves, did not seem to concern either themselves or the Grosvenors (with the possible exception of Sir Thomas Grosvenor, who, among other charges in the case brought against them in the Exchequer, alleged that they owed money in ground rents).[8]

Certainly Robert Andrews was a successful, and, by whatever means, a relatively wealthy man at the time of his death in 1763. His salary from the Grosvenor family was then £150 per annum,[61] but, besides his solicitor's business, he also held a post in the Excise Office and was the lessee of some revenues of the Duchy of Cornwall called the Post Groats, worth £400 per annum. Besides his residence in Grosvenor Street he also had a house in Acton, and his estate and effects were valued at £18,000.[62]

One of Robert Andrews' executors was his son-in-law and successor as the Grosvenors' London agent, Thomas Walley Partington, also a solicitor. Andrews' will established very complicated trusts, and the difficulty in carrying these out led to a case in Chancery in 1789, Andrews v. Partington,[63] in which certain legal principles were laid down on how long the number of persons eligible to claim a share in a settlement (in this case the number of Robert Andrews' grandchildren) could remain uncertain. The problem arose because Andrews' son, the Reverend Robert Andrews, had twelve surviving children at that time and claimed that he might have still more. The decision in Andrews v. Partington that a numerically open class of beneficiaries normally closes when the first member becomes entitled to claim his share (in this instance when the first grandchild reached the age of twenty-one) constituted an important legal precedent.[64]

Thomas Walley Partington, who was born in 1730, came from a prominent Chester family.[65] His father, Edward Partington, was an attorney who acted for the Grosvenors in that city.[66] Thomas Walley was admitted as a student to the Inner Temple in 1746[67] and in 1750 he was working as a clerk to Elisha Biscoe, a solicitor whose clients included a number of builders on the Grosvenor estate.[68] By 1753 he was associated with Andrews[69] and in the following year he married the latter's daughter, Elizabeth.[70] From 1757 he occupied a house in Brook Street and shortly afterwards also took over an adjoining house (the joint plot, later numbered 55, being on the site of Claridge's Hotel).[71] At the time of his death in 1791 he also had houses in Shepherd Street (probably the modern Dering Street near Hanover Square) and at Offham in Sussex. He does not appear to have been as directly involved in the development of the estate as his predecessors, but like Robert Andrews he had achieved relative prosperity when he died. According to the terms of his will his personal estate alone was worth at least £20,000.[72]

By 1779 Partington had formed a partnership with Edward Boodle,[73] who had at one time probably been his assistant (an Edward Boodle witnessed a Grosvenor estate deed in 1767).[74] After Partington's death Boodle became the London solicitor for the Grosvenors and occupied the premises in Brook Street which had been Partington's (they are entered in the ratebooks in 1789–91 as Partington and Boodle's).[71] The firm of Partington and Boodle, which became Boodle Hatfield and Company at the end of the nineteenth century, continued to occupy premises on the estate, in Brook Street until 1836 and then at No. 53 Davies Street, where its present offices are situated.[75] Thus a remarkable degree of continuity can be traced from Richard Andrews, who was appointed

* I.e., the difference between the total rent which he obtained by his sub-leases to builders and the rent which he had to pay to the ground landlord under his head lease.

receiver of the rents for Dame Mary Grosvenor's estates in Middlesex in 1700, to Messrs. Boodle Hatfield and Company, who are solicitors to the Grosvenor Estate at the present day.

The Estate Surveyor

Thomas Barlow, who was the estate surveyor when building commenced, was a carpenter by trade. Little has heretofore been known about Barlow but he emerges as one of the most important master builders working in west London in the early eighteenth century. The earliest known reference to his building work is in a deed of 1701 concerning a house, probably built by him, in Albemarle Street,[76] and he was also the builder of other houses in that vicinity.[77] His address at that time was in Maiden Lane, in Covent Garden,[78] where he was the building lessee of houses in Southampton Street in 1708 and undertook repairs to St. Paul's Church in 1714–15.[79] In 1715, however, he appears in a more significant role as 'agent' for Lord Scarbrough in negotiations with the 'Fifty Churches' Commissioners over the siting of a church near Hanover Square.[80] In view of Barlow's later position on the Grosvenor estate and the fact that Lord Scarbrough was the promoter of the development of the Hanover Square area[81] there must at least be a possibility that Barlow was responsible for the layout of that development. He was certainly deeply involved in the building operations there and appears to have been the builder of several of the houses with a distinctively Baroque appearance in St. George Street.[82] He was at one time owner of the freehold of the site of St. George's Church, but conveyed the ground to General William Steuart who in turn gave it gratis to the Commissioners.[83] Barlow was also active in the development of the Conduit Mead estate and built himself a house in New Bond Street where he lived until his death.[84] Barlow Place (formerly Mews) off Bruton Street is named after him.[85]

In a petition addressed to the Lord Chancellor Sir Richard Grosvenor stated that he had appointed Barlow on 10 August 1720 'to Lett Severall Feilds or Closes... to build upon' and that 'a Scheme or Plann of the Said Intended Building has been Drawn by the said Barlow'.[86] The purpose of this petition was to enable money to be freed from Dame Mary Grosvenor's account in Chancery in order to build sewers and to pay Barlow's expenses and salary. He was to receive £50 for the initial work he had undertaken and then £50 per annum 'besides his Reasonable Expences' (which generally amounted to £10 per annum).[87] He continued to act as estate surveyor until his death in January 1730,[88] but to what extent he exercised control over the operations of builders is difficult to determine. In one building agreement for a plot on the south side of Grosvenor Street and the south-east corner of Grosvenor Square it was stated that 'all and every of the houses which shall be built on ye said piece of Ground fronting Grosvenor Street aforesaid shall be built so as to range in their fronts in such manner as Mr Thos. Barlow the present Surveyor of the said Lunatick's Estate, or other the Surveyor or Surveyors... for the time being shall hereafter direct and appoint',[89] but this was an unusually explicit reference to Barlow, perhaps because the south side of Grosvenor Square was to be set back from the line of Grosvenor Street. As the author of the layout he appears to have been responsible for staking out plots on the ground and making some adjustments when building was under way, even correcting a 'grand mistake' in one instance.[90] The fact that several early leases were witnessed by the master of the Mount Coffee House (on the site of the present No. 80 Grosvenor Street), which was built by Barlow and was one of the earliest buildings on the estate to be completed (by November 1721), suggests that negotiations with builders may well have been conducted in that establishment.[91] One of Barlow's functions was the assessment of the value of houses in order that money held in Chancery could be made available to their builders on mortgage.[37] In general, however, neither the wording of agreements and leases, nor the surviving visual evidence suggest that Barlow exercised a very firm control over building operations, and when he died in 1730 it was not considered necessary to appoint a successor. Robert Andrews took over some of his functions and the post of estate surveyor remained vacant until the 1780's, when the assessment of fines on the renewal of leases posed new problems which led to the employment of William Porden.

Like Richard and Robert Andrews, Barlow was also directly concerned in the development. He was the recipient of the first building agreement (dated 8 August 1720, two days before his official appointment) covering the area bounded on the north by Grosvenor Street, on the west by Davies Street, and on the south and east by the boundaries of the estate (no. 1 on plan A in the end pocket), and he subsequently held all this land under one lease granted in July 1721. For this he paid the very low ground rent of £67 per annum, or *2s.* per foot frontage calculated on the frontage to Grosvenor Street only.[92] Within this area he built the Mount Coffee House and No. 75 Grosvenor Street (both now rebuilt) and some coach-houses and stables in Grosvenor Mews, developing the rest of his land by sub-leases to other builders or occupiers. In improved ground rents alone he obtained a profit of £280 per annum on this sub-development, which was substantially complete by the time of his death.[93]* He also took other parts of the estate under building agreements, including (jointly with Robert Andrews) the area bounded by Upper Brook Street on the south, Park Street on the west, North Row on the north and North Audley Street on the east (no. 55 on

* For the subsequent rise in value of this large leasehold plot see page 19.

plan A), the largest plot to be covered by a single agreement.[94] Building here had, however, hardly begun before his death.

Barlow was one of the founder-directors of the Westminster Fire Office in 1717[95] and was also one of the initial Vestrymen of the parish of St. George, Hanover Square, chosen by the 'Fifty Churches' Commissioners in 1725.[96] On his death in January 1730 he was described as 'a very noted Master-Builder'.[88] In a complaint brought in Chancery by his descendants against one of his executors it was stated that he left a leasehold estate which brought in about £600 per annum in ground rents and £400 in rack rents, several freehold houses and a personal estate of upwards of £1,000.[97] While there may have been some exaggeration in these figures there is little doubt that Barlow's career as a builder had been eminently successful. He left the bulk of his estate to his son, Richard, who died in 1740 'haveing greatly wasted and outrun his fortune'.[98]

The Layout

There was nothing remarkable about the terrain of The Hundred Acres either to pose difficulties or create opportunities for Barlow in devising his layout. The ground sloped gently from a high point in the north-west corner to the valley of the Tyburn in the east, the lowest level being in the south-east corner. The only topographical feature of any note was the remnant of one of the fortifications erected during the Civil War and known by the eighteenth century as Oliver's Mount.[99] Probably by then little more than a raised earthwork, it was, however, sufficiently recognisable to give its name to Mount Field and subsequently to Mount Street, Mount Row and the Mount Coffee House, and the development which began in 1720 was often referred to initially as 'the new buildings about Oliver's Mount'. So completely was it obliterated in the course of building that its exact location is difficult to pinpoint, but the evidence of a map of 1717 and some vague references in documents suggest that it stood near the junction of Mount Row and Carpenter Street, where a public house called Oliver's Mount was established.[100]

Barlow's layout of the Mayfair estate is an exercise in disciplined, straightforward town planning—a grid of wide, straight streets with a grand *place* in the centre—which makes no concession at all to the irregular boundaries of the land. The positioning of the main east-west streets, and consequently of the square which lies between them, links up with the layout of the Hanover Square area. Brook Street and Upper Brook Street are direct continuations of that part of Brook Street which joins the south side of Hanover Square, while Grosvenor Street and Upper Grosvenor Street are aligned with the axis of St. George's Church (which had, however, not been built although its site had been determined upon when the Grosvenor estate layout scheme was made). In Brook Street Sir Richard Grosvenor had to take leases of land in Conduit Mead, which lay between his estate and the Hanover Square estate, and enter into agreements with builders there—in one instance allowing a builder to have land on his estate on especially favourable terms—in order to prevent them building across the proposed line of Brook Street and thus blocking up this important line of communication with older established parts of the West End.[101] The reason for the positioning of Grosvenor Street is less obvious. Barlow knew that the street could not be extended as far as St. George's Church in order to provide a monumental 'vista-stopper', for the course of the narrow Maddox Street, which was to skirt the north side of the church, had been decided by 1718, and frontages to the street west of its intersection with St. George Street were being developed by the following year.[102] It is possible, though highly unlikely, that Barlow foresaw that the steeple of the church (the design of which had not even been decided) would provide an effective terminal point to the view down Grosvenor Street from the west, but, more prosaically, it may be that he simply chose a convenient position for the street parallel with Brook Street. From the wording of his own building agreement of August 1720 Barlow originally anticipated that Grosvenor Street would be extended as a sixty-foot-wide road as far as New Bond Street,[16] but in the event the street narrows at the eastern boundary of the estate. This awkward transition is effected by bringing forward the frontage of No. 80 Grosvenor Street where Barlow originally built the Mount Coffee House.

There are several references in documents to a grand plan in which the layout was expressed,[103] but this does not appear to have survived. A small sketch plan is folded loosely in a notebook in which Robert Andrews kept a brief record of agreements and leases;[104] several comments are written on it and it may have been a working copy of the grand plan. It is somewhat misleading, however, as a record of the intended layout, for it seems that some streets were added to the sketch plan at a date later than the original drawing. The best record of the layout as originally planned is the map of the whole of the Grosvenors' London property drawn in 1723 by John Mackay,[105] which shows Mayfair as set out for building (Plate 1). This part of the map has the measurement of foot frontages inscribed, suggesting that it may have been taken from Barlow's grand plan, and at the foot of the map the area is described as 'Grosvenor Buildings or the Fields Commonly called Oliver's Mount Fields; being Partly built and a Square And Eleven Principal Streets designed As per Plan...'. Few mews are shown, except in the area developed by Barlow himself, and the sites of these were probably worked out in the course of development. The evidence of this map suggests that alterations in the layout were made as building proceeded, particularly in the western part of the area. More streets were formed than originally intended, including Green Street, and the site of the projected chapel was altered. That some

of these changes were variations from the initial scheme is confirmed by documentary evidence.[106]

The extent of The Hundred Acres enabled Barlow to plan on a lavish scale. Grosvenor Square itself measures 680 feet × 530 feet between the building lines and covers over eight acres, its spaciousness increased by setting the houses in the square thirty feet back from the frontages of the streets leading into it (a device also used in Hanover Square, but not in Cavendish Square). The main east-west streets—Grosvenor Street and Upper Grosvenor Street, Brook Street and Upper Brook Street—were intended to be sixty feet wide and most of the remaining streets fifty feet. Even the mews were spacious, an impression now enhanced by the relatively recent widening of their entrances, which were originally left deliberately narrow to make the stable yards less obtrusive. Long, straight, unbroken lines of terrace frontage, so favoured by the early Georgians, abound, and would have been even more extensive if the original layout scheme had been scrupulously followed.

The Course of Development

The translation of Barlow's plan into the realities of bricks and mortar took over half a century to complete. The last leases, for sites in the north-west corner of the estate, were not granted until 1777,[107] by which time it was necessary to consider renewals of the earliest leases. The progression of the development was generally, and logically, from east to west, but the pace was by no means even. On the rudimentary evidence of the dating of estate leases (some leases being of large plots which were sub-let in smaller sites) there was considerable building activity throughout the 1720's, with 1725 and 1728 as the peak years, a slow-down from 1733 to 1735, a new surge to another peak in 1740, a considerable decline throughout the 1740's and early 1750's (only six leases were granted between 1741 and 1755), and a gradual development of the remaining unbuilt land over the next twenty or so years. The marked reluctance of builders to take sites near the north end of Park Lane and the western end of Oxford Street was probably due to the proximity of Tyburn gallows, situated at the present junction of Edgware Road and Bayswater Road, where public executions attended by vast and tumultuous crowds continued until 1783.

In general the frontages to Oxford Street and Park Lane were not regarded with any favour by either the officers of the estate or by builders. The whole development was at first noticeably turned inwards towards Grosvenor Square and away from the extremities of the estate, with the exception of the eastern boundary where it was clearly desirable to link up with existing streets. Although areas on the north side of Brook Street and Grosvenor Square extending as far as Oxford Street were taken under building agreements as early as 1723–5, the completion of buildings along the frontage to Oxford Street was in some cases delayed for over thirty years.[108]

In 1766 John Gwynn remarked disparagingly on 'that heap of buildings lately erected from Oxford-Road to Hyde Park Corner, whose back-fronts are seen from the Park'.[109] The wording of early building agreements for ground at the western edge of the estate suggests that this orientation was a matter of deliberate policy (although the layout shown on Mackay's map envisages buildings along the Park Lane frontage). Under these agreements ground rents were to be calculated by the extent of frontage along Park Street, and while it was usual to include provisions against the siting of coach-houses and stables along that street or in any of the main east-west streets, no such restriction applied to Park Lane.[110] In fact stabling was built there on a site now occupied by part of Grosvenor House.[111] One short terrace of houses facing the park called King's Row was built in the 1730's (on the site of the present Nos. 93–99)[112] but it was set back from Park Lane and quickly shielded from the road by a screen of trees (Plate 13a, b). Even in the 1750's when Norfolk (now Dunraven) Street was laid out the houses were built with their back elevations overlooking the park and their garden walls forming the Park Lane frontage (Plate 19b, c). In 1791 William Porden, the estate surveyor, remarked on the opportunity lost 'in originally laying out the ground of making a handsome front towards Hyde Park',[113] and it is not clear why Park Lane was so ostracized. Certainly in the nineteenth century it was a very busy road and was originally quite narrow: some stretches were widened in the course of building on adjacent land.[114] The park was concealed by a brick wall which was not entirely replaced by iron railings until 1828,[115] and, although a gate was provided at the cost of Sir Richard Grosvenor for the benefit of his tenants (Grosvenor Gate),[116] the prospect from ground level at least could not have been very attractive.

Building Agreements

Over the long period which was required to cover The Hundred Acres with buildings some ninety-three or more pre-lease building agreements were concluded with prospective undertakers,* the vast majority of whom were building tradesmen. The originals or counterparts of ninety of these agreements have survived among the Grosvenor Estate records, and the existence of three others is recorded although the documents themselves are lost.[117] There are a few plots for which no agreements have been found, but in at least two instances it is likely that no agreements were made before leases were granted —a frontage to Oxford Street taken by a brickmaker in

* The term undertaker is here used to mean someone who undertakes the development of a parcel of land under a building agreement.

exchange for an existing lease of a brickfield there, and 185 feet on the south side of Grosvenor Square leased to Robert Grosvenor.[118] The areas taken under building agreements are shown on plan A in the end pocket. They varied from single house sites to large plots covering several acres, the biggest being that taken by Thomas Barlow and Robert Andrews in 1725 (no. 55 on plan A). In most cases the agreements were made some considerable time before leases were granted of the land covered by them, and as soon as they had been signed they became negotiable documents. In 1728, for instance, Robert Grosvenor bought an existing agreement for a plot on the west side of Park Street (no. 61 on plan A) for thirty guineas 'and divers other good Causes and valuable Considerations',[119] and the houses subsequently built there became part of his trust estate. In a few instances agreements were surrendered and replaced later by others, but in most cases where the original undertaker was unable to fulfil his contract the benefit of his agreement was assigned to someone else.

Although the agreements do not follow a standard form they are generally similar in wording and indicate, at least on paper, a marked degree of laxity in the control of building operations. Under them Sir Richard Grosvenor or his successors (or in some cases Robert Myddelton, for the reasons indicated earlier) agreed to grant a lease or leases of the ground when building had reached a certain stage. This was usually expressed as within forty days of the first and second floors of the house or houses being laid, or within forty days of tiling-in. Sometimes it was specified that the street before the front of the house(s) should be levelled and paved to the middle before leases were granted, but more specific paving clauses were contained later in the documents.

When the ground taken included a frontage to a stable yard a stipulation was usually made that future lessees were to be granted the right of use of the stable yard and the horse pond, watering place, pump, water and dung place to be made available there on paying to the ground landlord a share of the costs of making the yard and its appurtenances proportionate to the amount of foot frontage to the yard. This requirement was invariably repeated later in the document, perhaps to emphasise the responsibility of the undertaker to ensure that such costs were met, and lessees were also required to pay their share of keeping the mews in repair on the same basis of assessment. Most stable yards were, however, situated entirely within the limits of the areas taken and in the majority of these cases no reference was made to them in agreements, the provision of mews presumably being at the cost (and possibly also the discretion) of the undertaker. Clauses relating to the use of such yards were, however, often inserted in leases, specifying that the lessee was to pay his share of the cost of making the mews, but not to whom the cost was to be paid.[120]

Clauses specified the term of years for which leases were to be granted and the ground rent payable for the whole ground taken under each agreement. These ground rents are discussed in detail on pages 17–19. As stated earlier, the leasehold terms not only varied from one agreement to another but were sometimes exceeded when leases were granted; and little attempt was made to provide a common starting or ending date for such terms, even at the beginning of the development. Under the first agreement of all the terms were calculated from Lady Day 1721, but the second and several subsequent contracts merely stipulated that they were to begin on the last quarter day before the date of each lease. From time to time, notably in the 1730's and in the 1750's, attempts were made to achieve some degree of uniformity in the dates on which leases would fall in, but the long delay before the development was completed nullified such efforts, and the last leases granted did not expire until 1864,[121] over sixty years later than the earliest ones.

Besides his ground rent each lessee was, in almost every instance, required to pay an extra rent if he allowed his premises to be used for certain noxious trades. This extra rent was usually fixed at £30 in the main streets, but was sometimes only £10 in the lesser ones, such as Mount Street. The list of such trades varied, being generally longer for plots fronting on to the principal streets, but some of the variations appear to have been arbitrary, and some leases contained longer or shorter lists than their parent agreements.[122] The most commonly restricted trades were:—butcher (both shop and slaughter-house), tallow chandler, soapmaker, tobacco-pipe maker, brewer, victualler, coffee-house proprietor, distiller, farrier, pewterer, working brazier and blacksmith. Occasionally in later agreements sugar baker and glassmaker were added, and in the leases of No. 88 Brook Street, No. 9 Grosvenor Square and a plot in Duke Street the occupations of roasting cook, boiling cook, silk dyer, hatmaker and 'scowerer of cloths' were also discouraged in this way.[123] More usually trades were omitted from the list, either in agreements or individual leases, particularly those of butcher (although slaughter-houses were generally still included), victualler, coffee-house keeper, farrier, pewterer, brazier and blacksmith. In some of the extensive back land of large plots only a common brewer or a melter of tallow was required to pay the increased rent.[124] However, in the whole area fronting north on Grosvenor Street and west on Davies Street, which was taken by the estate surveyor, Thomas Barlow, at the beginning of the development, no trades at all were restricted.[92]

The assumption implicit in this general policy was, evidently, that the extra rent would be a sufficient deterrent to the establishment of undesirable trades. The Grosvenors could hardly have been satisfied with the relatively insignificant additions to their income as compensation for the damaging effects of some of these trades if they had been conducted near to expensive houses. A tallow chandler was unlikely to prove a satisfactory neighbour for an earl or a marquis. A similar device had been used when building leases of Alexander

Davies's land at Millbank were granted in 1663 but there the penalty for noxious trades had been assessed at £200 per annum,[125] a sum more likely to discourage would-be practitioners of undesirable arts. In the eighteenth century, however, in this as in so many other matters on the estate, much seems to have been left to the good sense of builders and future tenants.

The agreements also stipulated that all leases were to contain 'Common usuall and necessary Covenants', a remarkably vague phrase to cover a crucial area of estate management, embellished in the first agreement to read, 'such common and reasonable Covenants and Agreements as are usually contained in Leases of Houses in London'. No doubt builders knew what to expect and the leases were somewhat more explicit (see below).

Although the clauses relating to the actual building operations varied in detail from document to document they followed in essentials a formula worked out in several early agreements. By this the undertaker was at his own costs within eighteen months to build, tile in and enclose on the ground floors (i.e., put in the doors, windows and internal shutters), or cause to be built, on the front of his plot, a good and substantial brick dwelling house or houses to range uniform in the fronts (i.e., follow a common building line with adjoining houses). Within twenty-four months he was to finish the house or houses and back buildings, put up good iron rails before the front and posts in the street, and do the rough and smooth paving work in the street. The work was to be completed 'as fully and amply in every Respect as if all the Particulars for Building had been herein expressly mencioned and Sett Down'. He was also to make the stables and back buildings as low as they conveniently could be and cover them with slate. The time allowed for completion was often varied, Barlow for instance being simply enjoined to proceed 'with all convenient speed', and was, in any case, rarely adhered to.[126] In some instances where agreements covered ground with more than one street frontage the undertaker was only required to build houses on the principal frontages, while other brick buildings, or brick walls where there were no buildings, sufficed for the other fronts (including Park Lane, as stated earlier).[127] In later agreements the type of paving to be used was more clearly indicated: footways up to the posts separating them from the roadways were to be laid with Purbeck stone, and the roadways before each plot with good rag or other paving stones to the middle.

What is perhaps most remarkable about these building requirements is their lack of precision, even by the relatively lax standards of the day.* In the absence of any further contracts (and the only others that have been found are between the principal undertakers and other builders taking plots from them or between builders and prospective purchasers) these agreements seemingly provided the only form of control in writing which the landlord and his officers had over the buildings to be erected on the estate. All that could be ensured under them was that a house would be of brick, would adhere to a uniform building line with its terrace neighbours, and being 'good and substantial' would presumably not fall down. Of course, it was also supposed to conform to the London Building Acts of 1707 and 1709 which required certain standards of construction, chiefly in order to prevent the spread of fires.† In only two instances was the amount of money to be spent on building specified—both, surprisingly, in Mount Street, where one undertaker was required to expend £300 within two years and another £200 within twelve months in erecting buildings 'for dwelling in'.[129] Under some agreements for Brook Street the houses to be built were required to be 'large'[130] while in Grosvenor Square (where the agreements tended to be slightly more comprehensive and will be discussed more fully below) it was sometimes stipulated that houses were to be not less than thirty feet wide by thirty feet deep. In general, however, throughout the long course of the whole development it was not considered necessary to modify substantially the terminology first employed, and the last agreement made in 1765 was hardly more explicit than those of 1720.

The undertaker had to guarantee that the leases offered by the ground landlord would be accepted, and on the execution of his lease, the lessee was to pay for the use of any sewer built in front of his plot, usually at the rate of six shillings per foot. At first this sum was paid to Sir Richard Grosvenor, but after his death in 1732 it was more usual to specify that the money was to be paid to whomsoever was entitled to receive it, and the phrase 'if he [the undertaker] doesn't build same' was occasionally inserted.[131] It was also usually stated in early agreements that a separate lease was to be granted of each house built, but this was often ignored and it became common practice to let large areas of ground under one lease after the total ground rent to be obtained from any particular plot had been secured by leases already granted, and in some cases even before.

The final clause in all but a handful of agreements required all disputes between the parties concerned, or between one builder and another, to be submitted to three named referees, or any two of them. Any decision made by them was to be accepted and obeyed within forty days. Exactly how this proviso worked out in practice is not known, but it may have made up for some of the deficiencies in the earlier clauses. In theory, at least, if the Grosvenors or their estate officers were not satisfied

* A model agreement of 1724 for developing the Cavendish-Harley estate in St. Marylebone, although also couched in general terms, contains more detailed provisions relating to the building work including the types of materials to be used; and an agreement of 1711 for building on the Bedford estate in Covent Garden also specified the storey heights and timber scantlings to be employed.[128]

† But the Acts were not always scrupulously observed, e.g. No. 72 Park Street where in the first three storeys the window frames are not set back the requisite four inches from the front of the reveals.

with the way building operations were being conducted they could submit a complaint to this panel of arbitrators. Unfortunately no record has survived of the way in which this procedure operated in practice—if it did at all—but it may be significant that provision for it was still being made in the last agreements concluded. One agreement stipulated that the parties concerned should act upon any decisions made in this manner 'without having recourse to Law or Equity',[132] and behind the employment of this device there may have been a desire to prevent the protracted lawsuits which so often arose in the course of building operations.

The referees who were chosen to adjudicate on disputes included some of the best-known architects and building tradesmen of the time. For agreements made between 1720 and April 1724 they were almost invariably Nicholas Dubois, James Gibbs and Thomas Barlow, although there is no indication that Dubois or Gibbs were in any other way connected with the development of the estate. Until his death in 1730 Barlow was always a member of the panel. Others who served as referees were Edward Bussey junior, surveyor; Benjamin Timbrell, carpenter; Joseph Stallwood, bricklayer; Edward Shepherd; Colen Campbell (for the last four agreements dated before his death in 1729); John James; — Barton, surveyor; Thomas Phillips, carpenter; Roger Morris; Robert Andrews; James Horne; Robert Scott, carpenter; John Phillips, carpenter; Thomas Walley Partington; William Timbrell, carpenter; and George Shakespear, carpenter.

Some agreements contained additional stipulations relating to the specific circumstances of a particular plot. In an agreement of 1723 with Edward Shepherd for an area on the north side of Brook Street with long frontages to Davies Street and Gilbert Street it was laid down that no stables or coach-houses were to be built in these 'cross streets' within two hundred feet of Brook Street.[133] Restrictions on the siting of stabling can be found in other agreements but were more frequently inserted in leases. Later agreements for the south-western area of the estate contained clauses reserving to the ground landlord the right to grant free passage to and from neighbouring estates along South Street or South Audley Street, with power to stop up the roads leaving only a footway.[134] Edward Shepherd, who contracted for part of the west side of South Audley Street as far as the southern boundary of the estate, received a concession granting him right of way into the adjoining property of the Dean and Chapter of Westminster which he held on lease, but this privilege did not extend to other nearby estate owners (such as Lord Berkeley and Sir William Pulteney) or their tenants without permission.[127] It is doubtful whether these conditions had any practical effect, but they were no doubt inserted in case undesirable developments on adjoining properties should require the restriction of communication with them. An agreement of 1720 for the eastern end of Brook Street made reference to the construction of arches and shores over the Tyburn brook to carry the roadway. One of the joint undertakers of this agreement also held adjoining land in Conduit Mead on lease and covenanted to continue Brook Street into that estate at its full width as far as his holding permitted.[135] When Augustin Woollaston, who may have been a brickmaker by trade, took land at the western edge of the estate in 1725 he had to contract to use any bricks which he might make from brick earth dug out of the ground there for his building operations on the estate, particularly the north side of Grosvenor Square, where he also held land under agreement.[136]

Even for Grosvenor Square itself, however, there were remarkably few extra provisions. The first agreements for the east and west sides in November 1724 and February 1725 were, indeed, hardly more explicit than those for other streets, but by March and April 1725 more clauses were being written into agreements for the other sides, and these were also inserted in leases of houses on the east and west sides. A share of the costs of making the enclosure in the centre of the square and maintaining the garden was to be paid, but the only additional requirements affecting the building operations were that an area eight feet wide from house front to pavement was to be made in front of each house, a ten-foot-wide pavement was to be laid with Purbeck stone, and the roadway from thence 'quite home to the said intended Square' was to be laid with 'common paving'. In fact the paving work around the enclosure was done at Sir Richard Grosvenor's initial expense and was subsequently added to the charge of laying out the garden, as stated earlier. A surprisingly late addition to such agreements (although contained in all leases or sub-leases of individual house sites in the square) was a clause granting to tenants the 'Liberty and Privilege in Common with other Tenants fronting on the said new intended Square of walking within the Garden designed to be made in the said new intended Square and of having and keeping a Key or Keys to the Gate or Gates thereof'.[137] Endorsements were added to some of the agreements for ground fronting on to the square stipulating that the houses erected should be at least thirty feet wide and thirty feet deep.[138] This condition was included in the last agreement (for the south side), but was still ignored in the case of No. 35, which, according to the dimensions given in the building lease, had only a twenty-five-foot frontage to the square.[137] Several other houses on corner sites in the square were also less than thirty feet in width.

Building Leases

In some cases, as has been indicated, some of the more notable deficiencies in agreements were corrected in the leases granted under them.[139] There were 460 such leases of plots ranging in size from individual house sites (and in one case part of a yard[140]) to extensive areas which were then sub-let in smaller building plots by their lessees.

Although by no means uniform, the leases generally followed a standard pattern. They were usually granted in consideration of buildings erected, in course of erection, or to be erected; the payment of rent; and the performance of covenants. Each was of a plot of ground and the building or buildings standing on it or to be erected there. Even in leases of individual house plots the phrase 'and all other buildings built or which may be built' on the same was often added, no doubt to cover stabling, offices or other out-buildings; but this phrase, if interpreted literally, gave the lessee complete freedom to cover the ground with whatever buildings he wished.

The term of years granted by such leases and the extra rent payable if undesirable trades were practised have been discussed above; the ground rents will be examined separately in the next section.

The 'common usual and necessary covenants' referred to in the agreements are set out fully in the leases themselves. The lessee undertook to pay the ground rent and the extra rent payable if he practised a noxious trade; to pay his share of the cost of making and keeping in repair the stable yard, if applicable; to finish the building within a specified time in a workmanlike manner; to put up rails and posts, and do the necessary paving work to the middle of the street; to build his stables or other buildings at the back of his plot to as low a height as possible; to maintain the premises in good repair; to surrender the buildings at the end of the leasehold term with their fittings intact; to allow to the landlord or his agents the right of inspection at least twice each year, and to put right any defects thereby discovered within three months. A further clause gave to the landlord the right of repossession in case of non-payment of rent in the usual manner of such leases.

The time limit laid down for completing buildings was usually six months but this was often varied. In leases of large areas containing a number of house plots a longer time was frequently allowed, and in one instance the lessee was merely required to finish his buildings 'with all Convenient Speed and as soon as may be'.[141] For houses in Grosvenor Square twelve or eighteen months were generally allowed. Many instances could be cited of houses which were not completed within the allotted span and there is no evidence of any attempt on the part of the Grosvenors or their officers to enforce such provisions rigidly. In one case, when a builder died after being in financial difficulties, partially built houses were standing in a deteriorating condition ten years after a lease of them had been granted to him, but Robert Andrews, acting for Sir Robert Grosvenor, agreed not only to remit the arrears of ground rent due but also to pay a small sum to the builder's principal creditor in return for an assignment of the lease in trust for Sir Robert.[43]

Additional covenants were included in leases whenever particular circumstances demanded. Often these were concerned with the siting of coach-houses and stables. In leases of plots which had their principal frontages on major streets such as Brook Street or Grosvenor Square and long return frontages to other streets such as Davies Street or Duke Street, a condition was often inserted that the building of stabling in the latter streets was either prohibited or only allowed if no entrance directly into the street from the stable was constructed, access being obtained from the mews at the rear.[142] Among the more unusual stipulations about the location of stabling was that contained in leases of sites on the south side of South Street in which it was stated that if lessees built stables on their plots they were not to keep dung in the street but were to 'sink a place...in the said Street...for the holding and keeping of such Dung and...cover the same over in a Safe manner even with the Surface of the said Street'.[143] In leases of plots with frontages on to stable yards, the use of the yard and its facilities was granted in common with other lessees of plots abutting on the yard.

The building leases for Grosvenor Square contained provisions about the square garden. In return for the privilege of 'walking in' the enclosure the lessee had to pay an additional annual rent (calculated at 9*d.* per foot frontage), the proceeds of which were to be used for maintaining the garden, watering the roadway in the square, and paying a gardener to look after the enclosure.

Ground Rent

Although the amounts of ground rent payable under individual leases differed widely, a general consistency can be discerned in the sums required under the various building agreements. The rent demanded for each piece of ground was either expressed as a rate per foot frontage on the principal front of the land (and occasionally on more than one front when the plot lay between two streets) or as a lump sum, which can sometimes be reduced to an equivalent rate per foot frontage.

In early agreements covering sites in Grosvenor Street and Brook Street the ground rents were usually 6*s.* per foot on the Grosvenor Street frontages and 5*s.* on Brook Street, the plots being generally 150 or 200 feet in depth.[144] For substantially larger pieces of ground on the north side of Brook Street, with back land extending as far as Oxford Street, however, the rate was increased. In an agreement for the area bounded by Brook Street on the south, Davies Street on the east, Gilbert Street on the west and Oxford Street on the north the ground rent charged was 9*s.* per foot, assessed on the Brook Street frontage, but the agreement was not carried out and when a new one was made with another developer this rate was reduced to 8*s.* per foot.[145] The latter rate was also paid for the remaining frontage of Brook Street as far west as Duke Street, with an equally extensive 'hinterland'.[146]

On the south side of the eastern part of Mount Street, where the southern boundary of the estate or the location of the parish burial ground prevented any great depth of

site, sixty to seventy feet being the average, rents of only 2*s*. to 2*s*. 6*d*. per foot frontage were asked.[147] Even on the north side, however, the figure was at most 3*s*., although the building plots (if not the house sites as eventually built) extended back for some 150 feet.[148] Mount Street was probably never originally intended to be more than a minor street, and the building of the parish workhouse on the south side in 1725–6 was in keeping with its lowly status.[149]

The ground rents for Grosvenor Square were not significantly different from those for Brook Street or Grosvenor Street. The first builder to take an extensive frontage to the square (the whole of the east side) was John Simmons, carpenter, in November 1724, and for 350 feet with a depth of 260 feet he agreed to pay £112 per annum, equivalent to slightly over 6*s*. per foot frontage.[150] For the same number of feet on the west side the undertaker's rent was £150, but his plot had greater depth and abutted at the rear on Park Street.[151] On the north side the rents ranged from approximately 8*s*. to 10*s*. per foot, but, as at the western end of Brook Street, the plots extended northwards for about 600 feet.[152] Most of the south side was let by Sir Richard Grosvenor to his brother Robert at only 2*s*. per foot frontage, but in the agreements which he made with builders Robert Grosvenor charged the equivalent of 10*s*. per foot frontage for sites which reached as far as the north side of Mount Street.[153]

To the west of Grosvenor Square the ground rents were more variable and, in view of the large areas often involved, were generally more favourable to builders than in the eastern part of the estate. For the extensive rectangle of ground between Upper Brook Street, North Row, Park Street and North Audley Street, for instance, Thomas Barlow and Robert Andrews were jointly charged only £150 per annum (apparently calculated as 5*s*. per foot frontage on either the Park Street or North Audley Street fronts, or 2*s*. 6*d*. on both).[94] Apart from the section of South Audley Street lying to the south of South Street, where the rents were equivalent to between 6*s*. and 9*s*. per foot frontage (and where houses of a high quality were built),[154] 5*s*. per foot for one frontage alone appears to have been the maximum amount charged here until the 1750's. It was not until June 1765 that a ground rent of a substantially different order was required when John Phillips, carpenter, had to pay £320 per annum for the last undeveloped piece of ground, the area bounded by Oxford Street, Park Lane, North Row and Park Street. This sum is equivalent to between 13*s*. and 14*s*. per foot if assessed on the long east–west frontage to Oxford Street, or to exactly £2 per foot on Park Street.[155]

The precise ground rent charged was no doubt often arrived at after negotiation with the builder or developer interested in a piece of ground. As early as 1721 Major Joseph Watts, who was one of the promoters and first directors of the Chelsea Waterworks Company,[156] had entered into an agreement to build on the whole site now occupied by Grosvenor House, and the rent charged had been 4*s*. per foot on the Park Street frontage (400 feet).[157] No building was then taking place so far westward and some five years later Watts appears to have wanted to reduce his commitment. Robert Andrews explained the situation to Sir Richard Grosvenor in 1726: 'Major Watts was this morning with Mr. Barlow and Me', wrote Andrews, 'about taking as much of the Ground He formerly held as would be sufficient for the building three houses upon. Mr. Barlow offered it for 10s. per ft. by Gros. Street front the whole depth into Mount Street but the Major woud have it for 6 and intends to write to You, to shew how reasonable it is for a person that has been so serviceable to the Family as he has been by projecting the Waterworks to have such a favour allowed him, of which I thought it proper to give You this informacion not doubting but You will easily make him sensible his Merrit is not so great in regard to his Services done the Family as he imagines.'[158] The rent now demanded by Barlow was in fact higher than the rate which he had been charging to the east of Grosvenor Square, and apparently no accommodation was possible for Watts did not develop any of the site. Andrews' letter also suggests that a somewhat more optimistic view of the ground rents obtainable in the western part of the estate was taken at this date than proved realistic in the event.

In 1734 Edward Shepherd, the architect and builder, who had already built several houses on the estate, made an offer of only 18*d*. per foot frontage for a very large plot between Park Lane and Park Street with a depth of about 600 feet from Oxford Street, the rent to be calculated on the north front alone. Andrews assessed the plot as worth 2*s*. per foot frontage on both the Park Lane and Park Street fronts: the difference was between £33 2*s*. 6*d*. as offered by Shepherd and £125 as computed by Andrews, who noted that 'there is no foundation to agree'.[159] Sir Robert Grosvenor duly turned down Shepherd's offer, but it was not until 1765 that the last part of this ground was eventually taken, the total ground rent received from it then amounting, however, to over £500.

Some parts of the estate were let to undertakers on particularly favourable terms in return for services rendered. The agreement with Major Watts in 1721 referred to above was no doubt the result of his role in promoting the Chelsea Waterworks Company which supplied the new houses with water. Another plot at the western edge of the estate was taken by Francis Bailley, carpenter, who was then building in Conduit Mead, in return for the assignment of some of his land there to Sir Richard Grosvenor to enable Brook Street to be carried through from Hanover Square to the Grosvenor estate. Bailley's rent was 5*s*. per foot frontage, 'being a cheaper price than the other ground thereabouts was... designed to be let for',[160] but he, like Watts, did not eventually build there. For similar reasons the triangular area now

bounded by Brook Street, Davies Street and South Molton Lane was also made available at a very low rent to two developers who had interests in Conduit Mead: parts of this site to the north of Davies Mews were not built over for many years.[135] We have already seen that in the very first agreement, made with the estate surveyor Thomas Barlow, for the extensive area to the south of Grosvenor Street and east of Davies Street, a ground rent of only 2*s.* per foot frontage on the Grosvenor Street front alone was required. No doubt this was partly in return for Barlow's services in laying out the estate and seeking builders to work there, but he was, of course, paid a fee for these activities, and another consideration in Sir Richard Grosvenor's mind may have been a desire to let Barlow have a piece of land on terms that would enable him to raise sufficient capital to develop it quickly and profitably, and thereby attract other builders to the estate. In 1730 the promoters of the Grosvenor Chapel were granted land adjacent to its site, on both sides of South Audley Street, at a rent of only 1*s.* per foot frontage in consideration of their 'hazard and expense' in building the chapel.[161] They were also allowed a five-year peppercorn term instead of the usual period of between two and three years.

The scale of ground rents on the Grosvenor estate was a good deal lower than that in nearby developments for which comparable evidence is available. In Albemarle Ground (the area of Albemarle Street, Stafford Street, Dover Street and Grafton Street) in the late seventeenth century rents ranged from approximately 5*s.* to 13*s.* 9*d.* per foot frontage for building plots varying from sixty-five to one hundred feet in depth, and the leases ran for only some fifty or fifty-one years.[162] On the Burlington estate (Cork Street, Clifford Street and Savile Row area), where building took place contemporaneously with the Grosvenor estate, the ground rents appear to have been calculated initially on the basis of 1*s.* per foot frontage for every ten feet of depth and varied between 7*s.* and 16*s.* per foot frontage for sixty-one- or sixty-two-year terms.[163] The calculation of the ground rent obtained from the development of Conduit Mead is complicated by the fact that some ground there was assigned to builders rather than leased to them. The total rent received for the twenty-seven or so acres was £1,076, or about £40 per acre. A report of 1742 estimated, however, that only two-thirds of the acreage had been let for rent, and if assessed on this proportion alone the figure was £60 per acre.[164] This compares with the final sum of £31 per acre secured in ground rents on the Grosvenor estate in Mayfair by its initial development,* and in Conduit Mead the leases were for less than fifty years.

All of these areas were much smaller than the Grosvenor estate, and in The Hundred Acres, where house building was being pushed some way beyond the existing urban limits, it was probably necessary to keep the ground rents at a low level in order to attract builders, particularly to the land near Hyde Park, where the rents were at first lower, in fact, than was desired or originally anticipated. In the event, however, several undertakers were able to obtain a handsome surplus in improved ground rents over the rent which they paid to the Grosvenors.

A remarkable example of the rise in value of such leasehold property occurred in the large area to the south of Grosvenor Street and east of Davies Street let to Thomas Barlow, the estate surveyor, in 1721 on a ninety-nine-year lease at £67 per annum. This was the largest piece of the Grosvenors' Mayfair lands to be let under a single lease and covered about six acres, now embracing, in terms of present streets and buildings, Nos. 55–81 (consec.) Grosvenor Street, Nos. 2–26 (even) Davies Street, Grosvenor Hill, Bourdon Street and Place, Broadbent Street, Jones Street and Nos. 25–31 (consec.) Berkeley Square. In this estate within an estate Barlow sub-let the land in building plots for at most eighty years (with one exception) and often for sixty or less, and from it he obtained some £280 per annum in improved ground rents over the £67 he had to pay, and £160 in rack rents. When Barlow's property was sold at auction in 1745 for the benefit of his descendants this very large plot fetched some £7,000. In 1792, however, when the whole area was again put up for auction, several of the sub-leases had already expired and others were shortly due to do so, giving purchasers the prospect of a considerable return in rack rents for the remaining twenty-eight years of the original Grosvenor lease, besides the possibility of renewals on favourable terms, and the sum realised amounted to over £58,000.[165]

Within the general framework of the ground rents laid down in agreements, the rents at which individual building plots were let varied widely and often bore no relation to the size or importance of the site. Sometimes the total ground rent required under an agreement was secured by leases of only a small part of the ground, and the remainder would be let (often in one lease) at a token rent, usually 3*s.* 4*d.* per annum.[166] Some huge pieces of land embracing two or three acres were let for such nominal sums, particularly between Oxford Street and the backs of house plots in Grosvenor Square and Brook Street. Even the rents of adjoining house sites could vary widely. To take one instance, No. 5 Grosvenor Square, with a forty-five-foot frontage, was leased to John Simmons, its builder, in May 1728 for £22 10*s.* per annum while No. 4, with a seventy-foot frontage, was leased to him in September of the same year for 4*s.* per annum, both for ninety-nine-year terms.[167] No doubt such variations were often made for the builder's convenience, to enable him to make a quick sale, possibly at an enhanced price, of a house at a low ground rent, or, as in Simmons's case, to enable him to create an improved ground rent which he could sell to raise money for his building operations.

* If the improved ground rents received from Sir Robert Grosvenor's trust estate are added the Grosvenors' total rental from their Mayfair lands amounted to £34 per acre.

Architects and Builders

The names of some 290 individuals who were connected with the building trade, either as practitioners of its arts and crafts or as suppliers of materials, are recorded in the documentary evidence relating to the development of the estate. These were the men who entered into building agreements, were direct lessees of the Grosvenors, or were sub-lessees of developers, and it can reasonably be assumed that there were also many more sub-lessees whose names have not been traced. While by no means all of them can have aspired to the description of 'master builders' they were nevertheless in business in a substantial enough way to be parties to various legal instruments, and must have been supported by countless journeymen, labourers and apprentices. Their activities on the estate were, of course, spread over the whole sixty-year period of its first development but the names of a substantial number of them occur in documents dating from the first decade, and it is not difficult to envisage Defoe's 'World full of Bricklayers and Labourers'.

A handful of these 290 can justifiably be called architects, although only two were actually so described. One of these was Colen or Colin Campbell, who described himself as Architect to the Prince of Wales when he was granted a building lease in 1726,[168] and the second was John Crunden, who was the building lessee of a terrace of houses in Hereford Street in 1777.[169] The others usually styled themselves 'esquire' or 'gentleman'. They included William Benson, whose architectural career had already been cut short before he appeared on the estate; Edward Shepherd; Thomas Ripley; Roger Morris; and Thomas Archer, who had a house built in Grosvenor Square but apparently not of his own designing. In the case of Shepherd and Morris, however, the line dividing them from an outstanding master builder like Benjamin Timbrell is indeed fine.

Any discussion of the role played by architects in the development of the estate must begin with the enigmatic presence of Colen Campbell. Sir Richard Grosvenor was a subscriber to all three volumes of *Vitruvius Britannicus* published in Campbell's lifetime and Eaton Hall is featured in the second volume of 1717, but no account of any dealings with Campbell has survived in the family archives, and if Sir Richard Grosvenor and his brothers had any views on architecture they remain obscure. Campbell was the lessee of two adjoining house plots in Brook Street in 1726 and on one of these he built the still-surviving house (No. 76) in which he lived until his death there in 1729 (Plate 33c; fig. 2e on page 107).[170] The ground on which these houses were built, however, was originally taken under a building agreement by Edward Shepherd, and it was as Shepherd's nominee that Campbell received his lease. In fact Shepherd had agreed to make the site available to Israel Russell, painter-stainer, and Campbell had subsequently obtained an assignment of Russell's agreement with Shepherd in 1725. Russell witnessed the lease.[168]

Although No. 76 and the now demolished No. 78 Brook Street are the only buildings which can with some certainty be attributed to Campbell, his involvement in the development of the estate was undoubtedly more extensive. We have already seen that in four agreements concluded shortly before his death he was named as one of the referees for settling disputes.[171] More directly, an engraving in the Gibbs Collection at the Ashmolean Museum shows the elevation and plan of 'Seven New intended Houses on the East Side of Grosvenor Sq^{r} as Designed by Colen Campbell Esqr 1725' (Plate 4b). The engraving was probably intended for publication, but the circumstances in which the design was made are a mystery. An agreement to undertake the development of the east side of the square had been signed by the builder John Simmons in November 1724.[150] Whether Simmons commissioned Campbell to provide a design, whether Sir Richard Grosvenor procured a design which he hoped Simmons would follow, this being the first side of the square to be taken by a builder (although no stipulation that any overall design had to be adhered to was made in the agreement), or whether Campbell's contribution was unsolicited is not known. Perhaps significantly there is some similarity between the east side as built by Simmons and Campbell's scheme. Simmons's façade was much plainer but it was nevertheless treated as a symmetrical composition with the ends and centre given additional emphasis (Plate 5). 'By this means', to quote Sir John Summerson, 'the block assumed the character of a single palatial building, and an important step had been taken towards a new conception of street architecture'.[172] Campbell's design was for seven houses, and Simmons's range, as viewed from the square, also appeared to consist of seven houses, but, in fact, contained an extra house on the south side with its entrance in Grosvenor Street. As in Campbell's design, the centre house as built was wider than the rest, but it had a frontage of seventy feet rather than sixty as shown by Campbell, and there were corresponding differences in the dimensions of the other houses. A reference in a letter by Robert Andrews in 1726 to a dispute with Simmons over sewers may be pertinent although it hardly clarifies matters. Andrews wrote, 'It was an unlucky misunderstanding at first but such a Genr! design as that is seldom ever carried on without oversights of that kind which makes it the more pardonable'.[158] Part of Simmons's composition survived in a little-altered state at No. 1 Grosvenor Square until *c.* 1936 and can be seen on Plate 8a.

There is another design by Campbell for Grosvenor Square, architecturally very similar, dating from 1725 in the Royal Institute of British Architects. This consists of an elevation and plans for three houses with a combined frontage of approximately 185 feet.[173] Again nothing is known about the history of the design. It is, however,

interesting to note that in April 1725 Robert Grosvenor was granted a lease by his brother of 185 feet of frontage on the south side of the square, but by August he was contracting with builders to sub-let the ground to them in building plots of such dimensions that the execution of Campbell's design would have been impossible.[174] Edward Shepherd took 180 feet on the north side of the square in 1725,[175] but he eventually built four houses there, three of them to his own rather grand design, which, although Palladian, cannot be related to Campbell's.

Two other designs attributed to Campbell in the R.I.B.A. have been associated with Grosvenor Square,[176] but they show astylar blocks in the manner of his Old Burlington Street houses or of his own house in Brook Street, and the dimensions do not fit any of the sides of the square.

One of the associates of Campbell who lived on the estate was John Aislabie, a former Chancellor of the Exchequer who had been discredited by the South Sea Bubble. In 1729 Aislabie concluded the purchase of No. 12 Grosvenor Square, on the north side, from its building lessee, John Kitchingman, a timber merchant, moving in during that year.[177] The house, which was demolished in 1961, had a Palladian façade (fig. 2a on page 106) and interior decorative features in the manner of Campbell.

Another member of Campbell's circle who had a house on the estate was William Benson, the architect of Wilbury House in Wiltshire, which was an early example of the Palladian revival. He had been made Surveyor-General of the King's Works in 1718, having manoeuvred Wren out of the office, only to be dismissed himself for incompetence in the following year.[178] Campbell was his Deputy Surveyor and Chief Clerk but also lost his position on Benson's disgrace. Benson was, however, well compensated financially and among other perquisites received the reversion of the office of Auditor of the Imprests.[178] In 1725 he and his brother Benjamin (who had replaced Hawksmoor as Clerk of the Works at Whitehall in 1718) jointly took an assignment of a building agreement for thirty-six feet of frontage on the south side of Grosvenor Street, where they had two narrow houses built (Nos. 45 and 46, now demolished).[179] William Benson lived in No. 45 from 1726 until 1752 and was succeeded as occupant by John Aislabie Benson, his son.[71] Whether Benson designed these houses, or what, indeed, they looked like is not known, and he is chiefly of interest in the history of the estate as a mortgagee of Sir Richard Grosvenor, to whom he lent £10,000 in 1732,[180] probably in connection with the extensive work then being undertaken at Grosvenor House, Millbank.

Of the architect-builders who worked on the estate, Edward Shepherd must rank as the most important, both in terms of the original extent of his work and of the amount surviving. He is first recorded on the estate in 1721 as the assignee of an agreement for a plot on the south side of Brook Street now occupied by part of Claridge's Hotel. In 1723 he was granted a lease of the house which he had erected (No. 47), and is there described as a plasterer, which accords with Vertue's account of his career.[181] In November of the same year he entered into an agreement to build on the north side of Brook Street between Davies Street and Gilbert Street,[133] and in the course of this development (and others on the estate) he progressed from calling himself a plasterer to firstly a 'gentleman' and finally an 'esquire'. It was for part of this ground in Brook Street that Colen Campbell was granted a building lease in 1726 in the circumstances described above, and, in view of instances where Shepherd obtained leases for building tradesmen who did work for him, it is possible that the two men were professionally associated in some way. Between 1726 and 1729 they lived within two doors of each other, Shepherd at No. 72 Brook Street and Campbell at No. 76.[71] Certainly by the end of the 1720's Shepherd had graduated from being a plasterer to being an assured if not outstandingly distinguished architect, and Campbell may have been his mentor.

In the absence of any evidence to the contrary it can be conjectured that Shepherd was responsible for the design of the elaborate interior of No. 66 Brook Street (now part of the Grosvenor Office), of which he was the building lessee in 1725 (Frontispiece, Plates 6c, 9a).[182] Four years later he assigned the house to its first occupant, Sir Nathaniel Curzon, and Curzon's account at Hoare's Bank records payments to Shepherd and his mortgagee but none to any other architect.[183]

His most remarkable design during these years, however, was for three houses on the north side of Grosvenor Square (Nos. 18, 19 and 20 in the modern sequence) which he united behind a Palladian façade of red brick above a rusticated, stuccoed ground storey with an attached hexastyle Corinthian portico as its centrepiece (Plate 5). The design was presumably in existence by April 1728, when an agreement with a bricklayer who was to work on the houses made reference to 'the modell plann or forme and elevation... which hath been made or drawn by the said Edward Shepherd'.[184] Originally the composition was symmetrical but within a few years it was made to seem unbalanced when the adjoining corner house (No. 21) was refaced to match its neighbour. Robert Morris wrote in 1734 that 'the same Architect did compose a regular Range for that whole Side, in which he has shown a Nobleness of Invention, and the Spirit and Keeping of the Design is not unworthy of the greatest British Architect; but the unpolite Taste of several Proprietors of that Ground prevented so beautiful a Performance from being the Ornament of that Side of the Square'.[185] That he had Shepherd in mind is suggested by his reference elsewhere to 'that Grandeur of Esqr; Shepherd's [range] on the North'.[186] The only other undertaker on the north side was Augustin Woollaston, a brickmaker, who received his frontage at the same time as Shepherd (March 1725),[187] but the first building leases

of his ground were granted in 1726,[188] some two years before those of Shepherd's houses.

No. 12 North Audley Street, which has an interior as fine as that of No. 66 Brook Street, was built on part of the 'hinterland' of Shepherd's ground on the north side of Grosvenor Square (no. 54 on plan A), presumably for its first occupant, Colonel (later Field-Marshal and Earl) Ligonier, who paid a rack rent to Shepherd for some five years before purchasing the house outright in 1735.[189] Although Shepherd was almost certainly the builder, there is a possibility that he was here working to another's designs, for on stylistic grounds there is a strong case for attributing the design of the interior, and in particular the splendid long gallery at the back (Plate 11), to Sir Edward Lovett Pearce, the Irish Palladian architect who provided a design (probably unexecuted) for a house for Ligonier near Dublin.[190]

Other large and apparently well-appointed houses by Shepherd in North Audley Street have been demolished but in South Audley Street more has survived of the range from No. 71 to No. 75 where he was the undertaker.[127]

Thomas Ripley's known work on the estate is confined to one house, No. 16 Grosvenor Street, for which he was the building lessee in 1724. He too had graduated in rank, from 'carpenter' in 1720 when he entered into an agreement to build on this plot to 'esquire' on receipt of the lease.[191] The first occupant of the house was Lord Walpole,[71] the eldest son of Sir Robert Walpole, and it was to the latter's influence rather than his own skill that Ripley owed his advance in the world. Ripley was also one of the first builders to take ground in Grosvenor Square, signing an agreement to develop the whole of the west side in 1725.[151] He was one of the parties to the arrangement with Sir Richard Grosvenor for the laying out of the square garden, but by the time building leases of his plot were granted in 1728 he appears to have relinquished all his interest under the building agreement to Robert Scott, carpenter, and Robert Andrews,[192] and there is no indication that he had anything whatsoever to do with the heterogeneous mixture of houses which made up that side of the square.

Roger Morris is first encountered on the estate in 1727 when (as a bricklayer from St. Marylebone) he was given possession of some ground in Green Street by Thomas Barlow and Robert Andrews, who were the undertakers for a larger area of which Morris's plot formed part. He built a house for himself at No. 61 Green Street, living there from 1730 until his death in 1749, and the building lessee of the neighbouring house on the west (formerly No. 60, but now joined to No. 61) was James Richards, who was the master carver of the King's Works and an associate of Morris.[193] In 1738 Morris, who had become master carpenter of His Majesty's Ordnance, built a large block of stables for the Second Troop of Horse Guards on the site now largely occupied by Green Street Garden.[194] To the east of the Guards' stables, on the west side of Park Street, he was also responsible in his capacity as developer for the erection of a terrace of narrow-fronted and apparently unremarkable houses between Wood's Mews and Green Street, all since demolished. The lessee of one of these houses was his kinsman, Robert Morris, the author of the favourable comment about Edward Shepherd's houses in Grosvenor Square quoted above, who lived in Park Street from 1739 until his death in 1754.[195]

The evidence relating to the part played by other notable architects is more fragmentary and in some cases entirely speculative. Nicholas Dubois, James Gibbs and, briefly in 1730, John James were named in several building agreements as parties to whose judgment disputes were to be submitted, and Isaac Ware witnessed the agreement with Thomas Ripley for the west side of Grosvenor Square, but none of these architects is known to have been involved in any building work on the estate. Henry Flitcroft is known to have undertaken alterations to No. 4 Grosvenor Square (the great centre house on the east side) for its second occupant, Lord Malton,[178] but his name also occurs in other circumstances in which his role is less clear. In 1728 he provided a mortgage of £400 on No. 12 Upper Grosvenor Street, which the master builder Benjamin Timbrell was then building for his own occupation,[196] and seven years later he witnessed an assignment of No. 6 Upper Brook Street (now demolished) from Edward Shepherd, who had built and briefly occupied the house, to Lord Gower.[197] Flitcroft was also associated with Timbrell in other enterprises, and, perhaps coincidentally, the widow of the Duke of Kent's son, whom Lord Gower was to marry in the year following his move to Upper Brook Street, had previously lived in a house built by Timbrell at No. 9 Clifford Street on the Burlington estate.[198] Later architects such as Sir Robert Taylor, James and Samuel Wyatt, or the Adam brothers, who certainly worked in the area, fall into a somewhat different category, for they were adapting or embellishing existing houses for clients rather than concerning themselves with the first development of the estate.

It is impossible to give details of the work of all of the building tradesmen whose names are known, and information about those who worked in the principal streets is contained in the tables on pages 172–95. Nevertheless the contribution of a few may be singled out. Prominent among the builders, if only by the continual recurrence of the name, was the family of Barlow. At least three generations of the family, which came from Forebridge, Stafford, worked as bricklayers on the estate, but lack of biographical information and the practice of giving the same Christian names to successive generations have made it impossible to determine exact relationships, or, in some cases, to be sure which member of the family was responsible for a particular building. There were four Williams, and probably two Johns and two Georges who were all involved in building work. The eldest William Barlow, sometimes described as William Barlow senior, was the son of Hugh Barlow of Stafford, husbandman, and was

apprenticed to a member of the Tylers' and Bricklayers' Company in 1705.[199] He himself took as apprentice in 1715 another William Barlow, son of George Barlow of Stafford, mason, and therefore perhaps his cousin,[200] and this may be the William Barlow, sometimes described as William Barlow junior, who built the two adjoining houses, No. 88 Brook Street and No. 9 Grosvenor Square.[201] William Barlow senior was extensively involved in the earliest building activity at the eastern edge of the estate and continued to be active until his death in 1743. He was appointed bricklayer to the parish of St. George, Hanover Square, in 1725, and in this capacity helped to build the workhouse on the south side of Mount Street.[202] He was also one of the four proprietors of the Grosvenor Chapel.[203] None of the houses of which he was the building lessee have, however, escaped rebuilding. His grandson, Sir George Hilaro Barlow, was created a baronet in 1803.[204] No relationship has been discovered between the Barlow family of bricklayers and Thomas Barlow, carpenter, who was the estate surveyor.

The position of Benjamin Timbrell as one of the foremost master builders working in the West End of London in the first half of the eighteenth century is well known,[178] but his work on the Grosvenor estate has not so far been recorded. He was the building lessee of some ten substantial houses there (including at least two in Grosvenor Square), of which No. 52 Grosvenor Street (Plate 8c; fig. 16 on page 136), No. 69 Grosvenor Street and No. 12 Upper Grosvenor Street survive in part. The latter was his own residence, where he lived from 1729 until 1751.[71] He was almost certainly involved in the building of other houses where he was not the direct lessee, and of the four proprietor-builders of the Grosvenor Chapel he is the most likely to have provided the design (fig. 7 on page 119). As one of the original vestrymen of the parish of St. George, Hanover Square, he often supplied plans for parish buildings, including the workhouse.[205] His son, William, also worked as a carpenter on the estate[206] and his daughter, Martha, married John Barlow,[207] the son of William Barlow senior.

With Thomas Barlow and Benjamin Timbrell, Thomas Phillips, carpenter, was one of the relatively few non-aristocratic vestrymen appointed by the 'Fifty Churches' Commissioners in 1725 to govern the new parish of St. George, and he also assisted in the design and execution of parish buildings including the workhouse (with Timbrell).[208] He had been employed, with Timbrell, as carpenter for the building of the church of St. Martin in the Fields and enjoyed a high standing in his trade.[178] On the Grosvenor estate he built houses in Brook Street and Grosvenor Square. From 1723 until his death in 1736 he lived in one of these houses, No. 39 Brook Street[209] (later partly rebuilt by Jeffry Wyatville), and his nephew, John Phillips, also a well-known master builder, lived there from 1741 until his death in 1775 or 1776.[210] John Phillips was the undertaker for the last area of the estate to be developed—in the north-west corner—and he was probably the builder of the two large, detached houses erected there, Camelford House and the house later called Somerset House, the latter apparently to his own design.[211]

John Simmons, carpenter, the builder of the east side of Grosvenor Square, was the son of John Simmons, citizen and cooper of London, and was himself a freeman of the Merchant Taylors' Company.[212] He was probably the John Simmons, joiner, who worked for Gibbs at the church of St. Mary-le-Strand.[213] Besides his considerable undertaking in Grosvenor Square he also built several houses in Brook Street, Grosvenor Street and Upper Brook Street. He had a house and workshop on the Grosvenor estate at Millbank,[214] and he was thus one of the few builders working on the Mayfair estate who did not live either there or in adjacent parts of the parish of St. George, Hanover Square. After his death in 1738 his widow, Elizabeth, continued his business until her own death in 1755. When their grand-daughter married in 1778 she was able to provide a dowry consisting of some property at Millbank and eight houses in Mayfair (including two in Grosvenor Square) which had been leased to John or Elizabeth Simmons and were then still owned by their descendants, having in the meantime been let on short-term leases at rack rents.[215]

Other builders who had a substantial impact on the development of the estate included Robert Scott, carpenter, who was also one of the proprietors of the Grosvenor Chapel (with Timbrell, William Barlow senior and Robert Andrews);[203] he was the builder of some ten houses in Grosvenor Street, Grosvenor Square and Upper Grosvenor Street, and of numerous other houses in the lesser streets where he was often joint lessee. Lawrence Neale, carpenter, who lived at No. 24 Upper Grosvenor Street (on part of the site now occupied by No. 93 Park Lane) from 1730 to 1745,[71] was responsible for over a dozen substantial houses, including three in Grosvenor Square. Richard Lissiman, mason, who was the son of a gunsmith from Colwall in Herefordshire and who died in 1733, was the building lessee of several houses in Grosvenor Street, including the important trio of Nos. 33-35 (consec.), and Upper Grosvenor Street.[216] Another builder who died at an early stage in the development was John Green, from whom Green Street almost certainly takes its name. He was drowned in 1737 when he fell into a well he was inspecting for the Marquess of Carnarvon at No. 43 Upper Grosvenor Street, a house which he had himself built some six years previously. He was then living in Green Street and was described as 'a very wealthy Builder'.[217] In the middle years of the eighteenth century the names of John Spencer, carpenter, and Edmund Rush, mason, appear regularly in the estate records, both as builders and developers of substantial areas in the vicinity of South Street, Portugal Street (now Balfour Place), Green Street, Norfolk (now Dunraven) Street, and the west end of Upper Brook Street where house-building was still in progress in the 1750's. Spencer

lived on the estate for several years, latterly at No. 60 Green Street (now joined to No. 61), but in 1771 he was declared bankrupt and quit his house, his subsequent movements being unknown.[218]

Building Methods and Finance

Sufficient evidence has come to light about the methods used by builders in the development of the estate to provide several specific examples of modes of building practice which were undoubtedly widespread in the eighteenth century. There are examples of co-operation between builders trained in different crafts, both directly in the few cases where specific contracts have survived, and indirectly in the granting of leases. The contracts are instances of what Sir John Summerson has called 'a remarkably efficient system of barter'[219] whereby the need for cash was reduced by offsetting one man's carefully costed work against that of another. In 1724 Edward Shepherd, who held under agreement the ground on which Nos. 66–78 (even) Brook Street were built, contracted with Thomas Fayram, mason, that he would procure a lease or assignment to Fayram of No. 68 Brook Street, then 'lately built but not finished', and in return Fayram was to pay him £606, half of which was to be in cash and half in mason's work, presumably at No. 66 and other houses in that range (see Plates 6c, 33c). The rate at which Fayram's work was to be measured was carefully set down, *viz.*—2*s.* per foot for Portland block, 1*s.* per foot for superficial plain work, 1*s.* 3*d.* per foot for the same moulded, 5*s.* per foot for white and veined marble chimneypieces and slabs, 2*s.* 6*d.* per foot for white and black marble squares, 1*s.* 6*d.* per foot for Portland paving, 1*s.* per foot for plain firestone hearths, 7*d.* per foot for Purbeck paving and 1*s.* 10*d.* per foot for Purbeck steps.[220]

An agreement drawn up four years later between Shepherd and Francis Drewitt, bricklayer, is even more informative. Shepherd, who was then in possession of a piece of ground on the north side of Grosvenor Square under an agreement of 1725, undertook to obtain for Drewitt a lease of No. 20, which was to be built according to Shepherd's plan and elevation, this being one of the houses forming his Palladian composition discussed above. Shepherd was to supply sufficient place and grey stock bricks at the rate of £3 5*s.* per rod,* and Drewitt was to do the bricklayer's work on two houses to be built by Shepherd in the square, presumably No. 19 and No. 21 (the latter being leased to Shepherd's brother, John, a plasterer).[221] For this Drewitt was to be allowed £1 6*s.* per rod including ornaments. He was to carry out the work according to Shepherd's plans and elevation and under Shepherd's direction. In return Shepherd was to do the 'Plaistering worke' on the front of Drewitt's house (namely the entablature, 'Rustick Story', cellar storey and the ornaments to the windows) at the lowest price customarily charged for such work. As soon as the respective work of each was finished the account was to be settled between them and Drewitt was to pay Shepherd the balance before he received the lease.[184] Drewitt, who signed documents with a mark, obtained £400 by mortgaging this agreement before the lease was granted.[222] The lessee of No. 18, the easternmost house in Shepherd's Palladian group, was Thomas Fayram,[223] with whom presumably a similar contract was made.

An unusually explicit reference to the barter system is contained in an agreement of 1755 between Edmund Rush, mason, who was principally responsible for the development of Norfolk (now Dunraven) Street, and Jacob Hancock, painter, who contracted to take a building lease of a plot on the east side of the street. The document states that 'Edmund Rush shall do and Perform or cause to be done and Performed all the Masons Bricklayers and Carpenters Works wanting and Necessary to be done in and about the building and Finishing the Carcass of the said Messuage or Tenement or other buildings to be Erected and built upon the said Peice of Ground...and whatever Sum of Money the same shall amount to... the said Edmund Rush doth hereby agree to Accept and Take out in Work and Business to be done by the said Jacob Hancock for the said Edmund Rush in his Trade or Business as a Painter'.[224] Other lessees of houses in the same range as Hancock's included a carpenter, a bricklayer, a mason, a carver, a plumber and another painter,[225] and similar arrangements were probably made with them, for Rush granted the lease in each case.

The mutual co-operation of several building lessees responsible for a long terrace range can often be assumed but surviving contracts between them are rare. One such is an agreement of 1742 between Elizabeth Simmons, the widow of John Simmons, on the one part, and Joshua Fletcher, mason, John Barlow, bricklayer, Lawrence Neale, carpenter, John Smith, timber merchant, and Robert Andrews, on the other. Elizabeth Simmons was in possession of 189 feet of frontage along the north side of Upper Brook Street to the west of No. 21, presumably as the result of an agreement made between her late husband and Robert Andrews, who was the head lessee of the ground, and she and the others mutually agreed to build seven houses there (Lawrence Neale being responsible for two). She covenanted to build her house 'with the same Expedition' as the others 'to the Intent that the whole of the said peice of Ground may be built upon and such Buildings carried up at one and the same time', and, moreover, she undertook to employ Fletcher, Barlow and Neale on the house in their respective trades, it also being stipulated that Neale was to obtain his timber from

* A clause was added at the end of the agreement substituting red bricks for grey, and for this change Drewitt was to make 'a reasonable allowance', presumably meaning that he was to pay for these at a higher rate. The houses were somewhat unusually faced with red bricks.

Smith's firm. For this work she was to pay them 'in ready Money', as she herself had no building skill to offer in return.[226] The seven houses, Nos. 22–28 (consec.) Upper Brook Street, were built, nearly though not quite as arranged (see table on pages 186–7).

Although the barter system could lessen the dependence of a builder on a supply of ready money, it could not eliminate the need for cash altogether. Some of the accounts of John Jenner, bricklayer, have survived among the records of a Chancery case which followed his death in 1728. These include bills from various tradesmen who had supplied materials or worked for him, with statements of what proportion of the account had already been settled. In only one is there a direct indication that part of the payment had been made in kind, Henry Huddle, carpenter, having done work amounting to £404, of which he had received £306 in cash and lime. One or two other instances of reciprocal arrangements can, however, be assumed from the system of accounting, for an account book kept by Jenner's executor contains entries of money received from Francis Commins, mason, partly in payment for bricklayer's work (presumably done by Jenner) on the same day as he, Commins, was ostensibly paid money for mason's work. Nevertheless for the most part Jenner and later his executor appear to have had to meet their commitments in cash.

The bills also provide evidence about the cost of materials and workmanship. For carpentry Huddle charged £7 per square (100 square feet on plan) for a house in Grosvenor Square, £3 per square for a house in Brook Street which Jenner built for 'Mr. Hogg' (presumably Thomas Hogg, lime merchant), and 45*s.* per square for coach-houses and stables. For 'Act of Parliament' bricks James Whitaker, brickmaker, received £1 per thousand. Daniel Wheatley, carver, submitted a bill in which his prices ranged between 3*s.* 6*d.* per foot for a frieze, 1*s.* 2*d.* per foot for bed moulding, 8*d.* per foot for door and window architraves and 3*d.* per foot for 'cornish'. He also charged £6 for thirteen fronts of Ionic caps (presumably to pilasters).[227]

Enrolments of many of the mortgages whereby builders raised money on the security of their leases, or in some cases of their pre-lease agreements, are in the Middlesex Land Register. The sum borrowed is not always stated, but there is sufficient evidence, nevertheless, to indicate the general pattern of long-term borrowing. The majority of mortgages were for amounts ranging between £100 and £500, chiefly at 5 per cent interest (the maximum allowable by law), although additional sums were often provided by mortgagees as building progressed. In 122 mortgages of building leases for streets other than Grosvenor Square between 1722 and 1760 the average amount borrowed initially from each mortgagee was £470. This rather high average figure is explained by a few instances in which substantial sums were involved. Richard Lissiman mortgaged No. 34 Grosvenor Street during the course of building for firstly £1,300 and then a further £1,125 from the same mortgagee.[228] Benjamin Timbrell borrowed at least £2,000 in two instalments on the security of a house on the site of the present Nos. 71–72 Grosvenor Street,[229] and No. 40 Upper Grosvenor Street was also mortgaged by its building lessee for a similar sum.[230] In Grosvenor Square, where the scale of operations was bigger, the loans were often of £1,000 and upwards. No. 38 was mortgaged for £3,500 by its building lessee, Israel Russell, painter-stainer, to a citizen and clothworker of London.[231] Nos. 12 and 25 were each mortgaged for £3,000,[232] and it can be assumed that similar or greater sums were borrowed for the building of other houses in the square where detailed record of the transactions has not survived.

The mortgagees came from a variety of stations in life, one of the largest sources of capital on the Grosvenor estate being, as we have already seen, the ground landlord. Among the many gentlemen and esquires were doubtless a number of solicitors and barristers, some of them identifiable by addresses in the Inns of Court. Widows and spinsters were prominent in providing the small sums necessary to maintain the essential flow of cash to builders, but a high proportion of mortgagees were tradesmen living or working in the several Westminster parishes. Among them were two apothecaries, a cordwainer, three fishmongers, a gingerbread baker, a linen-draper, two oilmen, a pattern-maker, a peruke-maker, a poulterer and a woollen-draper.[233] From slightly further afield were a brewer of St. Giles and a gardener of Chelsea,[234] while there were also merchants or tradesmen with City connexions, some of them members of various livery companies including the Clothworkers', Ironmongers', Goldsmiths', Cooks', and Farriers'.[235] There were also several instances in which builders obtained mortgages from timber merchants, brickmakers or even fellow craftsmen, but these were no doubt sometimes *post hoc* securities for materials supplied or work done. Few of the mortgagees were from outside London and most of these had addresses in the Home Counties. One of the most important was Philip Stone, a maltster from Shepperton, who lent money to several builders.[236] Richard Lissiman's mortgagee for No. 34 Grosvenor Street, mentioned previously, did hail from the provinces, however, being a gentleman from Hambledon in Hampshire. The clergymen mortgagees included Dr. John Pelling, the rector of St. Anne's, Soho, who advanced £2,000 to Edward Shepherd towards the building of No. 19 Grosvenor Square.[237] Among noble lenders were the Earl of Uxbridge, Baron Carpenter and the Dowager Lady Gowran; and Lady Mary Forester of Hampton Court lent £2,000 to Benjamin Timbrell.[238] At the other end of the social scale Richard Wood, a coachman, lent £100 on a mortgage of a house in South Street.[239] Institutional lenders are more difficult to identify, because the deeds relating to their loans were often executed in the names of individuals and do not mention the name of the firm or company concerned, but there is no evidence that they played a major role in the

supply of money to builders on the Grosvenor estate. A notable exception was the series of mortgages, amounting to £7,000 by 1743, obtained by Edward Shepherd from Christopher Arnold and Richard Hoare, goldsmiths, which were, in fact, loans from Hoare's Bank.[240]

Little is known about the majority of mortgagees apart from their names and sometimes their occupations, but John Aldred, a former seaman, is an exception. He had been captain of the 'Rochester', a man of war, and in 1710 was 'Commander of the Forces in Newfoundland'.[241] In 1731, when he was living in St. Marylebone, he began lending money to builders on the estate, and between then and 1734 he executed at least six mortgages for a total of £2,500.[242] In 1733 he took up residence in a new house at No. 15 Upper Brook Street (Plate 44b, far right, now demolished) of which he was already the mortgagee and lived there until his death in 1740 (see table on page 187).[243] He also had a country house in Buckinghamshire, and at the time of his death he was able to leave legacies of over £6,000, including £2,000 each to St. Bartholomew's and St. Thomas's Hospitals.[244]

Although much of the loan capital needed for the development of the estate was no doubt channelled through attorneys, scriveners were also very important in providing similar services. They not only acted as witnesses to transactions but were also sometimes parties themselves. James Swift of St. Martin-in-the-Fields, for instance, made several loans to builders, including £2,750 to Benjamin Timbrell and £2,000 to Thomas Knight, joiner, on mortgages of Nos. 28 and 47 Grosvenor Square respectively.[245] Whether he was using his own money or funds entrusted to him by his clients for investment is not known, but he also witnessed other mortgages,[246] as did several of his fellow scriveners.[247] The foremost member of this profession connected with the estate, particularly during the early years of its development, was John Hodson of St. Paul's, Covent Garden. He was probably an associate of Thomas Barlow, the estate surveyor, who had also lived in Covent Garden, and he witnessed both Barlow's agreement with Sir Richard Grosvenor for the large plot on the south side of Grosvenor Street and the resultant building lease.[92] He was also an executor of both Thomas Barlow's and his son Richard's wills.[248] No doubt profiting from this connexion he was able to extend his practice on the estate and witnessed a considerable number of building agreements and leases relating to it. He also provided a number of mortgages to undertakers and builders,[249] but in 1743 he suffered a fate more usually associated with his builder-clients when he was declared bankrupt.[250]

Evidence about other sources of funds apart from mortgages is less readily available. The accounts of John Jenner show that builders operated on an extensive system of short-term credit for materials and sometimes workmanship.[227] William Packer, carpenter, who was the building lessee of a house in Grosvenor Square, must have encountered financial difficulties for his lease was assigned in trust to creditors, and the deed of sale of the house contains a list of his creditors and their occupations. They included three timber merchants, a brickmaker, an ironmonger, a sawyer, two carvers, a turner, a joiner, a blacksmith, a painter, a lighterman, a butcher, a baker, a coal merchant, a carman and two victuallers including the proprietor of the Mount Coffee House.[251] Borrowing on the security of bonds and promissory notes was no doubt also a widespread practice, but little evidence of this has survived. There is, however, a reference to Robert Andrews lending £400 on a bond to Thomas Knight, the builder of No. 47 Grosvenor Square, before any mortgage of the property had been made,[252] and in 1743 Job Beasley, a servant to a resident of Putney, complained that he had purchased two promissory notes drawn on a builder who became bankrupt, but 'coming but Seldom to London', he had missed the declaration of the dividend.[253] Several mortgages must in fact have been executed to cover money already advanced and in many cases doubtless already spent.

One way to raise capital without borrowing was to sell annuities. This method would only be available to the large-scale undertaker with a considerable annual income, but there are examples of its use by builders on the Grosvenor estate. Thomas Barlow raised £1,500 by selling an annuity of £100 out of the rents and profits of his ground on the south side of Grosvenor Street,[254] representing a return for the purchaser of just over 6½ per cent.

When building was well under way it was possible for the larger operator to obtain cash by selling the improved ground rents which he had created in the course of development. There are several instances of this practice on the Grosvenor estate, where the level of rents required by the ground landlord was so favourable to undertakers. Unfortunately, as in the case of mortgages, much of the evidence occurs in the Middlesex Land Register, where the sums of money involved are only rarely stated, but from the available information the rate at which improved ground rents were bought varied widely. John Baker, esquire, was the purchaser in several such transactions, usually paying between sixteen and nineteen years' purchase, representing an annual return of about 5½ to 6 per cent on his investments. In April 1725 he paid £320 for ground rents of £20 per annum arising out of subleases of houses in Brook Street (sixteen years' purchase),[255] but in December of the same year he paid £142 10*s.* for rents amounting to £7 10*s.* (nineteen years' purchase).[256] In the following year he paid £635 for several houses on the east side of Duke Street let on subleases at rents totalling £35,[257] and two years later he paid Edward Shepherd £1,100 for a rent of £59 9*s.* from thirteen houses in James (now Gilbert) Street (both between eighteen and nineteen years' purchase).[258] In 1728 Henry Huddle, carpenter, paid a sum equivalent to twenty years' purchase to buy the rent for

which he was liable under a sub-lease of a plot in Mount Street.[259]

In some cases, however, the rate was twenty-one years or longer, giving a return of under 5 per cent. A document among the papers relating to John Jenner, referred to earlier, values the improved rents arising from his building activities at twenty-two years' purchase. This may well have been an optimistic assessment, for in 1729 Francis Commins, mason, paid £210 for £10 worth of rents from Jenner's executor.[260] In 1739 Abraham Crop, a merchant, bought a plot of ground on which a rent of £69 10*s*. had been secured for £1,459 10*s*.[261] Both these sums were equivalent to twenty-one years' purchase, and this was also the basis on which Robert Grosvenor paid John Simmons for the improved ground rents of houses on the east side of Grosvenor Square in 1731–2. In 1733, however, he bought the increased rent of the large centre house there at twenty-three-and-a-half years' purchase,[42] his willingness to pay this exceptionally high price being probably due to his wish to provide a stimulus to the whole development by the completion of such an important house.

The builder who was fortunate would find a purchaser for a house either before work had begun or when the building was only in carcase. In a few instances leases were granted to the first occupants of houses on the estate rather than to building tradesmen, but in only one of these cases has the contract which was presumably made as a matter of course between the respective parties come to light. This is an agreement of 1769 concerning the large house at the north end of Park Lane (later known as Somerset House, Plate 14b) which was leased to Viscount Bateman in 1773.[262] By this contract John Phillips, who held the land under a building agreement of 1765 (no. 92 on plan A), undertook to build a house and stables for Bateman at a cost of £6,500 plus an extra £500 for an abatement in ground rent. The document contains several detailed provisions relating to the building work including the dimensions of the timbers to be used.[263] At No. 48 Upper Grosvenor Street (fig. 2c on page 107), where the lessee, Colonel William Hanmer, was the first occupant, the builder of the house, Robert Phillips, bricklayer, was a party to the lease,[264] and it is known that a contract for building the house was made between Phillips and Hanmer. It apparently contained detailed specifications and was endorsed with accounts of the partial payments made by Hanmer as the work progressed.[265]

Two examples of large and imposing houses which were purchased before completion are Nos. 34 and 52 Grosvenor Street, both of which survive, albeit in altered states (Plates 8c, 9b; figs. 16–17 on pages 136–7). A building lease of No. 52 was granted to Benjamin Timbrell in November 1724,[266] and in March 1725 Sir Thomas Hanmer, the former Speaker of the House of Commons, agreed to pay Timbrell £4,250 for the house which was 'now erected or in building' and was 'to be finished in the best manner now used'.[267] Hanmer's accounts show that the payments were spread over eighteen months as building work progressed, and he moved in at Michaelmas 1726. As well as the purchase money Hanmer paid sums to other craftsmen for work in fitting up the house, and Timbrell allowed him a reduction of £60 from the stated price 'for the Staircase', presumably because Hanmer had employed Giovanni Bagutti, the eminent Italian plasterer, on the embellishment of the staircase compartment rather than entrust the work to Timbrell.[268]

A similar arrangement was made at No. 34 Grosvenor Street, for which Sir Paul Methuen paid £4,500 to its building lessee, Richard Lissiman, in 1728, some three years after Lissiman had been granted the lease.[269] Methuen held back £500 of the purchase money until certain works were completed and a memorandum was drawn up setting these out in detail. Among the specifications was the instruction that Lissiman should 'wainscoat the Staircase with Oak, in the same manner as the Staircase is wainscoated, in the house where Sir Thomas Hanmer now lives. And...cover all that part of the Staircase and Sealing above it, that is plaisterd, with Ornaments of Stucco, to the Satisfaction of Sir Paul; But with this Express condition, that Mr. Lissiman is not to be at any greater Expence for the same then [*sic*] forty pounds. So that if Sir Paul should be desirous to have it done very finely Mr. Lissiman shall be obliged to contribute forty pounds towards ye Charge of it, and no more'.[270] Surviving bills indicate that Methuen, too, made extra payments to craftsmen for work at the house, although there is no bill for plasterwork.[271]

A shortened version of one contract shows that shortly after receiving his building lease of the house on the west corner of Duke Street and Grosvenor Square William Barlow junior agreed to complete the house according to the requirements of Thomas Archer of Whitehall, esquire (the architect), after which Archer was to have the option of purchasing it for £1,600. Although all the provisions are not known Archer's general instruction seems to have been that the house should be finished in the same manner as No. 9 in the square, at the opposite corner of Duke Street, which Barlow had built previously.[272] Barlow borrowed £650 from Archer to complete the house, but in January 1727 he was declared bankrupt, and by November of the same year Archer was complaining that the house was still unfinished and was 'now in a ruinous and destructive manner, open and exposed to the wind and rain'.[273] In February 1728 Barlow's assignees in bankruptcy conveyed the house to Archer for an unknown amount.[274]

Undoubtedly the most unusual method of selling a house was the raffle held for No. 4 Grosvenor Square, the centre house on the east side with a seventy-foot frontage (the largest in the square). This imposing mansion was built by John Simmons and was valued at £10,000, but it was described by his widow as 'not being every Body's Money'. She devised a scheme to sell 39,999 tickets at 5*s*. 3*d*. each, with a free ticket for anyone who bought

twenty-four. The raffle, which was held on 8 June 1739, was won jointly by the wife of a grocer in Piccadilly and her lodger, who sold the house to the Duke of Norfolk. According to *The Gentleman's Magazine* the Duke paid £7,000, but the deeds seem to indicate that the price was only £4,725, a remarkably low sum for such a large house.[275]

The highest price known to have been paid for a new house on the estate was £7,500 in 1730 for No. 19 Grosvenor Square, which was described as 'the fine House... built by Mr. Shepherd the famous Architect'.[276] With a sixty-foot frontage and a handsome Palladian façade it was perhaps originally the grandest house in the square. In 1731 No. 7 Grosvenor Square was let to Lord Weymouth for seven years at a peppercorn rent for the first year and £396 per annum thereafter with an option to purchase the house within three years for £6,400, the price to include four coach-houses in the mews behind.[277] Other known prices paid to their builders for houses in the square were £5,250 for No. 18, £4,800 for No. 17, £4,200 for No. 12 and £3,400 each for Nos. 44 and 46.[278] No. 34, however, which was a smaller house on a corner site, sold for £1,750.[279]

Substantial sums were also paid for houses in other streets. The £4,500 paid by Sir Paul Methuen for No. 34 Grosvenor Street, a house with a forty-three-foot frontage, and the £4,250 paid by Sir Thomas Hanmer for No. 52 in the same street, with a fifty-foot frontage, have already been cited. No. 51 Grosvenor Street (fig. 2b on page 106), another imposing five-bay house next door to Hanmer's, was purchased in 1726 by Sir John Werden for £3,900.[280] According to a contemporary newspaper report the Hon. John St. John paid £4,000 in 1738 for a house with over forty feet of frontage which now forms part of No. 75 South Audley Street, and from the evidence of his account at Hoare's Bank Sir Nathaniel Curzon paid £3,000 in 1729 for No. 66 Brook Street (Frontispiece; Plates 6c, 9a), both of these houses being built by Edward Shepherd.[281] Another large house with a thirty-five-foot frontage on the site of the present No. 32 Grosvenor Street was sold in 1726 for £2,800 to Charles Edwin, a Welsh landowner who was later M.P. for Westminster.[282]

The £5,000 paid in 1740 by the second Baron Conway (later created Earl and finally Marquess of Hertford) for No. 16 Grosvenor Street, a house with a fifty-five-foot frontage, comes into a slightly different category. Although Lord Conway paid the money to Thomas Ripley, the builder of the house, he was not the first occupant, No. 16 having already been inhabited for some fifteen years by Lord Walpole, the son of Sir Robert Walpole, who was Ripley's principal patron, and other instances have been found where houses acquired an enhanced value after having been lived in for some years.[283]

Prices in the region of £1,000 appear to have been usual for smaller houses in the principal streets. The 'Fifty Churches' Commissioners paid £1,300 to its builder for No. 15 Grosvenor Street,[284] and No. 35 Grosvenor Street was sold for only £1,250[285] even though it stood next door to Sir Paul Methuen's grand house which cost him nearly four times that sum, and moreover was built at the same time by the same builder. Another house in Grosvenor Street, on the site of No. 65, was purchased by a widow in 1726 for £1,240.[286] On the north side of Brook Street to the east of Davies Street prices were significantly lower, two houses on the site of the present Nos. 52 and 54 with twenty-foot frontages selling for £500 and £550 in 1725.[287] In the lesser streets, with one or two notable exceptions, they tended to be lower still. In 1737 Captain Robert Booth paid only £180 to Edward Shepherd for No. 11 North Audley Street,[288] a house which still survives behind a later façade and which was even smaller than its twenty-two-foot frontage suggests. A house in James (now Gilbert) Street sold for £250 in 1726 and one in South Audley Street in 1730 for £275.[289]

Rack-rental values also varied widely. In auction particulars dating from about 1745 of the estate which had belonged to Thomas Barlow, the annual value of twenty-five houses on the south side of Grosvenor Street is given.[21] The average was £88, the highest being £220 for a house with a forty-two-foot frontage built by Benjamin Timbrell. Francis Salvadore, a merchant in the City, paid Edward Shepherd £250 per annum on behalf of the Portuguese ambassador for No. 74 South Audley Street,[290] and the Earl of Chesterfield paid £240 yearly for No. 45 Grosvenor Square (with an option to purchase the house for £4,200 which he did not take up).[291] There is, however, a remarkable contrast between the £396 per annum paid by Lord Weymouth for No. 7 Grosvenor Square and the annual rent of £24 which Richard Barlow, Thomas Barlow's son, paid Edward Shepherd for a house in North Audley Street.[292] Some houses built by John Jenner in Mount Row were valued at an even lower figure, for his widow stated that five of them were worth annually only £60 altogether.[293]

Perhaps understandably there is more clear evidence about the failures of builders than their successes, but some at least left their descendants in a comfortable if not vastly wealthy state. The example of Thomas Barlow, who was also the estate surveyor, is given on page 12. Thomas Richmond, a carpenter from Soho who built three houses in Grosvenor Square, left an estate consisting chiefly of leasehold houses worth over £8,000 at his death in 1739.[294] Edward Shepherd, although indebted to Hoare's Bank, was also in a basically sound financial position at the time of his death in 1747. His widow sold some of his property to clear his debts, and after a long series of disputes the bulk of his estate was sold at the end of the eighteenth century for over £13,000.[295] When Benjamin Timbrell died in 1754 his daughter claimed that he owned freehold land and houses to the annual value of £1,000 and leasehold ground on which he had built 'several large and magnificent Dwelling Houses', which, together with his money, stocks and other securities, gave him a personal estate of £20,000, but

that his executors were defrauding her of her share of the inheritance by claiming that he died in mean and low circumstances.[296] One is more inclined to believe her side of the story, but even a successful builder such as Timbrell could find his affairs severely compromised at times. John Green was described as 'a very wealthy Builder' at the time of his unfortunate demise in 1737[297] and when his son died two years later he was said to be 'possessed of a plentiful Estate',[298] but nevertheless the Grosvenors do not appear to have been able to recover the money owed by Green towards the cost of making the garden in Grosvenor Square.[36] It may be noted that, with the possible exception of Green, all of these builders had extensive interests outside the Grosvenor estate.

The bankruptcy records for the years 1720–75 show that commissions of bankruptcy were awarded against 38 of the 290 known builders or allied tradesmen working on the estate.[299] There is, however, evidence that many builders became insolvent without actually being declared bankrupt and that in several cases the assets of a builder at his death were insufficient to meet his liabilities. A document among the estate records dating from about 1738, with revisions made some years later, lists the amounts still owing from builders for the laying-out of the garden of Grosvenor Square.[36] This indicates that of the thirty-one builders or firms to take plots around the square, eight became bankrupt and at least another eight died either insolvent or with insufficient funds to complete the payments.* Of the eight bankruptcies, seven can be confirmed from other sources and there is little reason to doubt the basic accuracy of this record, which was intended to aid in the recovery of money owed to the estate. Typical of several marginal comments on the document is that beside the name of Francis Bailley which reads 'A prisoner many years and not worth a shilling', with the single word 'dead' added later, evidently to conclude the matter.

Some indication of the narrow margin under which builders operated is given in a letter from the builder Roger Blagrave's solicitor to Robert Andrews in 1744 or 1745. Blagrave, who built several substantial houses in South Audley Street, South Street and Park Street, had apparently made an addition to one of his houses which extended beyond the limits of his building plot and was consequently having difficulty in obtaining a building lease. His solicitor claimed that as a result Blagrave was unable to borrow money to complete the house and concluded, with no doubt pardonable overstatement on behalf of his client, that 'The Man has laid out all his Substance and many Years Constant Labour in these Houses and if he Cannot Obtain a Term in this peice must be inevitably Ruined and cannot get Money to pay his Journeymen another Weeks Wages and is really very Deserving'.[300]

Other Features of the Development

Of the two features often considered essential for the success of a large scheme of development—a church and a market—the Grosvenor estate initially provided only the former. In some ways this might have been considered the less needed, for the large new church of St. George, Hanover Square, was consecrated in 1725 and the Grosvenors assisted firstly the 'Fifty Churches' Commissioners and then the authorities of the new parish after its formation in 1725 in a series of ways. In 1723 they sold the freehold of one and a half acres near the southern boundary of their estate to provide a burial ground for the church.[301] The price of £315, or £210 per acre, if calculated on the normal basis of thirty years' purchase of an assumed ground rent of £7 per acre, was little more than the agricultural value of the land and was well below the potential value realized in the course of development. They later also sold the freehold of No. 15 Grosvenor Street at thirty years' purchase of the ground rent of £4 10*s*. to the Commissioners as a residence for the rector of St. George's,[302] and allowed a workhouse for the parish to be built in Mount Street on a ninety-nine-year lease.[303]

The provision of a chapel near the western boundary of the estate was, however, planned from the first,[105] and when the land for it was made available in 1730 to the three building tradesmen and Robert Andrews who were jointly to build it, the words of the agreement made it plain that spiritual considerations were subordinated to practical aims. The preamble stated that, 'As well for the Conveniency and Accomodation of the severall Tenants or Inhabitants of new Houses lately built... lyeing in and about Grosvenor Square... As also for the Encouraging and promoting of building in Generall upon such parts of the said Estate as yet remain unbuilt It hath been adjudged and thought proper to erect a Chappell'.[203] Sir Richard Grosvenor assisted the chapel's proprietors by granting contiguous building land in South Audley Street to them at very low ground rents, but apart from reserving pews for his family and servants he did not directly involve himself in its erection and management, even though it eventually became known as the Grosvenor Chapel (Plate 12b; fig. 7 on page 119). In 1732 he sold the fee simple of its site to the rector and churchwardens of St. George's as a means of resolving the problem that the vaults under the chapel could not be consecrated for burials unless the ground were held freehold by the parish.[304]

The burial ground and the sites of the rectory and chapel were the only parts of the estate sold freehold during the eighteenth century. Another Anglican proprietary chapel, St. Mary's, was, however, built in 1762 on leasehold ground at the south-east corner of Park Street and Green Street.[305]

* It should be noted that these failures did not necessarily arise from the engagements in Grosvenor Square alone, for the builders concerned also had commitments elsewhere.

The Grosvenors did not promote the development of a market on their estate until the 1780's when Grosvenor Market, occupying an inconveniently situated site at the north-east corner of the estate in the northern part of the triangle bounded by South Molton Lane, Davies Street and Davies Mews, was erected partly by speculative building and partly under contract.[306] It was not a success, for a rival market called St. George's Market had just been established to the east of James (now Gilbert) Street. This was on part of a large plot on the north side of Brook Street which had been leased in 1726 to Edward Shepherd for ninety-nine years, and in this lease the only trades listed as noxious had been those of brewer and melter of tallow.[307] The ground landlord therefore had virtually no control here, and in many other areas of the estate few trades were restricted and shops had been established from an early date. A petition by the builders of Grosvenor Market complained of such shops, particularly those of butchers, who, the petitioners thought, were defying their lease covenants, in Oxford Street, Chapel Street, North and South Audley Streets, North Row, Park Street, Davies Street, Mount Street and Duke Street.[308] Both the Westminster poll books of 1749 and a list of householders in the parish of St. George, Hanover Square, dating from *c.* 1790, show that a substantial proportion of the occupants of these and other streets were indeed tradesmen (see Chapter V).[309] Grosvenor Market nevertheless struggled on for some decades, but it gradually ceased to be a centre for retail trade, and the whole site was redeveloped in 1890.

Taverns and coffee houses were also, originally, extremely numerous, and the very first building to be completed on the estate was probably the Mount Coffee House at the eastern end of Grosvenor Street.[310] Although some attempt was made in early building agreements to restrict them to the mews or minor streets they were soon to be found in all parts of the estate except Grosvenor Square. In the main streets they were generally confined to corner sites where the entrance and sign could be sited less obtrusively in a side street or alley.[311] The death in 1739 of Mr. Fellows, master of the Three Tuns tavern in Grosvenor Street, was reported in *The London Daily Post*, where he was described as 'well known among the Builders; and is said to have died rich'.[312] Building workers no doubt provided a large part of the clientele of such places in the early years.

A supply of water was obtained from the Chelsea Water Works Company, which was incorporated under an Act of 1722 and which obtained a royal warrant in 1725 to build a reservoir at the eastern edge of Hyde Park to supply *inter alia* the new buildings about Oliver's Mount (Plate 2). Water for the reservoir came from a system of basins and canals connected with the Thames on the Grosvenors' Pimlico property, and at first had to be raised to the higher levels of Mayfair by horse power until pumping machinery was installed in 1742. The reservoir was converted into an ornamental basin with a fountain in the middle in 1835 and its (much diminished) site is now occupied by the fountain to the south of Grosvenor Gate.[313]

The Chelsea Company's supply was, however, by no means adequate at all times and for all purposes. In 1742 a man who was employed by the inhabitants of Grosvenor Street to water the roadway during the summer complained to the Westminster Commissioners of Sewers of irregularities in supply, 'the said Water not coming in sometimes for a fortnight together'. He sought permission to obtain the water which he needed from the common sewer flowing under Avery Row, and this request was granted.[314] Some houses had private wells, as is evidenced by the fate of John Green, the builder, who drowned when he fell into one at No. 43 Upper Grosvenor Street.

An ancient conduit pipe, which originally carried water from springs at Paddington to the City of London, ran under the north-west corner of the estate a short distance to the south of Oxford Street. Clauses were written into agreements and leases of plots in the area protecting the rights of the proprietors of the London Bridge Water Works Company (who had been granted a lease of the conduit system by the City Corporation) to have access to the pipes and any conduit heads. When the present No. 449 Oxford Street was being rebuilt in 1875 a conduit head was discovered underneath the former house on the site in a good state of preservation, and drawings were made of it. Another was situated further west, on the east side of Park Street near the corner with Oxford Street, and was housed in a building which belonged to the City Corporation, presumably by right of the medieval charters granting to the City the ownership of the pipes and other features of the system. In 1866, when this corner of Park Street and Oxford Street was first being redeveloped, the Grosvenor Estate paid £2,470 to the Corporation to buy the freehold of the ground on which the 'conduit house' stood.[315]

Conclusion

The development of the Grosvenor estate in Mayfair proceeded with great pace until 1740, and then in a more desultory fashion as the momentum of building slowed throughout the metropolis. In 1741 the builder Roger Blagrave was complaining about paying rates on several of his houses in South Street which were standing empty,[316] and of the thirty-eight builders on the estate who are known to have become bankrupt, nine suffered this fate during the years 1740 to 1742. In 1754 the parish Vestry drew attention to the unsatisfactory state of the western end of Upper Brook Street, where land on the south side had stood vacant for some time,[317] and the twenty-year gap between the dates when sub-leases were granted to the builders of No. 35 (1737) and No. 34 (1756)[318] suggests a considerable slackening in demand over this period. Nevertheless, despite the lapse of over

fifty years before building work on the estate was completed, the basic layout scheme was adhered to with little alteration, and on the whole the development can be accounted a success. Horwood's map of 1792–9 shows that some 1,375 houses were built on the estate, besides many other buildings such as coach-houses, stables, workshops, riding houses, chapels and a workhouse. The evidence of ratebooks suggests that there were few very long delays in filling houses once built and the presence among the early occupants of many people of rank and wealth indicates that fashionable society was well represented from the very start (see Chapter V).

Sir John Summerson has remarked that in the eighteenth century 'Ground landlords rarely found it practicable to dictate the architectural character of the buildings on their land. They might set out the lines of the streets and squares, but once the building agreements were signed the control of elevations was virtually out of their hands'.[319] This was certainly true on the Grosvenor estate. The Grosvenors commissioned the severely rectilinear layout and provided a good deal of practical assistance to builders but they appear to have eschewed any overall aesthetic control. The only notable case in which architectural uniformity was achieved was on the east side of Grosvenor Square, where a composite elevation with centre and wings was created by the undertaker John Simmons. Edward Shepherd did the same in a slightly grander style with three houses on the north side, but they were not even in the centre of the long range of thirteen houses there. In the description of the square in the 1754 edition of Stow's *Survey* the author remarks that the lack of uniformity in the houses had been criticized but concludes that 'they are so far uniform, as to be all sashed and of pretty near an equal Height'.[320] Much the same could be said of the other streets. The kind of overall architectural composition which John Crunden achieved in the 1770's with a small group of three houses in Park Street between North Row and Hereford Street (Plate 13c) was very much the exception, and, of course, in this case dated from the end of the development. Elsewhere the generality of plain brick façades no doubt provided a measure of homogeneity, and most houses appear to have been of three storeys with basements and garrets (an effect now largely obscured by the addition of one or more extra storeys to many houses), but the storey heights were by no means uniform and the width of frontages differed widely.*

An example of the suspicion with which building tradesmen regarded attempts to produce uniformity occurs in the agreement of 1742 to build a group of seven houses in Upper Brook Street, previously mentioned on page 24. Here the words 'that the said Houses shall have a continued Brick Facie through the same and the several Windows thereof shall respectively rainge with each other so as to make a regular Line of Building as to the said Facie and Windows' have all been struck through, the alteration being insisted upon by the several building tradesmen who were parties to the agreement before they would execute the deed.[226]

The most important houses were generally built in Grosvenor Square and the principal east-west streets, viz.: Brook Street and Upper Brook Street, Grosvenor Street and Upper Grosvenor Street. There were exceptions, notably Bourdon House in Davies Street, Roger Morris's own house at No. 61 Green Street, Ligonier's house at No. 12 North Audley Street, the range for which Edward Shepherd was undertaker at Nos. 71–75 (consec.) South Audley Street and the group of houses opposite at Nos. 9–16 (consec.), all of which survive in some form. Some of the larger houses built in Park Lane and the north-western corner of the estate at a late date also deviated from the general pattern, and, from the evidence of the social status of their occupants, the houses at the south end of Park Street with gardens extending to Park Lane were of some quality. Even some of the smaller houses in streets like North Audley Street, Duke Street or South Street—selling at about £200 to £300 or renting at approximately £25 per annum—were, however, by no means insubstantial. The house on the east side of North Audley Street which Richard Barlow rented from Edward Shepherd in 1733 for £24 had a yard or garden and a stable behind, and consisted of three storeys and a basement. The rooms above ground were 'wainscotted all round from bottom to top' and had Portland stone or marble chimneypieces.[321] Houses built by John Jenner on the south side of Mount Row, which was essentially a mews, were of low annual value, but an insurance policy on one of them for £200 shows that it had three storeys and a garret with four rooms wainscotted and four Portland stone chimneypieces.[322]

Some of the houses in Mount Row were sub-divided from the time of first letting, and, despite the reputation of Mayfair as a preserve of the rich, there was originally a good deal of accommodation for the less well-to-do, not least on the Grosvenor estate. There were a number of courts and passages, some of them opening out of the principal streets, and several of the mews had dwelling houses as well as stables and coach-houses built in them, particularly Adams Mews (now Row), Grosvenor Mews (now Grosvenor Hill, Bourdon Street and Bourdon Place), Lees Mews (now Place), Mount Row and Reeves Mews. In the northern part of the estate, where large blocks of land had been let under single leases with few restrictive covenants, streets like James (now Gilbert) Street and Bird (now Binney) Street were laid out in rows of narrow-fronted houses which had very little open space at the rear. These houses in the vicinity of Gilbert Street were rebuilt during the years 1822 to 1833 in the

* For instance, the plots on the south side of Grosvenor Street between Davies Street and the Mount Coffee House sub-leased by Thomas Barlow, the estate surveyor, had the following frontages (in feet): 17½, 19, 25, 36, 36, 24, 18, 20, 17, 19, 21½, 35, 28, 20, 35, 35, 42, 34, 34, 22, 26, 37, 19½.

first major redevelopment scheme to take place on the estate, but there is no evidence that any desire to raise the social *cachet* of the area lay behind the decision of the Grosvenor Estate to sanction this speculative venture by the builder Seth Smith.

Brown's Court, which lay between North Row and Green Street, and was one of several such alleys on the south side of North Row, is an example of the lower level of housing provided on the estate. The ground on which it was laid out was part of the large area bounded by North Row, North Audley Street, Green Street and Park Street which was leased *en bloc* in 1728 at a ground rent of four shillings per annum.[323] The lease stipulated merely that 'good and substantial' houses should be built on the main street frontages and the only restricted trade was that of a brewer. In 1730 John Brown, bricklayer, was granted a sub-lease of part of this ground[324] and by 1739[71] he had built nine tiny two-storey houses along a ten-foot-wide court entered from Green Street and North Row through even narrower arched passageways. Some of the houses had garrets and cellars but several had neither. Each house was virtually one room deep with a yard behind, and the small closet wings belonging to some of the houses shown in the ground plan of the court at the end of the eighteenth century (fig. 1) may have been additions. Brown's Court was largely, or perhaps completely, rebuilt in 1824[325] and was swept away during the redevelopment of the north side of Green Street at the end of the nineteenth century.

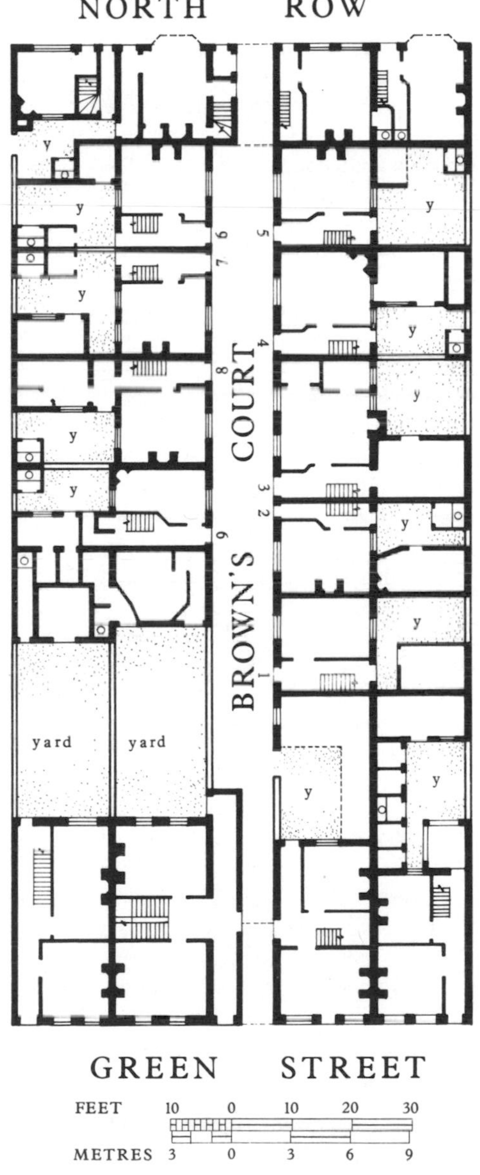

Fig. 1. Brown's Court with adjoining houses in Green Street and North Row. Ground-floor plan in *c.* 1800

Some idea of the unsatisfactory condition of that area of the estate which lay immediately to the south of Oxford Street at the beginning of the nineteenth century can be gleaned from a letter written in 1816 to Lord Grosvenor by Edward Boodle, his lawyer. He had been induced, he wrote, 'to be of a Committee of Inhabitants to go round a part of the Parish between the North side of Grosvenor Square and Green Street, and the South side of Oxford Street', and he had 'never experienced in one day more scenes of distress and misery than presented themselves to us in the course of that day's investigation'.[326] The first Duke of Westminster was later to make the improvement of this area one of his major philanthropic concerns, and in the late nineteenth century several blocks of working-class dwellings were erected to the north of Grosvenor Square and Brook Street. They replaced the run-down houses which were the legacy of the treatment of this part of the estate as a relative backwater from the start of development.

The extensive stabling required by the occupants of the larger houses—many had more than one coach-house—spilled out from the mews into the lesser streets. Some attempt was made to limit this by provisions in building agreements, but stabling with access directly into the roadway was built in South Street, Park Lane and Oxford Street among others, and parts of the frontages of the 'cross streets' (as the north-south streets were called) were taken up with either garden walls or the flank walls of coach-houses and stables. Several large blocks of stables and 'riding houses' were also built, usually for army regiments, the largest being that provided in the 1730's by Roger Morris for the Second Troop of Horse Guards between Green Street and Wood's Mews. The presence of such buildings does not seem to have been considered detrimental to the amenities of the estate; no specific restrictions appear to have been placed on their use, and care was taken in the leasing of adjoining plots to preserve their light:[327] for the stables built by Morris a plot on the south side of Green Street was even left vacant to be used as a 'dung place'.[328]

For the ground landlords the principal benefit of the development lay, of course, in the distant future when

the terms of the first building leases would come to an end, and renewals could be granted at greatly enhanced rents with premiums or fines payable on renewal. In the meantime, however, some years elapsed before their income from the new buildings even matched their expenditure. The agricultural rent received from the fields in Mayfair in the early eighteenth century was between £3 and £4 an acre,[329] or probably somewhat less than £400 for the whole estate there. Once the land had been turned over to the builders the income from ground rents did not begin to exceed this figure until 1725,[45] and it was during these early years that the Grosvenors were spending heavily in the promotion of their new development. If the account of Dame Mary Grosvenor's personal estate at her death in 1730 is taken at its face value, the money spent for this purpose up to that time exceeded the total income received from the speculation by over £4,500.[40] In 1732, however, Sir Richard Grosvenor was able to reap an early advantage from the whole project by borrowing £10,000 at 4 per cent interest from one of his tenants, the loan being made on the security of the newly created ground rents of houses in Brook Street, Grosvenor Street and Grosvenor Square.[180] As more and more houses were built the income gradually increased, and in 1743 this loan was repaid.[330] Eventually the ground rents received from the whole of The Hundred Acres amounted in 1768 (before any leases had been renewed) to £3,133 per annum, or £31 per acre,[331] plus £312 per annum received in improved rents from Sir Robert Grosvenor's trust estate.[332]

Because of the great extent of their landholdings in various parts of England and Wales, it is difficult to determine the effect of the development of Mayfair upon the Grosvenor family's finances, but there is little doubt that the reversionary value of the houses there as building leases began to fall in was a crucial factor in helping to preserve solvency at a difficult period. By the 1770's the affairs of Lord Grosvenor had reached a parlous state: besides his establishment at Eaton he maintained a racing stable at Newmarket costing over £7,000 a year and paid out another £9,400 annually in jointures, annuities and interest charges on mortgages (including £1,200 to his estranged wife). He had apparently been living beyond his means for some time and in 1779 his debts amounted to over £150,000.[73] On the advice in particular of his London agent, Thomas Walley Partington, he contemplated selling all of his estates in Middlesex with the exception of The Hundred Acres in Mayfair and Grosvenor Place in Belgravia. He prevaricated, however, much to the annoyance of Partington, who concluded one letter with remarkable frankness, 'Do my Lord recollect what I laid before you...and for Gods sake as you value your own peace of mind, resolve upon something before Lady Day'.[333] Eventually in 1785 his estates were conveyed to five trustees, viz.: his brother Thomas Grosvenor, the Right Honourable Thomas Harley, the bankers Robert and Henry Drummond, and Thomas Walley Partington, to sell some lands and use the money, together with the remaining rents, to discharge the debts.[334] Over the next twenty years the increasing income from fines and higher rents as leases were renewed in Mayfair helped to retrieve the situation (see page 38), and in the event none of the London estates had to be sold. With the management of the estate passing to trustees and the appointment of an estate surveyor to advise on policy with regard to lease renewals in the 1780's, however, a new stage in the history of the estate had effectively begun.

CHAPTER III

The Administration of the Estate 1785–1899

Between the completion of the first building development in *c.* 1780 and the accession of the second Duke of Westminster in 1899, which may be regarded as the start of the modern phase of the history of the estate, four members of the Grosvenor family held the property. During this period Baron Grosvenor was created Earl Grosvenor in 1784, and his son and great-grandson were respectively advanced to the Marquessate of Westminster (1831) and to a dukedom (1874), the latter being the only wholly new dukedom in the peerage of the United Kingdom (apart from those connected with the Royal House) to be created in the whole of the reign of Queen Victoria.[1] Two younger brothers of the second Marquess of Westminster also held distinct peerages, one as Earl of Wilton and the other as Baron Ebury, and in 1886 the Marquess's youngest son was created Baron Stalbridge.[2] Thus in the closing years of the nineteenth century four members of the Grosvenor family sat in the House of Lords, all of them being, moreover, closely related by the marriages of both the second Marquess and the first Duke to the almost equally resplendent dynasty of Leveson-Gower, possessors since 1833 of the Dukedom of Sutherland, plus (in 1846) the Earldom of Ellesmere. And in the House of Commons other members of the Grosvenor family sat in one of the two seats for the City of Chester from 1715 to 1874 without a break. For forty-two years of this period they held both the Chester seats, while other members of the family often represented other constituencies.[3]

This rapid social or dynastic advancement was matched by a corresponding growth in the wealth of the family, which was increasingly based upon the London estates. At a dinner party in 1819 the Chancellor of the Exchequer (Nicholas Vansittart) informed the American minister in London that the property-tax returns showed that Earl Grosvenor was one of the four richest men in England, with an annual income of 'beyond one hundred thousand pounds, clear of everything'.[4] At that time the enhancement of revenue from the Mayfair portion of the estate by the renewal of the original building leases was still at an early stage, and the development of Belgravia and Pimlico had hardly even begun. In the succeeding decades these two sources produced a torrent, and in 1865 the Grosvenors were described as 'the wealthiest family in Europe —perhaps... the wealthiest uncrowned house on earth'.[5]

Professional Advisers and Estate Staff

During the period covered by this chapter each of the four successive owners of the Grosvenor estate took an active part in the administration of their London properties, and this is described later. Their professional advisers were nevertheless influential. The most important of these were the successive partners in the legal firm of Partington and Boodle. After the death of Thomas Walley Partington in 1791 these were Edward Boodle (d. 1828),[6] and his nephew John Boodle,[7] who from 1806 had a house in Davies Street before removing first, in 1829, to his uncle's house at No. 55 Brook Street until 1836, and then to No. 53 Davies Street (now the Grosvenor Office).[8] The latter appears to have been used principally, or solely, as an office, John Boodle's residence from this time being in Connaught Square; and he also had a property called Heath Farm, near Watford. After his death in 1859 his effects were valued at 'under £14,000'.[9] Since at least 1838 he had been in partnership with his younger son, William Chilver Boodle, his son-in-law, Edward Partington, and his first cousin (Edward Boodle's son), Henry Mitford Boodle.[10] In 1858 they were joined by Henry Mitford's son, Henry Trelawny Boodle, both then living in Leinster Gardens, Bayswater.[11] Henry Mitford died at his house in Tunbridge Wells in 1878, leaving a personal estate of 'under £8,000';[12] Edward Partington, who lived at Gloucester Place, Hyde Park, died in 1883 leaving a personal estate of 'under £24,206',[13] and William Chilver Boodle, who had lived first in Connaught Square but latterly in Dover, died in 1887, leaving personal estate of 'under £11,694'.[14] The surviving partner, Henry Trelawny Boodle, was joined in 1897 by his two sons, Trelawny Frederick and Walter Trelawny Boodle,[11] and died at his house on Wimbledon Common in 1900 leaving effects valued at £48,892.[15] With the admission of G. F. Hatfield to a partnership in 1899 the name of the firm became Boodle Hatfield and Company.[11] Trelawny Frederick died in 1930 and his brother Walter Trelawny —the last of the Boodles to be connected with the firm— in 1931.[16]

Until the death of Edward Partington in 1883 the firm entered itself in the directories as 'Boodle and Partington, conveyancers'. Thereafter only the names of the individual partners appear, but in 1898 the entry becomes 'Boodle and Co., solicitors' and in 1899 'Boodle Hatfield and Co., solicitors'. It was in fact a firm of lawyers with many other clients besides the Grosvenors, and with one exception its members were paid by the Grosvenors by fee, not by regular salary. The one exception was Edward Boodle, whose financial difficulties led in 1807 to his borrowing several thousand pounds from the second Earl Grosvenor,[17] and in return the latter agreed to pay him

partly by fee and partly by a regular salary of some £250 per annum.[18] It follows, therefore, that none of the partners—not even Edward Boodle, who in 1808 was 'in high spirits' upon being offered the receivership of the estates of the late Lady Bath[19]—ever devoted the whole of his attention to the affairs of the Grosvenor estate. Henry Trelawny Boodle, for instance, as solicitor to the Marquess of Northampton, had at least one other client with property problems even more complex and probably time-consuming than those of the Grosvenors in Mayfair and Belgravia.[20]

The Grosvenors' advisers also included in the latter part of the eighteenth and throughout most of the nineteenth centuries a succession of 'agents'. The first recorded of these was John Boydell, a nephew of Alderman John Boydell, the engraver and print publisher who became Lord Mayor of London in 1790, and a brother of the Alderman's partner, Josiah Boydell. The Boydell family came from Shropshire and Flintshire, and another of John Boydell's uncles, Thomas Boydell, was in Earl Grosvenor's service at Eaton, evidently as steward. John Boydell is known to have been the Earl's London agent from at least 1787 until 1791, when he became insolvent. He lived at a house in Stratton Street,[21] and his functions included the management of the Earl's London household, the payment of tradesmen's bills, servants' wages and sometimes of expenses at Newmarket. At that time the Earl's financial affairs were in an extremely disordered state, and John Boydell seems to have got into the habit of accepting bills of exchange in his own name, partly, at any rate, in order to pay the Earl's more pressing creditors. In 1791 John Boydell fell ill and the Earl, feeling 'much uneasiness from the apparent irregular management of his Household affairs', discovered that many tradesmen's accounts had not been paid for five or six years. In the ensuing investigation John Boydell was declared insolvent, and the Earl paid his assignees in bankruptcy some £2,500. Both Edward Boodle and Josiah Boydell were active in these inquiries, and the former said of John Boydell that his 'errors appear to be of the head and not the heart'.[22]

The next agent was Abraham Moore, a London barrister who was appointed in 1796 after the manager of the family lead mines in North Wales had proved 'a most decided Knave', having 'gone off to America, loaded with more spoils than those of' Earl Grosvenor himself, whose income from this source in 1800 amounted to over £18,000.[23] At that time Earl Grosvenor was so deeply in debt that he had 'no regular disposable income at all but what is derived from Cheshire and North Wales',[24] and Moore's main function seems to have been (in addition to the management of the mines) the imposition of some sort of order on the Earl's embarrassingly disordered financial affairs. In 1809–12 he was paid a salary of £500 per annum, but he also received fees for the management of an election at Chester,[25] and like the Boodles he had extensive other commitments, regularly absenting himself from his chambers in the Temple for weeks at a time to practise on the Western Circuit, as well as to attend to such other matters as 'holding the Eton College courts'. His correspondence gives an impression of great efficiency, his constant orders to Edward Boodle, and more particularly to the steward at Eaton Hall and to the local manager of the Welsh mines, being followed up in the latter case by annual personal visits to Eaton during the Long Vacation.[26] But in the long run a part-time agent did not prove a success, for in 1821 it was discovered that Moore had been supporting his numerous financial transactions 'by a most ingenious fraud', thereby cheating the second Earl Grosvenor, who now described him as 'one of the greatest Scoundrels in existence', of very large sums of money.[27] Like his predecessor at the lead mines he too departed to America, where he died at Jersey City in the following year.[28]

After these débâcles the next agent was a man of altogether lesser status than Moore. This was Edmund Empy,[29] who seems to have been employed by Earl Grosvenor as a clerk at a salary of £50 per annum as early as 1802.[30] In 1808, when Moore and a mentor of the second Earl Grosvenor, John Hailstone, were chivvying Edward Boodle to re-organise his office, Hailstone reported to the Earl that 'you will see how we are driving on with Boodle. We have got a separate room in his house for *our* clerk, a measure which I was determined to carry at the point of the bayonet, for if this plan is effective it will depend on keeping our authority paramount and distinct.'[31] This clerk, employed by Earl Grosvenor but working in Boodle's office, was probably Empy, and from his installation 'at the point of the bayonet' in Boodle's premises evidently originates the arrangement whereby the salaried staff of the Grosvenor Office and the quite separate staff of the Grosvenors' lawyers were housed under the same roof—an arrangement which continued at No. 53 Davies Street until 1923, and is even now perpetuated by their occupation of adjacent premises which still share a common entrance at No. 53.

Empy did not have overall control of the administration of the Earl's affairs as had Moore. He seems indeed to have been only concerned with the London properties, where he was occupied with the collection of rents, the renewal of leases and the general maintenance of the estate.[32] The tone of letters addressed to him by the second Earl from Eaton suggests that even in London his position was a relatively subordinate one.[33]

Empy lived at No. 100 Park Street from 1823 to 1841,[34] when he seems to have retired; he died at Tunbridge Wells in 1845 or 1846.[35] He was succeeded by Abraham Howard, who is described as 'agent to the Marquess of Westminster' at the Grosvenor Office, No. 9 (now 53) Davies Street, and sometimes as a conveyancer. He lived at No. 2 Eccleston Square[36] where he died in 1864, leaving effects 'under £5,000'.[37] His successor, Frank Burge, from 1864 to 1870, was initially paid £300 per annum, later raised to £400. His duties were to keep the accounts

and letterbooks, enter up rentals and leases, and fill in in colour all lease plots on maps of the London estate. His office hours were from 10 a.m. to 4 p.m., and he was to attend the weekly Board meetings on Wednesday evenings; he was not to take any other employment.[38] In 1865 an auditor of the Marquess's London estates was also appointed, at a salary of £100, later raised to £300.[39]

Neither Burge nor the next agent, William R. Glennie (1871–92), were lawyers,[11] but Glennie had previously been in the employment of the second Marquess of Westminster since at least 1855, possibly as steward at Grosvenor House.[40] In 1885 he was receiving a salary of £600 per annum, and after his retirement in 1892, a pension of £400.[41] He lived at Berkeley Lodge, Wimbledon,[11] and at his death in 1902 he left effects valued at £8,860.[42] His successor, Charles Robert French, had also previously been in the family's service, again probably as steward at Grosvenor House, and in 1895 his salary was £480 per annum.[43] He remained agent until 1918, living at Evelyn Gardens, South Kensington; he died in 1922, leaving effects valued at £3,877.[44]

In addition to their lawyers and their salaried 'agents', the Grosvenors also employed a series of 'surveyors', all of whom were architects of some distinction with their own independent private practices, and whose works are discussed elsewhere. The first (after the death of Thomas Barlow in 1730) was William Porden (*c.* 1755–1822), who was appointed by the first Earl Grosvenor in or soon after 1784,[45]* when valuations of properties on the Mayfair estate for the renewal of the original building leases were beginning to require professional advice. He was paid a retaining fee or salary of £200 per annum, but he also charged a fee for other work for Earl Grosvenor, notably at Eaton Hall and Grosvenor House.[50] His successors from 1821 were Thomas Cundy I, II and III, who held the position of surveyor successively to 1890. Cundy II and III both received salaries varying from £300 to £500 per annum,[51] but their principal remuneration was by fee for the extensive works which they superintended for the Grosvenors;[52] and probably Thomas Cundy I was paid in the same way.† From 1890 to 1910 the estate surveyor was Eustace Balfour, whose partner in private practice was Thackeray Turner.

Thus throughout the whole of the nineteenth century (and indeed even later) the only full-time salaried staff employed by the Grosvenors for the administration of their Mayfair estate, not to mention the development of those in Belgravia and Pimlico, were the 'agents' and their clerical assistants. After Moore's defalcation in 1821 the importance of the post of agent was greatly and no doubt intentionally reduced, and its subordinate position is clearly seen in the fact that it was H. T. Boodle and not W. R. Glennie who gave evidence relating to the Grosvenor estate to the Select Committee of the House of Commons on Town Holdings in 1887.

In the management of their almost equally great wealth the Dukes of Bedford contrived a different system. Like the Grosvenors, they had very valuable London properties and large country estates, but they 'were advised firstly by a peripatetic chief agent, and secondly, by the local stewards of each estate'. All of them were full-time salaried employees, often they seem to have been lawyers, and at least one of the agents, Rowland Prothero, later Lord Ernle and President of the Board of Agriculture from 1916 to 1919, was a man of great distinction. From 1815 onwards they compiled annual reports on the condition of the estates, thereby providing successive Dukes of Bedford (and later, their grateful historians) with a bird's-eye view of the general situation.[54] In 1887 it was the steward of the London estates in Covent Garden and Bloomsbury who gave evidence—very ably—to the Select Committee on Town Holdings; and it is hard to resist the conclusion that the administrative system on the Bedford estate was in the nineteenth century better organised than on the Grosvenor.

The Estate in Trust, 1785–1808

Towards the end of the eighteenth century tenants on the Mayfair estate began to apply to Lord Grosvenor for the renewal of their leases. The first such applicant, in 1774, was Lord Grosvenor's own lawyer, Thomas Walley Partington, for the two houses which he occupied on the south side of Brook Street. Although the original leases did not expire until 1801 and 1804 they were nevertheless renewed to 1826 at the same low ground rent as hitherto, with no additional restrictive covenants and without a fine.

In the north-eastern portion of the estate virtually all of the original building leases had been granted for only eighty years instead of the more usual ninety-nine years, and in 1778–81 Lord Grosvenor evidently intended to renew the leases here for terms the expiry dates of which would correspond roughly with those in nearby areas of the estate. In 1778–9 he therefore employed (Sir)

* The exact year of his appointment is uncertain. In 1785, when he may have been working in James Wyatt's office,[46] he was appointed surveyor to the Vestry of St. George's, Hanover Square,[47] and by 1786 he was certainly in Earl Grosvenor's employment. But in a letter written by him in 1814 to the second Earl Grosvenor he stated that 'I have now been 30 years in the service of your Lordship and your Lordship's Father', which, if correct, means that he was appointed in 1784.[48]

In 1783–6 John Jenkins was also acting as surveyor for Lord Grosvenor in the erection of Grosvenor Market, and for works at Lord Grosvenor's houses at No. 45 Grosvenor Square, Millbank and Salt Hill. In 1787 the payment of his fees for the latter three items, amounting to some £100, was witnessed by Porden.[49] There is no evidence that Jenkins was concerned in the general management of the Grosvenor estate.

† One of Thomas Cundy III's daughters married a son of Henry Mitford Boodle.[53]

Robert Taylor and George Shakespear to make a detailed plan of the north-eastern portion, to estimate the repairs needed at each house, and to assess the value of the fines to be paid by the tenants in order 'to make up their present Terms 41 years from Michaelmas 1778'.[55]* In 1780 two leases, one in Grosvenor Street and the other in Davies Street, were renewed in conformity with this intention, and 'fines' or premiums were exacted for the first time; but the policy was abandoned soon afterwards. In Davies Street the extra rent payable if certain listed undesirable trades were practised was £60 per annum, whereas in Grosvenor Street it remained at the original figure of £30.[56]

With many more similar applications certain to be received during the next few years, the renewal terms to be offered would clearly require careful consideration, and this was probably the principal reason for Lord Grosvenor's appointment of a surveyor to advise him.

The extra revenue to be derived from the fines payable on the renewal of the Mayfair leases was indeed already being regarded as the salvation of the estate from the enormous debts which, as we have already seen in the previous chapter, had been incurred by the first Lord Grosvenor. As early as 1772, when he was wanting to borrow another £5,000, Partington was 'presuming to remind your Lordship that when you borrowed the last money you determin'd it should be *the last* you would borrow'.[57] By April 1779, however, the situation was worse, and with debts of over £150,000 Lord Grosvenor was compelled to mortgage all his estates to the Right Honourable Thomas Harley, the bankers Robert and Henry Drummond (with whom Lord Grosvenor had banked since 1765), and Partington, who, as trustees for all the creditors, agreed to 'advance to his Lordship a Sum sufficient to pay all his Lordship's Debts in London, at Newmarket and elsewhere'. In return Lord Grosvenor undertook 'to give up his racing System by Selling and disposing of his Horses as soon as the then next meeting should be over', and to order all his rents (except £1,000 per annum for the support of Eaton Hall, Chester, and Halkyn Hall, Flintshire) to be remitted to the trustees for the payment of family jointures and of the interest on his debts. Lord Grosvenor was to be allowed £4,000 per annum, and the residue was to provide a sinking fund for the discharge of the principal sums—'which Fund was to be assisted by Fines to be now received for renewing Leases in Middlesex'.[58]

But this arrangement was not strict enough to salvage Lord Grosvenor (who did not in fact sell his horses until 1796),[59] and in 1781 Partington was exhorting him to 'turn your thoughts to what passed in April 1779, when your Friends stepped forward to save your Lordship from impending disgrace—pardon the word, but I call it so, because you had numerous creditors who would have brought disgrace upon you, had you not satisfyed them by the Assistance of such Friends as I believe no Nobleman in such a situation ever met with; by their means every Debt was paid, and a Plan laid down to retrieve your affairs—Think my Lord how these Friends must feel at the present situation of your Affairs, and how hurt they must be to find their most friendly efforts ineffectual, and that instead of securing your Lordship they are likely to suffer great inconvenience themselves.'[60]

Even this and other 'fruitless representations' from Partington proved ineffective, however,[61] and in 1785 Lord Grosvenor was finally compelled to convey virtually all his estates to the same trustees as in 1779 plus his brother Thomas Grosvenor, upon trust to sell several properties, but excluding those in Mayfair.[62] The revenue shortly to arise from the renewal of the Mayfair leases was again thought of as an important factor in 'reducing the enormous Debt', and when these new dispositions were still in course of discussion, Partington urged Lord Grosvenor that 'in my humble opinion the sooner your Lordship appoints your Surveyor the better'.[61]

It was therefore in these extremely inauspicious circumstances that the renewal of many of the original building leases in Mayfair was commenced. In the history of any great estate this is the time when the initiative in determining the future character of the property returns to the ground landlord, and the decisions made are therefore of crucial importance. In the 1780's there were few, if any, precedents to follow, for many of the London estates originally developed under the leasehold system in the late seventeenth or early eighteenth centuries had since been broken up, and almost the only survivors of any size were those of the Crown and the Dukes of Bedford. On the former there seems, at any rate until 1794, to have been no settled policy respecting renewals or rebuildings.[63] Although on the Bedford estate in Covent Garden it had been the practice since the middle of the seventeenth century to require payment of a fine for renewal of leases, some of which prohibited certain trades without licence from the ground landlord, the impact of estate policy there was not great.[64] And the same seems to have been true further west on the numerous small estates in the northern part of the parish of St. James, where the falling-in of original leases was not responsible for any identifiable turn of the fabric towards neglect or renewal.[65]

So the Grosvenor estate authorities had to formulate their own policies with little guidance from elsewhere, and as the sole object of the trustees established in 1785 was to pay off the debts they naturally adopted a course which would bring in money quickly. This was by granting renewals at a low ground rent but subject to a large fine for such a term as would, with the remaining years of the existing original lease, make up a total term of sixty-three years.

* The very detailed plan made by Taylor and Shakespear forms the basis of fig. 4 on pages 110–11.

The first such lease granted by the trustees was in 1786,[66] and with some modifications in the ratio between the ground rent and the fine, this remained one of the basic features of estate policy in Mayfair for about a hundred years, and even then was not permanently abandoned. For the discharge of Lord Grosvenor's debts it proved eventually successful. Between 1789 and 1808 fines for the renewal of leases in Mayfair totalling over £180,000 were received,[67] and in the latter year the trust of 1785 was dissolved, the debts (with a few trifling exceptions) having been paid off. Some estates in Cheshire and Wales had had to be sold, but all those in London had been preserved intact.[68]

The authors of this policy were presumably Lord Grosvenor's surveyor and his trustees, two of whom, Robert and Henry Drummond, were bankers and therefore expert in money matters. The surveyor was William Porden, who held the post for some thirty-seven years before being finally superseded in 1821. Throughout this period he maintained his own private architectural practice, and (as previously mentioned) was paid a retaining fee or salary of £200 per annum by Lord Grosvenor. For valuations made for the renewal of leases he also received a fee of two guineas from the applicant, which was subsequently deducted from the fine payable to the trustees;[69] and for architectural work for Lord Grosvenor he also charged a commission of five per cent.[70] From 1796 until his death in 1822 he lived in Berners Street.

At first, as Partington had correctly foreseen in 1784, 'the money to be raised by renewing Leases' went 'but a little way' towards paying off the debts.[61] But in 1789 twelve leases were renewed, yielding fines totalling £6,581,[67] and this increase of business led at about this time to the establishment of a Board, the first known meeting of which was on 9 January 1789.

The records of the Grosvenor Board are contained in forty-six volumes of minute books extending from 1789 to about 1920. Throughout this period the Board dealt primarily with the renewal of leases, and also with any other matter affecting the estate. When the development of Belgravia, and later of Pimlico, began, the records became more voluminous, and later in the nineteenth century the amount of information recorded in each entry—which had at first been extremely sparse—became considerably more detailed. But throughout the whole period the method of entry remained basically the same: each item of business was entered, with the date, under the name of the applicant (or, in later years, of the address of the premises under consideration), generally on a new page, but sometimes, when space permitted, half way down beneath a short item of other completed business. Often in later years the entry for one item may extend over many pages and several volumes, and sometimes the chronological sequence of entries is confused by references back to a previous page or even volume where a blank space was deemed a suitable place to continue the record.

The names of those present at meetings were never recorded, but the members of the Board were, evidently, one or more of the partners from Boodle and Partington, the estate surveyor, the agent, and of course, whenever he desired to come, the reigning member of the Grosvenor family. The other trustees do not seem to have attended. The meetings were held weekly, until about 1838 at Boodle's office in Brook Street[71] and subsequently in 'the Board Room' at the Grosvenor Office at No. 53 Davies Street. In 1808 some fifty items of business were being considered at a single meeting, and the drafting of the minutes was evidently done by Lord Grosvenor's clerk and future agent, Edmund Empy.

The part played by the successive owners of the estate in the deliberations of the Board naturally varied according to the personal disposition of each holder of the Grosvenor family title. Often they were absent, 'out of town' or otherwise committed, but in general they seem to have attended assiduously when possible, and of course their wishes (sometimes conveyed in their absence in writing) overruled those of the other members of the Board. The first Earl Grosvenor made at least two decisions of some long-term importance, insisting in 1794 that in the renewal of leases the first claimant should be the owner of the existing lease,[72] and in 1791 (at Porden's instance) refusing to renew the leases of the houses on the site of the modern Nos. 93–99 (consec.) Park Lane in order to facilitate rebuilding at a later date.[73] He also provided the name for a 'Row of new buildings in the Road leading to Chelsea', and even concerned himself in such a trivial matter as the repair of a parish watch-house; but he wisely refused to interfere with the valuations which Porden made for the renewal of leases.[74]

Until 1808 the main object of the Board was to pay off the debts on the estate, and 'Lord Grosvenor's general terms' for renewal were therefore (as Edward Boodle informed an applicant in 1796) to extend 'the subsisting term to 63 years from the time of granting the renewal upon payment of a fine proportionate to the number of years to be added and calculated upon the rent or annual value after deducting the ground rents and land tax'.[75] The fine was payable immediately, but the new rent did not commence until the expiry of the original term. Whenever an application was received Porden would inspect the house and assess the annual value or rack rent, and also the appropriate ground rent which, until the debts were paid off, was kept very low in order to maximise the fine. The amount of the fine was then calculated, evidently by Boodle or Empy, and the terms sent to the applicant.

These calculations were based, at least as early as 1795, upon the published 'Tables of calculation', sometimes referred to as 'Smart's Tables'.[76] Commencing in 1707 John Smart, described as 'at the Town-Clerk's Office, London', had published several editions of Tables of Simple and Compound Interest, which were evidently used at first by the Grosvenor Board. In 1802, however, Francis Baily, the astronomer, published greatly improved

Tables for the purchasing and renewing of Leases,... with rules for determining the value of the reversion of estates after any such leases, which quickly ran through several editions and in 1811 were pirated (much to Baily's annoyance) by the architect William Inwood, whose compilation had by 1880 achieved twenty-one editions.[77]

The theory behind the tables was carefully explained by Baily. 'The sum paid down for the grant of a lease may be considered as so much money paid in advance for the annual rents, as they become due; or... it is such a sum given to the lessor as will enable him, by putting the money out to interest at the given rate, to repay himself the rack rent of the estate, or the yearly value of his interest therein, during the given term: all we have to do, therefore, in this inquiry, is to find out such a sum as, put out to interest at the rate required, will enable him to do this.'[78] This was done in his tables,[79] which gave the number by which the annual value was to be multiplied (referred to as the number of years' purchase) in order to obtain a lease for a given number of years, separate tables being provided for various rates of interest ranging from two to ten per cent.

On the Grosvenor estate, however, the leases being granted did not come into force immediately, but in reversion on the expiry of the subsisting term. In such cases the sum to be paid by the lessee for the addition of any number of years to the unexpired part of an old lease was equal to the difference between the value of the lease for the *whole term* (on the Grosvenor estate, sixty-three years) and the value of the unexpired part of this term already in the lessee's possession.[80] When this difference, expressed in years' purchase, had been calculated from the relevant table—that for five per cent was used on the Grosvenor estate at this time—the answer was multiplied by the annual value of the property after deduction of the ground rent and land tax, and provided the amount of the fine to be paid.*

During the course of negotiations for renewals countless calculations of this kind were made on the Grosvenor estate throughout the nineteenth century. The renewals were made for many years to the owner of 'the original lease from Lord Grosvenor's ancestor',[82] as the first Earl had decided in 1794.[72] This was often not the occupant, and the practice produced unsatisfactory results when the occupant had recently made improvements at his own expense. Thus in 1819 the Board minutes record that in the case of a public house in Grosvenor Mews (now Bourdon Street) the absentee head lessee had 'been in no respect a beneficial tenant to Lord Grosvenor, and should he treat for the renewal, it will only be to make a profit of the man who has been responsible for [the property]...; this system of giving an option to Lessees under such circumstances has been attended with considerable inconvenience to Lord Grosvenor, and is contrary to the practice of other large estates in London, who treat only with the occupier unless the original improver be living. On the Duke of Northumberland's estate the occupiers only are treated with.'[83]

In this particular case the head lessee refused to treat, and ultimately the renewal was granted to the occupant, but when the two parties were competing against each other, preference was given to the head lessee, even though the Board were fully aware that he would thus be able to continue to make a profit by charging the occupant a higher rent than that stipulated in the ground lease.[84] It was not until 1873 that a particularly extortionate example of this sort of practice, at No. 9 Upper Grosvenor Street, led the third Marquess of Westminster, on the strong recommendation of Thomas Cundy III, to renew to the occupant,[85] and two or three years later this was stated to be the usual practice.[86]

At first the rigidity of the system adopted by the Board for the assessment of fines met with hostility from some applicants. The Bishop of Gloucester, for instance, on being informed in 1795 that the fine for the renewal of the lease of his house at the corner of Davies Street and Grosvenor Street would be £3,010, 'expressed his surprize at the magnitude of the fine, and said he supposed it amounted to a prohibition to renew'.[87] But the fact that the calculation of the fines was made upon scientifically based published tables and could therefore be checked by the applicant meant that unless he was able to dispute Porden's valuation, he had no valid objection. And haggling over the amount of the fine was also generally useless, as the Marquess of Hertford, living in Grosvenor Street, found when he was politely informed in 1795 that 'however desirous Lord Grosvenor may be to meet his Lordship's wishes on all occasions, it is utterly out of his power to comply with them in this instance as the gentlemen who act as trustees of his Lordship's estates cannot without a flagrant breach of their trust submit to take £1,174 18*s*. 6*d*. less than the Tables of calculation warrant them in asking for the renewal'.[88]

The successful levy of fines did, however, depend upon the capacity of applicants to pay them, and when this capacity was much reduced by the financial crises of the later 1790's some modification of the Board's policy had to be made. Whereas the total yield from fines for renewals in Mayfair averaged £7,268 per annum between 1789 and 1792, it fell between 1793 and 1800 to an annual average of £3,183, and in 1794 nothing at all was paid.[67] In 1799 Samuel Stephens, a picture-frame maker and head lessee of a house in Brook Street, stated that 'from the difficulties of the times he is not able to raise money to pay the Fine

* *Example*. At No. 17 Grosvenor Street in 1800, John Morris, the applicant for a renewal, had one year unexpired in the subsisting term, and sixty-two years were therefore to be added. Baily's five per cent table shows that the value of a sixty-three-year lease was 19.075 years' purchase, and of the subsisting one-year term was 0.952. The value for adding sixty-two years was therefore 19.075—0.952 = 18.123 years' purchase. Porden valued the house at £240 per annum, which after deduction of his recommended ground rent of £18 and the land tax of £11 12*s*. was reduced to £210 8*s*. This latter sum, multiplied by 18.123, gives a fine payable of £3,813.[81]

for the renewal of the lease of his House' and therefore asked for a shorter-term repairing lease at a rack rent.[89] He was told that, 'as Lord Grosvenor's object must be to renew upon Fines', he could not have a lease at a rack rent so long as there was any possibility of renewing on a fine to any applicant who might present himself. Several such candidates did apply, but they all withdrew, and ultimately Stephens was granted a repairing lease at a rack rent, without a fine, for twenty-one or thirty-one years.[90] At about this time there were several other such cases,[91] and, again in 1799, one applicant to whom a thirty-one-year lease was granted was informed that Lord Grosvenor had now 'generally assented to the measures of granting repairing leases of such of the houses now nearly expiring as cannot be renewed upon a fine',[92] this being clearly preferable to allowing houses to stand empty.

Lord Grosvenor himself had not much helped his trustees in their efforts to pay off his debts. In 1791 he was borrowing yet more money,[93] and we have already seen that although he had agreed in 1779 to sell his race-horses he did not in fact do so until 1796, and three years later he was still active at Newmarket.[94] In 1798 his financial situation was critical once again, even his allowances to his son and his estranged wife being in arrears, and numerous creditors were hounding him for payment.[95] To one such the new agent, Abraham Moore, wrote, 'We literally have not the means of paying... at present. Lord Grosvenor's income is curtailed above one third during [the] continuance of the war and his London property rendered till the return of Peace incapable of improvement.'[96] In November 1798 Moore was 'almost destitute of means to support the ordinary expenses of Lord Grosvenor's reduced establishment',[97] and although his successful exploitation of the lead mines in North Wales yielded over £18,000 in 1800,[98] he had to tell Countess Grosvenor, whose allowance was again in arrears, that she would have to wait 'until I can turn some lead into money'.[99] In July 1801 he even had to borrow 'to prevent an execution going into his Lordship's house'.[100]

The full extent of Lord Grosvenor's debts at the time of his death on 5 August 1802 is not known, but in December 1804 the trust debt still amounted to over £108,000.[101] His son and heir, Robert, second Earl Grosvenor and later first Marquess of Westminster, was a very different man from his spendthrift father, and was evidently determined to discharge all the debts as fast as possible. This (as previously mentioned) he managed to do, with a few small exceptions, by 1808, when the trust of 1785 was dissolved, and completely by 1809.[102] Some lands in Cheshire and North Wales had been sold, but this astonishing recovery seems to have been largely due to the upturn of the national economy, which coincided roughly with the first Earl's death. This improved financial climate encouraged tenants to apply for the renewal of their leases, many of which had only a few more years to run, and was reflected in the receipt between 1801 and 1807 of fines from Mayfair totalling £114,553 (annual average £16,364) and from the North Wales lead mines between 1800 and 1804 of £139,460 (annual average £27,892).[103] It was also a remarkable testimony to the virtually limitless resilience of the Grosvenor family's vast resources.

The liquidation of the first Earl's debts in 1808–9 provides a convenient standpoint from which to examine the progress of the Mayfair estate during the previous twenty years. In general, this was the period when, mainly through the renewal of the original leases, the ground landlord began to exert his authority more strongly than hitherto. In those easy-going days, however, the extent of this control was still not very great, and only two major innovations seem to have been made.

The first of these, made in 1795, was to insert a clause in new leases requiring the tenant to insure his premises against fire.[104] After the burning of the Pantheon in Oxford Street in 1792 there was much public interest in the dangers of fire, and in 1793 the Duke of Bedford had started, in his repairing and building leases, to specify constructional preventive measures[105]—a policy not adopted on the Grosvenor estate until many years later. For some years after 1805 the second Earl Grosvenor's tenants were required to insure with the Globe Insurance Office, from which he had recently borrowed £30,000,[106] or by 1815 with 'some responsible Insurance Office'.[107]

The second innovation was, whenever reasonably possible, to insert in new leases of premises in certain of the 'best' streets an undertaking on the part of the lessee not to use the property for a 'Tavern, Coffee House or Public House or any Open or Public Shop nor for any Art, Trade or Manufactory whatsoever'.[108] This ban applied in Grosvenor Square, Upper Grosvenor Street, Upper Brook Street and Park Lane, and with some exceptions, in Grosvenor Street and Brook Street. It also applied to certain houses which backed on to Park Lane, notably the west side of New Norfolk (now Dunraven) Street and, at its southern extremity only, the west side of Park Street.[67]

The implementation within the best streets of the ban on 'any art, trade or manufactory whatsoever' was not always possible (except in Grosvenor Square, where commerce had never intruded), for by 1790 a substantial proportion of the houses in even some of these streets was already occupied by tradesmen, some practising the very trades listed in the original leases as having to pay the £30 surcharge on the ground rent. Thus in Grosvenor Street at least twelve out of some seventy-four occupied houses on the estate there, and in Brook Street some twelve out of forty on the estate, were in 1790 occupied by tradesmen, largely concentrated in both streets at the eastern ends.[109] So when Francis Grosse, a perfumer, applied to renew the lease of one of these houses in Grosvenor Street, no objection was raised, he agreeing in 1795 to accept the ban on a 'tavern, coffee house or public house or any open or public shop' in exchange for

the omission of 'nor for any art, trade or manufactory whatsoever'.[110] Similarly, there was no objection in 1799 to Samuel Stephens, the picture-frame maker of Brook Street previously referred to, and the Board minutes record that 'the clause prohibiting any open or publick Shop must be qualified so as not to restrain him from carrying on his own business'.[111] Even the lease of the Lion and Goat public house at No. 5 Grosvenor Street was renewed in 1800 without difficulty,[112] but some trades were regarded as obnoxious, Porden in 1818, for instance, advising the Board not to renew the lease of a tallow chandler in or very near Upper Brook Street.[113]

Sometimes it was evidently for financial reasons that leases were renewed to tradesmen in these best streets. Thus in 1802 No. 43 Brook Street, having stood empty for a year after the expiry of the original lease and the refusal of the head lessee to renew on fine, was leased by Lord Grosvenor's authority to Pellot Kirkham as a hotel, despite this use being 'contrary to the restrictions contained in the leases of the other houses that have been renewed in Brook Street'.[114] Three years later, in precisely similar circumstances, William Wake of Wake's Hotel, Covent Garden, was allowed to open a hotel nearby at No. 49 Brook Street (now part of the site of Claridge's Hotel), and in both cases Lord Grosvenor actually helped them by using 'his influence' to obtain magistrates' licences for the sale of alcohol.[115] Extensions of trade in the principal streets were evidently not undertaken lightly, however, for in 1805 a bookseller's application to take No. 51 Brook Street (also now part of the site of Claridge's Hotel), which had been empty for over a year, was refused, and the house remained empty for another two years before being ultimately let on fine to a private resident. But pressure for permission to use houses in this part of Brook Street as hotels was evidently very strong, and although an application made by the lessee in 1812 on behalf of a hotel keeper, James Mivart, to use this house as a hotel was personally refused by Lord Grosvenor, Mivart was nevertheless using it as 'a private lodging house' in the following year.[116] It is to these establishments of Wake's and Mivart's that Claridge's Hotel traces its origin.

By about 1835, when all the leases in these best streets had been renewed, the effect of this policy seems to have been to rid Upper Grosvenor Street and Upper Brook Street of any such trade as had insinuated itself there in the eighteenth century. In Grosvenor Street and Brook Street it largely prevented any further commercial incursions until many years later. Those parts of these two streets which lay outside the eastern boundary of the Grosvenor estate had evidently become largely commercialised during the eighteenth century, and (as mentioned above) trade had even gained a footing here within the estate, particularly on the north side of Brook Street east of Davies Street. Commercial pressure, expressed principally through difficulty in finding private residents willing to take houses adjoining or opposite to tradesmen, must therefore have been very strong here. The census of 1841 shows, however, that in Grosvenor Street there had been virtually no change since 1790 in the ratio of commercial and domestic occupation, while in Brook Street the slight increase of trade was due to the establishment of hotels.[117]

In all except these best streets the restrictive covenants which lessees were required to accept in their new leases on other parts of the estate were at first surprisingly lax. These were merely to pay the rent, maintain the premises, permit the landlord to inspect them and give notice to repair them within three months, and to surrender them peaceably at the end of the new term; and if the rent were in arrears, the landlord could resume possession. Undesirable trades were at first controlled in the same way as hitherto, by the payment of an additional annual ground rent (generally still £30) if the premises were used by a butcher, slaughterman, tallow chandler or melter, soap maker, tobacco-pipe maker, brewer, victualler, coffee house keeper, distiller, farrier, pewterer, working brazier or blacksmith—this list being virtually identical with that contained (wholly or in part) in the original building leases. In 1799, however, a complete ban was placed on all these listed trades, plus that of hotel keeper, and this ban was also extended, by an important new proviso, to include any 'other noisome or offensive Trade or Manufactory whatsoever',[118] thus applying to the whole of the estate a restriction only a little less severe than that in the best streets already referred to.

Hitherto, throughout the greater part of the estate the ground landlord's control had rested primarily—at least until individual leases were renewed—upon the clause in the original lease requiring the £30 surcharge on the ground rent for the practice of some or all of the trades listed above. Numerous trades were left unrestricted, and in 1806, for example, Lord Grosvenor was unable to prevent the conversion to an upholsterer's shop of No. 76 Grosvenor Street (where in any event the original lease of the whole large block in which it stood had omitted all restriction on specified trades).[119] Even tallow-melting had not everywhere been restricted, which perhaps explains why in 1819 the estate authorities allowed it to continue at a site in Chandler (now Weighhouse) Street in the mistaken belief that the original lease did not prohibit it there.[120] But generally, where the appropriate restriction existed in the original lease, a threat to enforce payment of the surcharge seems to have secured the suppression of such nuisances as those caused by butchers, slaughtermen, blacksmiths and tallow chandlers.[121] Sometimes this took a long time. In the case, for instance, of John Holland, a tallow-melter in South Audley Street, who had renewed his lease in 1795,[122] Edward Boodle had in 1800 'perceived a most offensive smell proceeding from the house', but threats to enforce the £30 surcharge, followed by demands for its payment (with six years of arrears) and refusal to renew his lease when it should next expire seem to have produced little lasting improvement

until 1817, when the Board was informed that 'since Mr Holland has been spoken to, the work has been carried on... in such a manner as not to be offensive'.[123]

No example of the £30 surcharge being actually paid has been found, and both this and the ban imposed in 1799 upon any 'noisome or offensive Trade or Manufactory whatsoever' seem to have been used primarily as reserve powers to secure reasonable neighbourly conduct rather than interpreted literally. Thus Robert Mansbridge, a 'spruce beer brewer' had the lease of his house in Brook Street renewed in 1800 without difficulty, but when two years later he asked 'that the prohibitory clause respecting a brewhouse might be struck out of his lease, being fearful that it would affect him', he was told by the Board that 'as he had exercised his profession on the premises for many years unmolested, he had no occasion to be under apprehension for the future while he conducted it as he had hitherto done, but that the clause could not be dispensed with because it would leave him or his successors the liberty of making a brewery of a very different kind, to the essential inconvenience of his neighbours'.[124] And another reserve power—that of threatening to refuse to renew the lease when it should come up for negotiation—was sometimes used to abate nuisances which did not actually contravene the existing covenants—e.g. the beating of 'beds and feathers' on the roof of a house adjoining Grosvenor Square,[125] a steam engine off Oxford Street[126] or a house of ill-fame in New Norfolk (now Dunraven) Street,[127] or in Brook Street 'the constant disturbance... suffered particularly in the night from the violent kicking and plunging of Lord Penrhyn's horses'.[128]

The treatment of public houses reflected the different policies pursued by the first and second Earls, and also the changing social conditions on the estate. In 1793 there were some seventy-five pubs on the estate (excluding those in Oxford Street),[129] and the first Earl seems not to have objected to the renewal of their leases, even in the case of those in the best streets.[130] At first the second Earl reluctantly continued this policy, an applicant in Upper Grosvenor Street being informed in 1809 that 'Lord Grosvenor would not be sorry to see the public house discontinued as such, though his Lordship would not insist upon it'.[131] Starting around 1815, however, he refused to renew the leases of any public houses in the best streets,[132] and elsewhere he also sometimes refused to do so.[133] But pubs were a valuable source of revenue, and between 1815 and 1824 several large London brewers, including Meux, Reid and Company, Combe, Delafield and Company (both now part of the Watney's chain) and Whitbread's, were competing against each other for renewals. Meux, Reid had already acquired the sub-leases of several houses on the estate, but Lord Grosvenor refused to treat with them until and unless the head lessee had declined to do so.[134] Combe, Delafield and Meux, Reid both rejected Lord Grosvenor's first terms out of hand,[135] but ultimately, after receiving some encouragement from the Estate,[136] Meux, Reid negotiated nine new leases on payment of a fine of upwards of £7,000,[137] one of the advantages of treating with a brewer being his greater capacity to repair and even occasionally to rebuild his premises. By 1828, on the eve of the Beer Act of 1830, the total number of licensed premises on the estate had declined at most very slightly (if at all),[138] the suppression of some pubs being partly counterbalanced by the establishment of new hotels, particularly at the eastern ends of Brook Street and Grosvenor Street.

During Porden's reign as surveyor (*c.* 1784–1821) rebuilding was hardly ever made a condition for the renewal of a lease, and very little took place. Such little as tenants did undertake was evidently regarded by the Board as either an 'improvement' or as normal maintenance work.[139] Sometimes such 'improvements' were considerable, but in general the Board did not interfere, provided that they did not contravene the lease in question and were not injurious to the estate or the neighbours.[140] At the western ends of Upper Brook Street and Upper Grosvenor Street the building of projecting awnings and balconies which interfered with the neighbours' view of Hyde Park was gradually controlled by the insertion of special restrictive covenants in new leases,[141] and when Lady Cunliffe, living in New Norfolk (now Dunraven) Street wanted to block up five or six windows she was told that she would 'be liable to the expence of opening and restoring them at the expiration of her lease'.[142] Outgoing tenants' liabilities for dilapidations were carefully enforced, sometimes by a Court order.[143]

But although there was little actual rebuilding, Porden did initiate three long-term improvement schemes, all of which ultimately had a happy outcome. In 1791 he persuaded Lord Grosvenor not to renew the leases in King's Row (now the sites of Nos. 93–99 consec. Park Lane) so that in due course 'a handsome front towards Hyde Park' might be built in place of the original tumbledown agglomeration here.[144] This policy was maintained on a number of occasions,[145] and after Porden's death his aim was achieved—for the most part in 1823–8 (Plate 19a). Similarly, improved lines of frontage for the north side of Berkeley Square and the west end of Bourdon Street, projected by Porden in 1800–3, were implemented shortly after his death.[146]

His third scheme achieved a quite different object from that intended. In 1789 he had suggested that Green Street might be extended eastward from North Audley Street to Duke Street. But unfortunately he made this suggestion immediately after the lease of a substantial part of the ground needed had been renewed for sixty-three years, and so when the property was put up for sale in 1792 Lord Grosvenor's trustees had to buy up their own lease at a price of 1,500 guineas—despite the enormous debts then encumbering the estate.[147] In 1795 the land was leased on a short-term basis to the St. George's Volunteer Corps, but the arrangement did not prove a happy one,

for in 1798 several of the officers—including 'Major Harrison the coal merchant and Captain Gunter the confectioner'—refused to pay Lord Grosvenor his rent 'until their demands on his Lordship are paid'.[148] After the return of peace in 1802 the ground was leased (determinable on six months' notice) for upholsterers' workshops, but in 1818 Porden recommended that the cost of buying up the rest of the ground needed would be too great, and that therefore 'the proposed opening should be given up, and the neighbourhood continued to be occupied (as it now is) by workshops etc, which although not the most respectable in appearance, Mr. Porden states to be of great value'.[149] Shortly afterwards, however, the site was sold (with other adjacent ground) to the Church Building Commissioners,[150] and St. Mark's Church was built upon it in 1825–8.

Generally, during the years between 1785 and 1808 the first and second Earls Grosvenor, their Board and their trustees began to make some impact upon the evolution of the estate. Primarily this was done through their policy of, whenever possible, renewing leases on fine to provide terms of sixty-three years to come. The fact that leases could nearly always be renewed on these terms whenever the lessee chose to apply meant that the expiry dates of these renewed leases varied greatly from one house to another.* In 1794 Lord Grosvenor did decide that no lease should be renewed if the existing one had more than fifty years to run,[151] but even this rule could be subject to exceptions.[152] The Estate was therefore committing itself far ahead, but without any long-term policy, for the making of the leases of adjacent sites co-extensive with each other seems only to have been done at the lessee's request, and even then evidently as a favour.[153] The result of this practice was to make simultaneous rebuilding on adjacent sites much more difficult, and hardly any such reconstruction in fact proved possible until the 1880's and 1890's, when the effects of a less haphazard and more flexible policy in the granting of the third generation of leases began to produce approximately simultaneous expiry dates, notably in Mount Street and parts of South Audley Street. In many other parts of the estate, however, the original individual plots have never been merged, and in some cases the original houses still stand on them.

The Free Estate, 1808–45

Robert, second Earl Grosvenor, and from 1831 first Marquess of Westminster, held the family estates from 1802 until his death in 1845. He had inherited them from his father unentailed, but still subject to the trust created in 1785 for the payment of massive debts. These he had, as we have already seen, virtually discharged by 1808, when the trust was dissolved; thereafter he was the absolute master of all his numerous properties.

At the time of his succession in 1802 the second Earl was aged thirty-five. In his marriage, the Grosvenors' 'old luck with heiresses had not deserted them', his wife being Eleanor, only surviving daughter and heiress of Thomas Egerton, first Earl of Wilton. He had sat in the House of Commons since 1788 as a supporter of Pitt, but after the latter's death in 1806 he joined the Whigs. In later years he supported the Reform Bill, and in 1831 was raised to the rank of Marquess of Westminster. A near-contemporary, writing in 1865, described him as 'An admirable man of business, an honest politician, his character was deformed only by a thrift, always more or less apparent in the family, which in him rose to a mania ... the thrift which gives rise to stories such as those told of the Marquess is unusual, and has done much to lower the great popularity of the house'.[154]

Within a year or two of his succession he began to use his vast wealth to the full—or if not quite to the full, with more purpose than his father in recent years. While still paying off the old debts he bought more lands in Cheshire 'very desirable to him' for some £30,000,[155] and in 1804 he began the rebuilding of Eaton Hall on a huge scale to Gothic designs by Porden.[156] In 1806 he bought the Agar Ellis collection of pictures for 30,000 guineas, having previously spent £20,000 on a suitably impressive house in which to house it and his own family. This was Gloucester House in Upper Grosvenor Street, hitherto occupied by George III's brother, the Duke of Gloucester, until his death in 1805.[157] Renamed Grosvenor House, this now became the family's principal London residence. Old Grosvenor House at Millbank was pulled down in 1809,[158] and No. 45 Grosvenor Square, where Earl Grosvenor's father had lived in preference to Millbank, was sold. After spending large sums on alterations and redecorations Earl Grosvenor moved into the new Grosvenor House in 1808.[159]

After this tremendous initial burst of expenditure the pace slackened somewhat, but in later years he continued to buy pictures, enlarge Grosvenor House, and above all, buy more land—notably the Pulford estate in Cheshire (1813, £80,000), the Shaftesbury estate in Dorset (1820, £70,000, much enlarged in later years), the Stockbridge estate in Hampshire (1825, £81,000) and Moor Park, Hertfordshire (1827, £120,000). He also kept up his father's racing stud.[160]

The growth of the Earl's income was, however, well able to support these outlays. Between 1768 and 1782 the rental of the Mayfair estate only had been about £3,450

* Thus the building leases of two adjacent houses granted in 1730 for 99 years would both expire in 1829. One lessee might apply for a renewal in 1790, when he still had 39 years unexpired. He would be granted a reversionary term of 24 years to give him a total of 63 years to come, and his new lease would expire in 1853. But his neighbour might not choose to apply for a renewal until 1820, when he had only 9 years of the original term unexpired. He would be granted a reversionary term of 54 years, and his new lease would not expire until 1874.

per annum, but by the time of the second Earl's succession in 1802 it had risen to £5,550. This modest increase was largely due to the expiry around 1801 of a number of the original leases granted only for eighty years, and to the grant of a few short-term leases on rack rents. But by far the greater part of the yield from the estate at this period took the form of fines, which (as previously mentioned) amounted between 1789 and 1808 to over £180,000. After 1808 there is a gap in the records of fines received, but the yield no doubt continued high, for many leases were being renewed.

By 1820 the rental had risen to over £8,000, but in the following year it bounded up to nearly £20,000.[161] The reason for this was that the increased reversionary ground rents due on leases renewed on fine in previous years now became payable for the first time, the original ninety-nine-year leases granted in 1721 having now expired. This was, of course, a continuing process, reflecting the rate of building and the grant of leases a century earlier; and there were also a great many original leases still to be renewed at greatly enhanced rents. So by 1825 the Mayfair rental rose to over £41,000,[161] and by 1835 to some £60,000.[162] Nor was this and the unrecorded fines anything like all, for it was in these years that the large-scale development of the great estate in Belgravia and Pimlico began to yield a much increased crop of ground rents. The Earl's expenditure, colossal as it was, was not therefore excessive in relation to his resources, and although he had between 1826 and 1829 to mortgage his estates for £130,000, he was still able to repay the whole amount in 1835–6.[163] When he died in 1845 he left his estate with no encumbrances other than those providing for his family.

As well as being thrifty he was, indeed, 'an admirable man of business' (at least until his latter years), and being dissatisfied with the existing administration of his properties he began in 1807 to attempt to reform the workings of Edward Boodle's office. In this uphill struggle—started evidently in anticipation of the forthcoming dissolution of the trust of 1785—he was assisted by his friend John Hailstone, the geologist, whom he had first met at Trinity College, Cambridge, in the 1780's. Boodle, it appears, was in financial difficulties of his own, and he was also dilatory beyond belief, some of his clients not having received any bills for his services since 1780. This must have adversely affected Lord Grosvenor's affairs, relying so heavily as he (even with the active Abraham Moore as his agent) and his forbears did, almost of necessity, upon the firm of Boodle and Partington. So for some years, and particularly during the Earl's frequent absences from London, Hailstone concerned himself with introducing a semblance of efficiency into the management of the Grosvenor business in Boodle's office in Brook Street.

In February 1807 Boodle was complaining of 'great fatigue and headache owing to his exertions', possibly caused by an 'experiment' made by Hailstone, which a few days later was said to have 'failed intirely. At the rate he is capable of travelling the business would not be finished in the next generation.' A year later Hailstone was reporting that 'Our operations have certainly wrought an evident change for the better in Mr. B. who now seems to exert himself in good ernest'[164]—a reference, probably, to the installation of Lord Grosvenor's own clerk, Edmund Empy, in Boodle's office (see page 35). This seems, indeed, to have been the only enduring success of the whole campaign, for Hailstone continued to refer sarcastically to Boodle as 'the energetick', and in February 1808 he concluded that 'It is equally impossible to drive him beyond his easy amble as the bold P out of his curvets'.[165]

'The bold P' was, of course, a facetious reference—habitual in this correspondence—to the Earl's surveyor, William Porden, who was also a victim of this early attempt at the introduction of 'business efficiency' methods. From his house in Berners Street Porden himself had at first joined in the game of making fun of Boodle, describing him (in a letter of 1803 to the Earl) in his rather incongruous capacity of an officer in the volunteers as 'armed cap-a-pie, in Sash and Gorget, and Kavan-Hullar Beaver, going, to be comfortably inspected in a heavy Rain'.[166] But pleasantries of this kind soon ceased, for Porden too was incurably dilatory. In 1807 Hailstone wrote that 'I seldom miss a day but I walk to the House [Grosvenor House] and sometimes spur the bold P. till he is ready to lash out at me'.[167] In 1808 Lord Grosvenor, at Eaton, was exasperated with Porden because there was no mason working there, the last having departed after 'a tiff' with Porden—'this, you know, must be the effect of P. rages'. Two years later he was 'out of all Patience at Porden's delays about things here', and soon afterwards Hailstone was told that 'if you can give any elastic Vigour in Brook or Berners Street, you will do great things'.[168] Indeed, of all the professional men employed by the Earl, only the agent, Abraham Moore, escaped criticism—at least until his massive embezzlements were discovered in 1821.

It is, however, easier to get rid of an architect than of the family solicitor, and so Edward Boodle survived until his death in 1828, while Porden was eventually superseded in September 1821.[169] By then he was aged about sixty-six, and in addition to his exasperating dilatoriness there had in the past been disagreements with the Earl about his fees[170] and possibly also about matters of estate policy. Porden was certainly not the man to have day-to-day charge of the impending development of Belgravia, and he died a year later at his house in Berners Street, in September 1822.[171] His successor, Thomas Cundy I, an architect and builder of Ranelagh Street (now Beeston Place and the eastern end of Ebury Street), where he owned several leasehold houses,[172] at once initiated a rebuilding policy in Mayfair—possibly at the Earl's behest—but he died in 1825 without having had enough time to make any great impact there. He was succeeded by his son, Thomas Cundy II, who held the post for over

forty years and whose influence upon the fabric of the Grosvenor properties in Mayfair—greater, perhaps, than that of any single other architect except Edmund Wimperis—may still be seen, in one way or another, in many of the main streets on the estate.

Porden's departure coincided with the discovery of Abraham Moore's defalcations, and although Porden was in no way involved in Moore's crimes, this simultaneous change of architect and agent does seem to have inaugurated a new and more autocratic régime. Having to rely upon a new surveyor, a new agent (Empy) of substantially lower status than his predecessor, and the irremovable Edward Boodle, Lord Grosvenor was evidently very much in personal command of his estates in the remaining years of his life. And there is no doubt that he liked to have his own way, for his daughter-in-law said of him that 'When Lord Grosvenor is possessed of an idea one might just as well talk to the winds'.[173]

But if the day-to-day administration of the Grosvenor estates in London in the first two decades of the nineteenth century does not seem to have been very efficient, the basic principle of management adopted in *c.* 1786—renewal for long terms on fine—was sound; and its long-term as well as its financially immediate effects were beginning to become apparent, as the hard-pressed Edward Boodle pointed out in 1814 in a letter to Lord Grosvenor. In 1809 the fourth Viscount Grimston (later first Earl of Verulam) had in the normal way been granted on fine a reversionary term of sixty-three years to come on his house, No. 47 Grosvenor Square, only to find, four years later, that 'a radical defect in the original building of the house' required its complete rebuilding, which he duly undertook at a cost of £12,900.[174] This prompted Boodle to make one of the rare general comments to be found in the records of the Grosvenor Office: 'it is, I confess, highly gratifying to me to witness the good effects of that system of renewal which was peculiar to your Lordship's Estate, altho' it has been since adopted by other considerable Proprietors of Ground and houses in this Metropolis. Lord Grimston has furnished a striking instance in favor of it, by having followed his renewal with completely rebuilding his House, and upon a very improved Plan. While this system shall be pursued the Estate will be kept not merely in good heart and condition, but will keep pace in modern improvements with all the Neighbouring property, and having from its situation so much the advantage of all the adjacent Estates, will preserve its consequence as long as Hyde Park remains unbuilt upon.'[175]

Under the second Earl the detailed application of the 'sixty-three year reversionary renewal on fine' policy was frequently altered. This was particularly evident in his decisions about the ratio between the rent and the fine. During the course of the nineteenth century this ratio was reversed, the low rent and high fine of the early years being gradually replaced by a high rent and a low fine. The change was not a smooth one, however, and its ups and downs evidently reflected disagreements between the current possessors of the estate on the one hand and their legal and professional advisers on the other.

The latter always advocated high fines and low rents, by means of which (to quote Messrs. Boodle in 1845) the tenant 'has a larger Interest in the House and is more likely to improve the Property':[176] or (to quote Porden in 1821) 'the making the Rents on renewal too high, causes the Property to be neglected near the expiration of the lease'.[177] The attitude of the current possessors varied, however. Generally, they favoured higher rents and lower fines, but although they could and did overrule their professional advisers, there were other factors—notably their own expectation of life—to be taken into account.

Connected with the ratio between rent and fine was the question of how long before the expiry of a lease the current possessor of the estate was prepared to treat for its renewal. As we have already seen, the first Earl had at first renewed to any of his tenants willing to pay a fine, but the effect of this had been to commit the estate far ahead without any long-term policy and to create wide divergences in the expiry dates of such renewed leases. In 1794 he had therefore decided not to renew when the existing lease had more than fifty years still to run,[178] and the second Earl reduced the period still further, by 1815 to thirty years,[179] and by 1823 to ten years.[180] Subsequently, however, he reversed this policy, by 1834 his rule being not to renew when the unexpired term had more than twenty years to run,[181] and at this level it remained until his death in 1845.[182]

In the years prior to 1808, when the first Earl's debts were being paid off, the reversionary rent fixed at each renewal was kept extremely low in order to maximise the fine; generally it amounted to only about one tenth of the annual value of the property. After 1808 it was fixed at 'one fifth (or at most one fourth) of the improved annual value of the house',[183] and in 1816 the ground rent was sometimes as much as one third of the annual value.[184] In 1821 Porden was resisting an applicant who wanted the rent to be well over half the total value—'he should be absolutely required to pay half in Fine and half in Rent, which will bring our practice back to nearly what it was, till lately'—and he asked Lord Grosvenor to make this a standing order. But 'His Lordship thinks otherwise at present'.[185] Shortly afterwards this upward movement of the rent went even further, an applicant for stables in North Row having to be told that 'he must pay a fine of at least $\frac{1}{5}$ part' of the annual value.[186]

In order to understand why in the early 1820's the second Earl favoured high rents and lower fines it is necessary to bear in mind that by greatly reducing the length of time before the expiry of a current lease in which he was prepared to treat for its renewal, he had postponed a great many such renewals. At that time he knew that about one third of all the original leases on the Mayfair estate were still unrenewed, and that most of

them would expire during the next decade or so. As in 1820 he was aged fifty-three, he seems to have thought that it was in his own best interests to charge a high rent and a low fine on such renewals in order to maximise his future income when the old leases expired—hence his disagreement with Porden, concerned with the long-term standards of upkeep of the estate.

Later on, however, his interests changed. By 1835 almost all the original leases had been renewed at greatly increased rents,[162] and his own expectation of life had, of course, diminished. Relatively few more renewals were to be expected before his death, and in any case he might not live to enjoy the benefit of the enhanced reversionary rents arising from them. So in the last decade of his life it was better for him to have higher fines and lower reversionary rents, for thereby he had the immediate use of the fines, either as capital or, invested, as income. By 1834, therefore, he was encouraging applications to renew by extending the period in which he was prepared to treat from ten to twenty years before the expiry of the existing lease, and at some unknown date he reverted to his earlier ratio of one quarter rent and three quarters fine—much to the satisfaction, no doubt, of Cundy and Messrs. Boodle.[187]

His son, the second Marquess of Westminster, reversed this policy immediately after his succession in 1845. In order to facilitate rebuilding he inaugurated a more flexible leasing policy (though still normally based on the sixty-three-year term) and he therefore reduced the period for renewal negotiations in anticipation of the expiry of existing leases from twenty to ten years, where it remained for the rest of the century and beyond. Contrary to Messrs. Boodle's advice, however, he raised the proportion of the rent from one quarter to one half.[188] In 1845 he was aged fifty, and just as his father had done at the same age, he favoured higher reversionary rents, payable within not more than ten years. By this means he evidently hoped to enjoy both the fine and at least some years of the enhanced rents. By the time of his death in 1869 the rental of the Mayfair estate had risen from some £60,000 in 1835 to £80,000 in 1870.[189]

In 1866, however, the 'half rent, half fine' formula was changed to two-thirds rent and one-third fine[190]—a change possibly caused by tenants' inability to raise capital in that year of financial crisis. This policy was continued by his son, the third Marquess (later first Duke), who succeeded to the title in 1869 at the age of forty-four.[191]

But whatever variations were from time to time made, it was always an essential object of successive owners to keep the estate, as Edward Boodle phrased it, 'in good heart and condition'. In the early years of the nineteenth century this had been comparatively easy, for the value of all individual properties on the estate were rising. Thus, to take one of many examples, Porden valued Colonel (later Field-Marshal) Thomas Grosvenor's house at the corner of Grosvenor Street and Grosvenor Square at £300 per annum in 1797, £360 in 1803, and £500 in 1808, and his reports in these years constantly refer to 'the general increase in the value of property'.[192] But after reaching a peak in about 1812 a decline began, and from 1814 to at least his retirement in 1821 he was often reporting that 'the value of property is falling'.[193] Tenants often had such difficulty in paying their fines that they were allowed to pay them in two six-monthly instalments (with interest), and B. F. Hardenburg, the sculptor, was even permitted to pay his over a five-year period without interest.[194] This fall in values corresponded in date with the slump of 1811–16 in London building, but its continuance after building had picked up again may perhaps have been due to competition from the great new residential districts then being built in Tyburnia and on the Portman and Crown estates in St. Marylebone.

The existence of these new rivals for aristocratic patronage may have prompted a more positive attitude to rebuilding on the Grosvenor estate in Mayfair. This new policy was started very shortly after the appointment of Thomas Cundy I as the new surveyor in the autumn of 1821, and he was instrumental in enforcing it: but it may equally well have originated with the Earl himself, who, with the vast increase of the 1820's in rents from the Mayfair estate, could now well afford to forgo a little of this extra revenue by encouraging rebuilding.

From 1822 onwards applicants for the renewal of dilapidated properties were encouraged, or occasionally required, to rebuild, and in such cases they were also required to do so in accordance with 'a plan approved by Lord Grosvenor's surveyor' (i.e. Cundy).[195] Usually the term granted did not exceed sixty-three years, and despite the lessee's rebuilding expenses, he still often had to pay a fine as well as a ground rent, even in such streets as Upper Grosvenor Street and Park Lane, where rebuilding would no doubt be costly.[196] In South Street and on the north side of Berkeley Square, however, where a number of 'first rate' houses were built in the 1820's, terms ranging between ninety-six and ninety-nine years were granted, those in South Street being also subject to a fine.[197] Some of these houses still survive (Plate 24c).

Thus the foundations of the Grosvenor rebuilding policy, by which large parts of the estate were in later years to be transformed, were laid in the early 1820's by the second Earl and Thomas Cundy I. In the next two decades some rebuilding took place, notably in Green Street, Bourdon Street and around South Street, while in the Weighhouse Street area substantial redevelopment was undertaken by the builder Seth Smith, some sixty-three small houses being built there between 1822 and 1833. But when the original houses were still in good condition, the second Earl and first Marquess was generally content, until almost the end of his life, to pursue in renewal negotiations the old policy of adding to the existing term to give sixty-three years to come, without requiring rebuilding or even alterations to the front.[198] And he would probably have agreed with Messrs. Boodle's verdict of 1845 upon the satisfactory results of

this policy: 'very few renewals which have been negociated have gone off [i.e. proved abortive] and for many years not a single House has been on hand [i.e. untenanted], and the Marquess of Westminster's name as a Landlord has obtained that Opinion with the Public that nearly every person would give more for a Lease on His Lordship's Estate than on any other'.[199]

But Thomas Cundy II was evidently not so satisfied, and in May 1844 he had an interview with the Marquess, who agreed 'to Mr Cundy's suggestion for improving the appearance of the houses in Grosvenor Square by the addition of stucco work to the fronts with porticos, window dressings, cornices and balustrades to such of the houses as may be thought to require it'. In future, in terms for the renewal of leases of houses in the square, stipulations to this effect were to be included, and a design was to be submitted by the applicant.[200]

Before anything could be done, however, the first Marquess died, on 17 February 1845; and it was to be under the aegis of his son, the second Marquess, that the transformation of the outward appearance of the estate was to be commenced.

The Estate Entailed, 1845–99

Richard Grosvenor, second Marquess of Westminster (1795–1869), had married the youngest daughter of the first Duke of Sutherland. He had represented Chester or one of the Cheshire constituencies as a Whig from 1818 to 1835,[2] but after his father had presented him in 1831 with Motcombe House, near Shaftesbury, on the Dorset estate, he had spent most of his time there in simple domesticity, surrounded by his wife and their numerous children. Daily family prayers, the instruction of his elder children in Latin verse and the works of Shakespeare, and other such preoccupations had formed the routine of this 'deeply serious... high-principled, reserved' man,[201] who after his death was said by *The Times* never to have risen 'to the height of his opportunities'. He was, however, considered to have administered 'his vast estates with a combination of intelligence and generosity not often witnessed... His gift of a fine Park to the city of Chester' being regarded as 'an instance of almost princely munificence.'[202]

But within his family, and even in a wider circle, he had an evidently well-deserved reputation for parsimony, an attribute which, although originating in his youth,[203] was perhaps aggravated by the terms on which he had inherited much of the family wealth. His father—equally renowned for his thrift—had left a will of such complexity that it took the family solicitor, John Boodle, two hours to read.[204] By it the London estates were entailed to trustees for the use, firstly, of his eldest son, the second Marquess, for life, and then for life to his grandson, Hugh Lupus, the future third Marquess and first Duke; and the trust so established had, moreover, been extremely strictly drawn.[205] Finding himself thus restricted, the second Marquess's frequent lectures to young Hugh Lupus, about his 'idleness, listlessness and weak moral character' had evidently been intensified, and when in 1856 the latter had asked his father for financial help in addition to the income of £8,000 per annum already settled on him, the second Marquess had refused. 'With only a life interest in this strictly curtailed property I am sorry I cannot aid you.'[206] Nevertheless he did contrive to buy yet more lands, paying for them out of his own income from the settled estates, at a total cost of £195,000.[207]

At about the time of his death in 1869, his rents from the Mayfair estate alone amounted to *c.* £80,000 per annum.[189] Between 1845 and 1864 receipts from fines or premiums payable to the trustees on the renewal of leases amounted to £108,538. About half of this appears to have been used to discharge family encumbrances created by the first Marquess, but in 1864 there remained £55,584, the income from which (invested at three per cent) was payable to the second Marquess.[208]

Hugh Lupus, third Marquess and first Duke of Westminster (1825–99) was in some respects similar to his father. He, too, served his political apprenticeship in the House of Commons (as Liberal M.P. for Chester, 1847–69), married firstly a Leveson-Gower—his first cousin, a younger daughter of the second Duke of Sutherland, who bore him a large family—was deeply religious, and was regarded with some awe by his sons. But he was not known for thrift or parsimony. Although he never gambled he revived the Grosvenor racing stud (winning the Derby four times) and between 1870 and 1880 he rebuilt Eaton Hall, which once more became the family's out-of-town headquarters, at a cost of some £600,000.[209] He was a vigorous supporter of a variety of philanthropic causes, and unlike his father, he remained to the time of his death active in politics, where his admiration for his friend and neighbour, Gladstone, did not prevent his opposing both Gladstone's abortive Reform Bill of 1866 and the Irish Home Rule Bill of 1886. But despite the first of these disagreements it was Gladstone who recommended the Marquess for a dukedom in 1874—apparently for little other reason than the deep respect in which he was almost universally held; and although the second rift lasted longer, the old friendship was ultimately renewed.[210] The Duke, in fact, managed somehow to personify the generally prevalent idea of how a great rich nobleman should conduct himself, and after his death it was admiringly said of him that 'He could pass from a racecourse to take the chair at a missionary meeting without incurring the censure of the strictest'—a remarkable tribute at any time, but particularly so in the Victorian era.[211]

The Duke's biographer, Mr. Gervas Huxley, states that the settled properties of which he had become in 1869 the new life-owner 'were valued at close on £4,000,000, after deducting the capital value of all

encumbrances, and consisted of the whole of the London estates and part of the Cheshire, Chester, and Halkyn estates. He also inherited the absolute ownership of Eaton Hall, Halkyn Castle, and the bulk of the Cheshire, Chester, and Flintshire properties', with a capital value of some £750,000. 'The Dorset and Wiltshire properties owned by the second Marquess were unsettled and had been left to his widow for her lifetime', with remainder respectively to her younger son and her son-in-law.[212]

Only two important additions to his own personal estates were made by the third Marquess and first Duke—Reay Forest in Sutherlandshire, which he leased from his relatives the Dukes of Sutherland, and where he used Lochmore Lodge for his summer holidays; and Cliveden, Buckinghamshire, which he inherited in 1868 from his mother-in-law, the Dowager Duchess of Sutherland.[213] In 1893, however, he sold Cliveden to William Waldorf Astor for £250,000 to enable him to make provision for his children—fifteen in all, eleven by his first wife, who died in 1880, and four by his second—of whom eleven were still living in 1893.[214]

On the settled estates (which included the London properties) the entail created by the first Marquess could be broken when the first Duke's son, Victor Alexander, Earl Grosvenor, came of age. This was done in 1874, the estates being resettled[215] upon the first Duke and his son successively for each of their lives, and then upon Earl Grosvenor's eldest son as tenant in tail male.[216] Earl Grosvenor died in 1884, and soon after the succession of his son to the dukedom in 1899 the estates were once again disentailed and resettled (see pages 67, 79).[217]

During the time of the third Marquess and first Duke the rental from the Mayfair estate alone rose from *c.* £80,000 per annum in 1870 to *c.* £116,000 in 1882, and to *c.* £135,000 in 1891.[218] Between the resettlement of 1874 and the Duke's death in 1899 receipts from the fines or premiums payable to the trustees on the renewal of leases in Mayfair amounted to some £650,000. From this at least £200,000 was spent on improvements to the Duke's settled estates in both Cheshire and London, some of the very large mortgages incurred by the Duke were paid off, and provision was made for various members of the Duke's family. The running balance was placed on deposit and in the 1890's the interest therefrom was paid to the Duke as income.[219]

With the accession of the second Marquess in 1845 it is clear that the administration of the Mayfair estate became much stricter than hitherto. Ever since the precipitate flight of Abraham Moore, the agent, and the supersession of Porden, the surveyor, in 1821, the first Marquess had kept matters very much in his own hands; but by 1845 he was aged seventy-eight, and chiefly in Belgravia he had sometimes allowed building to proceed without formal leases or contracts, transferred ground rents from one contract to another, and through a casual system of record keeping generally got into a muddle, principally in his dealings with Thomas Cubitt. Within six months of his father's death, therefore, the second Marquess obtained a private Act of Parliament to set these matters right; and power was also obtained for the trustees established by the first Marquess's will to enter into contracts for the granting of leases—a power not adequately provided for in the will.[220]

The main object of the second Marquess's stricter management was to preserve and enhance the overall value of the estate, and—in the days before the statutory protection of buildings of historic or architectural interest—this of necessity involved the periodic rebuilding of outworn portions of the fabric. Rebuilding therefore became for the first time an integral part of estate policy. But rebuilding could generally only be undertaken when individual leases expired, for the purchase of subsisting leases was expensive and only rarely undertaken at this date; and as hitherto virtually no attempt had been made to make the leases of adjoining sites expire simultaneously, it followed that at first rebuilding could only be done on individual sites. Co-ordinated rebuilding over several adjacent sites would only become possible later, when the effect of renewing leases of adjacent sites for comparatively short terms all expiring contemporaneously had had time to make itself felt.

The second Marquess took an active interest in the architecture of his estates, and such evidence as exists suggests that he favoured co-ordinated schemes of rebuilding.[221] The old policy of renewing to applicants for such a term as would, with their subsisting leases, give them sixty-three years to come, was therefore no longer followed as a matter of course. Instead, both he and his successor considered each site in relation to its neighbours, and although they sometimes continued the old policy, they more frequently refused to renew beyond the date of expiry of the longest subsisting lease in any particular range of houses. At that date, when all the leases would expire at about the same time, the rebuilding of the whole range could at last be considered. Thus, for instance, at Nos. 1–8 (consec.) Upper Brook Street, the subsisting leases granted between 1810 and 1824 under the old haphazard policy expired at various dates between 1873 and 1887, but by short renewals of varying lengths granted between 1859 and 1876 they were all made to expire in 1886 or 1887.[189]

The increased flexibility of this policy made it possible in due course to phase the rebuilding of large parts of the estate over a number of years. Rebuilding entailed sacrificing the immediate in favour of the long-term interest of the estate, since the ground rents were lower than the receipts which would have been obtained on rack rents, and usually there were no fines. It also entailed much administrative work for the estate officers, and some social disturbance for the adjacent residents. It was therefore important that not too much rebuilding should take place at any one time, and these factors were clearly in the

second Marquess's mind when he stated in 1867 that 'I do not wish any new work to be taken in hand beyond what is now marked out but shall renew the Leases as they occur at short periods as we have done before, in order to give future opportunity for blocks being formed for local improvements'.[221] Thus to revert to the example of Upper Brook Street, Nos. 1-8 were not in fact rebuilt in 1887, for in 1881 the lease of No. 5 had been extended by the first Duke to 1906. In the early 1880's a considerable amount of rebuilding was already in progress or in prospect, notably in Mount Street, Oxford Street and the artisans' dwellings around Brown Hart Gardens, and between 1881 and 1886 the leases of the other seven houses in Nos. 1-8 Upper Brook Street were all also renewed to 1906, thereby merely postponing the opportunity to rebuild.[218]

The reign of the second Marquess was therefore more one of preparation for than of actual rebuilding, and what did take place was mostly on individual sites—notably three separate blocks of artisans' dwellings in Bourdon Street, and one in Grosvenor Market, ten mansions in Grosvenor Square, and a number of houses at the east ends of Brook Street and Grosvenor Street. But in the mid 1860's he was at last able to carry out two large schemes, one in Belgravia and one in the north-west corner of Mayfair, where the original building leases granted in the latter part of the eighteenth century were now expiring. In Belgravia he rebuilt part of Grosvenor Place and extended it southward (as Grosvenor Gardens) to Victoria Station (opened in 1860), both the layout, which included the formation of two triangular gardens, and the very large new houses being designed by Thomas Cundy III. In Mayfair the rebuilding of Hereford Street, parallel with and set back from Oxford Street, also to designs by Cundy III, began in 1866. By that time it was already well known that the Marquess was 'determined to pull down and rebuild on his estates whenever he has an opportunity'.[222]

But although his opportunities for such wholesale clearances had been very limited, and even rebuilding on individual sites had been restricted in scope, the second Marquess did nevertheless make very considerable alterations in the outward aspect of his Mayfair property, and the stamp of his taste, as executed chiefly by Thomas Cundy II, is still very apparent in many surviving buildings there. This imprint was made by requiring tenants, as a condition for the renewal of their leases, to execute precisely specified modifications to the then still Georgian elevations of their houses.

As we have already seen, the idea of 'improving the appearance of the houses in Grosvenor Square by the addition of stucco-work to the fronts with porticos, window dressings, cornices and balustrades to such of the houses as may be thought to require it' had already been suggested by Cundy II to the first Marquess in 1844;[200] but the latter had died a few months later. This suggestion was evidently at once approved by his successor, for in May 1845 Cundy's clerk was measuring the fronts of the houses on the south side of Grosvenor Square, the occupants being informed that the new Marquess was 'anxious to obtain a correct design for some proposed improvements'.[223] He was, however, intending to go much further than Cundy had suggested, for in November 1845 he sent John Boodle two very important 'instructions for future renewals' of leases. Firstly, in all future leases there was to be a covenant requiring 'no alteration of the frontage without permission from the Grosvenor Estate Office'; and secondly, all houses of four or more windows' width were 'to have a Doric Portico with fluted or plain Pillars carried out to the end of the area railing'.[224]

The elevational alterations which, in negotiations for the renewal of leases of houses in the principal streets, tenants were now usually required to execute, were generally designed by Cundy II. The applicant had to sign a bond, often of over £1,000, to ensure the due performance of the works, which generally included the addition of a Doric open porch and sometimes a balustrade in front of the first-floor windows (both in Portland stone), cement dressings to the windows, and a blocking course, balustrade or moulded stone coping at the top. Sometimes an additional storey was to be built, plate glass might be required for all the windows, and occasionally also works of improvement in the domestic offices in the basement. Attached to the bond there was usually a detailed specification of the works and a copy of Cundy's design.[225]

The effect of this policy, which was vigorously pursued throughout the whole of the second Marquess's reign from 1845 to 1869, was to make the principal streets on the estate, hitherto purely Georgian in appearance, look increasingly like those of South Kensington (see page 133). Over twenty examples of fronts entirely designed or altered by Cundy II (latterly assisted by his son Thomas Cundy III) still survive. These are chiefly in Brook Street, Upper Brook Street and Grosvenor Street, and originally, before later rebuildings, there were many more, notably some dozen in Grosvenor Square alone, for the south range of which he produced in 1849 a complete scheme of 'suggested alterations'.[226]

Tenants or builders engaged in the complete rebuilding of individual houses also found it convenient to have Cundy as their architect, or at least for him to provide the elevation, for they knew that his work would be acceptable to the Marquess; and sometimes it was made a condition of rebuilding that Cundy should design the new front.[227] Thus in Grosvenor Square (Plate 25) he and/or his son did ten houses. Four of these were for tenants (Nos. 18, 20, 21 and 30, all demolished), another four for the builder C. J. Freake (No. 4, which still survives, and Nos. 10, 26 and 40, all demolished), and one each for the builders Wright Ingle (No. 42, demolished) and Sir John Kelk (No. 2, demolished). Ingle also employed him at the still-surviving Nos. 11 Upper Brook Street and 20 Grosvenor Street, as did Kelk at No. 128 Park Lane.

For the prolific local builders John Newson and his son George John Newson he did Nos. 14, 23 and 24 Grosvenor Street and Nos. 48–50 (even) Brook Street, all of which still survive, as well as others now demolished.

The Cundys did not always have a free hand, however, for the Marquess sometimes rejected even their designs. At No. 21 Grosvenor Square, for instance, he refused to allow Venetian windows, despite the evident wishes of both Cundy III and the tenant (who was of course paying for the new house there);[228] and when in 1848 Cundy II produced 'for the Marquess's consideration' two drawings showing the existing elevation and 'his proposed elevation' for all the houses on the north side of Brook Street east of Davies Street, it was recorded that 'the Marquess does not approve the proposed plan, and Mr Cundy takes it away'.[229] Subsequently, however, four houses in this range (Nos. 48, 50, 56 and 58, all still surviving) were rebuilt to elevational designs by Cundy, but presumably in a different manner to that originally proposed.

The elevational alterations required by the second Marquess involved the tenants in considerable expense, but there is little evidence that they objected on this ground. When the works were very extensive, as in the case of Miss Mary-Anne Talbot at No. 24 Grosvenor Square, which had a long flank elevation to Upper Brook Street, the fine was reduced or remitted to suit the financial convenience of the tenant; but the full annual value of the house was nevertheless expressed in the ground rent, which was raised from £13 (on a lease granted in 1792) to £460, in exchange for a renewal of only thirteen and a quarter years to come (1855–68).[230] She and her sister were, however, very wealthy women, for in 1862 they were able to sell their Portobello estates in North Kensington for building for over £100,000.[231] At the still surviving No. 15 Upper Grosvenor Street Arthur Ward was required in 1862 to provide a porch, balcony and window dressings (designed by Cundy) in exchange for a reversionary extension of only ten years, from 1871 to 1881; but he had to pay a fine of £1,125 and (from 1871) a rent of £215 instead of £50.[232] For tenants as rich as those in the best streets of the Grosvenor estate, the cost of the Marquess's 'improvement' requirements were almost trivial. Porches were fashionable and popular, and the records of the Metropolitan Board of Works show that quite a number of them were erected voluntarily by tenants, sometimes without the approval of the Grosvenor Board. Many of these have been lost through later rebuildings, but at least one, badly designed in 1867 by Henry McCalla, architect, still survives at No. 68 Grosvenor Street.[233]

In one case, however, the Marquess's requirement to erect a stone balcony at first-floor level was resisted on stylistic grounds, though unsuccessfully. This was at No. 41 Upper Brook Street (now demolished), where Sir Henry Meux, the brewer, had in 1851 commissioned Samuel Beazley to make extensive alterations. The Marquess's intention was to make the house correspond outwardly with its neighbour, No. 42, which had an elegant iron balcony erected in previous years. Beazley had therefore designed a similar iron balcony for No. 41, but nevertheless the Marquess (down at Motcombe House in Dorset) rather perversely instructed Cundy to insist on a stone balcony, and this was duly put up, not without much mutual acrimony. Beazley died shortly afterwards,[234] and when the lease of No. 42 came up for renewal a few years later Cundy and his master were able to have the offending iron balcony there replaced by one of Portland stone corresponding to Meux's at No. 41.[235]

Obedience to the Marquess's architectural commands was, indeed, almost unavoidable, and the only known example of successful defiance was provided by a woman. This was Mrs. Gwynne Holford of No. 36 Grosvenor Square, who, having signed a bond for £1,000 to comply with his behests and paid a fine for renewal, then refused to do the work (for what reason is not recorded). Ultimately in 1869 she was excused, on forfeiture of £300 of her bond. But this reprieve was granted not by the implacable second Marquess but during his last fatal illness by his son and heir; and it may be doubted whether the father would have been so lenient.[236] In later years, when this formidable lady applied for another renewal, the first Duke and Thomas Cundy III wisely required her only to insert plate glass in the windows, but she died in 1881 before the completion of negotiations.[237]

The extensive up-dating of the plain old Georgian fronts and the complete rebuilding of some houses were only the most apparent and most immediately effective manifestations of the altogether stricter régime inaugurated by the second Marquess. His control was, of course, mainly exercised through the covenants contained in his leases, which were much more carefully drawn than hitherto. But whilst he could make the immediate execution of elevational alterations a condition for the grant of a reversionary lease, the new covenants which he inserted into such leases did not become operative until the expiry of the subsisting term. Many of the existing leases on the estate still had long terms to run, moreover, and often there was therefore no opportunity to renew them on stricter terms during his years in charge. Thus as late as 1876 the tenant of a house in Norfolk (now Dunraven) Street held under a sixty-year lease granted in 1820 did not have to obtain the first Duke's consent to make alterations because 'at present the old lease is in force'.[238] And although immediately after his succession in 1845 the second Marquess began to refuse to renew when the existing lease had more than ten years to come,[239] there was nevertheless a time lag of varying length but seldom less than of about a decade before many of his leasing innovations could take effect.

The single most important of these innovations was the covenant requiring 'no alteration of the frontage without permission from the Grosvenor Estate Office'.[239]

Commencing in 1845 this clause has been inserted in all subsequent Grosvenor leases, the phrase 'no alteration of the frontage' being soon extended to any part of the exterior of a building, any additional or substituted building, or any change in the 'architectural appearance', this last including even the enclosure of the sides or front of projecting porches.[240]

As the existing leases which did not contain this clause gradually expired this new covenant gave the second Marquess and his successors a vice-like control over the outward appearance of the buildings on their properties which has never been relaxed, and which has in some considerable measure been responsible for the high visual quality of many parts of the Grosvenor estates in London. With the passage of time this instrument of control was, moreover, refined still further. In 1851 the Marquess approved a design by Cundy II for area railings 'for general adoption', and a specimen of it was made 'for the inspection of the lessees'.[241] Beginning in 1854 all leases contained a covenant requiring stucco-work to be painted once every seven years and all wood and ironwork twice.[242] A few years later the stucco was required to be painted 'of a stone colour', and the work was to be done in every leap year, thus ensuring 'that houses were kept clean simultaneously and the general appearance was good'.[243] In 1866 'Words [were] to be added to the forms of lease to prohibit alterations to chimney pots',[244] and soon afterwards tenants were required to clean and repoint the brickwork every seven years.[245]

But the outward appearance of the buildings was not the only field in which the Grosvenors' control was greatly extended in the middle years of the nineteenth century. In his later years the first Marquess had begun to require his tenants to contribute a fair share to the repair of party walls—hitherto sometimes a troublesome cause of dispute—and to notify the Estate Office of any assignments of head leases.[246] His successor at once began to stipulate a right for his officers to make a schedule of fixtures in all leased premises,[247] in order to prevent the removal of such fixtures at the end of a lease, some of them, particularly chimneypieces, being of considerable value.

More important than these purely administrative changes, however, were those innovations concerned with the uses to which any particular property might be put. We have already seen that in the 'best' streets in the latter part of the eighteenth century a ban had been placed, wherever reasonably possible in the then existing circumstances, upon 'any art, trade or manufactory whatsoever'. In Grosvenor Square always, and in the other 'best' streets sometimes, the second Marquess extended this ban to professional use as well, doctors and surgeons being the main target for exclusion; and he also prohibited his tenants in these 'best' streets from doing or permitting anything which 'may be or become a nuisance or annoyance' to either himself as ground landlord or to the adjoining tenants.[248]

Elsewhere on the estate leases had since 1799 contained a list of prohibited trades followed by 'or other noisome or offensive Trade of Manufactory whatsoever'. In the second Marquess's time this list of prohibited trades—now considerably longer*—was at first concluded with the greatly strengthened formula 'or any other trade or business that shall be a nuisance or annoyance to the neighbourhood'.[250] By the 1860's, however, this phrase had become even more stringent as 'any other trade, business or occupation which in the judgement of the Marquess of Westminster shall be deemed objectionable or a nuisance to the neighbours'.[251]

With control of this nature there was in practice hardly any difference between the phraseology of the lease of a mansion in Grosvenor Square and that of a coach-house in a mews: the Marquess, and later the first Duke, could and did specify precisely for what purpose any building might be used. Thus some leases for premises in Brook's Mews granted in 1887 forbad the practice there of 'any art, trade, business' or even profession, and required the tenant to use them 'as a private dwelling house only and the said demised coach house and stable as a private gentleman's coach house and stable for horses only, and the rooms over the same...for the lodging of servants or others to be employed in or about the said demised premises and for no other purpose'. When, as sometimes happened, mews premises were to be used for purposes other than 'a private gentleman's coach house and stable', a manuscript addition was inserted into the standard printed lease which came into general use in the 1880's. Thus a lease of 1891 of other premises in Brook's Mews banned all trades, businesses or professions except that of jobmaster and horse-dealer; and a few years later a similar lease contained the usual ban, followed by an exception in favour of the business of the Stohwasser and Winter Puttee Legging and Military Equipment Corporation Limited.[252]

The granting of exceptions such as these had of course to be made judiciously. It was all very well to ban hog-skinners, catgut-spinners, horse-boilers and such like

* In 1887, when the list reached its maximum extent, a tenant in Brook's Mews undertook not to use the premises as a forge, place of public entertainment or museum, and not to carry on any of the following trades: butcher, pork butcher, fishmonger, slaughterer, knacker, horse boiler, hogskinner, cat gut spinner, cart-grease or varnish maker, melter of tallow, soap boiler, melter of fat, tripe boiler, tripe seller, sausage maker, sugar baker, fellmonger, dyer, scourer, alehouse keeper, beerhouse keeper, tavern keeper, licensed victualler, gambling or betting house keeper, brass or iron founder, blacksmith, whitesmith, coppersmith, working brazier, pewterer, tin or iron plate worker, packing-case maker, undertaker, coffin maker, glass maker, farrier, goldbeater, beater of flax, hemp or feathers, beater of carpets, bone boiler, cork burner, chimney sweeper, dealer in soot, dealer in second-hand clothes, boots or shoes, dealer in old iron or marine stores or any other trade, business or employment 'which shall be dangerous or a nuisance or annoyance' to the adjoining tenants and occupiers.[249]

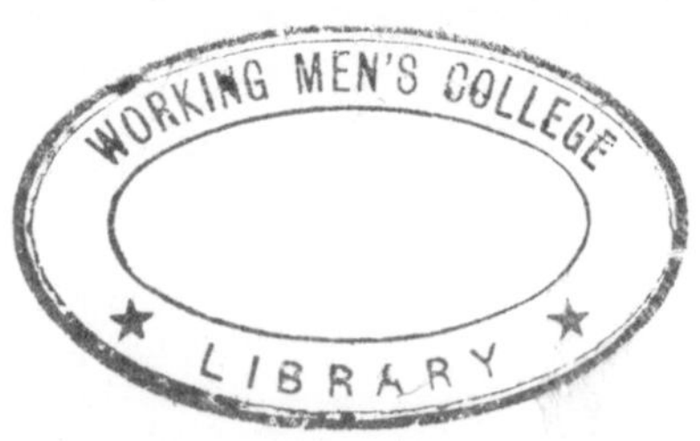

from the estate, but not even its most august residents could do without butchers or fishmongers, nor their servants without licensed victuallers, all of which trades were in general also prohibited, but of which there had always, of necessity, been quite a number of practitioners. So exceptions in their favour had to be made, although, as we shall see later, this did not prevent the first Duke from making a great reduction in the number of licensed victuallers. But subject only to the limitation of having to allow for the basic human requirements of all the residents, the ground landlord's control of the use of all premises had, well before the end of the nineteenth century, become complete and total. And later additions to the lease covenants, such as the prohibition of the display of goods for sale on the pavements, the exhibition of bills or placards, or the keeping of 'living fowls' were all relatively minor.[253]

The new restrictive covenants contained in mid nineteenth-century Grosvenor leases were not, however, the only means of control. No regular inspections of the properties on the estate were made at that time (except immediately prior to the grant of a new lease), because it had been found that the system of usually exacting a fine on renewal gave the tenant 'the greater interest during the term' and thus provided 'a guarantee against breaches of the covenants of his lease'.[254] But despite the lack of inspection, the Grosvenor Board (meeting weekly at 3 p.m. on Tuesdays or Thursdays 'except when Marquess in town')[255] seems to have known what was going on, and frequently required tenants to conform. In 1858–61, for instance, Lord Chesham made unauthorised alterations to the rear of his new house, No. 20 Grosvenor Square, and after being told to remove them a compromise was reached;[256] and in 1864 George (later Viscount) Goschen was made to stop building an unauthorised conservatory at his house at the corner of Park Lane and Mount Street.[257]

The Board was, in fact, well informed—sufficiently so to know in 1853 that 'in all the modern stables there are water closets', but that in those held under old leases privies were still prevalent, and that therefore new leases of stables should require the formation of properly drained water closets.[258] In 1869 it knew of the existence of nineteen slaughter-houses in Mayfair, Belgravia and Pimlico, all prohibited under the terms of the respective leases. All of them were, however, 'in commercial neighbourhoods', and after enquiries had been made among the neighbours it was found that only four were a nuisance. The owners of these were told to stop, but, in the days before the freezing of meat, slaughtering had to be done near the point of consumption and at least one slaughterman was subsequently reprieved provided that he 'uses every precaution to prevent nuisance'.[259] In the more delicate purlieus of Grosvenor Street, however, Colonel Augustus Meyrick was in 1865 prohibited from keeping a cow, despite his lawyer's opinion that 'some gentlemen like to keep a cow in London'.[260] But prostitutes presented a more difficult problem, here on the Grosvenor estate as elsewhere, and although the existence of brothels in Gilbert Street and Chapel (now Aldford) Street was known to the Board, no effective action seems to have been taken against them.[261]

Commencing in 1864, when extensive rebuilding in Grosvenor Place and Gardens in Belgravia was in progress, a clerk of works was employed 'to inspect the building works generally over the Estate'. His salary, and also the considerable fees due to Thomas Cundy III (although the latter did not succeed his father as surveyor until 1867) were paid out of a new Improvement Account, opened at the same time. The receipts paid into this account came mainly from the proceeds of the auction sales of the old materials and fixtures of houses about to be demolished, of which there were quite a number at that time. In 1864, for instance, the proceeds of the sale at two adjoining houses in Grosvenor Square (about to be rebuilt by C. J. Freake as a single house) amounted to £843. Payments out were mostly to the St. George's Vestry for road, pavement and sewer works executed on behalf of the Estate, principally no doubt at Grosvenor Place and Gardens. From time to time, when expenditure exceeded the income from the sales, the Marquess transferred additional funds from his private account.[262]

The rebuildings in Grosvenor Place and Gardens and in Hereford Street, Mayfair, in the mid 1860's were the forerunners of the very extensive rebuildings which took place in Mayfair in the 1870's, 80's and 90's. These operations, and the antecedent demolitions, caused much disturbance to adjoining occupants. In 1861 the second Marquess therefore began to prohibit the dusty noisy work of demolition during the London social 'Season', when all important personages were sure to be in residence in their town houses. In that year C. J. Freake, about to rebuild No. 26 Grosvenor Square, was required to demolish the old house in August and September after the Season was over,[263] and in 1865 Sir John Johnstone had to demolish No. 30 in February and March before it had begun.[264] Soon afterwards the cleaning and pointing of brickwork was interdicted in the months of May, June and July,[265] and in 1875 Sir John Kelk was forbidden to commence work on No. 3 Grosvenor Square until 1 August as 'it is the rule of the estate that no works of this nature should be commenced during the London season owing to the annoyance which would be caused to the neighbours'.[266] It was not, indeed, for nothing that the second Marquess, who had inaugurated this policy, now continued by his son, was known (to quote *The Building News* in 1865) to be 'determined to have none but tip-top people on his estates'.[222]

Rules of this kind were required in order to minimise the upheavals caused by the colossal rebuilding programme executed under the auspices of the third Marquess and first Duke during his thirty years' reign (1869–99). This rebuilding was probably larger in scope than any carried out on any other London estate (except, perhaps,

that of the Crown) in the whole of the nineteenth century, and at the time of writing (1976) large parts of the existing fabric of the Grosvenor estate in Mayfair date from these years. It included the whole of Mount Street, Duke Street, Aldford Street and Balfour Place; almost all of South Audley Street north of South Street; all of the north side of Green Street and a quarter of the south side; almost all of the south side of Oxford Street from Davies Street to Park Lane; most of the west side of North Audley Street and the south side of Bourdon Street; substantial parts of Park Street and several mews (Adams Row, Balfour Mews, Mount Row and North Row); part of the north side of South Street; the Carlos Place quadrant on an improved frontage, and the realignment of the north end of Davies Street; three new churches, two schools, new Vestry offices, a library and a dozen blocks of artisans' dwellings.

Notably absent from this list are the houses in the principal streets. Half a dozen of the mansions in Grosvenor Square were in fact rebuilt in these years (Nos. 3, 27, 33, 34, 41 and 39 'practically') and the great block of Claridge's Hotel reared itself in Brook Street; but in Grosvenor Street and Upper Grosvenor Street there was hardly any rebuilding and none at all in Upper Brook Street. It was in these streets, principally, that the second Marquess's policy of elevational improvements to designs, usually by Thomas Cundy II, had been most rigorously applied. Because the houses here were generally in the hands of wealthy tenants they were already in good order, and although the first Duke's procedure in renewing leases in the principal streets, as elsewhere, was to make the terms of all the houses in any single range expire at approximately the same time, rebuilding was nevertheless often postponed when that time arrived, as at Nos. 1–8 Upper Brook Street, previously mentioned—presumably because the Duke wished to limit the amount of rebuilding going on at any one time and felt that the claims of other lesser streets were more urgent.

The first Duke inherited the long-term results of the second Marquess's leasing policy and was able to rebuild whole ranges to a single design. Almost all his rebuilding was done in this way, rather than on individual sites, and it is because so little rebuilding took place in his time in Brook Street, Grosvenor Street, Upper Brook Street and Upper Grosvenor Street that so many of the original houses there, though often greatly altered, have survived. When in his early years (1899–*c.* 1914) the second Duke turned his attention to these four 'best' streets, there had been a partial reaction away from renewal in whole ranges, and he often favoured individual refronting or rebuilding. So by the chance of this change of fashion they, or at any rate their individual sites, survived again, and although in later years a number of blocks of flats or offices have been built, these four streets still retain in some measure—and certainly more than anywhere else on the estate—the domestic flavour of the original development.

The first Duke's preference for rebuilding in ranges rather than on individual sites provided architects on the estate with new problems and opportunities, and this is at any rate one reason why the buildings erected in his time are so strikingly different from those built under his father. But their own architectural tastes also differed, and these differences reflected current changes in Victorian fashion. Whereas the second Marquess had liked and required the Italianate stucco widely prevalent in London in the 1850's and 60's, his son was a supporter of the Queen Anne Revival and a fervent admirer of the new 'South Kensington' red-brick and terracotta manner. Throughout the whole of his reign he championed the new modes and materials, and only two months before his death in 1899 he commented on a proposal in Duke Street 'the more red brick the better'.[267]

This difference in taste extended to the architectural embellishment of existing buildings. In 1856, for example, the second Marquess had required the applicant for a reversionary lease of No. 14 Grosvenor Square to erect an open Doric porch, remove the iron balcony at first-floor level and substitute three stone balconettes and add a square attic storey. This had not been done because the tenant later decided not to renew, but in 1878 the first Duke required a dormer attic instead of a square one, and the retention of 'the present character of the brick front'.[268] Stone or stucco porches, balconies, balustrades and window dressings were, in fact, now becoming things of the past, and it is hardly an exaggeration to say that all important surviving Georgian brick fronts without these embellishments are so because they did not have their leases renewed during the second Marquess's time—Nos. 76 Brook Street and 36 Upper Brook Street are cases in point. The tastes of the second and third Marquesses were indeed so different that in dealing in 1899 with an application to renew the lease of No. 55 South Audley Street, now the sole survivor of three houses built in white brick in 1859 to designs by Cundy II (fig. 14b on page 134), the Duke commented that he 'objected to the appearance' of this trio 'and would not consent to any arrangement for perpetuating it'.[269]

It was also presumably for reasons associated with the Duke's personal taste in architecture that, despite the enormous volume of rebuilding, Thomas Cundy III was hardly employed at all in Mayfair. He had succeeded his father as estate surveyor in 1867 and held the post until his resignation in 1890, aged seventy. Although he worked extensively on the Belgravia and Pimlico estates, where he designed churches and schools and (as previously mentioned) the new houses in Grosvenor Gardens and Place,[270] his work on the Mayfair estate consisted chiefly of planning for future rebuilding, routine administration, repairs and embellishments. The only row of houses designed by him there was that in Hereford Gardens, the rebuilding of which had started in the days of his father, Thomas Cundy II, and of the second Marquess, and he also did a number of commercial buildings in

Oxford Street. The records of the Grosvenor Estate Board contain hints of several disagreements between the Duke and Cundy,[271] and the stuccoed domestic buildings of Cundy's private practice in South Kensington are unlikely to have been to the Duke's taste.[272] This, doubtless, was the reason for Cundy's virtual exclusion from design work in the predominantly brick purlieus of Mayfair.

Cundy's successor as estate surveyor, Eustace Balfour,* was appointed by the Duke in 1890.[274] He was a brother of the future Prime Minister, a grandson of the second Marquess of Salisbury, and his wife, besides being a daughter of the eighth Duke of Argyll, was also a niece of the Duke of Westminster.[275] In architectural matters his well-mannered brick and stone fronts were entirely acceptable to both the first Duke and to his grandson and successor the second Duke, and he (and/or his partner, Thackeray Turner) worked extensively on the Mayfair estate, particularly in the south-west corner around Aldford Street and Balfour Place. He seems to have resigned in 1910 owing to bad health, and died in 1911, aged fifty-seven.[276]

Numerous other architects were of course employed in the Mayfair rebuildings during the first Duke's time, but before discussing the various ways in which they obtained their commissions it is necessary to examine the mechanics of the whole process. The general leasing policy continued to be to renew for comparatively short periods coterminous for all the houses in any particular range. In 1889 fear of the possibility of leasehold enfranchisement, then much in public debate, made the Duke and his Board decide not to renew (except in the case of rebuilding) for more than twenty years,[277] and in the 1890's this was generally reduced to ten years.[278] Under the deed of resettlement of 1874 the Duke's trustees now had power to accept surrenders of existing leases,[279] and this was sometimes done with the co-operation of an intending building lessee, who bought up the existing leases and then surrendered them to the estate as part of his rebuilding contract. In 1882 the Settled Land Act enabled trustees to spend capital money on improvements,[280] and at about this time the Grosvenor trustees occasionally bought outstanding leases themselves to expedite rebuilding. Thus in 1880 they bought a number of leases for the site of St. Mary's Church, Bourdon Street, and in the 1890's those of several in Mount Street, Park Street and Green Street,[281] the capital being repaid to the trustees by the building lessee or his nominee on the completion of rebuilding, and allowed to him by a reduced ground rent.[282]

From about 1876 onwards the Duke also began, in blocks where he intended to rebuild, to refuse applications for renewals. Many such applicants held leases with up to ten years still to run, and thus, at any rate in theory, they had some warning of their impending forced disturbance. Generally they were told that at the end of their term their property would be rebuilt, 'required for estate purposes', or 'probably wanted for improvements'. Between 1876 and 1899 nearly one hundred and fifty such applications were refused.

By all these means the Duke was able to obtain an increasingly tight yet flexible grip on his estate, and the final years prior to rebuilding provided an opportunity to decide the future character of a range or block about to be redeveloped—a process in which Cundy III was much involved. In 1877, for example, he was already planning the new frontage line for Charles Street (now Carlos Place), while in the block bounded by Green Street, Park Street, Wood's Mews and Norfolk (now Dunraven) Street he was required in 1880 to plan the future rearrangement of the plots.[283] In 1884 the Duke approved his preliminary plan for the adjoining block to the east and decided that 'there shall be no shops in Park Street but small private houses, and that a model lodging house shall be built in the mews at the rear of Green Street, with an open space to Green Street westward of Hampden House. Rebuilding to be carried out gradually as opportunity arises'—most of which was in due course effected.[284] Shops at the west end of Mount Street and in Green Street were to be eliminated in favour of 'small private houses' when rebuilding took place, and they were also intended to go at the eastern end of Brook Street,[285] but elsewhere they were encouraged—'The Duke wants shops in South Audley Street'.[286]

Rebuilding leases granted by the second Marquess in the 1850's and 60's for private houses had generally been for seventy-seven years, but under the first Duke the normal term was increased to eighty years for commercial properties as in Oxford Street, and to ninety years for private houses in and around Grosvenor Square.[287] In the mid 1880's ninety years became the normal term throughout the whole of Mount Street, and in some premises where terracotta was required to be used an extra six months at a peppercorn rent was granted in addition to the normal allowance of one year.[288] Negotiations for a building lease culminated in the signature of a building contract containing detailed specifications, to which in 1888 Cundy III suggested adding a clause requiring fireproof construction. In 1890 the specifications were tightened up by Eustace Balfour.[289]

From the mid 1870's onwards it was the practice, whenever possible, to treat first of all with the occupant for both the renewal of leases and the grant of rebuilding leases. In the case of private houses to be rebuilt individually there was seldom any difficulty. Thus Dr. Joseph Walker, in occupation of part of No. 22 Grosvenor Street and in possession of the whole of the adjoining No. 21, a lodging house, accepted terms for the rebuilding

* As commander of the London Scottish Royal Volunteer Corps (a position to which he had risen from the ranks) from 1894 to 1902 he was often referred to as Colonel Balfour.[273]

of both houses in 1898–9, the lodging-house keeper evidently having no wish to treat; or Sir John Kelk, wanting a house in Grosvenor Square, bought the lease of No. 3 and after being granted a renewal, proceeded to rebuild it completely (now demolished). The Duke's policy in such cases was to 'let to a gentleman for his own occupation' rather than to a speculator,[290] and if the occupant under an expiring lease did not wish to rebuild, a rebuilding lease was generally offered to some other gentleman known to be looking for a site in the locality. No. 41 Grosvenor Square was rebuilt by C. H. Wilson, M.P., in this way in 1883–6, and No. 27 by the Earl of Aberdeen in 1886–8 (fig. 22 on page 150). There was seldom if ever any shortage of takers.

When—as more usually happened in the first Duke's time—a whole range of private houses was to be erected simultaneously, building was invariably done by a speculator of known substance, generally a builder. Thus, for example, Matthews, Rogers and Company built Nos. 2–11 (consec.) Green Street (1891–5), Daw and Son Nos. 14–22 (even) Park Street and 68 Mount Street (1896–7) and Higgs and Hill Nos. 2–12 (even) Park Street (1897–*c.* 1900, now partly demolished). Usually each rebuilding site was offered by the Board to a reputable speculating builder, but occasionally a speculator applied for a site and got it, as in the case of J. T. Smith at Nos. 106–116 (even) Park Street and 19 Green Street (1887–8), or of Holloways at Nos. 40–46 (even) Brook Street (1898–9). Similarly in November 1890 Trollopes applied for and obtained the very important site of Nos. 6–9 (consec.) Mount Street, 1–8 (consec.) Carlos Place and 1–15 (odd) Mount Row, and in the following year they obtained the site of Nos. 45–52 (consec.) Mount Street by competitive public tender—apparently the only occasion when this method of selection was used in those years.*

But when shops, and particularly a whole range of them, were to be rebuilt, there were very considerable problems, which were closely examined in 1887 by the Select Committee of the House of Commons on Town Holdings. The shopkeepers naturally feared the loss of their goodwill through enforced removal, and (to quote from H. T. Boodle's evidence to the Committee) the Estate Board therefore generally recommended 'that the occupier, if he is capable of rebuilding, shall be the person to rebuild, so that the question of disturbing him does not arise'. In certain cases, moreover, the Duke had 'found it practicable to allow old tenants to rebuild, even when the new elevations form part of one general design ...two or three of them adjoining combine and employ the same architect and builder'.[291]

This had indeed happened during the time of the second Marquess at Nos. 489–497 (odd) Oxford Street, which were rebuilt in 1865–6 with elevations in the French style by Thomas Cundy III (Plate 27b). Here the individual shopkeepers who were the rebuilding lessees combined together to employ a single builder, Mark Patrick and Son, and even agreed among themselves to reduce the number of original plots in order to obtain wider frontages for their shops. This block has been demolished, but another with similar elevations by Cundy survives at Nos. 407–413. Here in 1870–1 Peter Squire, manufacturing chemist and chemist in ordinary to the Queen, was the rebuilding lessee for four old shops and houses, one of which had hitherto been in his own occupation, and which he rebuilt as two—now Nos. 411 and 413 Oxford Street. Shortly afterwards his neighbour, a fruiterer, was the rebuilding lessee for the adjoining two shops and houses (Nos. 407 and 409). This completed the short range between Binney Street and Duke Street, and at about the same time the adjoining range (also short) to the west was rebuilt, the building lessee for No. 415 being T. B. Linscott, a confectioner, for the centre portion J. M. Macey, a builder, and for the western portion the trustees of the Association in Aid of the Deaf and Dumb, who built a church there (all now demolished). Macey built all three portions, No. 415 and the church (Plate 29c) under contract with the respective lessees, and the centre evidently as a speculation on his own account.

Linscott had at first been 'rather reluctant to rebuild', but the Duke and his advisers had insisted that it was 'absolutely necessary that his house should be pulled down'. Some years later, however, H. T. Boodle said that 'whenever he [Linscott] sees me, he thanks me for having been firm, and having advised him to rebuild. He says, his profits are a great deal more than they had been for years; it has immensely improved his business, and he sees how short-sighted he was in wishing to retain the old house.'[292] With this encouraging example several other Oxford Street tradesmen became building lessees in later years, notably a linen draper in 1875–6 at Nos. 431 and 433, who had previously occupied the adjoining shops, and Thrupp and Maberly, the coach-builders, who in 1884–7 rebuilt their own premises (now demolished) between Lumley and Balderton Streets.

This procedure, in which each tradesman/rebuilding lessee acted on his own individual account, negotiating terms with the Grosvenor Board and then employing a builder to put up the new house and shop, was at first employed elsewhere on the estate. In 1875, for instance, W. J. Goode began the rebuilding of his own shop at

*Other examples of ranges of private houses built by speculators include: Charles Fish, 51–54 (consec.) Green Street, 1882–3; Robert Edis, 105–115 (odd) Park Street and 25–31 (consec.) Green Street, 1891–4; Trollopes, 34–42 (even) Park Street, 1895–9; Colonel Bird, Balfour Place, east side, 1891–4; W. H. Warner, the block bounded by Mount Street, Balfour Place, Aldford Street and Rex Place, 1891–7; William Willett, 39–47 (odd) South Street, 1896–8; William Cubitt and Company, 94–104A (even) Park Street, 1896–8, and 55–59 (consec.) Green Street, 1897–8; Bywaters, 16–19 (consec.) Dunraven Street, 1897–8.

Nos. 18–19 South Audley Street, and in 1882 Henry Lofts, an estate agent with offices in Mount Street due to be rebuilt soon, was the rebuilding lessee for Nos. 34 Berkeley Square and 130 Mount Street, which adjoined each other. But in the mid 1880's a substantial frontage of over ninety feet on the south side of Mount Street was leased in two blocks to two local businessmen for rebuilding to designs prepared by the same architect, Ernest George (Plate 34b). This site had hitherto been occupied by part of the St. George's Workhouse, which was now removed to Pimlico, and simultaneous rebuilding by more than one lessee was therefore relatively easy to arrange, there being no occupants with claims to be considered. The two lessees were W. H. Warner, Lofts's partner in the firm of Lofts and Warner, and Jonathan Andrews, a builder with premises on the north side of Mount Street soon due for demolition.

This precedent was followed, in more elaborate form, in the rebuilding of most of the rest of Mount Street east of South Audley Street during the ensuing decade. On the south side of Mount Street the Grosvenor Board arranged for the rebuilding of Nos. 125–129 (consec.) by four local shopkeeper-lessees in 1886–7 (Plate 34c); Nos. 116–121 (consec.) by four shopkeepers and a surgeon, all local (1886–7); Nos. 94–102 (consec.) in 1889–91, and Nos. 87–93 (consec.) Mount Street (Plate 34a) and 26–33 (consec.) South Audley Street (1893–5), each by five local shopkeepers or businessmen.

On the north side of Mount Street similar consortia were formed at Nos. 1–5 consec. (1888–9, Nos. 1–3 now demolished), and at Nos. 27–28 Mount Street and 34–42 (consec.) South Audley Street (1888–9). And the same procedure was followed in parts of other predominantly commercial streets, notably in South Audley Street, at Nos. 61–63 consec. (1889–91) and Nos. 64–68 consec. (1891–3); in Duke Street at Nos. 55–73 odd (1890–2); and in Oxford Street at Nos. 385–397 odd (1887–9). Generally each group of lessees employed a single building contractor—Perry Brothers, for instance, at Nos. 87–93 (consec.) Mount Street and 26–33 (consec.) South Audley Street, or Kirk and Randall at Nos. 55–73 (odd) Duke Street; but when one of the lessees was himself in the building trade, he was sometimes allowed to do the building on his own site. Thus at Nos. 94–102 (consec.) Mount Street Bywaters were the contractors for four of the lessees, but the fifth, Andrews, being a builder, was permitted to do his own construction work provided that 'the bricks and terra cotta are obtained from the same source as the other houses so that the colour may be alike';[293] and similarly at Nos. 116–121 (consec.) Mount Street W. W. Weir, an upholsterer, was allowed 'to build his own house', he being 'experienced in building works'.[294]

The administrative labour required to establish and supervise these tradesmen's consortia and their architects (who will be discussed later) was very considerable and could only have been attempted on such a large rich estate as that of the Grosvenor family. Even there it evidently placed considerable strain on the Duke's advisers, for when a private resident whose lease had only four more years to come applied in 1884 for a renewal he was brusquely told that 'the matter could not be pressing and must await more pressing renewals'.[295] This, perhaps, was one reason why, despite the Duke's evident wish to treat so far as possible with commercial occupants, commercial sites were nevertheless quite often offered to speculators, just as sites for residential ranges always were. This practice, which entailed much less work for the estate staff, was first adopted in the 1870's when Thomas Patrick, of Mark Patrick and Son, builders, became the rebuilding lessee of Nos. 443–451 (odd) Oxford Street (1876–8), his architect being J. T. Wimperis. It was continued at Nos. 57–60 (consec.) South Audley Street, where James Purdey, the gunmaker, who had not hitherto had any premises on the estate, began in 1879 to buy up the subsisting short-term leases with a view to rebuilding. This was done in 1881–2, Purdey taking the prominent corner with Mount Street for his shop while the rest of the building was used as residential chambers—a successful speculation evidently, for in 1892 he rebuilt the adjoining No. 84 Mount Street and signed a contract to rebuild No. 31 Green Street (both private houses).

In South Audley Street Purdey had clearly been allowed to rebuild because the previous occupants preferred to sell their old leases to him and remove rather than undertake to rebuild for themselves; and lack of applications to rebuild from occupants may sometimes have been the reason why commercial sites were offered to speculators. But this was at any rate not altogether the case on the west side of Duke Street, where in August 1886 Boodle invited J. T. Wimperis, the architect, to treat for the site now occupied by Nos. 54–76 even (Duke Street Mansions).[296] As previously mentioned, Wimperis had already acted as Patrick's architect at Nos. 443–451 (odd) Oxford Street, and in 1884–6 he had at his own suggestion acted as both architect and lessee for the building of chambers and one shop at the corner site of Nos. 56 South Audley Street and 44 Mount Street (Plate 33d). In August 1886 Boodle undoubtedly knew that one of the occupants of the Duke Street site, E. L. Armbrecht, a chemist, wanted to rebuild,[297] but the building contract and subsequently the new lease for the whole range were nevertheless granted to Wimperis. The Board's allegedly unfair treatment of Armbrecht was subsequently investigated at great length by the Select Committee of the House of Commons on Town Holdings. Boodle's defence of his conduct was no doubt legalistically sound, but his assertion that, if Armbrecht had been allowed to rebuild, the erection of a block of artisans' dwellings at the rear of the site would have been 'obstructed' was not very convincing, and the suspicion remains that Wimperis got the contract in preference to an occupant because he was known from previous experience to be efficient and because he could,

as both lessee and architect, undertake the whole range single-handed.[298]*

But despite the criticism implied in the Select Committee's enquiries, the Grosvenor Board continued to offer commercial sites to speculative builders. In 1891 the site of Nos. 25–29 (consec.) North Audley Street, after being refused by several other firms, was taken by Matthews, Rogers and Company, the first of a number of speculations undertaken by them on the Grosvenor estate. Four of the five shops which they built here were sold on completion to Mount Street tradesmen disturbed by rebuilding there. Trollopes in 1893–5 built Nos. 75–83 (odd) Duke Street (Plate 35b), half as a speculation and half under contract with a dressmaker whose previous premises on the opposite side of the street were to be demolished; and the same firm also built Nos. 10–12 (consec.) Mount Street in 1894–6 under a similar arrangement for No. 10 with a firm of auctioneers previously occupying other premises in the street about to be rebuilt. Holloways were the lessees for the adjoining Nos. 14–26 (consec.) Mount Street in 1897–8 (Plate 34a; fig. 20c)—evidently at Boodle's suggestion[300]—and in 1898 Bywaters accepted an offer of the site of Nos. 31–38 (consec.) North Audley Street, they having previously built the adjoining No. 30 under contract with a firm of saddlers who had negotiated a rebuilding lease.

When the amount of contemporaneous rebuilding of ranges of residential property is also taken into account, it is clear that a very considerable volume of speculative building was proceeding on the estate, particularly in the mid 1890's. The Board was therefore concerned that this work should be of good quality, and in 1896 it drew up 'a list of builders whose names may be put down as reliable in case any building sites offer'. These were Stanley Bird, Colls and Company, William Cubitt and Company, Higgs and Hill, Holloway, Lucas Brothers, Matthews, Rogers and Company, Mowlem and Company, Sprake and Foreman, George Trollope and Sons, and William Willett.[301] In the distribution of its favours among these firms the Board attempted to be fair, and so when Trollopes applied for a vacant site in Balfour Mews the Board decided that 'Messrs. Trollope have already had far more sites [on the estate] than any other builders in London and their application cannot be acceded to'. The allocation of important work was not, however, necessarily confined to these firms—Daw, for instance, who was not on the list, was granted the site in Balfour Mews.[302] But the Board was nevertheless very careful about what firms should be allowed to build on the estate, and whenever a lessee who was not himself a builder invited tenders for the rebuilding of his premises, he was required to consult the Board about the names of the firms to be invited to tender. Failure to do so produced an admonishment—'The names ought to have been sent in the first instance before any of the builders were asked to tender'.[303]

These administrative mechanics of the Duke's rebuilding were one of the chief subjects which interested the members of the Select Committee of the House of Commons on Town Holdings in their prolonged examination of H. T. Boodle in 1887. But they were not in the least interested in the architects who designed the new buildings. Who these architects were, and how they were chosen, is however a matter of importance in the history of the estate.

The architects known to have worked on the estate during the first Duke's time included several of the foremost practitioners of the day—for instance, W. D. Caröe, Ernest George, J. J. Stevenson and Alfred Waterhouse—and many of the others were drawn from the middle ranks of the profession. The hacks, who proliferated in the late nineteenth century, did not in general get much work here. The relatively high standard of design which therefore resulted may be largely attributed to the discriminating influence of the Duke himself and of his advisers.

This influence varied with each building or range of buildings, and there was never any set procedure in the selection of architects. Sometimes there is no evidence about how the choice was made, but the Duke's influence and authority must generally have been strong, even when not directly exerted. All designs had to be submitted to the Board, and in most cases they were closely examined by the Duke himself, who often only approved them after considerable modification. After about 1875 all prospective rebuilding lessees knew that the Duke would insist on red brick in the Domestic Revival manner, and even when they were allowed to choose their own architect, their choice must have been greatly affected by this knowledge.

In 1887 their choice was still further circumscribed. The Board minutes record that 'With regard to the architects for rebuilding plots, the Duke wishes the following names to be selected from by the rebuilding tenants: one architect to be employed for each block of buildings. Mr. Norman Shaw, Mr. [J. T.] Wimperis, Mr. [R. W.] Edis, Mr. [T.] Chatfeild Clarke, Mr. [J. T.] Smith, Mr. [Thomas] Verity, and Mr. Ernest George'.[304]

In practice this list was not exclusive,[305] and was changed from time to time (see page 147). In 1894 it consisted of J. MacVicar Anderson, Ingress Bell and Aston Webb, A. J. Bolton, H. C. Boyes, W. D. Caröe, T. Chatfeild Clarke, T. E. Collcutt, R. W. Edis, Ernest George and Peto, Isaacs and Florence, C. E. Sayer, J. J. Stevenson and J. T. Wimperis.[306]

The way in which this list of 'approved' architects was used varied greatly. In cases—comparatively rare—when a private gentleman wanted to rebuild a single house for his own occupation, he was generally allowed to choose

* On the expiry of his lease at Lady Day 1887 Armbrecht took temporary premises on the east side of Duke Street on a yearly tenancy, but in 1890 he was accepted by the Board as one of the rebuilding lessees for Nos. 55–73 (odd) Duke Street.[299]

for himself, subject to the Duke's approval. Sir John Kelk, for instance, seems to have done so in the appointment of John Johnson at No. 3 Grosvenor Square (1875–7, demolished), and it was evidently the lessee, C. H. Wilson, who chose George Devey for No. 41 Grosvenor Square (1883–6, demolished). Both these appointments were made before the existence of the 'approved' list, but its existence did not prevent Lord Windsor from selecting Fairfax B. Wade, who was not on it, for his large house at No. 54 Mount Street (1896–9, Plates 36a, 37), overlooking the garden of Grosvenor House—a choice which evidently pleased the Duke, who firmly overruled his Board's objections to Wade's elevational designs.[307] Similarly, when Lord Ribblesdale proposed Sidney R. J. Smith—likewise not on the list—for No. 32 Green Street (1897–9) the Duke consented and appointed Smith as architect for the adjacent sites in Norfolk (now Dunraven) Street and North Row as well (Plate 36b).[308] But when the Earl of Aberdeen announced that he did not intend to have an architect at all for the rebuilding of No. 27 Grosvenor Square (1886–8, demolished), the Duke insisted that there should be one, and the appointment was evidently made by him or by Boodle, the choice being J. T. Wimperis, who, it may be noted, had recently had several other commissions on the estate.[309] Even for private gentlemen the safest course was perhaps that adopted by Dr. Joseph Walker at Nos. 21 and 22 Grosvenor Street (1898–9), who attended the Board 'and, of course, leaves the question of architect to the Duke. After he has left the Board, it is suggested to ask the Duke if he would allow Mr. Balfour [the estate surveyor, probably present at this meeting] to be the architect.'[310]

But most of the private houses built in the first Duke's time were, as we have already seen, built in ranges by speculating builders, and in these cases the architect was almost always appointed by the Duke himself or by the Board with his approval. When, for instance, the builders Higgs and Hill were in 1896 offered terms for the site of Nos. 2–12 (even) Park Street, they were told that A. H. Kersey (not on the list) was to be the architect.[311] In the same year Boodle, at a Board meeting at which the Duke was evidently not present, successfully suggested H. O. Cresswell as architect for Nos. 94–104A (even) Park Street, Boodle being under the impression that Cresswell was on the approved list, although no record of this has been found.[312]

Boodle seems, indeed, to have had his own share of influence in the choice of architects. In 1886 he approached J. T. Wimperis about the site of Nos. 54–76 (even) Duke Street, and it was he who proposed in 1891 that the Board should 'communicate with Col. Edis as to any clients of his who might be desirous of rebuilding' on the large L-shaped site at the north-west corner of Park Street and Green Street. R. W. Edis had already rebuilt Nos. 59 and 61 Brook Street in 1883–6 (one being intended for his own occupation)[313] and he was also one of three architects on the 'approved' list of 1887 who sometimes acted as speculator as well as architect for large sites on the estate.* At Boodle's corner plots Edis ultimately took on the whole site himself, and between 1891 and 1894 he designed and built Nos. 105–115 (odd) Park Street and 25–31 (consec.) Green Street. This was evidently successful from his point of view, for in 1894–6 he was clamouring for more building sites. But the Board would not oblige him. He had 'seriously departed' from the estate specification, and it was therefore decided that 'he should not be offered further sites'. Furthermore, 'The Board do not think it expedient that an architect should speculate on the estate, as architects are wanted to design and supervise the buildings of others'.[314]

A not very different practice adopted by two large firms of builders, who liked to use their own 'tame' architect, was not, however, objected to. At four sites where rebuilding was undertaken by George Trollope and Sons in the 1890's, his brother, John E. Trollope, of the firm of Giles, Gough and Trollope, was the architect (Nos. 6–9 consec. Mount Street, 1–8 consec. Carlos Place (Plate 34d) and 1–15 odd Mount Row, 1891–3; Nos 45–52 consec. Mount Street, 1891–3; the Barley Mow, Duke Street, 1895–6; and Nos. 34–42 even Park Street and 53 Mount Street, 1895–9); but at another site the Duke required him to use someone else (Nos. 75–83 odd Duke Street, W. D. Caröe, 1893–5). Similarly Matthews, Rogers and Company agreed in 1891 to rebuild Nos. 25–29 (consec.) North Audley Street to designs by the Duke's nominee, Thomas Verity, who was probably insisted upon because there was a public house (the Marlborough Head) to be rebuilt at the adjoining No. 24 and Verity had already done another public house on the estate, the Audley Hotel (1888–9), to the Duke's hard-won satisfaction. But in all their subsequent work on the estate Matthews, Rogers and Company were always allowed to use 'an architect in their own firm', M. C. Hulbert.[315]

By far the most prolific architect of private houses was, however, the new estate surveyor appointed in 1890, Eustace Balfour, who seems to have been able to get whatever work he wanted and then, sometimes, delegate it to his partner in private practice, Thackeray Turner. As early as 1891 he is recorded as declining to act as architect at Nos. 2–8 (consec.) Green Street because 'he would like to transfer his services to the Portugal Street site'.[315] In this south-western part of the estate he (and/or Turner) did so much work during the 1890's that Balfour Place (formerly Portugal Street) and Balfour Mews were named after him. It included Nos. 1–6 (consec.) Balfour Place

* The other two were J. T. Smith, lessee and architect for Nos. 106–116 (even) Park Street and 19 Green Street (1887–8), and J. T. Wimperis, lessee and architect for Nos. 56 South Audley Street and 44 Mount Street (Audley Mansions, 1884–6) and for Nos. 54–76 (even) Duke Street (Duke Street Mansions, 1887–8).

(1891–4); the whole block bounded by Mount Street, Balfour Place, Aldford Street and Rex Place (1891–7, see Plate 35a); Alfred Beit's mansion at No. 26 Park Lane (1894–7, demolished), where Balfour's employment by Beit as architect was made one of the conditions of the contract for the rebuilding lease (Plate 38a); Nos. 14–22 (even) Park Street, 68 Mount Street and stables on the west side of Rex Place (1896–7); and the east side of Balfour Mews (1898–9). Elsewhere on the estate the firm of Balfour and Turner did No. 10 Green Street (1893–5) and St. Anselm's Church, Davies Street, of 1894–6 (Plate 38b), and in 1897–8 Balfour was diplomatically—and successfully—asking for Nos. 21–22 Grosvenor Street and 40–46 (even) Brook Street (1898–9).[316]

In the choice of architects for the rebuilding of shops and commercial premises there was very wide variety of practice. In the 1860's and early 1870's, as we have already seen, both the second Marquess and the third Marquess and future first Duke required their tenants in Oxford Street (which was the first commercial street to be extensively rebuilt) to use elevational designs supplied by the estate surveyor, Thomas Cundy III; and sometimes the tenants employed obscure architects of their own to design the internal disposition of their buildings. Nos. 407–413 (odd) Oxford Street are cases in point. But the Duke's success in 1875 in persuading W. J. Goode to start the rebuilding of a large shop in South Audley Street to designs by Ernest George in the red-brick manner of the Queen Anne Revival (Plate 32) seems to have aroused his architectural ambitions. So when the next phase of commercial rebuilding began in the later 1880's he often nominated architects whose work reflected his own tastes.

The first such nominee was J. T. Wimperis, who had already done two jobs on the estate—Nos. 443–451 (odd) Oxford Street (1876–8) and Nos. 34 Berkeley Square and 130 Mount Street (1880–2)—his selection as architect in both these cases having been made by the building lessee. Subsequently he had applied successfully to be both lessee and architect for Nos. 56 South Audley Street and 44 Mount Street of 1884–6 (Plate 33d), and in 1886 he was invited by the Board to act in the same dual capacity at Nos. 54–76 (even) Duke Street (1887–8).[317] Thomas Chatfeild Clarke, who had also been responsible for the design of various buildings erected in Oxford Street since 1883, was invited to design Nos. 385–397 (odd) Oxford Street (1887–9), despite the objections of one of the rebuilding lessees, who wanted to have someone else: in 1890 it was decided that he should be the architect for Nos. 64–68 (consec.) South Audley Street (1891–3), which were about to be rebuilt by local tradesmen, this commission being subsequently extended to the adjoining Nos. 69 and 70, designed by his son Howard Chatfeild Clarke in 1898–1900.[318] In 1889 'Mr. Boodle suggests and the Duke approves of Mr. Caröe being the architect' for a group of tradesmen in the rebuilding of Nos. 55–73 (odd) Duke Street (1890–2), and in 1892 the Duke nominated Caröe for the nearby Nos. 75–83 (odd) Duke Street, to be rebuilt by Trollopes and one shopkeeper (Plate 35b).[319] Thomas Verity and (after his death in 1891) his son Frank were the Duke's selections for Nos. 24–29 (consec.) North Audley Street (1891–3), probably (as we have already seen) because this range included a public house, Thomas Verity having already done the Audley Hotel satisfactorily. But for his death Thomas Verity would probably also have been appointed for the Barley Mow at No. 82 Duke Street (1895–6), which went instead, on Boodle's suggestion, to John Trollope with Trollopes as builders, despite the objection of the publican-lessee, who wanted 'a Mr. Frampton, a friend of his, to be the architect'.[320] And although Auguste Scorrier, hotel keeper and prospective lessee for the rebuilding of the very important Coburg (now Connaught) Hotel at the corner of Mount Street and Carlos Place, ultimately got the man he wanted, he was made to understand that the choice was not his to make. After he had been imperiously informed in November 1893 that 'the architect had not been decided upon by the Duke' his solicitors, displaying a finesse which was on this occasion conspicuously absent in Boodle's office, politely suggested that the Duke might make his selection from one of three architects, namely Lewis H. Isaacs of Isaacs and Florence, William J. Green and E. T. Hall. As neither Green nor Hall seems ever to have designed a hotel, whereas Isaacs had done the Victoria in Northumberland Avenue and the Imperial at Holborn Viaduct, the Board took the hint and in January 1894 'the Duke appoints Mr. Isaacs the architect'.[321]

Sometimes the Duke's influence in the choice of an architect is apparent, even though he did not act directly. At Nos. 104–111 (consec.) Mount Street (1885–7) W. H. Warner, the estate agent and one of the rebuilding lessees, took the lead in submitting designs by Ernest George. He may well have done so because he knew from W. J. Goode's experience in South Audley Street in 1875 that George's work would be acceptable; and so it proved, after the Duke had required the height of the proposed buildings on this north-facing site to be reduced to admit more light to the houses opposite (Plate 34b).[322] After 1887 groups of shopkeepers who were negotiating for the rebuilding of a range to one design were sometimes sent the Duke's list of 'approved' architects, from which they were to choose.[323] Ernest George and Peto were probably selected in this way for Nos. 1–5 (consec.) Mount Street (1888–9, Nos. 1–3 demolished), and Thomas Verity almost certainly so at Nos. 27–28 Mount Street and 34–42 (consec.) South Audley Street (1888–9).

At what turned out to be the largest range of buildings by a single architect on the whole of the Mayfair estate the Duke's influence was rather more uncertain. This range, by A. J. Bolton, consisted of the new Vestry Hall on the south side of Mount Street (1886–7, now demolished, site occupied by No. 103), Nos. 94–102 (consec.) Mount Street (1889–91), Nos. 87–93 (consec.) Mount Street and 26–33 (consec.) South Audley Street

and the new public library (1893–5). In 1883 the Vestry of St. George's arranged with the Duke to buy the freehold of part of the old workhouse for the site of the new Vestry Hall, and then 'invited the competition of four architects' for the new building. Bolton was chosen by the Vestry,[324] but the Duke, who was himself a vestryman, evidently did not much like the design, and Bolton was required to call at Grosvenor House, where the Duke 'told him of his wishes and requested to have an altered elevation'.[325] By 1887, however, when he opened the new Vestry Hall on 23 April,[326] the Duke's opinion of Bolton's work had perhaps changed somewhat, for when both the Vestry clerk and Bolton himself asked in 1888 that 'the latter, who acted for the Vestry building, may be the architect for the proposed new houses' at the adjoining Nos. 94–102 (consec.) Mount Street, the Duke agreed. He did, however, stipulate—rather in vain, as it turned out—that 'he would like a repetition of the houses' (not in fact themselves identical) by Ernest George at Nos. 104–111 (consec.); and in 1892 he appointed Bolton architect for the rebuilding lessees at Nos. 87–93 (consec.) Mount Street and 26–33 (consec.) South Audley Street, stipulating in this case—with more effect—that Nos. 94–102 Mount Street 'are to be copied'.[327] By this time Bolton had won a competition for the design of the public library in Buckingham Palace Road, Victoria, also on the Grosvenor estate, where the Duke had presented a freehold site gratis,[328] and in April 1891 the St. George's Library Commissioners asked the Duke for a site for a library in Mayfair. Here he agreed to grant them a ninety-year lease, but before the building contract was exchanged 'the question who is to be the Architect selected by the Duke' was discussed at a Board meeting in his absence, when it was 'felt that, as Mr. Bolton is building all the adjoining houses, his Grace may possibly select him, although he is understood not to have altogether approved of his [Bolton's] design for the Free Library in Buckingham Palace Road'. Despite his evidently still only qualified approval of Bolton he did ultimately agree, 'if the Vestry so desired'.[329]

Bolton's original appointment in 1884 for the first stage of this range—the Vestry Hall—was undoubtedly due to the Vestry, and the Duke's displeasure at the choice (mentioned above) was manifested again in 1887 when Bolton's name was not included on the first list of 'approved' architects. Perhaps in this case it would have been difficult, though certainly not impossible, for him to have resisted the Vestry's decision, but other cases show that even shopkeepers were sometimes allowed their own free choice. In 1880 William Lambert, surveyor, was the choice of James Purdey, the gunmaker, for Nos. 57–60 (consec.) South Audley Street (1881–2), and in 1889–91 he acted for the completion of this range (Nos. 61–63 consec.) by other commercial lessees. Edwin Hollis, a pork butcher, was allowed to have J. S. Moye for Nos. 399–405 (odd) Oxford Street (1880–2, demolished), and Thrupp and Maberly had Henry S. Legg at Nos. 421–429 (odd) Oxford Street (1884–7, demolished) despite Thomas Cundy's objection that he did 'not consider that Mr. Legge [*sic*] will be very suitable as he knows nothing of him'.[330] At Nos. 125–129 (consec.) Mount Street (1886–7) it seems likely that the four shopkeeper/rebuilding lessees chose W. H. Powell themselves, for in August 1885 the Board received letters 'from and on behalf of Mr. Powell...giving testimonials as to his fitness to be the architect for some of the rebuilding tenants in Mount Street'.[331] At that time there was as yet no list of 'approved' architects, but Powell's name did not appear on it in 1887 or in later years.* Similarly the four shopkeepers and a surgeon who were the rebuilding lessees at Nos. 116–121 (consec.) Mount Street (1886–7) seem to have chosen J. T. Smith themselves. When Smith submitted an elevation on their behalf in 1885 'his Grace did not approve of it as he thought the buildings very high and too elaborate in decoration'. But he later agreed to a revised version, 'though it appears to me to be overdone and wanting in simplicity',[333] a view which many others may still share, but which the Duke does not seem to have held very strongly, since in the following year he allowed Smith to be the lessee and architect for private houses at Nos. 106–116 (even) Park Street and 19 Green Street, and in 1887 included him in the 'approved' list.

When E. McM. Burden, a Duke Street chemist about to rebuild Nos. 78 and 80 there (1887–8), submitted designs by his brother, R. H. Burden, in 1886, he was 'told that the Board do not think the drawing good enough for the site, but the Duke will decide'. R. H. Burden 'had not had experience in street architecture', and ultimately on Boodle's suggestion J. T. Wimperis, who was then in course of rebuilding the nearby Nos. 54–76 (even) Duke Street, was called in to revise Burden's designs.[334] Such ducal dislike of commercial lessees' architectural tastes was probably the reason for the compilation of the 'approved' list in 1887, but even in later years complete freedom of choice was sometimes still allowed. Thus Walton and Lee, auctioneers, were allowed in 1893 to nominate H. C. Boyes for No. 10 Mount Street, although he was not on the list of 1887. This choice was evidently considered to be satisfactory, for in 1894 Boyes became the architect (for Trollopes) for the adjoining Nos. 11 and 12 as well, and his name was put on the revised list of that year.[335] In 1896 Holloways, the builders, negotiating for the rebuilding of Nos. 14–26 (consec.) Mount Street (Plate 34a; fig. 20c), successfully asked that Read and Macdonald (never on the list) 'whom they can highly recommend, may be the architects'.[336] And a firm of saddlers was allowed to have Henry S. Legg (likewise never on the list) at No. 30 North Audley Street (1896–7), despite Eustace Balfour's recommendation of Ernest

* Perhaps because he subsequently migrated to Natal, where he died in 1900.[332]

George; and when the adjoining Nos. 31–38 (consec.) were rebuilt a year later by the contractors Bywaters, Legg was again the architect, this time at the instigation of the Board.[337]

In addition to the rebuilding of private houses and shops there were two other categories of buildings in which the Duke's philanthropic temperament prompted him to take an active personal interest. These were artisans' dwellings and public houses.

During the second Marquess's time (1845–69) several small blocks of artisans' dwellings had been built on the Mayfair estate—St. George's Buildings and Grosvenor Buildings, Bourdon Street (1853 and 1869), by the St. George's Parochial Association (Plate 30a, b), and Bloomfield Flats, Bourdon Street (1856) and Oxford House, Grosvenor Market (1860, demolished), by a local builder, John Newson.[338] The Grosvenor Estate did not initiate any of these schemes, but between 1866 and 1875 the second Marquess and his successor, the first Duke, were both intimately involved in much larger projects in Pimlico, first in conjunction with the Metropolitan Association for Improving the Dwellings of the Industrious Classes, and later with the Improved Industrial Dwellings Company. In Mayfair the latter also built Clarendon Flats (formerly Buildings), Balderton (formerly George) Street in 1871–2 (Plate 30c), and in 1880 the Duke was already considering with the Company a very large scheme for improved dwellings between Grosvenor Square and Brook Street on the south and Oxford Street on the north, to be implemented when the existing leases expired in 1886.[339] Thus this project was in existence well before the tremendous public outcry of 1883 about the prevailing conditions of working-class housing, and between 1886 and 1892 nine blocks of dwellings were built in that area (Plate 31). They and Clarendon Flats provided accommodation for some two thousand people, this being seven hundred more than the scheme displaced, and the Company was bound in its contract with the Duke 'to offer to the persons who are now residing...upon that portion of his estate, the opportunity of occupying the dwellings as they are from time to time erected'.[340] The Duke himself paid the cost of laying out a large garden in what is now Brown Hart Gardens—later converted into a roof 'garden' above the Duke Street Electricity Sub-station (Plate 31b). His annual rental for the whole area redeveloped fell from £2,193 under the old leases to £502 under the new ones granted to the Company.[341]

The Duke's policy towards public houses reflected a more severe side of Victorian philanthropy; and it also exhibits more clearly than in any other aspect of the estate's administration the vast powers which he possessed as ground landlord. We have already seen that the second Earl and first Marquess (1802–45) had begun to try to reduce the number of pubs, and that in 1828, on the eve of the Beer Act of 1830, there were around seventy-five on his Mayfair estate. At about the time of the accession of the third Marquess (later first Duke) in 1869 there were still about forty-seven pubs and beer shops there,[342] and encouraged no doubt by the changes of 1869–72 in the licensing laws he decided to make a further drastic reduction in their numbers. In the ensuing years the great majority of applications to renew pub leases, whether from publicans or from great brewers like Watney's or Meux, were rejected outright. In 1874, for instance, Hanbury's were peremptorily informed that they could not have a renewal of the Swan in Oxford Street because 'on public grounds it is essential to reduce the number of public houses on the estate',[343] while Watney's in 1879 were told that the site of their Coach and Horses in Grosvenor Mews (now Bourdon Street) was 'already promised for the Parochial Institution'.[344] By 1891 no less than thirty-nine pubs and beer houses had been abolished on the Mayfair portion of the estate alone, and only eight still survived.[345] Today there are only five.

The motive for this massacre was, of course, the promotion of temperance,[346] and in *c.* 1884 a branch of the Church of England Temperance Society was established in the parish with the Duke's blessing.[347] In the newly rebuilt artisan quarter around Brown Hart Gardens he provided a drinking fountain, and he would have liked to establish a 'cocoa house' there too, had not the proposed lessee replied that he did not 'see much chance of making cocoa rooms in the place spoken of pay'.[348] Pubs did, however, pay, and their wholesale diminution was only achieved 'at a great pecuniary loss' to the Duke.[346] The Board could indeed state, in answer to a question about the Duke's policy towards pubs, that 'the question of loss does not influence the Duke in deciding upon this or any other matters affecting the good of the tenants or the improvement of London'.[349]

The mere abolition of pubs was, however, only one of the formidable prongs with which the Duke assailed the drink interest, for the surviving few were subjected to a regimen of controlling discipline of almost Spartan intensity. In the rebuilding of pubs the lessees had their architects chosen for them, of course, and at the Hertford Arms, 94 Park Street (now demolished) the tenant had to build his pub (to H. O. Cresswell's design) in a wholly domestic manner outwardly indistinguishable from the adjoining range of private houses.[350] At the corner of Mount Street and South Audley Street Watney's were only allowed to rebuild the Bricklayers' Arms (now the Audley Hotel) in 1888–9 on condition that they surrendered the lease of another nearby pub, and in the new building there was to be no entrance from South Audley Street. Even such a favoured architect as Thomas Verity had his first designs returned with the comment that 'His Grace thinks that the elevation...is too gin-palace-y in Mount Street'.[351]

Beginning in 1871 the Marquess (later Duke) also sought to reduce the hours of opening. These were certainly long—on weekdays, 4 a.m. to 1 a.m. (except Saturdays, midnight), and on Sundays 1 p.m. to 3 p.m. and 5 p.m. to 11 p.m. Sunday opening was, however,

what particularly offended the Duke, and at first he admitted 'that there would be difficulties in London in reducing the hours, however desirable'.[352] But in 1880 he decided that he would, in renewing leases, 'prohibit the houses being opened on Sundays except for drinking off the premises from 1 to 3 o'clock'.[353] This draconian decree was sometimes relaxed to facilitate the exchange of leases, and by 1895 Sunday drinking on the premises between 1 and 3 o'clock seems to have been generally allowed. But in that year he refused to allow F. W. Bevan, the licensee and rebuilding lessee of the Barley Mow in Duke Street (who was risking his own capital of over £4,000 in rebuilding by an architect and contractor both chosen by the Duke), to open on Sunday evenings; and although he subsequently did allow off-the-premises trade on Sunday evenings[354] he still had all the publicans completely at his mercy, thanks to the ingenious drafting of his pub leases.

These, in the list of prohibited trades, *included* that of licensed victualler, but a 'conditional licence' was attached, by which the Duke granted consent, personal to the lessee, to practise the trade of licensed victualler, provided that 'the said trade or business be respectably conducted to my satisfaction', that the peculiar Grosvenor restrictions on Sunday opening be observed, and that 'I or other the landlord for the time being may revoke this licence at any time if in my or his absolute discretion there shall have been a breach of any or either of the above conditions'.[355] With this power to revoke his own licences whenever he, at his sole discretion, might think fit, the Duke had much more power over the pubs on his estate than the licensing authorities themselves.

The control of pubs shows in its most extreme form the full extent of the Duke's authority over his estate. But there were other fields in which it was at any rate in theory not much smaller, although practical difficulties sometimes prevented its full use. It should, however, be noted that the Duke usually exerted his power to achieve objects generally congenial to at least the wealthy residents for whom the estate primarily catered. His control, through his leases, over the use to which individual buildings might be put is a case in point and has already been discussed. The results of this can still be clearly seen in Mount Street, where prior to its complete rebuilding in the 1880's and 90's, shops, private houses and apartments let 'to people coming up to town' were all mixed together. The Duke's policy, which could only be implemented at the time of rebuilding, was to have all the shops east of South Audley Street and only private houses to the west. 'Our experience', Boodle stated in 1887, 'is that tradesmen like what they call "a market". They like all the shops to be together, and private gentlemen naturally like their houses to be together without shops.'[356] Similarly the grandees residing in Upper Grosvenor Street (of whom the Duke himself was one) probably liked his decision in 1873 that 'professions as well as trades and businesses should be excluded from Upper Grosvenor Street,... without, however, interfering with professional men under existing leases.'[357]

Policies of this kind could, however, only be implemented gradually, and elsewhere trade was now so long established that its removal, however desirable it might be thought to be, was sometimes abandoned. In 1880, for instance, a tailor at No. 62 Grosvenor Street was refused a renewal because 'businesses are being excluded from Grosvenor Street as the leases expire',[358] but Collard's, the piano makers at No. 16 were granted an extension without difficulty in 1888;[359] while in Brook Street some attempt seems to have been made to eliminate shops,[360] but Claridge's Hotel was allowed to be rebuilt there in the 1890's. The eastern end of Brook Street was, indeed, becoming steadily less residential in character, while in Grosvenor Street the Alexandra Ladies' Club was admitted to No. 12 in 1887;[361] and discreet new businesses, notably that of 'Court dressmaker', were even allowed, provided that there was 'no show of business except a small brass plate, and the door to be kept shut except for ingress and egress'.[362]

Sometimes the Duke's requirements must have been irksome even to residents in the best streets. His liking for plate glass in the windows of private houses was not always popular, and his idiosyncratic fondness for stucco-work to be painted orange, as he himself had the Grosvenor Office at No. 53 Davies Street done in 1883 ('like that at the bottom of Waterloo Place') must have been vexatious to some tastes.[363] For railings he seems to have changed in the mid 1870's from stone colour to 'chocolate or red', but in later years the new red brick 'Queen Anne style' houses had to have their railings and window frames painted white.[364]

More usually, however, his actions did probably enjoy considerable support among his tenants. His objection to building work during the London Season, his preference for wood blocks—quieter but more expensive than granite—for the repaving of Oxford Street, and his strict control of advertising on his portion of the same street, are obvious instances.[365] In the 1870's and early 1880's the disfigurement of the estate by the erection of telegraph and telephone posts and wires was vigorously opposed, the proprietors being required to sign an acknowledgment that their installations were held on sufferance only, subject to three months' notice to quit.[366] When the new electric lighting companies obtained power in 1883 to put up posts and wires, subject to the control of the local authorities, the Board thought that 'a combination should be effected with other landlords to require all the electric wires to be put underground'.[367] And well-founded complaints from tenants were often taken up—against 'the uproarious conduct' of the children at the Ragged School in Davies Mews, or the constant standing of carriages outside the Grosvenor Gallery, or, from the Duchess of Marlborough against a dentist in Grosvenor Street whose activities were visible from her house opposite, and whom the Board politely

requested 'to put up a muslin curtain to prevent his dentistry patients being seen'.[368]

Nor was such concern confined to outward and visible (or audible) matters. From the 1870's onwards it became common for the Board, in the renewal of leases, to insist that water closets should be externally lit and ventilated instead of (as was sometimes hitherto the case) from the staircase.* The installation of lifts—first recorded in 1884[370]—produced a new type of problem through the frequent complaints of neighbours about the noise of their operation. In the mews behind the great houses extensive works of modernization were often required, particularly when Eustace Balfour was the estate surveyor (1890–1910), the following being a typical requirement —'Modernise the stabling as regards accommodation for a married coachman and one helper, providing at least four rooms (every room to have a fireplace) and a separate w.c. for the use of the helpers. The helper's room to be approached directly from the staircase, and to be kept quite distinct from the coachman's quarters...'[371] In many mews the old narrow entrances were widened by the demolition of corner houses, and in conjunction with the Vestry urinals *à la mode française* were provided for the army of outdoor servants who worked there—'the Duke was most anxious for a great many more urinals being erected in the Parish and in London generally'. And when Lord Manners's coachman complained that the urinal in Reeves Mews 'could be seen into from his upper windows', the Board acted with as much promptness as it had in the case of the Duchess of Marlborough and the dentist in Grosvenor Street.[372]

In addition to the extensive rebuildings and the general maintenance of the estate, a number of important other improvements were made during the first Duke's time. Communication between Berkeley Square and Grosvenor Square was greatly improved by the demolition of some projecting property of the Duke's at the east end of Mount Street (*c.* 1880), and by the widening and realignment of Charles Street (now Carlos Place, *c.* 1891). Several other streets were widened during the course of rebuilding, notably Duke Street, North Audley Street, South Audley Street north of South Street, and Mount Street, the land given up by the Duke for this last alone being worth £50,000.[373] Several short new streets were formed or realigned and widened—Red Place, Carpenter Street, Rex Place and Balfour Mews—and in 1898 the important realignment of the north end of Davies Street, first mooted in the 1830's,[374] was at last achieved, thereby providing greatly improved communication between Berkeley Square and Oxford Street.[375] When the Metropolitan Board of Works made improvements at Hyde Park Corner—some distance from the Grosvenor estate—at the public expense, the Duke of Westminster was the only landowner to make a voluntary contribution (of £3,000) to the cost, 'in consideration of the additional value that was given to his property'.[376] And when in 1890 the disused burial ground to the east of the Grosvenor Chapel was converted by the Vestry into a public garden the Duke, who had envisaged this improvement as long ago as 1874, began, and continued for the rest of his life, to pay £100 per annum towards the cost of its upkeep.[377] It was not indeed for nothing that the chairman of the Royal Commission of 1884–5 on the Housing of the Working Classes said publicly that he did 'not think that anybody on the Commission would be disposed to doubt the excellent management of the Westminster Estate'.[378]

In 1899, the last year of the Duke's life, there was a marked decline in the volume of rebuilding on the Mayfair portion of the estate. A phase of reduced activity was beginning, and his own tremendous impact upon the area had probably exhausted itself. In 1887, when this impact had not yet made itself fully felt, Boodle had stated before the Select Committee of the House of Commons on Town Holdings that the Duke's aim was 'to have wide thoroughfares instead of narrow, to set back the houses in rebuilding so as to obtain broad areas and a good basement for the servants...He also wishes to have effective architecture, to insist upon good sanitary arrangements in houses, to promote churches, chapels, and schools, and open spaces for recreation'. All this he had done chiefly 'because he desires better houses, and he is a great lover of architecture and likes a handsome town, and he would sacrifice enormously to carry that out on his estate'.[379]

By insisting so often upon rebuilding he undoubtedly had sacrificed the very considerable extra income which he could have obtained by leasing at rack rents. Boodle stated that 'rebuilding involves a loss of about two-thirds of the income'.[380] In Mount Street the total new ground rents amounted in 1898 to £8,343 per annum,[381] but if no rebuilding had taken place the rack rental from this one street would have been worth about £20,000 a year.[382] In 1897 the rental of the estate was actually said to have 'diminished, owing to the pulling down'.[383] The Duke's decision to go ahead with rebuilding on a large scale cannot therefore have been an easy one.

Yet despite the rebuildings the rental of the Mayfair estate nevertheless rose (as we have already seen) from *c.* £80,000 per annum in 1870 to *c.* £135,000 in 1891. About two thirds of this increase took place before the most intense phase of rebuilding began around 1886; and it should, of course, be remembered that although in rebuilding the Duke forfeited about two thirds of what he could have obtained by rack renting, his income still rose, because the new ground rents were substantially higher than the old ones.†[380]

* Even in Mayfair it does not appear that a constant supply of water was provided until 1893–4.[369]

† Some examples of the new ground rents, measured in square feet: stables, 7*d.*–9*d.*: Duke Street, 9½*d.*: houses in Aldford Street and Balfour Place area, 1*s.*: Mount Street east of South Audley Street, 1*s.* 3*d.*–1*s.* 6*d.*: Green Street, 1*s.*–1*s.* 8*d.*: public houses, 1*s.* 4*d.*–1*s.* 6*d.*

The extent of his sacrifice was therefore a matter of degree. But it was certainly one which no other London landlord made on the same scale, and the fact that he did make it gave substance to Boodle's claim that 'the Duke certainly takes the lead in the improvement of London'.[384] Nor should his success in the re-creation of 'a handsome town' on his estate be decried. It was an age when the quality of municipal street improvement was at its lowest ebb, and Mount Street was a vastly different kettle of fish from Shaftesbury Avenue or Charing Cross Road.

If the Duke had reason to be satisfied, so too did his rebuilding lessees, for according to Boodle they 'almost invariably' got their money back, and 'with a very large profit'. There was never any shortage of applications for sites, and the case (previously mentioned) of T. B. Linscott, the Oxford Street confectioner who had at first been 'rather reluctant to rebuild' but whose business had subsequently grown very rapidly, was 'usual in good thoroughfares'.[385] According to the estate agent W. H. Warner, who had no axe to grind in the matter, probably not a single one of the Mount Street lessees was 'dissatisfied with his bargain'.[386]

Throughout the 1880's and 90's the Board received numerous requests from architects and builders for sites, most of which were refused, occupants being (as we have seen) generally preferred. Those favoured few whose applications were successful, such as Edis or Trollopes, were almost always anxious to have more sites—a sure testimony to the financial success of their operations on the estate. Except in Balfour Place and Balfour Mews, where the market was sluggish for S. G. Bird in 1894 and for W. A. Daw in 1900,[387] speculators never seem to have had any difficulty in finding tenants or purchasers for their new buildings, and the high prices which they demanded were sometimes noted with interest by the Board, £16,000 for No. 68 Mount Street (W. A. Daw, ground rent £150) and for No. 78 Mount Street (W. H. Warner, ground rent £116), being cases in point.[388] The new houses in Green Street, although less expensive than those at the west end of Mount Street, were also evidently much sought after. In 1892 the Hon. Alfred Lyttelton bought one of them from the builders, Matthews, Rogers and Company, for £7,000, but sold it soon afterwards for £8,600 to F. Leverton Harris, who in turn re-sold it in 1896 for £12,600—an appreciation of eighty per cent in the course of four years.[389]

The market in Grosvenor Square was buoyant too. In reference to 'houses which have been rebuilt on a ground-rent, and afterwards sold for sums far exceeding the cost of building them', Boodle cited one house which 'cost 12,000*l*., and was sold for 18,000*l*.', and another which 'cost 18,000*l*. and was sold for 23,000*l*., and was afterwards sold again for 35,000*l*.'. No. 42, rebuilt as a speculation by the builder Wright Ingle in 1853–5 at a cost of less than £20,000, was sold in 1886 (without any addition to the original seventy-seven-year lease) for £30,000.[390] In 1878 Holland and Hannen were thought to have made a profit of about £8,000 in selling No. 39 to the Marquess of Lothian for £23,500 after having 'practically had to rebuild the house';[391] and in the 1890's Matthews, Rogers and Company's speculations in refurbishing Nos. 11 and 13 were probably correspondingly successful.

But although the Duke himself, his rebuilding lessees and the speculative builders were all probably pleased with the changes made on the estate, there were other people who were not. There were some who merely did not like the Duke's taste in architecture. When the renumbering of the houses in Grosvenor Square was in contemplation, the Earl of Harrowby took the opportunity to complain to the Vestry 'that the character of the Square has much deteriorated of late and its Appearance has been destroyed by the recent erection of houses like public institutions'. The Earl's own architectural tastes were probably rather old-fashioned, but this did not, however, prevent his expressing a deeper and more general source of grievance when he continued that 'Anyhow, ordinary courtesy should have led the Grosvenor Estate Board to have consulted the old and existing tenants of the other houses, though recent experience has unfortunately shown that their interests are no longer consulted by the Estate Board in the arrangements with the new builders'.[392]

It was during the very years that the renewal of the Mayfair estate was being so vigorously carried through that the leasehold system, of which the Grosvenor estate formed such a conspicuous example, was first seriously criticised. During the 1880's several abortive 'leasehold enfranchisement' bills were discussed in Parliament,[393] both the Royal Commission of 1884–5 on the Housing of the Working Classes and the Select Committee of the House of Commons of 1887 on Town Holdings examined the workings of the system in some detail, and the Duke himself was from time to time attacked in the press and in a number of pamphlets.[394] Great urban landlords, and dukes in particular, were being challenged for the first time, and the death duty clauses in Sir William Harcourt's Finance Act of 1894 only added to their tribulations.[395] Public attitudes towards them, hitherto ignored, suddenly became important to them in the new political climate emanating from the Reform Act of 1884. Boodle did battle on the Duke's behalf in the correspondence columns of *The Times*, and the Marquess of Salisbury (the sometime Prime Minister) helpfully suggested to his nephew Eustace Balfour, the Grosvenor estate surveyor, 'that the number of the Duke's houses might be ascertained to disabuse the public mind as to the Dukes of Bedford and Westminster owning practically the whole of the area within the County of London'.*[396]

* The Grosvenor Board had 'no objection' to having such a count made, but considered (the science of public relations having not yet been invented) that 'it may be doubtful in which way it should be utilized'.[396]

The most pungent critic of the leasehold system in general and of the Duke in particular was Frank Banfield, whose series of articles in *The Sunday Times* was published in book form in *c.* 1888 under the title *The Great Landlords of London*. In his chapter on the Grosvenor estate he attacked the Duke for sometimes giving preference to speculative builders before occupants, and for compelling prospective lessees in businesses with valuable goodwill to rebuild at their expense but to his architectural taste. 'I like fine streets as much as any one, but I object to see numbers of Englishmen forced to tax their capital so heavily and perilously merely to suit the dictatorial architectural caprices of a millionaire Duke.' He also asserted that 'tenants do not receive that consideration which is their due', being often left in ignorance 'right up to the end of their lease, whether they can renew or not', and criticised the estate (in the person of H. T. Boodle) for its 'take it or leave it' attitude when offering rebuilding terms, and for the unreasonable stringency of some of the lease covenants.[397]

In reference to this last he cited the case of a butcher in Mount Street, Edgar Green of No. 117, who was one of the lessees for the rebuilding of Nos. 116–121 (consec.) and who in his lease had had to 'sign away the right to hang carcases' in front of his shop window. When he had nevertheless displayed meat outside, Boodle had asked him to desist, but had also invited him 'to make an application to the Duke for leave to hang a moderate quantity of meat in the window in front if he wished to do so instead'. Green had then attended a meeting of the Board to put his case, and the Duke had said he would 'call and see the shop on his way home' to Grosvenor House. Subsequently he wrote to Boodle that 'I think Butcher Green's exhibition of prominent carcases of sheep may be permitted as an ornament to the street, as I have told him'.[398]

This case shows that, on occasion, the autocratic powers possessed by the Estate were used with discretion; but generally the criticisms made by Banfield and others were criticisms of basic features of the leasehold system itself. It was (at any rate on the Grosvenor estate) the function of the head lessee to improve, by building or rebuilding, the ground let to him on a long lease at a low rent. But whereas at the time of first development the prospective lessee was free to accept or reject the terms offered by the ground landlord, at the time of rebuilding he already often had a considerable amount of capital vested in the site in the form of goodwill, and in negotiation for terms the scales were therefore weighted against him. Boodle might claim with justice that no advantage was 'taken of a tradesman's good will, created by his own industry, so as to exact high terms from him', but he did also admit that 'in many cases of rebuilding it is impossible to let the old tenants rebuild. The tenants would not be equal to it . . . Great care has to be taken as to who rebuilds.' In the eyes of the Estate the tenant had a moral right to be 'fairly considered' at the expiry of his lease, and every effort was made to minimise the disturbance of rebuilding 'by endeavouring to find accommodation for the tenants displaced in the neighbourhood, as far as possible'; but 'if the necessities of the estate for public improvement require that he should go, he must go'.[399]

The Duke's rebuilding programme did undoubtedly cause a great deal of disturbance and some resentment. E. L. Armbrecht, the Duke Street chemist previously referred to, for instance, wrote to the Duke inviting him 'to imagine our positions reversed. Were your Grace a dispensing chemist, and I the Duke of Westminster, what would you then think of your landlord if, in the full knowledge that you had given the best of your life to the development of a business, I did not scruple to confiscate interests acquired at such a cost.'[400] And Thrupp and Maberly, coachbuilders in George (now Balderton) Street, complaining of the way in which they had been treated by Boodle in the matter of loss of light through the building of Clarendon Buildings opposite, asked the Duke to 'infuse into the managers of the Estate more urbanity and consideration of the feelings of others. We suppose it tends to save time to refuse to discuss matters, to say, "This is my plan, that is our form of lease, not a word shall be altered, you have only to accept or reject". But such a course is not a pleasant one to tenants.'[401]

Compulsory displacement, loss of business and a sense of grievance were all part of the price that had to be paid under the leasehold system for the Duke's improvements; but Boodle was able to make a good case for his contention that these improvements would not have been made at all if the estate had been divided into a multitude of small ownerships. In support of this he cited the case of Bond Street, where most of the tenants 'have leases perpetually renewable by right, and these leases in point of duration are practically equivalent to separate freeholds. No grand improvement, such as widening the street, is, therefore, made on a comprehensive scale, and Bond-street is, and will remain, unless the Metropolitan Board of Works steps in at an enormous cost to the ratepayers, one of the most inconveniently narrow thoroughfares in London.'[402]

Yet despite this disadvantage Bond Street nearly a century later still keeps its standing among the commercial streets of the West End; and this shows that it was not only due to the Duke's rebuilding policies and the general efficiency of his property management that the Grosvenor estate in Mayfair retained and has continued to retain its pre-eminence among the great estates of London. From the time of its first development in the eighteenth century it has always enjoyed immense advantages of topographical position. At first it was a natural refuge for the *beau monde* in westward retreat from the once fashionable but soon crowded and declining streets of Covent Garden and Soho. Then the proximity of Hyde Park came to be regarded as an added attraction—as was not the case in the early eighteenth century. Still

more important, the existence of the park on the western boundary of the estate dammed up further migration directly westward. Thus Mayfair is one of the few areas of London to benefit from the outward movement of the well-to-do without later suffering from it. No surface railway or railway constructed on the cut-and-cover principle has ever been built either on or even near the Grosvenor estate there, nor has it ever had undesirable neighbours of lesser social distinction, whose mere existence in adjacent streets might have detracted in course of time from its own *bon ton*. It has, in fact, had good fortune as well as natural advantages. With strict management and a determined programme of renewal as well, it is hardly surprising that in the first Duke's time it was generally regarded as the first among the big estates in London.[403]

CHAPTER IV

The Estate in the Twentieth Century

The death of the first Duke of Westminster on 22 December 1899 was, in retrospect, as great a landmark in the history of the Grosvenor estate as the death of Queen Victoria thirteen months later was to be in the history of the nation. In the palmy days of the late nineteenth century dukes had still been able to do pretty much as they pleased with their own, just as Imperial Britain had with her Empire; and if ominous rumblings could sometimes be heard, little attention was as yet paid to them.

But in the early years of the twentieth century dukes and all landed aristocrats found themselves on the defensive for the first time, and after Lloyd George's budget proposals of 1909, the Parliament Act of 1911 and the war of 1914–18 they were in full retreat. As early as 1873 it had been said of the great estate owners of London that 'Their position of affluence is independent of virtue or vice, prudence or folly. They exist; that is their service. It was the sole service of most of their ancestors.'[1] Views of this kind were not widely held in the 1870's, but fifty years later they seemed almost commonplace; and after the lapse of another fifty years the mere survival of so many great urban estates, even in attenuated form, provides in itself a notable tribute to the tenacity and adaptability of their owners and managers in the conduct of the great retreat.

The reign of the second Duke of Westminster, Hugh Richard Arthur, extended from 1899 to 1953. He was the grandson of the first Duke, his father having died in 1884, and at the time of his succession he was still a minor, about to go out to the South African War, where he served until 1901.[2] In their general mode of living there could hardly be a greater contrast between the peripatetic second Duke and his staid Victorian predecessor; and since his death he has in general attracted a bad press. *The Times* obituaries virtually restricted themselves to praising 'his business acumen', the efficiency of the administration of the Grosvenor estates, and his breadth of vision in extending his domains to Southern Africa and British Columbia.[3] But the politician and diarist Henry Channon described him more frankly as 'magnificent, courteous, a mixture of Henry VIII and Lorenzo Il Magnifico, he lived for pleasure—and women—for 74 years. His wealth was incalculable; his charm overwhelming; but he was restless, spoilt, irritable, and rather splendid in a very English way. He was fair, handsome, lavish; yet his life was an empty failure...'[4] Other comments of this kind could be cited, and it is therefore worth noting that immediately after the Duke's death Sir Winston Churchill, who was then Prime Minister, issued a statement publicly acknowledging their long friendship. 'As a companion in danger or sport he was fearless, gay, and delightful...Although not good at explaining things or making speeches, he thought deeply on many subjects and had unusual qualities of wisdom and judgment. I always valued his opinion. His numerous friends, young and old, will mourn and miss him, and I look back affectionately and thankfully over half a century of unbroken friendship.'[5]

Soon after his return from South Africa the new Duke married for the first time, and the estates were resettled.[6] After the first Duke's death estate duty assessed at over £600,000 had become payable (more than 90 per cent of it arising from the London properties), and for the first time in the history of the estate sales were resorted to to meet taxation. In 1902 Watney's, the brewers, bought the freehold of property in Victoria Street in the vicinity of the Stag brewery. In 1906 Westminster City Council purchased land adjoining the railway near Victoria Station, and St. George's Hospital bought that part of its site at Hyde Park Corner which stood on the Grosvenor estate. The last instalment of duty on the London estates was paid in that year.[7]

Immediately after the first Duke's death all rebuilding and improvement schemes not already commenced had been stopped, 'having regard to the money required for estate duties',[8] and very little rebuilding took place until 1906. By that time property values on the estate were falling for the first time within living memory—a matter of some surprise, perhaps, for modern readers apt to associate Edwardian Mayfair with limitless opulence—and although there was a recovery in rebuilding in the years 1906–14, the volume of work in progress at any one time has never approached that of *c.* 1886–96.

Hitherto, values on the estate had risen steadily by about ten per cent per decade,[9] but they had begun to fall in about 1901.[10] Three years later the Estate Board admitted that the market was 'bad',[11] and in 1905 the Duke was informed that for some time past the number of applications for the renewal of leases had declined. Some houses in the hands of lessees were unoccupied,[12] and in 1906 Sir Christopher (later Lord) Furness, in tentatively applying for the renewal of No. 23 Upper Brook Street, stated that he was 'undecided as to whether to take a fresh house in some other part of London, as the neighbourhood was becoming so depressing by reason of so many notice boards and empty houses'.[13]

This depreciation lasted until at least 1909 and particularly affected the larger houses. In that year the value

of houses in Grosvenor Square was said by an experienced estate agent to have fallen by 50 per cent since about 1901, and there were no less than ten houses—a fifth of the whole square—to let, 'whereas seven or eight years ago it was very difficult to purchase a house' there.[14] And for the renewal of the lease of Hampden House, Green Street, the Board was forced in negotiations with the Duke of Abercorn to reduce its terms from a rent of £1,000 and a premium of £25,000 in 1904 to a rent of £850 and a premium of £10,000 (plus works estimated at £2,400) in 1909.[15]

The fall in values certainly extended throughout the whole of the West End.[16]* Fears aroused by Lloyd George's budget programme of 1909 also had their effect, the Duke of Abercorn's agents forecasting in that year that the depression 'seems likely to become more acute, especially in view of prospective legislation'.[17] But the Estate's own leasing policy, practised by the first Duke and at first continued by his successor, of generally renewing for very short terms, often of only ten years or even less, was also a contributory cause. Although renewals of up to sixty-three years were still occasionally granted,[18] they were now very much the exception, and by 1904 both occupants and the speculative builders who often took houses for modernisation followed by a quick sale, were all complaining of the difficulties caused by short leases. Occupants pointed out that family trust money could not be invested in short leases, that it was becoming increasingly difficult to sub-let houses for the Season,[11] and that if they only occupied their houses for six months of the year they could 'get a flat at Claridge's for £3 10s a day', which was not more than the cost of running a house.[19] Speculators, such as William and Haden Tebb, clamoured for extensions of their terms, laying all the blame for their inability to sell upon the fact that 'people will not purchase a short leasehold, no matter how attractive and up to date the house may be'. The Tebbs had bought eight houses in the best streets 'at the top of the market' in 1900–2 for a total of over £61,000, all except one of them on leases of less than ten years. By 1906 they were glad to sell one of them (No. 41 Upper Brook Street) at a loss of over £7,000, while at No. 6 Upper Grosvenor Street, on which they had spent £8,500, the caretaker reported that 'Mr. Tebb would sell for £3,000 or almost give the house away.'[20]

At first the Board had ignored such complaints, and although (as previously mentioned) it admitted in 1904 that the market was 'bad', the estate surveyor, Eustace Balfour, still thought that values would continue to rise, as hitherto, at about ten per cent per decade.[9] In the following year, however, the Board was uncertain whether values would in future rise or fall, and there were also fears that 'the attractions offered on the Portman Estate and the Portland Estate on the north side of Oxford Street may depreciate the value of houses on the Grosvenor Estate'. In the spring of 1905 the Duke was therefore advised to grant longer renewals[21] and in May he agreed.[22] Less than two years later this decision was reinforced by political forebodings occasioned, evidently, by the accession of the Liberal government, the view of G. F. Hatfield, the Duke's solicitor, in January 1907 being that 'having regard to future legislation it would be well to get houses occupied for long terms.'[23]

Renewals for sixty-three years to come were now, once more, often granted, particularly in the principal streets, and in 1910 the Board stated explicitly that 'generally, 63 years leases should be granted wherever possible as the lessee will be more likely to look after and improve the property'.[24] This reversal of policy had very important results, for some houses now listed as of historic or architectural interest might well not have survived into the era of statutory protection but for the long renewals granted after 1905. Cases in point include No. 34 Grosvenor Street (renewed in 1905), No. 59 Grosvenor Street (1910) and No. 76 Brook Street (1911).

These long renewals were granted subject, usually, to the payment of a fine or premium, and almost always subject to extensive works of modernisation. Sometimes such works were accepted in lieu of a premium (as at No. 59 Grosvenor Street, for instance), and were evidently on occasion much needed. In 1905, for instance, a prospective lessee of No. 22 Norfolk (now Dunraven) Street, stated that 'the house is uninhabitable. The drainage is rotten: there is no lavatory that could be passed [by the local authority], being in the middle of the house; there is no hot and cold water and no bathroom.'[25] And in 1910 No. 21 Grosvenor Square (built to designs by Thomas Cundy II and his son in 1855–8) was said to have 'no gas or electric light and no bathrooms...There are no W.C.'s in the house except on the back staircase, and they are small and inconvenient. There is no serving room and no lift from the kitchen.'[26]

Externally, no alterations were generally demanded, except in the case of a number of important houses, which were refronted in stone. This was first done by the builder John Garlick, who in 1901–2 took No. 18 Grosvenor Street as a speculation and included a new stone front in his improvements.[27] At almost the same time, in 1902, No. 45 Grosvenor Square was refronted in Portland stone for the tenant by Edmund Wimperis and Hubert East (Plate 44a). From 1905 the process gathered pace: Garlick, for example, in that year provided No. 47 Upper Grosvenor Street, which, again, he had taken as a speculation, with a new brick and stone front designed by R. G. Hammond. The Board thought the new elevation to be 'a great improvement',[28] and in 1906, in the course of negotiations for a long renewal of the lease of No. 75 South Audley Street, the Duke's solicitor, G. F. Hatfield, suggested

* See, for instance, *Survey of London*, vol. XXIX, 1960, page 13 n. for difficulty in disposing of private houses in Cleveland Row, St. James's, in 1905.

that the lessee, the banker H. L. Bischoffsheim, might be required to refront in stone. Ultimately he agreed to do so,[29] and the same stipulation was subsequently made in the renewal of the leases of the adjoining Nos. 73 and 74 South Audley Street (Plate 44c). Several other houses, chiefly in Upper Grosvenor Street (Plate 44d), were similarly treated (or completely rebuilt with stone fronts) between 1905 and 1916, but after the war of 1914–18 the practice was generally discontinued, probably on grounds of excessive cost.

The change of leasing policy made in 1905 to renewals for long terms had important repercussions on rebuilding policy, which were carefully considered by the Board. In the words of the Duke's solicitor, the estate at that time had been for some decades 'divided into blocks, and it is the custom to renew the leases of all the premises in the various blocks for periods which make them coterminous, so that the whole of any particular block may be pulled down and rebuilt at the same time'.* This procedure was not in practice followed as effectively as this statement suggests, but in so far as it was pursued, it provided a number of advantages. These were that large sites 'for public and other purposes' could be provided, inconvenient boundaries could be rectified and rights of light and air settled, streets could be widened and new thoroughfares formed, and blocks could 'be treated architecturally as a whole, thus giving scope for a more effective design'. But there were also disadvantages. Sometimes there was 'a good house in a block which does not require rebuilding, and its removal with the block is a loss to the estate', leasing problems often arose, and 'Many people do not care to live in a house forming part of a block of houses all built on the same plan, but would prefer a house built to suit their own requirements, and according to their own design.' Ultimately it was therefore decided that 'no hard and fast rules applicable to the whole [estate] can be carried out with advantage'. Many 'houses might be rebuilt separately without detriment...', and 'each district and each house or existing separate leasehold in each district should be considered and dealt with individually. In this way, it is believed that the estate can be further developed, the present rentals maintained, and the general welfare of the estate improved.'[12]

Thus when rebuilding recommenced in 1906 a more pragmatic approach than hitherto was adopted. On the one hand, there were to be no more great schemes such as those executed by the first Duke in Mount Street, Carlos Place, Balfour Place and Mews, or in the 'artisan quarter' to the north of Grosvenor Square; and on the other hand, individual rebuildings were not to be encouraged, at any rate if the estate surveyor, Eustace Balfour, had his way, 'The experience that we have had as to individual rebuilding' being, so he informed the Board in 1907, 'so disastrous from the point of view of general improvement that it is only in cases of special necessity that I now advocate it.'[31] Instead, Edmund Wimperis (who after Balfour's retirement due to ill health in 1910 held the post of estate surveyor until his resignation in 1928) prepared in 1911 a ten-year rebuilding programme. This marked out fifteen blocks, or more accurately groups of generally up to about a dozen adjacent properties due for successive redevelopment year by year.[32]

Under these new dispositions a substantial amount of rebuilding took place between 1906 and 1914, and, after the interruption caused by the war of 1914–18, more of Wimperis's programme was completed in the 1920's. Commercial buildings were almost always built in ranges, and generally consisted of shops with flats or offices above, H. T. Boodle having noted as long ago as 1880 that 'flats should be encouraged for the upper classes as well as the working classes as they are found of great use'.[33] Examples of this type of development include Nos. 375–381 (demolished) and 439–441 (odd) Oxford Street (both 1906–8), Nos. 16–20 (consec.) North Audley Street (1908–9, originally shops with a hotel above), Nos. 39–42 (consec.) North Audley Street (1908–9), and Nos. 4–26 (even) Davies Street and 55–57 (consec.) Grosvenor Street (1910–12, Plate 47a). Houses were sometimes built in ranges, sometimes in pairs, and sometimes individually. Ranges include Nos. 37–43 (odd) Park Street (1908–10, Plate 46b), Nos. 80–84 (even) Brook Street and 22–26 (consec.) Gilbert Street (1910–13, Plate 45d), and Nos. 44–50 (even) Park Street and 37–38 Upper Grosvenor Street (1911–12, Plate 46a). Pairs were built at Nos. 2 and 3 Norfolk (now Dunraven) Street and Nos. 49 and 50 Upper Brook Street (both in 1907–8) and there were also about twenty-five individual rebuildings in Grosvenor Square and the principal residential streets. All the ranges, for both commercial and residential use, were undertaken as speculations by reliable builders such as Higgs and Hill, Matthews, Rogers and Company, or William Willett, but whereas individual houses had hitherto been usually rebuilt by an intending resident for his own occupation, many of them were now taken by builders as speculations, there being, evidently, fewer private gentlemen willing to build for themselves. Nos. 19 Upper Grosvenor Street (1909–10) and 75 Grosvenor Street (1912–14), for instance, were rebuilt as speculations, and so too were all four of the houses in Grosvenor Square rebuilt between 1906 and 1914.

In two different places on the estate advantage was taken of the upheavals caused by rebuilding to form a private communal garden in the centre of a block. In 1910, in one of his last reports to the Board, Balfour had advocated the gradual rebuilding of the rectangle bounded by Green Street, Park Street, Wood's Mews and Norfolk (now Dunraven) Street, the clearance of the stables and garages in the centre and the formation of 'a large common

* It may be noted that a similar policy had been followed on the Crown Estate with similar results.[30]

garden'.[34] This idea was subsequently executed by Edmund Wimperis, and although rebuilding in the block was not completed until *c.* 1924, it was sufficiently far advanced by 1914 for the garden for the use of all the residents to be laid out to Wimperis's designs (Plate 47b). The cost was paid by the trustees of the estate, the garden being viewed as an improvement, and its upkeep was provided for from a small private rate levied on the residents. The proposal to form this garden 'resulted in largely increased ground rents being obtained' for the houses shortly to be built around it,[35] and Wimperis therefore had no difficulty in persuading the Board to approve the formation of a similar, though smaller, garden in the centre of the block bounded by South Street, Waverton Street, Hill Street and South Audley Street. The almost complete rebuilding of three sides of this block was about to begin in 1914, and a garden, again designed by Wimperis, was formed here in 1915–16.[36]

During the years 1906 to 1914 the choice of architects for new buildings was nearly always tacitly surrendered by the Duke and the Board to the lessees. Plenty of work nevertheless still came to the estate surveyor. The silversmith John Wells, for instance, probably chose Balfour and Turner for the rebuilding of Nos. 439 and 441 Oxford Street (1906–8) in order to minimise the possibility of disagreements with the Board during his absence in New York, where he had other business interests.[37] Wimperis and/or his partners in private practice designed many of the new houses around the Green Street and South Street gardens, the large range comprising Nos. 4–26 (even) Davies Street, 55–57 (consec.) Grosvenor Street and the adjoining flats between Davies Street and Grosvenor Hill known as The Manor (1910–12), and he also had a number of other important commissions. On one occasion—at the prominent corner site of Park Lane and Oxford Street—the Board clearly favoured an architect of whom it approved (Frank Verity) and when in 1907 Higgs and Hill presented unacceptable plans for Nos. 37–43 (odd) Park Street the Board asserted that it 'should have been consulted first before an architect was employed'. Higgs and Hill were told that 'it is customary to submit to the Board a few names of architects for approval',[38] but some years previously they had had much trouble at Nos. 2–12 (even) Park Street with an architect—A. H. Kersey—nominated by the first Duke,[39] and this time they were determined that the architect should not 'be their master'. Mr. Higgs therefore produced a list of ten architects acceptable to him, from which the Board struck out five names, and Higgs and Hill then chose one of the survivors—W. D. Caröe.[38] This was a sensible compromise, but the case of Ralph Knott—the architect chosen by the lessee for the refronting of No. 21 Upper Grosvenor Street—whose designs were ultimately accepted by the Board despite strong dislike of them,[40] shows that there was now marked reluctance to use the Estate's authority in the choice of architects. In 1909 the Board informed an inquirer that 'more liberty is now given to the lessees to select their own architects',[41] and the sole occasion where the old authority was unequivocally asserted was in the building of the present Nos. 44–50 (even) Park Street and 37–38 Upper Grosvenor Street (Plate 46a). This site overlooked the garden of Grosvenor House, and the Duke required the lessee, the builder Willett, to employ Detmar Blow as architect.[42]

In general, however, the second Duke was not so assiduous in attention to the management of his estate as his grandfather had been. His restless mode of living and his dislike of London[43] precluded his regular involvement in administrative matters, and he appears to have only seldom attended the meetings of the Board. He seems to have accepted Hatfield's statement, made in 1905, that 'legislation is constantly curtailing the rights of the landowner and extending the power of the Public Authorities over all new buildings, thus reducing the necessity for street widening and such like improvement at private expense';[44] and even when the chance of making such an improvement did arise, as in the redevelopment of the block bounded by Green Street, Park Street, Wood's Mews and Norfolk (now Dunraven) Street, he 'left the question of dealing with this block to the Board'.[45] He did, however, make statements of broad intent from time to time, as, for instance, in 1907, when he 'in a general way expressed a wish for the erection of small houses on his estate';[46] and he was frequently consulted on matters which concerned himself, on controversial matters of taste, and on matters of policy.

In the building of Nos. 44–50 (even) Park Street and 37–38 Upper Grosvenor Street, mentioned above, the Duke was consulted in the choice of architect because of the proximity of the site to the garden of Grosvenor House. His appointment of Detmar Blow may perhaps have been due to his liking for the pleasing appearance of Blow's earlier No. 28 South Street (Plate 45a),[47] and it was possibly this liking which had led in turn to the Duke's commissioning Blow in about 1911 to design a hunting lodge for him at Mimizan in the Landes country between Bordeaux and Bayonne.[48] The Duke's own architectural tastes always, indeed, inclined towards 'the traditional', and in her *Memoirs*, Loelia, Duchess of Westminster, stated that he was 'most decidedly... a lover of old buildings'.[49] As we shall see later, these deeply rooted preferences led him to preserve several fine houses on the estate, but it is nevertheless doubtful whether he was as actively interested in current architectural matters as his grandfather had been. He did not, for instance, distinguish between the character of Blow's work and that of C. S. Peach, architect—with much assistance from Eustace Balfour—of the Duke Street Electricity Sub-station, whom he also explicitly desired to be given work on the estate, but whom Balfour considered to have 'no artistic perceptions'.[47] And it was perhaps from this lack of knowledge that sprang the Duke's modest reluctance to impose his own tastes on others.

This reluctance sometimes led to difficulties with the members of his own Board, particularly in such matters as the rival merits of large or small window panes. Balfour's view was that it was 'impossible to get good architecture with large panes',[50] but small panes were unpopular with many lessees, and when Knott's client at No. 21 Upper Grosvenor Street threatened to abandon her contract 'if the small panes are insisted upon' the matter was referred to the Duke, who 'saw no objection' to large panes.[51] Similarly at No. 20 Upper Grosvenor Street the Countess of Wilton (who was said by her builder, G. H. Trollope, to be 'very difficult') 'talked about throwing up the terms if she could not have large panes', and appealed from the Board to the Duke, who decided that 'a subdivision of the panes is not to be insisted upon'. Balfour could only lament that 'if permission is given there is no knowing where such windows will stop',[52] and thereafter all serious attempt to impose small panes on reluctant lessees seems to have been abandoned.[53] In the renovation and enlargement of Bourdon House, Davies Street, where he was himself in 1910 the architect for the Duke, he was, however, very careful to provide panes of the correct 'period' size.[54]

At No. 6 Upper Brook Street the uncertainty and unreliability of the Duke's decisions in architectural matters had a very unfortunate outcome. In the latter part of the eighteenth century this house had been virtually rebuilt, with extensive interior embellishments, to designs evidently by Samuel Wyatt (fig. 8a on page 121). Balfour thought it 'interesting architecturally, being probably an "Adams house"'[55] and in 1912 Wimperis said that it had 'the most distinctive front of any in the neighbourhood, and that it certainly ought to be preserved'.[56] In that year Lord Elphinstone was granted a sixty-three-year lease and was about to start renovating when he discovered that the stone front was structurally unsound and must be rebuilt.[57] The Board then required him to rebuild the front in Portland stone 'to the same design as at present', and in consideration of his extra cost agreed to grant him a ninety-year lease.[56] But the members of the Board refused to allow him to erect a projecting porch, it being their unanimous opinion that the character of the front would be destroyed by such an addition. Lord Elphinstone then wrote personally to the Duke, who informed the Board that Elphinstone 'would not have the porch'.[58] Four months later, however, the Duke happened to meet Lord Elphinstone in Paris, 'which reminded him of the porch. His Grace was rather inclined to let him have it, but did not wish to go against the opinion of the Board.'[59] At about the same time Wimperis noticed that the new front was not being rusticated in accordance with the previously existing work, and as this was 'an essential characteristic of the design ... its repetition should be insisted upon', at an extra cost of only about £25. But Lord Elphinstone regarded rustication as 'a continual eyesore' and asked that the whole matter should be placed before the Duke once more.[60] When this was done the Duke decided that the rustication should not be insisted upon, and in the light of this the Board resolved that it was not worth while to attempt to prevent the erection of a porch, the justly exasperated Wimperis considering 'that as the previous design is not to be followed, the addition of a porch is not important'.[61] Thus the original far-sighted intention to reproduce Wyatt's design was largely frustrated: and in 1936 the Duke seems to have raised no objection to the total demolition of the house by a speculator.

The loss, largely unrecorded, of this fine house was far from being the only such case on the estate during the second Duke's long reign, the similar fate of Grosvenor House and a number of the mansions in Grosvenor Square providing other obvious examples. It must be said, however, that during the early decades of the twentieth century there is little evidence to suggest that the surviving Georgian buildings or their often fine interior embellishments were greatly admired by the Grosvenor Estate's lessees or tenants. It was not until 1944 that public opinion on this subject was sufficiently strong for buildings of architectural or historic interest to be listed to ensure their statutory protection under the Town and Country Planning Act of that year. The losses of such buildings on the Grosvenor estate were matched all over London and throughout the country and should therefore be considered in the context of the times.

The Duke himself was, indeed, personally responsible for the preservation of several of the finest houses on his estate, despite the loss of income which sometimes resulted therefrom. In 1907 he finally refused (after first consenting) to allow the rebuilding of Nos. 9–16 (consec.) South Audley Street, contrary to Balfour's advice that this range should be demolished, and that the Duke would 'get a larger income if the premises are pulled down'.[62] In 1908 he refused—again ignoring Balfour's recommendation—to allow the demolition of No. 44 Grosvenor Square because of its historical associations, this being the house to which the news of the Battle of Waterloo was brought to the Prime Minister, Lord Liverpool, on 21 June 1815, and where in 1820 members of the Cabinet were to have been assassinated at dinner by the Cato Street Conspirators;[63] and when, a few months later, a large Georgian mural painting was discovered, concealed behind canvas, on a former staircase wall in the same house, he granted the lessee a remission of rent in consideration of the expense and inconvenience of preserving it.[64]

After the Duke's death No. 44 Grosvenor Square was demolished in 1968, the mural being, however, removed to the Victoria and Albert Museum.[65]

At Camelford House, which with Somerset House and other adjoining property formed part of a large and very valuable site at the corner of Park Lane and Oxford Street, the Duke's attempt to preserve was similarly frustrated, though much more quickly. Here the Duke had in November 1909 approved negotiations with J. Lyons and Company for the demolition and rebuilding of both Camelford

House and Somerset House, but immediately afterwards he revoked this decision and authorised an offer of terms for Camelford House to Mrs. Beatty, wife of Captain (later Admiral of the Fleet, Earl) Beatty. When his solicitor, G. F. Hatfield, went to see the Duke 'his Grace stated that it would be a pity to pull the house down, particularly having regard to No. 40 [Somerset House] having historical associations.* His Grace was told that... if the rebuilding did not take place, there would be a loss of about £6000 a year. His Grace stated that on a big estate like the Grosvenor something had to be sacrificed for sentiment and association...'[67] Unfortunately, however, Mrs. Beatty declined the terms, and as no other prospective occupant appeared, Camelford House was demolished in 1912.

At No. 11 North Audley Street the Duke's intention to preserve has, however, been maintained to the present time. The house itself is not of outstanding quality but the adjoining No. 12 is one of the very finest examples of Georgian domestic architecture on the whole estate, and the two houses share a unified façade and have from time to time been occupied as one. In 1883 the first Duke had decided to renew the leases of both Nos. 11 and 12, despite his intention to rebuild most of the rest of North Audley Street, the Duke's view, in the case of No. 12, being that 'it will be a pity to pull down the house owing to the beautiful room etc.'.[68] In 1913, however, the Board thought that an adjoining site in Balderton Street would be greatly improved if that of No. 11 were added to it, and with the second Duke's approval the lease of the house was therefore purchased by the Estate for this purpose. This had no sooner been done than the Duke began to have doubts about allowing its demolition. 'He was told that the object of purchasing the lease was that the house might be pulled down', but he nevertheless insisted that 'this ought not to be done and gave instructions accordingly'. Six months later the Board, still anxious about the site in Balderton Street, decided that 'the Duke be asked again about this house', but in the ensuing interview with Hatfield he reiterated that 'the house should be neither let or pulled down', and in 1914 he brusquely dismissed a suggestion for a skating rink here.[69] After standing empty for some years No. 11 was subsequently occupied by the Duke's daughter, Lady Ursula Filmer-Sankey,[70] before being reunited with No. 12 in 1948-9.

Thus Nos. 9-16 (consec.) South Audley Street and No. 11 North Audley Street all owe their survival directly to the second Duke, and it was through no lack of effort on his part that No. 44 Grosvenor Square and Camelford House have been demolished. Other decisions of his also show his concern for old buildings. During the pre-war years he affixed plaques on a number of houses commemorating the former residence of such distinguished occupants as Warren Hastings and Benjamin Disraeli,[71] and at the latter's house, No. 93 Park Lane, permission was refused for the addition of a bow window on the Park front, the house being regarded as 'somewhat historical'.[72] When asked for his views on the matter in 1912, he refused to countenance a proposal to demolish the church of St. George's, Hanover Square, and to build a new parish church on the site of the Grosvenor Chapel in South Audley Street.[73] And for various different purposes he was also responsible for the thorough renovation, at the Estate's own expense, of several important houses—Bourdon House, Davies Street (1909-11), Nos. 53 Davies Street (1922) and 66 Brook Street (1925-6), and No. 9 South Audley Street (1930-2).

Immediately after the outbreak of the war of 1914-18 the Duke joined the armed forces, serving at first as a temporary Commander, R.N.V.R., with armoured cars in France, and subsequently in North Africa, where he was awarded the D.S.O. in 1916. In the following year he was appointed personal assistant to the Controller, Mechanical Warfare Department, at the Ministry of Munitions.[2] At about this time Grosvenor House was taken over by the Government at the Duke's invitation, and after the return of peace he made his London home at Bourdon House, Davies Street.

Until the war the Grosvenor estates had survived largely intact. Small pieces of the Belgravia and Pimlico properties had been sold to pay estate duty after the first Duke's death; but after 1906 hardly any more land had been sold for some years, the Thames Bank Distillery site (1909) and several small pieces required by the London County Council, all in Pimlico, being relatively minor exceptions.[7] The second Duke had, however, bought a large estate in Rhodesia,[74] and very large mortgages and family charges dating from the first Duke's time were still outstanding.[75] It was probably in order to meet some of these liabilities that the second Duke had sold one of his outlying properties, Halkyn Castle, Flintshire, and the surrounding estate, in 1911-12.[76] But he had steadfastly refused to sell his London properties, despite half a dozen offers made for them in 1914[77] and despite the example of the Duke of Bedford's sale of his Covent Garden estate in that year.

Between 1917 and 1923, however, the Duke made massive sales, and for the first time these included substantial portions of the London properties. During this period many other landed proprietors were also selling their estates, and of the years 1918-21 it has been said that 'Such an enormous and rapid transfer of land had not been seen since the confiscations and sequestrations of the Civil War, such a permanent transfer not since the dissolution of the monasteries in the sixteenth century'.[78] The Duke of Westminster's contribution to this process was, firstly, the sale of the western portion of the Eaton estate in Cheshire for some £330,000 between 1917 and 1920, followed, between 1920 and 1923, by portions of the Pimlico properties, mainly in the vicinity of Victoria,

* Warren Hastings had lived there from 1789 to 1797.[66]

which raised some £1,100,000.[79] In 1921 two of the most famous pictures in the Grosvenor collection (Gainsborough's *Blue Boy* and Reynolds's *Mrs. Siddons as the Tragic Muse*) were also sold for £200,000.[80] By that year mortgages and family charges of over £900,000 had been paid, and the remaining encumbrances amounted to some £400,000.[81] After 1923 no more sales were made for several years, the only notable exception being that of No. 75 South Audley Street in 1925, on very favourable terms for the Duke, to the Egyptian Government for its London Legation (now Embassy).[82]

Throughout the whole of the war the routine management of the estate had been largely left in the hands of the Board, but in addition to his decision to sell part of the Eaton lands the Duke had made one other disposition of far-reaching importance. This was the appointment of the architect Detmar Blow to his personal staff in 1916.

Blow was then aged about forty-nine, and prior to the outbreak of war in 1914 he and his partner, Fernand Billerey, had had a flourishing private practice. As a young man and a very accomplished draughtsman, Blow, while drawing the church in Abbeville, had been befriended by the aged Ruskin, who had taken him on a tour of France and Italy and subsequently introduced him to Morris and Burne-Jones. In England he had learnt the technique of building at first hand by apprenticing himself to a working mason, and in 1892 he had won the R.I.B.A. Pugin Studentship.[83] Later in the 1890's he had been associated with Philip Webb in several commissions,[84] and he was a close friend of Lutyens,[85] who was two years his junior. Much, indeed, of Blow's work at this time had close affinities with that of Lutyens, particularly in his use of local materials, his gift for graceful scholarly design in the 'traditional' manner, and his insistence on the highest standards of building craftsmanship—all to be seen in his country house work, on which his early fame chiefly rested.

In 1905 Blow entered into partnership with the French architect Fernand Billerey (1878–1951). Billerey was the son of the official architect of the Department of Eure in Normandy, through whose life-long friendship with an English industrialist he had obtained a fluent command of English. He had studied in Paris, immersing himself in the Beaux-Arts tradition and learning drawing from Rodin before winning a scholarship for travel in Italy and Greece. According to family tradition, he worked at some point as an assistant at the Church of the Sacré Coeur in Paris, and had first met Detmar Blow in Italy.[86] But by September 1902 Billerey was in London in Blow's office, where he was evidently working for him as an assistant.[87] At that time Blow had chambers at No. 9 King's Bench Walk, and it was from this address that the partnership of Blow and Billerey began to function from 1905.[88]*

Hitherto Blow's practice had been almost exclusively in the country, No. 28 South Street, on the Grosvenor estate, 1902–3, being the only notable exception. Between 1906 and 1914, however, most of the partnership's chief commissions were in the West End of London, either for the design of large new houses such as No. 9 Halkin Street or No. 10 Smith Square, or for extensive interior embellishments, as at No. 10 Carlton House Terrace or the Playhouse, Northumberland Avenue. The style of some of this work was markedly different from Blow's earlier 'English Renaissance' manner, and years later the comment was made that 'his more formal style may be said to have dated from the association' with Billerey.[89] Just as Lutyens and so many contemporaries were becoming increasingly enthusiastic about the English classical tradition, so the new partnership of Blow and Billerey turned for inspiration, at any rate in London, to the corresponding French tradition, which was also enjoying growing popularity. This is particularly apparent in two commissions executed on the Grosvenor estate, Nos. 44–50 (even) Park Street and 37–38 Upper Grosvenor Street of 1911–12 (Plate 46a), and the façade of No. 46 Grosvenor Street of 1910–11 (fig. 25 on page 156), both very different in manner from Blow's earlier No. 28 South Street (Plate 45a), and in both of which Billerey's hand is unmistakably evident. Billerey was, in fact, 'a very, very good architect' in the opinion of such a discriminating critic as Professor Goodhart-Rendel,[90] who described the work of the partnership in these years as 'French architecture in London, architecture of the highest order, and of the kind which leads an Englishman to despair. It must take not a lifetime, but generations of inherited experience to produce the easy certainty with which Mr. Billerey has grouped the houses in Park Street, has modelled the galleries in "The Playhouse", has turned the vault over the staircase of No. 10 Carlton House Terrace.'[91]

Between 1905 and 1914 the partnership of Blow and Billerey was one of the most distinguished architectural practices in London. In 1914 it was, at all events, prosperous enough for Blow to buy a farm near Painswick in Gloucestershire, where he designed and built himself a very beautiful house (never fully completed) in the traditional 'Cotswold' manner, and into which he moved in January 1917. In the ensuing years he acquired by successive purchases an estate of over a thousand acres there.[92]

After the outbreak of war, however, the practice diminished greatly. Billerey went off at once to become an officer in the French army, in which he served as an interpreter for the duration,[86] and one of the few remaining commissions left for Blow was the restoration and embellishment of Broome Park, near Canterbury, for Earl Kitchener, who spent many 'happy hours' there 'with

* But according to the obituary notice of Blow published in *The Times* in 1939 'It was the late Mr. John Tweed, the sculptor, who introduced Blow to Mr. Billerey when he was looking for a partner.'[89]

his architect and friend, Mr. Blow...'.[93] In June 1916, however, Kitchener was drowned when H.M.S. *Hampshire* disappeared while *en route* for Russia, and it was at this unpropitious moment in his fortunes that, a few months later, Blow was invited by the Duke of Westminster to become, in effect, his private secretary.

At that time the Duke had known Blow for some years. His liking for Blow's No. 28 South Street (1902–3) had evidently led, as we have already seen, to his commissioning Blow to design and build the lovely single-storey hunting lodge at Mimizan. In 1908 he had appointed Blow as architect for Nos. 44–50 (even) Park Street and 37–38 Upper Grosvenor Street, which overlooked the garden of Grosvenor House; and in 1911 Blow and Billerey had worked for the Duke in the layout of formal gardens at Eaton Hall.[94] Thus at the time of this strange appointment—the immediate occasion for which was the departure to the war of the Duke's previous private secretary, Colonel Wilfred Lloyd—Blow and the Duke were already well known to each other, and their sixteen years of close association now about to begin, was evidently tinged with an element of personal friendship which was often acknowledged by the Duke with great generosity. But for Blow his employment with the Duke nevertheless meant, virtually, the end of his career as a creative artist whilst still at the height of his powers.

At the time of Detmar Blow's appointment in 1916 Edmund Wimperis had been the estate surveyor for six years. This was still a part-time appointment, and in association with a succession of partners he also conducted a flourishing private practice, the offices of which were conveniently situated in South Molton Street, some two minutes' walk from the Grosvenor Office in Davies Street. By 1916 his ten-year rebuilding programme of 1911 was already in process of execution, and his provision of private communal gardens for some of the residents of new houses in Green Street and South Street had proved very successful.

When war broke out in August 1914 another stage in Wimperis's rebuilding programme was about to be implemented, Matthews, Rogers and Company having contracted to rebuild almost the whole of the block surrounded by Upper Brook Street, Blackburne's Mews, Culross Street and Park Street. In October 1914, however, the contract had been placed in abeyance for the duration.[95] Wimperis had been quick to realise that, as the Board admitted, 'the conditions which the War had imposed had revolutionised the circumstances dealing with property...',[96] and in 1915 he drew the attention of the Board to the success of a tenant who had 'converted stabling in Aldford Street into a little house making it the best bijou house in London'. Wimperis was 'convinced that was the type of thing for which there was a great demand',[97] and in the 1920's he was able to prove his conviction in Culross Street, where several decrepit small houses and stables were rebuilt or refurbished (Plate 50a, b) and provided with a small communal garden on the lines of those in Green Street and South Street. The age of the mews house in a fashionable district had arrived.

It was also Wimperis who persuaded the Board itself to undertake, on occasion, the cost and risk of refurbishing obsolescent houses after their leases had expired. Hitherto this work had always been left to building speculators, who had taken a short lease, made improvements and relied on a quick sale for their profit. In 1918 the Board discussed 'the advisability of spending money on houses to be let as a general policy', and Wimperis urged, in relation to No. 10 Upper Grosvenor Street, that 'he would prefer that the Duke should spend money and take the risk of finding another tenant rather than a speculator should make a profit'.[98] This particular case does not seem to have been successful, but at No. 58 Park Street in 1919 the Estate, at Wimperis's instigation, spent some £570 on improvements, chiefly to the basement, and at once found a tenant willing to accept terms based on an annual value enhanced by £100. Subsequently Wimperis commented that 'I have in the past so often advocated a policy by the Grosvenor Estate of spending sums of money on improving premises that are in hand in order that His Grace the Duke of Westminster may himself reap the benefit of the improvement, that I wish to draw attention to the success of this policy in the case of No. 58 Park Street.'[99] In the 1920's this practice was adopted on numerous occasions elsewhere on the estate.

Thus when Detmar Blow entered the Duke's service Wimperis had already proved, and was to continue to prove, his worth as the estate surveyor. But with the benefit of hindsight it is easy to see that the involvement of two successful architects, both in their prime, in the management of the estate might lead to trouble, and this was not long in coming. Some mutual dislike perhaps already existed, for at No. 46 Grosvenor Street in 1910 Blow, having obtained the Board's approval for the proposed new façade there, had built it to a different design, and Wimperis, as estate surveyor, had stopped the work for a while until matters could be sorted out; similarly at Nos. 44–50 (even) Park Street and 37–38 Upper Grosvenor Street friction had arisen in 1910–12 through Blow's changes of intention. In 1920, however, Wimperis was protesting at Blow's frequent interferences and 'personal assumption of my responsibilities', and eventually he offered his resignation.[100]

By this time it was Blow who had the Duke's confidence, and although Wimperis's resignation was not accepted, he was clearly the loser in this trial of strength. He remained as estate surveyor for some years, and although his duties were not re-defined (as Blow had in the spring of 1920 promised that they should be) they seem in fact to have been largely restricted to routine matters such as dilapidation claims, the drawing of lease plans and the approval of plans of works to be done by lessees.[101] He was not, for instance, consulted when the future development of Park Lane was under discussion.[102] Some architectural work for the Estate still came his way, however,

for instance in Culross Street, the renovation of the Grosvenor Office at No. 53 Davies Street and of Nos. 55 and 57 (1922), and of the adjacent No. 66 Brook Street (1925–6), to which his own office as estate surveyor was then removed. But a growing proportion of his time was spent (in partnership with W. B. Simpson, and later also L. Rome Guthrie) on his own private practice. During these years this included several important new buildings on the estate—e.g. No. 38 South Street (1919–21, Plate 45c), Mayfair House in Carlos Place (*c.* 1920–2), the flats in Park Street known as Upper Feilde at No. 71 and Upper Brook Feilde at No. 47 (1922–4 and 1926–7, Plate 49a, b), Nos. 49–50 Grosvenor Square (1925–7) and No. 64 Park Street (1926–7). He resigned as estate surveyor in 1928,[103] but still practised privately in the 1930's. He died in 1946.[104]

After his victory over Wimperis, Blow was left in a position comparable with that of trusted minister in the court of an autocratic, pleasure-loving monarch: a not too fanciful analogy with Cardinal Wolsey and Henry VIII has, indeed, been suggested. It was Blow's wish 'to try and interest the Duke of Westminster in his Estate',[100] but the 1920's were the days when the Duke had two large yachts (the *Flying Cloud* and the steam yacht *Cutty Sark*) and a second hunting lodge in France (at St. Saens in Normandy) and his restlessness was such that during the whole course of his married life with his third wife he only once spent three consecutive weeks in the same place. Thus, while he 'enjoyed dictating the grand strategy and taking tremendous decisions' about his estates, regular personal involvement in their management was impossible;[105] and as, shortly before Wimperis's subjection, the Duke had decided that Boodle Hatfield's duties should be confined to purely legal matters,[106] Blow was left pretty much the master of all he surveyed.

He lived on the estate—at first at No. 31 and then at No. 9 Upper Grosvenor Street, and latterly at No. 3 Carlos Place. He was named as an executor of the Duke's will. He was one of the witnesses at the Duke's third marriage in 1930. When the Duke was in London he had frequent access to him; when the Duke was abroad he sometimes had power of attorney to act for him in certain matters, and when one of the Duke's trustees was out of the country he was granted similar power. He introduced his own personal methods of business procedure, entries in the series of Board Minutes, commenced in 1789, being, for instance, virtually discontinued. He advised the Duke in financial matters as well as in architectural matters, and after Wimperis's resignation he also acted as estate surveyor.[107] So it was not without reason that a builder anxiously trying to get a document signed by the Duke (who was then 'travelling about') informed the London County Council, 'I have sent the paper on to Mr. Blow, who acts for the Duke in all matters.'[108]

The period of Detmar Blow's ascendancy lasted from about 1920 until 1933. By chance, these were the final years in which great urban landlords could still treat their estates much as their forebears who had laid them out had been accustomed to do, as their own private property, broadly subject only to the landlord's covenants contained in their own leases, to the limitations of their own family settlements and to the statutory building regulations administered by the local authority and the district surveyors. Public overlordship by planning had barely started—town planning control in this part of London did not begin until 27 May 1935.[109] The zoning of land use, the redevelopment of outworn buildings, the style and aesthetics of architectural design, and the preservation or destruction of the historic fabric—all these were still, as they had always hitherto been, private matters for decision by the ground landlord and/or his advisers. On the Grosvenor estate Detmar Blow's years of eminence provided, both in their achievements and in their limitations, a fitting swansong for these traditional modes of private administration by which the estate had been hitherto managed.

These were years of much uncertainty for great urban landlords, who peered anxiously into the future to foresee what it might hold for them in the new social situation brought about by the war. On the Grosvenor estate it had not been clear, even before the war, whether the maintenance of an aristocratic residential enclave in Mayfair was still feasible, and in trying to move with the times the Board had sometimes been opposed by the tenants. In 1914, for instance, numerous objections from adjoining residents had compelled the Board to refuse to allow W. E. Hill and Son, the violin makers, to lease No. 75 Grosvenor Street (at the less fashionable east end of the street) and a private resident was not found for the house until 1917;[110] and even in socially less exclusive Park Street in 1912 the Board, after receiving similar protests, had to break its promise to allow a house agent at No. 88, one of the chief objectors being a dentist at No. 82, who stated that his patients 'would feel that he was losing caste if he had a business next door to him and they would drop off'.[111]

The Duke's own intentions were, moreover, still often unpredictable. We have already seen that he had attempted, at considerable financial sacrifice for himself, to keep Camelford House near the corner of Park Lane and Oxford Street, but that after Mrs. Beatty had declined his terms, the house had been demolished. A public outcry ensued when it became known that the new building was intended to have shops on the Park Lane frontage, but the Duke's reaction was that he did 'not see why from any sentimental feeling or moral obligation he should be prevented from carrying through a scheme which he believes would be of advantage to the estate'.[112] Nor did 'his inability to adapt himself to any change whatever', to which Loelia, Duchess of Westminster, refers,[113] prevent his abandoning Grosvenor House itself to the demolition contractors shortly after the war. Indeed, whatever may be thought of Grosvenor Estate policy towards the buildings on the Mayfair estate

in the years between the wars, bedrock conservatism or absolute resistance to change had little part in it. And in matters of social policy the Duke was similarly pragmatic, as in 1917, when he overruled his Board's advice and gave permission for negotiations for the establishment of offices for the Japanese embassy in Upper Grosvenor Street, hitherto an exclusively residential preserve.[114]*

After the war of 1914–18 both the social and architectural problems confronting the Grosvenor Estate were, indeed, more perplexing than at any previous time, for the imponderable questions of the social future were matched by equally baffling questions about the future of 'modern architecture'. Writing in 1931 Sir Edwin Lutyens pointed out that 'Forty years ago steel construction was in its infancy. Reinforced concrete was untried. Motor cars, aeroplanes, and most of the mechanical contrivances that play so large a part in life to-day were unheard of.' 'It is inevitable and right', he continued, 'that these things should influence architecture, the machines no less than the materials',[116] but the practical question for the administrator of a great urban estate was the form which this influence should take. This was particularly difficult in the case of the Grosvenor estate, for, to quote Mr. Christopher Hussey writing in 1928, 'No residential area of the West End has preserved so nearly or so long its original character' as it had; and he, at all events, had no doubt that the success of the Estate in meeting this challenge was largely attributable to the influence of Detmar Blow.[117]

After the war only two large new private houses for single-family occupation were built—No. 38 South Street and No. 15 Aldford Street, both in 1919–21; but the impending demise of the great town mansions was not as clearly apparent then as it is now, for even as late as 1936 an extra storey containing servants' bedrooms was built at No. 25 Grosvenor Square, which was to be occupied 'as a single family dwelling house'.[118] Despite the obscurity of the future, flats (and the conversion of large houses into flats) became the main residential building form of the 1920's, the design of the new blocks—notably those by Wimperis and/or his partners in Park Street, and at the south-east corner of Grosvenor Square and in Carlos Place—generally comparing favourably with that of others being erected elsewhere in London. But relatively small new private houses were also provided, obsolescent stables and coach-houses in, for instance, Mount Row, Shepherd's Place, Lees Place, Blackburne's Mews and Culross Street, being replaced by modest dwellings, each intended for single-family occupation (Plate 50c, d)—a policy which often involved for the Duke the sacrifice, in the general interest of the estate, of the highest price obtainable for a particular site.[119]

Unlike the reign of the first Duke, that of the second was not marked by the provision of artisans' dwellings on the Mayfair estate. This did not, however, betoken any lessened awareness of the problem of working-class housing, for which the Duke made very generous provision elsewhere, evidently in part at the instigation of Detmar Blow.[120] In Pimlico he leased land at a peppercorn rent to the Westminster City Council—indeed he offered more land than the Council required;[121] and on his Millbank estate in 1928 he not only granted a similar lease to the Council of land worth £200,000, but through his trustees he also provided over £113,000 towards the cost of the flats to be built on the site.[122]†

Such changes as did take place in Mayfair reflected the Estate advisers' slow and careful reactions to social forces emanating from outside the estate's own boundaries. One of these advisers, writing in 1934 in defence of their recent policies, pointed out that 'Trade and business has, for many years, tended to move westwards'. With the advent of motor traffic, streets such as Grosvenor Street and Brook Street had become 'noisy and somewhat congested, and it was found that the houses nearest to Bond Street gradually became unsuitable for private occupation. When the advisers to the Estate had quite satisfied themselves that this change was in no way temporary but permanent, and that houses ceased to be occupied by private families, and that it was more than unlikely that they would be so occupied again, then they had to consider what should be allowed to be done with such premises, at the same time bearing in mind that some of the houses would in all likelihood remain in private occupation for a considerable time. Great care was, therefore, taken as to these changes of user. The first changes would be from purely private to professional occupation. That is, a house might be used by a doctor or a surgeon or a dental surgeon, but not by a veterinary surgeon. As time went on it was found advisable to allow quiet businesses such as dressmaker or milliner, and after a further lapse of time and experience, shop fronts were permitted in certain cases... The point is that the inevitable changes of user were throughout most carefully watched and controlled by the Estate's advisers in the interests of the Estate's tenants and the public generally.'[124]

The success of flexible attitudes of this kind in achieving a smooth transition into the hurly-burly of the 1920's and 30's was matched by corresponding flexibility in leasing policy, a notable innovation here being the Estate's willingness to buy out existing leases in order to expedite rebuilding or other change. In Detmar Blow's time some £361,000 was spent on the purchase of over fifty buildings, the money being provided by the Estate trustees out of capital.[125] That the management of the estate during these years was a success is attested by the facts that, in the mid 1920's, only half of one per cent of the buildings on it were unoccupied, and that the income from it was rising.[126]

* The negotiations ultimately proved abortive and the house, No. 10, was never in fact taken by the embassy.[115]

† Between 1929 and 1934 he sold the rest of the Millbank estate to a property company for over £900,000.[123]

But Blow's principal and most lasting impact on the estate was, of course, in the field of architecture. Here two of the most distinguished architects of the day—Lutyens and Billerey—were commissioned to act as consultants. It was altogether characteristic of the traditionally personal methods of estate management of which the second Duke and Blow were among the final exponents that these two artists should, evidently, have owed their employment to their personal connexions with Blow—long-standing friendship in the case of Lutyens, professional partnership in the case of Billerey; and the results of their work still adorn the estate, although that of Billerey was very substantially modified in the course of building.

After Edmund Wimperis's status as estate surveyor had been greatly diminished in 1920, the valuations and routine reports were often done by specially commissioned independent firms of surveyors such as Hillier, Parker, May and Rowden.[127] Relatively little rebuilding took place for some years after the war, however, and so it was not until 1923, when the Duke finally decided to permit the redevelopment of the Grosvenor House site, that any important problem of architectural design arose. After a number of false starts the redevelopment of the site was taken over by an experienced speculator, and the Estate called in Lutyens to act with Blow in looking after the Duke's interests.

Although Lutyens's functions were supposed to be restricted to considering and ultimately approving the design to be submitted to him by the lessee, he did nevertheless, in close conjunction with Blow, prepare revised elevations of his own, no doubt to the annoyance of the lessee's architects, the ubiquitous Messrs. Wimperis, Simpson and Guthrie, who provided the plans and structural workings. What were in appearance virtually Lutyens's designs for the new Grosvenor House were duly executed in 1926–30 (Plate 48c).

Although doubtless inevitable, such great changes as this in the face of London aroused protest and dismay. But the Duke, at all events, was satisfied with the new Grosvenor House, and it was doubtless due to his and/or Blow's influence that Lutyens was commissioned by Westminster City Council in 1928 to act as architect for the very large housing scheme (previously referred to) then impending on the Duke's Millbank estate. On the Belgravia properties Lutyens was responsible for the elevations of Terminal House, Grosvenor Gardens (1927).[128] In Mayfair he was again employed in 1928 by the Estate for a site almost as important as Grosvenor House, that of the proposed new Hereford House, a massive building in Oxford Street to contain a department store and flats above. Here the lessees, Gamages (West End) Limited, had their own architects, C. S. and E. M. Joseph, but the building had to be erected 'to the satisfaction of Sir Edwin Lutyens and Mr. Blow as... Estate Architects' and, rather as at Grosvenor House, this resulted in Lutyens being in effect the author of the executed elevations.[129] At about the same time he acted in a similar capacity for shops and flats at Nos. 8–10 (consec.) North Audley Street, where the elevation is substantially his.[130] At the Estate's expense he also improved elevations for No. 8 Upper Grosvenor Street and provided a shop front at No. 138 Park Lane.[131] He was consulted over Aldford House (1930–2, architects G. Val Myer and F. J. Watson-Hart) and Brook House (1933–5, architects Wimperis, Simpson and Guthrie), and may have contributed to the elevations of the former (Plate 49d).[132] For all his work on the Mayfair portion of the estate executed between 1926 and 1933 his fees, paid by the Duke's trustees, amounted to over £12,000, some three-quarters of which were in respect of Grosvenor House.[133]

In view of the success of his work for the Duke it is perhaps surprising that it was not Lutyens, but Billerey, who was awarded what must have seemed at the time to be the greatest prize of all—the preparation of elevational designs for the coherent rebuilding of Grosvenor Square. The first conception of this bold idea almost certainly originated with Detmar Blow, as did the appointment of Billerey as architect; and it was through no fault of either of them that the scheme ultimately miscarried.

At the end of the war Billerey had returned to London to resume private practice, until about 1924 nominally at least still in partnership with Blow, and thereafter independently. In 1923 he had been employed by the Estate for preliminary work at Grosvenor House, and subsequently he had received several other very small routine commissions. In these post-war years Grosvenor Square presented perhaps the most intractable of all the problems confronting the Estate. The market for the rebuilding of its enormous houses had gone for ever, and those on the four corners suffered increasingly from the noise of motor traffic. When rebuilding was resumed, therefore, the first blocks of flats in the square were erected in the mid 1920's at the south-east corner, at Nos. 48 and 49–50 on either side of Carlos Place, to designs by, respectively, Wills and Kaula, and Edmund Wimperis and Simpson.

There was evidently some vague intention in the Duke's mind that the style of these two blocks should be repeated elsewhere in the square as opportunity arose,[134] but Wimperis resigned as estate surveyor in 1928, being succeeded by Blow, and in May 1929 Billerey was already concerning himself with the future of the square.[135] By this time the question of the general elevational design was becoming pressing, for the leases of Nos. 19, 20 and 21 at the western end of the north range were due to expire shortly. During the ensuing years Billerey produced a succession of elevational designs for the rebuilding of the north and south sides of the square,[136] and by September 1932 Blow had (in addition to overcoming numerous other difficulties) evidently persuaded the Duke to accept Billerey's proposals for the north range.[137] In January 1933 he finally approved on the Duke's behalf the now

urgently needed elevations for Nos. 19–21.[138] But two months later he relinquished all his duties with the Grosvenor Estate.

If Billerey's designs for the north range, and his less fully developed proposals for the south side, had been executed unaltered, the new Grosvenor Square would have provided a fine example of the Beaux-Arts manner adapted to twentieth-century requirements. But this was not to be. The lease of No. 38 on the south side had already been renewed for a long term in 1928, thereby effectively precluding the complete rebuilding of this range within the foreseeable future. Immediately after Blow's sudden departure the Estate destroyed the simple elegance of Billerey's proposed treatment of the roof of the north range by permitting the insertion of a second range of attic windows at Nos. 19–21,[139] and this (plus a further increase in the height of the roof and other modifications) was continued in the subsequent rebuilding of the rest of this range, finally completed in 1964 (Plate 54b). On the south side the Estate authorities in 1934 failed to impose Billerey's designs in the rebuilding of Nos. 35–37; and although Billerey, acting for other clients at Nos. 45–47, was still attempting in 1938–9 to provide a coherent design,[140] his chances of success were much reduced by Blow's departure from the Estate Office. On the east side complete rebuilding had been blocked by the renewal of the lease of No. 4 in 1931 for a long term, and Billerey is not known to have produced any designs for this or the western range. The rebuilding of neither the south nor the east side has ever been completed, the nineteenth-century fronts still surviving at Nos. 38 and 4 respectively. Those portions which have been rebuilt, in imitation of Billerey's elevations for the north range, merely exemplify by comparison the rare quality and accomplishment of his work. Blow's original conception, and Billerey's designs for its realisation, have both been forgotten, and amongst the architectural critics the new Grosvenor Square has become the object of such epithets as 'grandiose', 'uninspiring' and 'unimaginative'.

Detmar Blow left the Duke's service in March 1933. He died at his home in Gloucestershire in 1939, aged seventy-one.[89] His departure was a considerable loss for good architecture on the estate, for thereafter neither Lutyens nor Billerey received any commission of any importance from the Grosvenor Office. Blow's successor as estate surveyor was George Codd, hitherto an assistant surveyor in the office, who held the post until shortly after the war of 1939–45.

Frederick Etchells was one of the few architects still consulted from time to time by the Estate after Blow's resignation. As early as 1923 he had been employed to prepare models for the Grosvenor House schemes;[141] at the Estate's expense he directed extensive alterations at No. 14 Culross Street in 1927 (Plate 50b), and in 1933 he prepared plans for the rebuilding of No. 4 Mount Row (now demolished).[142] The Estate authorities continued to consult him on a number of small matters until 1935, but his fees for any one item seldom exceeded ten guineas. After Blow's resignation he did his best, though unsuccessfully, to prevent Codd from making further alterations in 1936 to Billerey's design for the centre portion of the north range of Grosvenor Square.[143]

By 1930 the Duke was over fifty years of age, and had no son of his own. Very large liabilities for estate duty were certain to occur after the Duke's death, and these, it was then thought, could only be met by sales of land. But if such sales were to be made quickly and on a large scale after the Duke's death, the market would inevitably be depreciated. The need to mitigate such an unfavourable situation and also to mitigate the impact of any future tax on ground rents provided some of the reasons why at about this time the Duke's advisers began to recommend the gradual sale of a few particularly valuable sites, the proceeds being of course available for investment.[144]

The implementation of this policy began in 1929 with the sale of part of the Millbank estate,[145] but the Duke was extremely reluctant to sell any part of Mayfair or Belgravia,[146] and it was not until 1930 that he agreed to do so. In 1930–2 the freeholds of the Connaught Hotel, Mayfair House (both in Carlos Place), Claridge's (Brook Street), Fountain House (Park Lane), Nos. 139–140 Park Lane, No. 32 Green Street and Nos. 415, 417 and 419 Oxford Street were all sold. There were also other sales in Pimlico (notably of the Victoria Coach Station site) and in Millbank.

There was, however, a new alternative to outright sales. Under the Settled Land Act of 1925 life tenants of settled land (such as the Duke) had been empowered to grant 999-year leases.[147] From the Grosvenor Estate's point of view, it was felt that this procedure would be advantageous because it would continue the mutually beneficial relationship between lessor and lessee, while by means of the covenants to be inserted in the leases, the maintenance and use of buildings on the estate could still be controlled.[148] Accordingly it had for the first time been employed in 1928 on the site of the present Fountain House, Park Lane, mentioned above. Here the lessees, the Gas Light and Coke Company (who ultimately bought the freehold outright), agreed, in exchange for a 999-year lease, to pay a large capital sum and a substantial rent, and to rebuild to designs to be approved by the Duke's architect.[149]

A number of similar leases were subsequently granted elsewhere on the estate.

During the war of 1939–45 the estate suffered severe damage by enemy action, and after the return of peace the problems with which it was faced were more difficult than ever before. A number of buildings had been totally destroyed, very many others severely injured, and even those which had survived with little or no damage were in urgent need of maintenance, which had perforce been largely suspended during the war. For several years after

1945 building licences had to be obtained before any substantial work could be started, and it was not until 1955, for instance, that the partially completed rebuilding of Grosvenor Square could be recommenced. In order to encourage the costly processes of restoration and/or improvement, the Estate's policy was to grant long leases, subject to the requirement that repairs, improvements, conversions or reconstructions should be carried out to the satisfaction of the Duke's staff. The expiry dates of these leases were arranged by blocks, to fit in with a comprehensive plan for the whole of both the Mayfair and Belgravia properties.[150]

Just when the estate was beginning to recover from the effects of the war the incidence of massive estate-duty payments, consequent on the death of the second Duke in 1953, postponed all plans for the future. During the latter part of his long reign he had instructed his chief agent, Mr. George Ridley, to 'go out into the world and seek investments in the Empire', and by a series of purchases he had extended the Grosvenor estates as far afield as Southern Africa and Australia. Shortly before his death he had bought Annacis Island in British Columbia, where he planned a great industrial estate, while at home he had initiated large schemes of afforestation in Cheshire, the Lake District, County Durham and in Scotland. On his estates in Scotland, too, the very substantial improvements which he had made there, and his support for the west coast fishing industry, had provided much local employment in the inter-war years. In a leading article *The Times* said of him that for more than half a century he had been 'the biggest private landlord in this country and probably in the world', and that 'It was in the management of his vast estates that his life found its best expression and achievement.'[151]

After his death it was reported in *The Times* that for years the Treasury had been taking ninety-five per cent or so of his income in taxes. Immediately after his death his estates in Britain were nominally valued at over £10 million, but the final figure upon which estate duty was assessed was very much larger,[152] and in 1971 *The Daily Telegraph* reported that some £17 million had been paid.[153]

Because he left no son, the resettlement made by the Duke in 1901 came to an end on his death in 1953, and subject to various family charges which he had created, he had been free to bequeath the settled estates as he wished. In order, if possible, to obviate for his descendants the recurrence of the enormous duty to which the estate would be liable on his own death, the Duke by his will divided the benefit of the bulk of the income from the Grosvenor properties among several members of the family. The heir to the title as third Duke was an elderly reclusive bachelor invalid, for whom financial provision had already been made. The income was therefore divided, in different proportions, between, firstly, the third Duke's heir-presumptive, his cousin, Colonel Gerald Hugh Grosvenor, who succeeded as the fourth Duke in 1963; secondly, the latter's brother, Lieutenant-Colonel Robert George Grosvenor, who became the fifth and present Duke in 1967, the fourth Duke having had no son; and thirdly, their respective eldest sons, if any. Each of these beneficiaries was to receive part of his share of the income absolutely, but whilst the benefit of the income was thus divided, the bulk of the estates was to be held 'in fee simple' by trustees. The days when the reigning Duke, as tenant for life, was pretty much the director of the whole of the family fortunes, were, in fact, ended, and in order to preserve the totality of the estate, which had always been one of its strengths, the management of the whole vast concern was now handed over to very able professional trustees acting for all the beneficiaries.[154]

The sales made to pay the duties arising from the second Duke's death included a number of estates in the provinces and some of the family pictures.[155] In London the whole of the Pimlico properties to the south of Buckingham Palace Road were also sold, but in Mayfair virtually no more sales have been made since as long ago as 1933, apart from that of the new Grosvenor House, which was sold in 1935 under an option to purchase granted to the building lessee in 1925. In 1934 the second Duke had, indeed, categorically refused to sell the freehold of Aldford House, Park Lane,[156] and he would no doubt have been pleased by the successful resistance made after his death by his trustees to extreme pressure to sell the freehold of the site of the proposed new United States Embassy on the west side of Grosvenor Square. Here they finally agreed to give the site subject to one proviso—the return of 'the Grosvenor Family's 12,000 acres in East Florida confiscated by the American nation at the time of the War of Independence', a property which probably included Cape Canaveral (sometime Cape Kennedy). The American Embassy in London therefore remained, it is said, the only one in the world of which the United States Government did not own the freehold.[157] The Duke's desire to preserve the Mayfair estate intact was, indeed, evidently so strong that it had even extended to the repurchase of four sites previously sold or donated—those of the Vestry Hall in Mount Street, sold to the St. George's Vestry in 1883–5 and repurchased in 1930; of St. Anselm's Church, Davies Street, given by the first Duke to the Ecclesiastical Commissioners in 1893 and repurchased in 1939 after the demolition of the church; of the Connaught Hotel, Carlos Place, sold in 1930, and of No. 32 Green Street, sold in 1931, both repurchased after the war of 1939–45.

After the vast estate duties arising from the second Duke's death had been paid off, the trustees initiated a great expansion of the Grosvenor estates, which by 1967 had achieved a 'remarkable growth of assets'.[158] No duties were payable in 1963 on the death of the third Duke, who had no interest in the estate, and after the death of the fourth Duke in 1967 the senior trustee was still able to say that 'The management of the estates will go on as

before and nothing is likely to cause any disintegration or fragmentation of the estates.'[155]

The new system of management inaugurated after the second Duke's death represented a fundamental departure from the previous administrative arrangements, which for more than two centuries had hitherto been, in the last resort, directed by the successive heads of the Grosvenor family. But the post-war years have, of course, also witnessed another equally fundamental innovation in the history of the estate—the assumption by the local authorities and the state, under successive Town and Country Planning Acts, of many of the functions hitherto discharged by the ground landlord. Town planning control, as we have already seen, had begun in Mayfair and in much of the rest of London in 1935, but its full impact did not make itself felt until after the war. For the Grosvenor authorities, with their long tradition of successful private management, this was a very difficult transition to make, and in 1934 the second Duke's advisers had even attempted, unsuccessfully, to have the estate excluded from planning control on the ground that the Estate Office already provided adequate supervisory machinery.[159] Accustomed as they were to making their own decisions in the best interests of the estate, the new planning legislation and its implementation by the local planning authority in the early post-war years often seemed, indeed, when viewed from the Grosvenor Office, to generate more heat (in the form of frustration and delay) than light.

After the war the Estate had wished the Mayfair portion of its properties to be used primarily for business purposes, while the Belgravia portion should be preserved as a primarily residential counterpart. This concept for the future character of Mayfair gave rise to considerable disagreement with the London County Council as the planning authority. After the devastation of the City of London by bombing, many of the large houses in Mayfair, hitherto in single residential occupation but at that time vacant, had been subdivided and converted wholly or partly to office uses, and numerous temporary planning consents of widely varying duration were granted for this purpose. In the altered social conditions of the post-war period the large tall ground- and first-floor rooms of many Mayfair houses were, in the Grosvenor authorities' view, no longer well suited for domestic occupation, but could readily find a new use as 'prestige offices'. By 1960 offices and private residential property each occupied about one third of the total floor space in the area, but the County of London Development Plan of 1951 had intended that ultimately most of Mayfair should be restored to residential use. This policy evoked a protest from the Grosvenor Office, which regarded the discouragement of offices as 'contrary to good estate management',[160] but it was nevertheless upheld and even strengthened by the Minister. When the Development Plan was reviewed in 1960 'it was decided that some houses should have their temporary office consents extended to December 31, 1990, others should be extended for shorter periods, and the remainder should have their temporary office consents extended until December 31, 1973, in order to give Westminster City Council time to formulate a policy for their future use.'[161]

Soon after the accession of the fifth and present Duke in 1967 the Grosvenor trustees (of whom the Duke himself was one) commissioned their own study of the future of their London estates, which was prepared by Chapman Taylor Partners and their fellow consultants and published in 1971 under the title *The Grosvenor Estate Strategy for Mayfair and Belgravia*. In his foreword to this work the chairman of the trustees acknowledged that during the previous twenty-five years or so 'The responsibility and the initiative for urban planning has shifted from the owner of a house or a street or an estate to the community—to its elected representatives and to their officers.'

In deciding to commission this study the trustees had felt that the post-war rebuilding phase being over, future developments or redevelopments should only be made in the context of a comprehensive planning framework. They were also much concerned at the deterioration of the environment, primarily caused by the intrusion of an ever-growing volume of motor traffic. The moment of publication of the *Strategy* proved extremely timely, for the shift of responsibility for urban planning from private to public hands, which had hitherto seemed (in the words of the chairman of the Estate trustees) 'both absolute and permanent', was then being modified by more conciliatory attitudes on the part of the public authorities. 'More recently a better balance has emerged: although the power of ultimate decision rests, as it should, with the community, the process by which that decision is reached welcomes the participation of everyone who is affected by it. This new attitude towards planning revives the estate owner's responsibility to look beyond the problems of the moment to the medium and longer term influences on his property—to the shape of the square, the pattern of the streets, the scale of the buildings.'[162]

The *Strategy* was also timely in that its preparation coincided with the designation in 1969 of most of the Grosvenor estate in Mayfair as a Conservation Area. This new planning concept had been created by the Civic Amenities Act of 1967, the object of designation being 'to preserve the character or appearance of areas of special architectural or historic interest, as distinct from individual buildings, to control development in such areas and to stimulate and encourage measures to improve the environment'.[163] In an area such as Mayfair (or Belgravia) conservation was clearly to have an important bearing upon future planning policies, and the *Strategy* took full account of it.

The planning objectives of the *Strategy* were 'to preserve what is of architectural value, to enhance the inherent character of the Estate, to relate street formation

to environmental qualities and to establish a balanced mix of uses, including a full range of residential accommodation, confining redevelopment of high intensity to appropriate districts close to public transport facilities'.[164] The basic idea for the realisation of these aims was that 'A structure of high intensity development on the peripheries' should shield 'the conserved inner areas or hinterland' of the estates in both Mayfair and Belgravia.[165] Numerous detailed proposals for this purpose were put forward, the most important for Mayfair being the comprehensive redevelopment of the whole of the Oxford Street frontage from Davies Street to Marble Arch, and 'an active improvement policy' for most of the rest of the estate.[166] Through traffic was to be diverted from the internal roads on to the boundary roads of Oxford Street and Park Lane, the eight-lane carriageway of the latter, it was hoped, being eventually sunk below ground level; and the number of vehicular entry and exit points to and from the estate was to be reduced.[167] As the amount of redevelopment envisaged was 'likely to be relatively small' (except in the vicinity of Oxford Street), considerable emphasis was placed upon the maintenance and improvement of 'the existing character and the ambience of the environment'.[168] The mixture of office and residential uses, often uneasily combined within a single building, was to be sorted out, increased residential use in the mews or in Aldford Street being counterbalanced by more offices in streets bearing a greater volume of traffic, such as Park Street or Davies Street.[169] The first Duke's *chef d'œuvre*, late Victorian Mount Street, was to be 'preserved and maintained as long as economically possible', and the range of erstwhile stables and coach-houses on the south side of Bourdon Street was to be converted into a shopping arcade.[170] The conservation policy was, in general, to be 'largely one of infill in scale and in character with existing buildings'; and whenever redevelopment did become necessary, the *Strategy*'s authors 'strongly advise against imitations of former styles whether Georgian or Victorian'.*[171]

The *Grosvenor Estate Strategy* of 1971 is one of the most important privately commissioned planning studies yet to appear, and its reception in the press was generally favourable. *The Guardian*, for instance, commented that 'what shines through the Strategy is its real concern for the environment and an understanding of it'; and *The Observer* thought that 'almost everything that is said seems to be more or less right and aimed at making a happier, better place to live and work in. Above all, perhaps, the conclusions appeared to have been generated primarily by human considerations rather than financial ones.'[172]

An opposite view was, however, taken in *Official Architecture and Planning*, where it was stated that 'It is depressing, but probably inevitable, that the primary objective of the effort should be the realisation of the full development potential of some of the most distinctive parts of central London'.[173] This verdict must have been discouraging for the authors of the *Strategy*, who had intended it to provide 'a link of unity' between the public authorities and the Estate.[174] A link it is nevertheless proving to be, despite the strains to which all links are sometimes subject. Since its publication in 1971 detailed discussions have taken place between Westminster City Council, the Greater London Council and the Estate, and in 1973 the City Council decided that, subject to certain modifications, the *Strategy* 'would be one of the material considerations to which the Council will have regard in determining planning applications for the Mayfair and Belgravia areas...'[175]

These modifications, which were also sought by the Greater London Council, have been agreed to by the Estate, and include a smaller increase of offices and a greater increase of residential accommodation than had been envisaged in 1971; and the resolution of the vexed question of the 'temporary office permits' problem, it being agreed that some premises would revert to residential use and others would continue as offices during the life of each particular building. The Estate also undertook to increase its stock of low-income housing and for this purpose leased an important site in Pimlico to the Peabody Trust.[176] Recently the size of the hinterland of the Oxford Street area proposed in 1971 for comprehensive redevelopment has been greatly reduced by the exclusion of Green Street, Binney Street, Gilbert Street and the east side of Duke Street (parts of which had at first been intended for redevelopment) and the blocks of 'artisans' dwellings' built in this neighbourhood in 1886–92. These blocks are now to be retained, some of them are to be modernised, and the loss of residential accommodation caused by the conversion of some of the lower floors into shops will be balanced by new residential accommodation to be provided in Weighhouse Street. Nearby, the reconstruction of Bond Street Tube Station to serve both the existing Central Line and the new Fleet Line is already in progress. Here the London Transport Executive, the Grosvenor Estate and the developers, Metropolitan Estate and Property Corporation Limited, are co-operating in the building of a larger and more efficient station than that originally envisaged. Above the station there will be several shopping levels and floors of offices, and the completion of the scheme in about 1980 will mark the achievement of the first phase of the

* It may here be noted that the architectural assessments contained in the *Strategy* should be treated with caution. The classification on page 22 of buildings 'by four historical periods and three grades of architectural quality' (a classification in no way connected with that in the Secretary of State for the Environment's list of buildings of special architectural or historic interest) contains a number of errors, of which the identification of Nos. 91–103A (odd) Park Street, by Wimperis and Simpson 1913–*c*. 1922, as '1700–1800 Georgian' provides one example. Nor will the authors' sweepingly unfavourable judgments upon most of the twentieth-century buildings on the estate be universally accepted.

comprehensive redevelopment of the south side of Oxford Street which the Estate had first proposed in 1971.[177]

During the preparation of the *Strategy* (which was started in 1968) and during the ensuing years of prolonged discussions with the public authorities about the acceptance and/or modification of its proposals, the Estate had submitted itself to a 'self-imposed stand-still on major commercial and residential redevelopment in the interest of strategic planning', its view being that 'individual schemes cannot be properly assessed in isolation and must relate to an overall strategy to ensure that the correct overall land use balance is achieved'.[178] Adaptation to the exacting demands of post-war planning was not, however, the only new problem confronting the Estate in these years, for under the Leasehold Reform Act of 1967 some tenants acquired the right in certain circumstances to buy the freehold of their houses. The exercise of this right would have frustrated many of the policies pursued by the Grosvenor Estate over very many years, but for the Estate's success in obtaining the insertion of a safeguarding clause in the Act. This provided that when the Minister of Housing was satisfied that 'in order to maintain adequate standards of appearance and amenity and regulate redevelopment' in any area owned by a single landlord, it was 'likely to be in the general interest that the landlord should retain powers of management', he was to grant a certificate to that effect. This certificate had to be approved by the High Court,[179] and in 1973 the Grosvenor Estate became the only landlord with a significant holding in central London to obtain final approval for such a management scheme. The approved scheme related only to Belgravia,[180] but application has recently been made for another for Mayfair. The whole episode provides striking public recognition of the 'general benefit'[179] which, even in the age of public planning, can still arise from the Grosvenor Estate's administration of its London property.

CHAPTER V

The Social Character of the Estate

At Michaelmas 1726 Sir Thomas Hanmer, baronet, Member of Parliament for the County of Suffolk and ex-Speaker of the House of Commons, vacated his town residence at No. 12 Old Burlington Street, and his household moved into a new house at No. 52 Grosvenor Street for which the price was £4,250 (Plate 8c; fig. 16 on page 136). Sir Thomas himself was then still at his country seat at Mildenhall in Suffolk and his housekeeper supervised the move in good time for the master's return to town in November for the new London Season. Sir Thomas had only lived in Old Burlington Street, where he was also one of the first occupants, since about 1723, but his new house in Grosvenor Street was much larger and no doubt better fitted to accommodate his retinue of some fourteen servants.[1] In being so soon prepared to move to another newly developing district further to the west, where he would inevitably be once more surrounded by the noise and clutter of building operations, he was following the lead of his compeers, for several of his new neighbours belonged to the titled ranks of society. The Earl of Arran lived on one side of him and on the other was Sir John Werden, baronet, father-in-law of the second Duke of St. Albans who was also living here at about this time, while two doors away at No. 50 the first Earl of Uxbridge was a new arrival.[2]

An indication of the attraction of the new suburb around Grosvenor Square for the social élite can be gathered from the standing of the first occupants, i.e. householders, of the houses in the principal streets, viz. Brook Street and Upper Brook Street, Grosvenor Street and Upper Grosvenor Street, and the square itself. A full list of these occupants is given in the tables on pages 172–95, but it should be noted that they were not all resident at the same time, as the houses were erected over several years. Of the 277 houses built in these streets, 41 were first inhabited by peers and seven more by persons who were created peers or succeeded to peerages while living on the estate, making 48 (17.3 per cent) in all. A further 69 houses were first occupied by other persons of title, i.e. the wives, widows, sons or daughters of peers; baronets and knights (or their widows); and foreign nobility. Thus, in all, the initial householders of 117 of the 277 houses (42.2 per cent) belonged to the titled classes of society. The proportion was naturally highest in Grosvenor Square itself, where of the 51 houses 16 were taken by peers (31.4 per cent) and 19 more by other persons of title, making 35 (or 68.6 per cent) in all. In these principal streets 54 of the first occupants (19.5 per cent) sat in the House of Commons at some time during their residence on the estate, 19 of them living in Grosvenor Square. Several of these M.P.'s also come into the category of persons of title and a few were Irish peers, who did not sit in the House of Lords and were thus eligible for election to the lower House.

The gathering momentum of the migration of fashionable society to the new estate can be seen from the number of members of both Houses of Parliament who had their town addresses there. In 1733 30 members of the Commons (5.4 per cent of the whole House) and 16 peers who could attend the Lords (8.3 per cent of the upper House) lived on the estate. By 1741 the numbers had increased to 45 (8 per cent) and 31 (16.3 per cent) respectively, and by 1751 to 49 (8.8 per cent) and 39 (23.3 per cent).[3]

On the whole the aristocracy and the gentry lived in the broad belt across the centre of the estate formed by the principal streets referred to above, but a few lived elsewhere, notably at the south ends of Park Street and South Audley Street, and later in Norfolk (now Dunraven) Street and Hereford Street, and, much later, in Park Lane. It was generally in these streets that the large households were concentrated, such as that of Sir Thomas Hanmer, already mentioned, or of Baron Conway (later Marquess of Hertford), who in 1746 had twenty-two servants at No. 16 Grosvenor Street. His steward kept a 'Grosvenor Street House Account' which shows that his annual expenses there amounted to little short of £3,000, of which £345 or only about 12 per cent was accounted for by his servants' wages, most of the remainder being spent on the payment of tradesmen's bills.[4]

The house account also itemised some of the travelling costs, including the carriage of trunks to London from other places, chiefly the Conways' seat at Ragley Hall in Warwickshire, and in these streets the comings and goings of the London Season must have been particularly marked. The influx of carriages into town at the beginning of the parliamentary session (in the eighteenth century usually in November, December or January) was quite noticeable. *The World* in January 1790 reported that 'London is now almost at the fullest:— every avenue yesterday was crowded with carriages coming into town.'[5] In the first half of the eighteenth century the parliamentary sessions generally lasted into the early summer, but in the latter half they usually extended into June, July or occasionally even August. Whenever it occurred, the commencement of the summer recess was soon followed by the departure of many of those residents who also had country houses. In September 1734 Mrs. Delany, who was then living at

No. 48 Upper Brook Street, remarked with characteristic independence to Dean Swift, 'The town is now empty, and by most people called dull; to me it is just agreeable, for I have most of my particular friends in town.'[6] It was during these uncomfortable, dusty months that the builders and upholsterers were called into the grand houses to prepare them for the next social round.

Even within those streets where the momentum of life must often have been regulated by the social calendar there were, however, a number of incursions from the world of trade. Victuallers established themselves, generally on corner sites, at the Mount Coffee House, the Three Tuns and the Red Lion in Grosvenor Street; the Barley Mow, the Cock and Bottle and John Dickins's coffee house in Upper Brook Street; and the Oval and the Wheatsheaf in Upper Grosvenor Street. Other first occupants known to have been tradesmen included an apothecary and a shoemaker on the north side of Brook Street, a grocer at the corner of Brook Street and Davies Street, and a cheesemonger and a tailor in Upper Brook Street; while William Campbell, upholsterer, had established himself in Grosvenor Street by 1727.[7] In a somewhat different category were the building tradesmen who occupied the houses they built in the main streets, sometimes for lengthy periods.

If trade made inroads into the principal streets, however, it dominated the lesser ones. The Westminster poll books of 1749[8] give a useful though imperfect guide to the occupations of many of the inhabitants of the estate at a time when such evidence is generally unavailable. In Westminster there was a particularly wide franchise, for the right to vote was vested in male householders paying 'scot and lot', i.e. the parish rates; of course the large class of women householders and the much smaller one of peers were excluded, and not all of those eligible to vote actually did so. The Westminster by-election of 1749–50 was, however, 'one of the most fiercely contested elections in the first half of the eighteenth century' and there was a very high poll. Charges of malpractice were brought, and the high bailiff was accused of 'allowing many votes by people who did not pay scot and lot and refusing those of others who did, and of having declined to produce the parish books showing who the legal voters were.'[9] Whatever the substance of these allegations the record has to be treated with caution. It consists of a meticulously written account of the names and occupations of the voters and the streets in which they lived. Some of the names in the poll books do not appear in the ratebooks but a close comparison is not always possible because of the loss of some ratebooks for the period of the poll. Nevertheless by correlating the two sources for certain streets and using only those names which can with reasonable certainty be confirmed as the occupants of the houses, a generalized picture can be built up.

In Mount Street, for instance, there were 116 houses entered in the ratebooks; 91 householders were seemingly qualified to vote and 66 of them did so. Of these 66 only nine described themselves as gentlemen or esquires, and one other (a schoolmaster) can be considered to belong to the professional classes. Excluding two coachmen and a turncock, 53 of the remainder (or 80 per cent of those who voted) were tradesmen. Thus almost one half of the ratepaying inhabitants of Mount Street were certainly tradesmen and the actual proportion was undoubtedly higher. Not only would many of the non-voting male householders have been engaged in trade, but so also would some of the female ratepayers, including the landlady of the Wheatsheaf tavern, and, quite possibly, a number of milliners; while at the poll the landlord of the Swan described himself as a gentleman. Of the 53 tradesmen who voted, 20 (37.7 per cent) belonged to the building and decorating trades; 14 (26.4 per cent) were purveyors of food and drink, including three victuallers and three chandlers; and 13 (24.5 per cent) were concerned with clothing or other wearing apparel.*

North Audley Street is a much shorter street with direct access from Grosvenor Square, but there the predominance of the trading element was just as pronounced. Of 36 householders paying rates 27 were eligible to vote and 25 did so. Of these 25 only five were gentlemen, esquires, or, in the case of Sir John Ligonier, a knight; one other was a schoolmaster but the remaining 19 (76 per cent of those who voted) were tradesmen. Five of them were builders or decorators, including a cabinet-maker; eight supplied food and drink, including three victuallers; and six worked in the world of clothing and fashion, including a staymaker and two peruke-makers.

In Davies Street, where most of the houses had been standing for twenty years or more, the pattern only varied slightly. Of 55 householders, 51 were entitled to vote and 44 of them did so. Three were gentlemen or esquires, and there were also a surgeon, a cook and a beadle, but 38, well over half of all the ratepayers in the street, were tradesmen. Of these 38, some five (13.2 per cent) were connected with building or decorating; 21 (55.3 per cent) were in the food and drink trades, including the resident victuallers of six taverns in the street and three chandlers; and six (15.8 per cent) supplied clothes, materials or wigs.

South Audley Street had its fashionable element, particularly at the south end, but over the whole street the tradesmen were still apparently dominant. Of 66 householders, 49 were eligible to vote and 38 exercised their franchise; 13 of these 38 were gentlemen or esquires and there was also one chairman, but the remaining 24 (63.2

* The occupations of the 53 tradesmen who voted in Mount Street were: (building and decorating trades) bricklayer, carpenter (6), carver, glassman, glazier, mason (3), painter (2), plasterer, plumber, smith, turner, upholsterer; (food and drink trades) baker, brewer, butcher (2), chandler (3), corn chandler, distiller, greengrocer, poulterer, victualler (3); (dress trades) breeches-maker, cutter, dyer, framework-knitter, laceman, linen-draper, peruke-maker (4), shoemaker, tailor (2); (other trades) apothecary, coachmaker, dealer in horses, lampman, saddler and snuffman.

per cent of the voters) were all tradesmen. Five of the 24 (20·8 per cent) pursued building or allied occupations; 14 (58.3 per cent) worked in the food and drink trades; only one, a peruke-maker, was concerned with clothing and fashion, but it is possible that some of the many single female householders were milliners. One at least was in trade, for Elizabeth Jones was the licensed victualler of the Albemarle Arms.

Some of the less salubrious areas of the estate lay immediately to the south of Oxford Street where land had been parcelled out in large blocks at low rents with few restrictive covenants in the original building leases. Two of these enclaves where building had progressed sufficiently by the mid eighteenth century for a coherent pattern of occupation to be established were the hinterlands behind the north side of Grosvenor Square between North Audley Street and Duke Street, and behind the north side of Brook Street between Duke Street and Davies Street. Here developers had laid out several narrow streets, viz. George (now Balderton), Queen (now Lumley), Brown and Hart Streets (now combined into Brown Hart Gardens) north of Grosvenor Square; and Bird (now Binney), James (now Gilbert) and Chandler (now Weighhouse) Streets north of Brook Street. The ratebooks show that by 1749 some 150 houses had been built in these streets and along the south side of Oxford Street. Several of them were let to tenants who did not pay rates and were thus ineligible to vote; against one such entry in the ratebooks where the ratepayer's name was left blank the collector had noted 'takes in vagabonds for Lodgers'. Nevertheless 92 ratepaying occupants of these streets did vote in the election of that year. Eleven were gentlemen, some of these being landlords like John Taylor who lived in one house in James Street himself and let half a dozen others to tenants; six fall into the general category of servants, including two coachmen and two chairmen; and 71 (77.2 per cent of the voters) were tradesmen. The remainder included a schoolmaster, a surgeon, a yeoman and a gardener. Of the tradesmen 26 (36.6 per cent) worked in the building trades, 22 (31 per cent) supplied food and drink including no fewer than eight victuallers, and 11 (15.5 per cent) were concerned with dress.

The impression created by the occupations of the voters in these streets could also be found in other parts of the estate. There were, however, some differences in the distribution of trades. Building workers were understandably most numerous in those parts of the estate where development was still in progress, in the streets to the north of Brook Street and Grosvenor Square, in the south-west corner around South Street and Chapel (now Aldford) Street, in Park Street and Green Street, and, more surprisingly, in Mount Street. Those involved in some capacity with horses or carriages, the wheelwrights, farriers, stable-keepers and coachmen, tended to live in the mews where there was clearly a good deal of residential accommodation. But, at this period, by no means all mews dwellers belonged to these or allied trades; in Grosvenor Mews, for instance, there were also victuallers, chandlers, builders, servants and a chimney-sweep among others. There was, however, no obvious concentration of food retailers and the numerous victuallers who presided over some 75 taverns or licensed coffee houses[10] were scattered throughout the estate. The chandler, that eighteenth-century Jack-of-all-trades, could also be found almost everywhere outside the five main streets.

The poll provides less evidence about the inhabitants of the principal streets, both because the presence of numerous peers and female householders (the latter accounting for over a third of the ratepaying occupants of Upper Brook Street alone) meant that fewer of them were eligible to vote, and because, of those who could have voted, a lower proportion exercised their right. Westminster tradesmen appear to have been more assiduous in using their political rights than the titled classes or country gentlemen. Many of these may indeed have been out of town, although the poll was taken during a parliamentary session. For comparative purposes the examples of Brook Street (that part on the Grosvenor estate only) and Upper Brook Street may be cited. There were then 94 houses already erected in the two streets and the householders of 54 of them were eligible to vote, but only 33 did so. Of these 33, gentlemen, esquires, 'honourables', knights, baronets, a general, a physician and a clerk account for 20, and the remaining 13 (39·4 per cent of the voters) were tradesmen, a surprisingly high number (considering that there may have been others who did not vote) for these august thoroughfares. They included two victuallers and a 'coffee man', all in Upper Brook Street at corner sites, two apothecaries, a linen-draper, a tailor, a wine merchant, a cheesemonger, a saddler, a smith, a glassman, and the master carpenter John Phillips at No. 39 Brook Street.

Thus by the mid eighteenth century, when the estate was still by no means completely built over, a coherent picture of its social composition had begun to emerge. It was that of a fashionable core of streets and a grand square occupied by the *beau monde*, encroached upon to a limited degree by residents engaged in trade, who in turn were to be found in overwhelming preponderance in the surrounding streets. Just as some tradesmen lived in the preserves of the socially distinguished, so also there were small coteries of the fashionable gathered in the outlying streets, and except in Grosvenor Square there was no strict segregation. The houses of the upper classes dominated physically by their size and by their large plots with long gardens extending to mews stabling at the rear, but they account for only about a quarter of the building fabric of the estate. The tradesmen, who formed such a substantial element of the population, evidently varied greatly in wealth and status, there being no doubt a considerable difference between, for instance, John Edmonson, saddler, of Upper Brook Street, who was listed in Mortimer's *Universal Director* of 1763, and the chandlers

of Grosvenor Mews; and the gulf between the tradesmen of North Audley Street and the nearby inhabitants of Brown's Court or Parr's Buildings off North Row must have been almost as great as that between a well-established tradesman and his fashionable clientèle. Many of these tradesmen would have relied greatly on the patronage of the rich and titled inhabitants, as Lord Conway's household accounts testify; and in the case of the peruke-makers, of whom there were at least sixteen on the estate in 1749 (four of them in Mount Street), their dependence must have been almost complete.

Over fifty years ago Mrs. Dorothy George commented that 'Eighteenth-century London inevitably suggests the brilliant society which made up the world of politics and fashion. This small world of statesmen and politicians and placemen, of wits and rakes and fops, was so self-sufficient, so conscious that it was the only world that counted, that it imposes its point of view on us...We know little of the artisans and labourers, the shopkeepers and clerks and street-sellers, who made up the mass of the population.'[11] The nature of the evidence is such that it could hardly be otherwise, but at least sufficient can be gleaned from very fragmentary information to suggest that the impression generally prevalent that this part of Mayfair was the almost exclusive province of the well-to-do and the well-connected is in some respects highly misleading. Fortunately the somewhat crude outline of the social composition of the area that can be drawn from such evidence as that provided by the poll books of 1749 can be filled in by more detailed and reliable evidence in later years.

A Survey of Householders in *c.* 1790

The end of the eighteenth century was a quiet period in the history of the Mayfair estate. The building operations begun in 1720 had finally come to an end in the 1780's, and rebuilding on any significant scale did not start until the 1820's. A stable pattern of occupation therefore established itself in these years, and this is well illustrated by a detailed survey of the 'inhabitants' which was compiled in 1789–90 by the authorities responsible for collecting the assessed taxes in Middlesex.[12]

Though its provenance must connect it with taxation the real purpose of this survey remains unknown. It covers the whole of the parish of St. George's Hanover Square, street by street, listing the 'inhabitants' with their status or occupation and a wealth of other detail besides.* The term 'inhabitants' here seems to have been synonymous with the resident householders, but it also included non-residents who had businesses on the estate or let houses there to tenants. All householders were included (which was not the case with the poll books, previously discussed), but no information was given about the size of households or of the population as a whole.

The total number of these 'inhabitants'—excluding as far as possible non-residents and double entries—was 1526. These can be divided according to rank or occupation as shown in the accompanying Table.

The figures in this Table confirm the impression, already hinted at by the 1749 poll books, of a very heterogeneous population in which trade and commerce predominated. The residents of rank and fashion, who

Householders in *c.* 1790

Status or occupation of 'inhabitants'		*Number of 'inhabitants'*		*% of total*
Persons of title		129		8.5
M.P.'s (both with and without titles)		35		2.3
Professional		112		7.3
Trade		890		58.3
Food and drink	288		18.9	
Dress and fashion	173		11.3	
Building	164		10.7	
Transport (including stable servants)	142		9.3	
Other trades	123		8.1	
Domestic servants		48		3.1
No occupation		343		22.5
less 'inhabitants' with dual status or occupations		−31		−2.0
		1526		100.0

* The headings under which the information sought by the survey was listed are as follows: 'House Number'; 'Inhabitants'; 'When Inhabited'; 'Furnished Houses'; 'Empty Houses'; 'Inmates Ground Floor'; 'Pays No Taxes'; 'Roman Catholics'; 'Widows and Spinsters'; 'Peers and Members of Parliament'; 'Army, Navy and Placemen'; 'Occupations'; 'Observations and Remarks'. The remarks usually include the sign of licensed premises, the nationality of aliens and sometimes the names of employers.

in this area might be expected to be numerically preeminent, are, however, not very easily identifiable in the survey, their presence being partly concealed in the 'no occupation' category, which includes 63 esquires and 24 gentlemen, and nearly 200 women. A better guide to the proportion of residents of rank and fashion is probably provided by *Boyle's Court Guide*, first published in 1792. Its 410 entries for the Grosvenor estate suggest that about a quarter of all householders on the estate belonged to this class.

The location of the various classes showed hardly any changes since the mid century. For those who could afford it Grosvenor Square was still the 'best address'—indeed one of the best in London. Of its 47 householders in 1790 thirty-one were titled, and these included three dukes, six earls (of whom one was Lord Grosvenor) and a viscount. Only slightly less fashionable were Upper Brook Street and Upper Grosvenor Street, which Mrs. Anne Damer, house-hunting in Mayfair in 1795, coupled with Grosvenor and Berkeley Squares as the 'ne plus ultra'.[13] In Upper Brook Street (where Mrs. Damer settled in 1799) 49 householders out of a possible 55 are listed in the court guide for 1792 and in Upper Grosvenor Street, 42 out of a possible 48. Brook Street and Grosvenor Street, always more vulnerable to commercial pressure than their extensions west of the square, were rather less exclusive, particularly towards their eastern ends. In Brook Street just under a quarter of all the householders were tradesmen and by 1805 the estate surveyor, William Porden, thought that the eastern half of the street was 'of such a mixed character of Houses as not to be thought an eligible situation for Persons of Rank'.[14] The newer developments in Hereford Street, Norfolk Street, Portugal Street and the south-west end of South Street were, however, all popular with fashionable residents. In South Audley Street the two facing groups of houses at the south end (Nos. 9–16 and 71–75 consec.) retained their fashionable *cachet* against commercial encroachments, as did the large houses overlooking the park at the south end of Park Street, and some of the houses on the south side of Green Street.

Titled people of all types accounted for 8.5 per cent of the 'inhabitants' listed in the survey. They included 37 peers (including Irish and Scottish peers), 18 baronets, 15 'honourables', and 39 'ladies'. Heading the list of peers was the Duke of Gloucester, one of George III's brothers, whose large detached house in Upper Grosvenor Street was later to become the London home of the Grosvenors. In addition to the Duke of Gloucester there were five non-royal dukes living on the estate. Foreign nobility was represented by the Hanoverian minister, Baron Alvensleben, at No. 37 Grosvenor Square, and the Duke of Orleans (Philippe Egalité) at No. 2 South Street, a house at the corner with Park Lane.

Several of the householders whose names appeared in the court guide were professional men. They included 'placemen' who were not also tradesmen; members of the armed forces; attorneys and lawyers; medical men (but not apothecaries) and architects. The 'placemen', of whom there were 32, were mostly either civil servants like Timothy Caswall of Davies Street, one of the Commissioners of the Salt Tax, or court officials, like Thomas Dupuis of Park Lane, the King's organist. Among the armed forces the Army was represented by fifteen officers and a surgeon, the officers ranging in rank from captain to general; the Navy's complement was two admirals, three captains and a surgeon. Three civilian surgeons were among the twelve householders who were medical men, the others being physicians, a dentist, a 'man midwife' and a chiropodist described as 'Operator to their Majesties for the Hands and Feet'. Another eight householders were attorneys, two of them being Earl Grosvenor's own lawyers, Edward Boodle and Thomas Walley Partington of Brook Street. Only two householders were described as architects, one being John Crunden, who occupied a house of his own designing in fashionable Hereford Street, and the other the little-known George Stoddart of South Street. Rather surprisingly the financial world had only one representative, George Brooks of Green Street, a founding partner in the banking firm of Dixon Brooks and Company, established in 1787 in Chancery Lane.[15]

More than half the householders on the estate in 1790 earned their living by trading in goods and services. Some 120 different trades were represented, ranging from muffin-makers to 'herald painters', but the main areas of activity were those concerned with food and drink, building, dress and fashion, and transport. The standing and scale of business of individual tradesmen evidently varied greatly. Twelve of them claimed to have the patronage of Royalty, the names of several appeared in the court guide, and the wealthy and fashionable inhabitants of Grosvenor Square naturally dealt with high-class purveyors, some of whom enjoyed metropolitan reputations. But at the other extremity were those who must have relied for their trade on the unfashionable but more numerous inhabitants of the lesser streets and mews.

The main shopping streets in 1790 were Davies Street, Duke Street, Mount Street, North and South Audley Streets, Oxford Street and Park Street—Mount Street being probably the most fashionable. The survey does not identify individual shops (except for a few occupied separately from the rest of the house), but as most tradesmen seem to have used their homes as their place of business, a good many ground-floor front rooms must have been turned over to trade. Some of them were fitted up with shop windows, as is shown on a plan of the east end of Brook Street in 1778–9 (fig. 4). Tradesmen had not at first needed the permission of the ground landlord to install shop windows, but from the 1760's estate leases contained a clause prohibiting the erection of bow windows[16]—evidently an attempt by Lord Grosvenor and his advisers to limit the proliferation of shop fronts.

The largest of the four main commercial groups were the food and drink trades, in which 288 tradesmen (some 19 per cent of all householders) were employed. Within this group the most numerous in a single occupation were the 74 licensed victuallers, of whom 73 occupied named licensed premises on the estate. Thus the number of public houses had hardly altered since 1750. Some losses in the older streets had been made up in the newer developments like Norfolk Street, but their distribution was as widespread as before, and among the principal streets only Grosvenor Square, Hereford Street and Portugal Street had none at all.

After the victuallers came the butchers, with 55 traders including poulterers and a tripeman. They were heavily concentrated in the north-east corner of the estate, particularly in St. George's and Grosvenor Markets (both exclusively food markets), where 35 butchers had their stalls. Their concentration in these two markets may have been the result of an attempt by Earl Grosvenor to take what was often an offensive trade out of the main streets. But even in the markets the butchers were not immune from complaints. In 1801, for example, a resident of Brook Street complained that on market days the stable yard behind her house was so crowded with cattle belonging to the butchers in St. George's Market that her carriage could not be 'aired' without running the risk of being 'gored by the bullocks'; and her neighbour objected to being disturbed in the morning by the bleating of sheep and calves.[17]

Less numerous than the butchers, but far more widely distributed, were the 43 chandlers whose main customers were the poorer inhabitants. Other householders in the food and drink trades included 28 greengrocers and fruiterers, 20 grocers, 18 bakers, 10 cheesemongers, 7 dairymen (including a cowkeeper in Green Street), and 6 fishmongers, one of whom was said to hawk his wares about the streets.

Slightly over 10 per cent of the householders were employed in what may broadly be termed the building industry. Apart from the regular building tradesmen—carpenters, bricklayers and the like—this group includes craftsmen and tradesmen associated with the decoration and furnishing of houses, principally upholsterers and cabinet-makers. Also included are four surveyors (none of them well known), but not the two architects previously mentioned. The carpenters, numbering 56, were by far the most numerous of any of the individual categories in this group. Many of them had their premises in the streets to the north of Grosvenor Square: in George Street, for example, where 14 of the 33 householders were employed in the building trades, there were seven carpenters. The most prominent member of the trade living on the estate was William Clarke of Little Grosvenor Street, described as carpenter to the 'Board of Works'. In addition to the carpenters there were 21 bricklayers, 12 masons, 11 plasterers, 9 glaziers, 6 plumbers and 2 slaters, but only one 'builder', William Rutledge of Mount Street.

Upholstery and cabinet-making was the best represented of the various furnishing trades, with 12 practitioners, some of them very well known. In Berkeley Square there was John Linnell, who had extensive workshops on the site of the present No. 25. Nearby at No. 70 Grosvenor Street lived Charles Smith, 'Upholsterer to their Majesties', while in Mount Street, which was soon to become a popular address with high-class furniture-makers, were to be found the cabinet-maker Edward Rawlings and the upholstery firm of Elward and Marsh, the latter much patronised by the Prince of Wales. (It is perhaps an indication of the standing of this firm that one of the partners, William Marsh, lived in a house in the fashionable part of South Street.) Altogether 29 building tradesmen had premises in Mount Street (20 per cent of all the householders there), numerically more than in any other street on the estate.

The dress and fashion trades employed a further 173 'inhabitants', many of whom lived in Mount Street, Oxford Street and Park Street. Twenty different types of tradesmen are represented in this group, including tailors, breeches-makers, mantua-makers, glove-makers, milliners, haberdashers, linen drapers, perfumers, hairdressers and peruke-makers. Tailoring and shoemaking, which together engaged 77 householders, were the most widespread of these activities. On the other hand dressmaking and millinery, trades chiefly practised by women (who were, of course, often not householders), are certainly under-represented.

The 142 householders who derived their livelihood from the trades grouped under the heading 'transport' included 30 stable-keepers, 27 coachmen and 23 coachmakers as well as smiths, farriers, wheelwrights, saddlers, horse-dealers and coach-brokers. The large number of stable-keepers suggests that there was a substantial demand for commercial stabling in the area in addition to the private requirements of residents who kept their own horses and carriages. A few of the coachmen were in the employment of particular individuals, but the majority seem to have worked on their own account. The coachmakers included John Barnard of Park Street, coachmaker to the King, and Murdoch Mackenzie of the 'Rhedarium for the sale of coaches' which occupied the former Guards' stables built by Roger Morris between Green Street and Wood's Mews. Advertisements for the Rhedarium offered coaches and horses for sale by commission, 'neat Carriages of every kind to let for any space of time', 'Stallions to cover', and stables 'for gentlemen's horses to stand at livery'.[18] For new or inexperienced horsemen who might wish to improve their technique there was a riding academy in Queen Street, and a riding master in Park Street. Supplementing the horse-drawn transport were eight chairmen, one in the service of the Duchess of Devonshire, but the rest evidently self employed.

The remaining 123 tradesmen were employed in trades unconnected with any of the four main categories. These

included fifteen coal dealers and twelve apothecaries, as well as stationers, chinamen, chimney-sweeps, tobacconists and watchmakers. Another twenty-one were the sole representatives of their trade on the estate, among whom were a piano-maker in Duke Street, a gunsmith in Mount Street, and a printer in Queen Street.

Apart from a few coachmen and other stable-servants, who traditionally lived over the mews stable, there were 48 householders engaged in some form of domestic service 'living out', evidently in their own houses. At first sight this may seem a surprisingly large number; but, as we have already seen, some families employed small armies of servants, more than could possibly be accommodated under one roof. (Lack of adequate servants' quarters in the original Georgian houses was one of the reasons why extra storeys were often added in the nineteenth century.) Married servants with families were no doubt obliged, and may have preferred, to provide their own accommodation. Many of the servants 'living out' were in the employment of the nobility resident both on the estate, like Lord Petre and Lord Abercorn, and elsewhere, like Lord Clive and Lord Powis. Lord Clive's porter had a house in Little Grosvenor Street which was only a few minutes' walk away from his lordship's own house in Berkeley Square, but a rather longer journey faced the Earl of Powis's cook on setting out from Green Street for the Earl's house in Portland Place. Domestic servants whose duties were specified in the survey included four porters, four valets and three cooks. Four of the Duke of Gloucester's pages had their own houses as did his cook, all within easy walking distance of Gloucester House. Lord Petre's butler, who shared his employer's Roman Catholic faith, lived in Green Street, not far from his master's mansion in Park Lane. Also included in the total number of domestic servants are three stewards, one combining the duties of steward to the Earl of Tankerville (who had extensive estates in Northumberland) with the business of a coal agent.

The survey of 1790 also provides information about the number of furnished houses and the number of sub-divided houses. Although there were probably more furnished houses than the 29 listed in the survey, they nevertheless represented only a small proportion of the 1400 or so houses on the estate. As the customers for these furnished lettings were most likely to come from the upper classes such houses were to be found almost exclusively in the fashionable streets. One upper-class occupant of a furnished house was the third Earl of Rosebery at No. 73 South Audley Street. The provision of furnished houses at this time was often in the hands of upholsterers and cabinet-makers, several of whom appear in the survey in the role of furnished-house proprietors. In Grosvenor Street the cabinet-makers Mayhew and Ince and the upholsterer Richard Taitt had a furnished house apiece, both however awaiting tenants in 1790, while at No. 65 Brook Street, a furnished house occupied by an 'esquire', the proprietor was the New Bond Street upholsterer Charles Elliott. But the ownership of furnished lettings was not confined to the professionals, for private owners would often let their town houses for brief periods while they themselves were away. Thus in Park Lane the second Earl of Warwick was enjoying possession of Camelford House during the absence abroad of Lord Camelford. Lord North, the former Prime Minister, used regularly to let his house at No. 50 Grosvenor Square while he occupied Downing Street: but 'conscious on how frail a basis his administration reposed, [he] would never let it for a longer period than one year. In consequence of this principle it annually changed possessors, and being frequently taken by newly-married couples, it obtained the name of Honeymoon Hall.'[19] Lord North's presence in his own house in 1790 did not deter the compilers of the survey from including No. 50 amongst the furnished houses. The demand for furnished houses, particularly by 'Families who spend but a short time in London', was soon to outstrip the supply and led naturally enough to the opening of several private hotels on the estate, one of the first of these being Kirkham's in Brook Street, which opened in about 1802.[20]

The sub-divided houses identified in the survey are those where one of the householders was said to inhabit only the ground floor; and almost all of these householders were tradesmen. Only 33 houses sub-divided in this way are listed, all of them in streets where commercial occupation predominated. There were also a few other houses apparently in joint occupation, and the occasional comment that an 'inhabitant' occupied one or more rooms provides further evidence of divided occupancy, which was doubtless far more widespread than the survey shows.

The London Season in 1841

We have already seen that as early as the 1730's and 40's many of the residents in the principal streets of the Grosvenor estate, and of course many more in other correspondingly fashionable parts of London, only spent part of each year in town, their seasonal movements being prescribed by those of the Court and by the dates of the parliamentary sessions. In the eighteenth century the number of people participating in this fashionable minuet between town and country cannot be even approximately calculated, but in the nineteenth century detailed information about the London Season was published for many years in *The Morning Post*, and this has been analysed for the year 1841.*

* This year was chosen in order to obtain supplementary material from the census of 1841. This census was preferred to those of 1851, 1861 and 1871 because the information contained in *The Morning Post* gradually becomes less detailed.

The Table opposite shows week by week the movements into and out of London of what *The Morning Post* called the 'Fashionable World'. Over four thousand movements are plotted, of which at least 15 per cent relate to residents on the Grosvenor estate in Mayfair; but the total size of the seasonal migration into and out of the capital must in reality have been substantially larger than that shown in the Table, because it may confidently be conjectured that many movements of both the 'Fashionable World' and its imitators were not publicly reported.

The year 1841 was not altogether a typical one because the general election by which the Tories displaced the Whigs was held in the latter part of the summer, but this serves to emphasize the extent to which the seasonal migration of the *beau monde* was influenced by the dates of parliamentary sittings. At the beginning of the year most people of fashion were out of town, either at home, visiting, or at Brighton. At the end of January there was the biggest influx of the year, for the opening of Parliament, and there then ensued a brief pre-Easter season,[21] marked by numerous dinners and soirées, the opening of the opera season, and the first royal levée. On 31 March, for instance, it was reported that Lady Compton Domville had held 'a very brilliant assembly' at No. 5 Grosvenor Square. 'The five spacious saloons in that superb mansion were most brilliantly illuminated.' Dancing 'to Weippert's band' had commenced at 11.30 p.m. and at 1.30 a.m. 'a most sumptuous supper' was served. And a day or two later Lady Anne Wilbraham had held 'a soirée dansante' at 'the family mansion in Lower Brook Street' (No. 68), at which 'Above 200 of the leading fashionables in town honoured her Ladyship with their company, as also the chief members of the corps diplomatique'.[22]

Early in April the adjournment of Parliament for the Easter recess and the removal of the Court to Windsor were accompanied by a substantial exodus, and Brighton filled up. With the reassembly of Parliament on 20 April, the Queen's return from Windsor, the first royal drawing-room, the reopening of the opera after Easter, and the first ball at Almack's there was a very large influx which marked the commencement of the main Season. Numerous arrivals at addresses principally in Belgravia, Marylebone, St. James's, Pall Mall and streets off Piccadilly, as well of course as Mayfair, were reported. The house agents did a brisk business in the letting of furnished houses 'for the Season', and the private hotels filled up, Mivart's and the adjacent Coulson's (formerly Wake's) in Brook Street being the most notable on the Grosvenor estate. Every Monday *The Morning Post* carried a column entitled 'Fashionable Arrangements for the Week', and on a single evening there were three separate receptions at various houses in Grosvenor Square alone. Other chronicled events included the Royal Academy exhibition, the Queen's levées, drawing-rooms and state balls, the Derby at Epsom, and Ascot races, the latter attended then as now, by the Queen from Windsor.

The prorogation of Parliament on 22 June and the imminence of a general election set off a gradual drift away from London. On 6 July Lady Compton Domville 'gave her farewell fête' in Grosvenor Square, the last ball at Almack's was held on the following night, and there were no more 'Fashionable Arrangements' in *The Morning Post*. Some emigrants went off on foreign tours, and it was reported that 'The fashionable departures for the German spas this season have been unusually numerous'.[23] There was also much visiting about from one country house to another, and Harrogate, Brighton, Goodwood races, yachting at Cowes, and shooting in Scotland all attracted their wealthy patrons.

But even at this 'dead' time of year fashionable London was never entirely empty. There were always some arrivals to report, and although the pattern of seasonal migration in the summer of 1841 was greatly distorted by the general election and the parliamentary session of 19 August to 7 October, which occasioned a considerable but short-lived influx, it is clear that even the most socially distinguished members of the 'Fashionable World' were often in London out of season. Such visits were, however, frequently of short duration, and the autumnal attractions of Buxton, Brighton, Leamington and Worthing, of racing at Newmarket, and above all of the hunting field, ensured that (after a brief influx in early December for the Smithfield Club's cattle show and annual dinner) London's social year had a quiet end, the twelve days of Christmas being generally celebrated out of town.

In addition to listing the arrivals in and departures from London *The Morning Post* also published 'changes' from one out-of-town address to another. Taken together all this information reveals the peculiarly peripatetic existence of the 'Fashionable World', while other records indicate the resources needed to sustain such a mode of life. The case of two earls and their families, both resident in Grosvenor Square, may be taken as examples.

The first Earl of Verulam had a town house at No. 47 Grosvenor Square and a country seat at Gorhambury Park, near St. Albans. The family estates in Hertfordshire and Essex were estimated in 1882 to contain some 10,000 acres yielding £14,000 per annum.[24] In 1841 the Earl was aged sixty-five; his wife was some nine years younger, and the youngest of their nine children was aged sixteen. On the night of the census (6–7 June) the Earl and Countess, two of their sons and one daughter were all resident in Grosvenor Square, where they were attended by seven male and eight female servants.[25] At Gorhambury House there were on the same night another seven female servants and one male servant, plus half-a-dozen other male servants in the adjoining stables.[26]

Towards the end of January the Earl had come up to Grosvenor Square from Gorhambury, where he was joined by the Countess, who had been visiting one of their married daughters, the Countess of Craven, at Combe Abbey near Coventry. Their eldest son, Viscount Grimston, M.P., still a bachelor, also joined them at

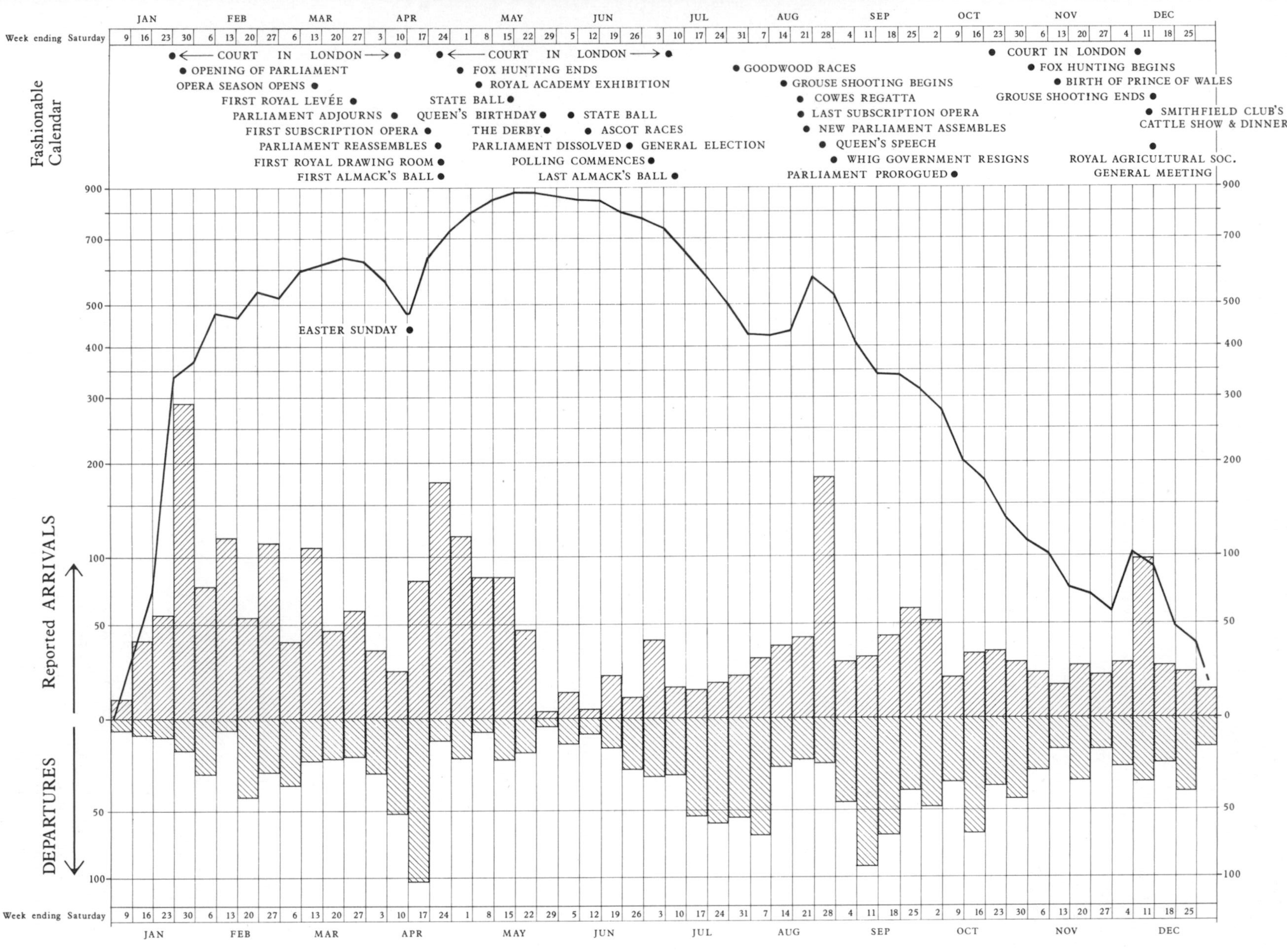

SEASONAL MIGRATIONS OF THE 'FASHIONABLE WORLD' IN 1841

This figure plots over 4,000 movements into and out of London of members of the 'Fashionable World', as reported in *The Morning Post* in 1841. Movements of single individuals or of married couples or of whole families are all expressed as one movement. Thus the total number of persons arriving and departing was in reality substantially larger than that given here.

The hatched columns show the total number of arrivals and departures reported in each week. Sometimes there was a time lag of up to ten days between the date of a movement and its publication.

The heavy black line shows the cumulative total of arrivals after subtraction of departures. The departures were not so fully reported as the arrivals, and to correct this shortfall the departures have been multiplied by a factor of 1.6.

Grosvenor Square from Ireland, all these arrivals coinciding with the opening of Parliament. In March the Earl and Countess went to the Duke of Rutland at Belvoir Castle, back to Grosvenor Square, and thence (with Lord Grimston and their youngest daughter) to Earl and Countess Amherst at Knole, Kent. Their return to Grosvenor Square in early April was soon followed by a visit by the Countess and her unmarried children to Longford Castle, Wiltshire, to stay with another of their married daughters, Viscountess Folkestone. By mid April the Earl of Verulam was at Newmarket, and a week later his family was back in Grosvenor Square. In mid May he and the Countess, with Lord Grimston and their unmarried daughter, were at Gorhambury for the races, but were back in town by 6 June. In the latter part of July the Earl and Viscount Grimston were visiting Mrs. Warde at the Squerryes, Westerham, before going to Buckhurst Park, Sussex, and ultimately to the Duke of Richmond at Goodwood. Meanwhile the Countess was entertaining her son-in-law and daughter, the Earl and Countess of Craven, at Gorhambury. At the end of August both the Earl and Countess of Verulam were in Grosvenor Square, but early in September the Earl and his son Viscount Grimston went off to the Marquess of Abercorn's shooting lodge in Inverness-shire, while the Countess and her youngest daughter went to Gorhambury. A few days later, however, the Countess and one of her sons were in Grosvenor Square on their way to Longford Castle again. By 24 September the Earl and Viscount Grimston were back at Gorhambury from their Caledonian foray, and a week later they too went on to Longford Castle. In mid October the Earl was said to be 'still at Newmarket', while the Countess, Viscount Grimston and her unmarried daughter left Grosvenor Square for visits to Mrs. Warde at the Squerryes and Earl Amherst at Knole. By the end of the month the Earl was back at Gorhambury before joining his wife at the Squerryes. In mid November they were at Gorhambury entertaining the Earl and Countess of Clarendon and 'a large circle of nobility and gentry around'. In December Viscount Grimston went to visit the Marquess of Abercorn at Baron's Court in Ireland, and on his way back to Gorhambury shortly before Christmas he stayed for a few days with his sister the Countess of Craven.

The second Earl of Wilton was a younger and considerably richer man than the Earl of Verulam. He was a younger son of the first Marquess of Westminster, having inherited his title from his maternal grandfather by special remainder. In addition to his town house at No. 7 Grosvenor Square he had a country seat at Heaton House, near Manchester, and a hunting lodge at Melton Mowbray. His estates, chiefly in Lancashire, Yorkshire and Staffordshire, were variously estimated in 1882 to be worth £31,000 or £65,000 per annum.[27] In 1841 he was aged forty-one, and by his wife (a daughter of the twelfth Earl of Derby) he then had four young children, the eldest of whom was aged eight. On the night of the census he, the Countess and two of their children were resident in Grosvenor Square, where they were attended by seven male and nine female servants.[28] At Heaton House on the same night there were a clerk, a housekeeper, three female servants and two grooms, while the residents in the cottages of the surrounding park included a gamekeeper and eight gardeners.[29] Egerton Lodge at Melton Mowbray was shut up for the summer, the only residents being an elderly couple evidently acting as caretakers.[30] The Earl's two younger children were at Walmer Castle, the official residence of the Lord Warden of the Cinque Ports, the Duke of Wellington, who was a friend and frequent correspondent of the Countess of Wilton. The Duke himself was not at Walmer, where the staff looking after the two children consisted of a housekeeper, one male and five female servants.[31]

Towards the end of January the Earl of Wilton had come up to Grosvenor Square from Eaton Hall, Chester (the home of his father the Marquess of Westminster), and left for Melton Mowbray for the hunting immediately after the opening of Parliament. A week or two later he was back in Grosvenor Square, but in mid February both he and the Countess were at Melton. In the first half of April they were successively at Belvoir Castle with the Duke of Rutland, Grosvenor Square, probably with the Duke of Wellington at Stratfield Saye, Melton Mowbray and Grosvenor Square again, before going with their children to Tunbridge Wells, perhaps staying in a rented house. In the latter part of April the Earl and Countess were both back in Grosvenor Square, but the Countess soon returned to Tunbridge Wells. Most of May seems to have been spent in Grosvenor Square, though the Earl was at the Derby at Epsom at the end of the month. Early in June the Countess took two of her children to Walmer Castle, but she was back within a few days to give 'a splendid entertainment' in Grosvenor Square, followed by a dinner party early in July. Soon afterwards she was for a few days at Heaton House—her only visit of the year—and then went (probably with her children) to a house near Ryde in the Isle of Wight. In due course she was joined there by the Earl, who was Commodore of the Royal Yacht Squadron, but by the end of August they were both at Grosvenor Square, where they gave a dinner for the Duke of Wellington. Mid September saw them once more at Ryde, and on 24 September *The Morning Post* reported that 'The Noble Earl purposes a cruise of a few weeks in his yacht, and will then go to Melton Mowbray for the hunting season'. This cruise seems to have taken in a visit to Walmer Castle, whence in early November he and the Countess returned by yacht to Ryde, and thence back to Grosvenor Square. On 9 November the Earl, 'unattended', arrived at Heaton House for his only and very brief visit of the year, and during the rest of the month there were visits with the Countess to Ryde, to the Duke of Beaufort at Badminton, and in early December to the Duke of Wellington at Stratfield Saye. By mid December they were at Grosvenor Square *en*

route for Melton Mowbray, but on 22 December they were back in town *en route* for Stratfield Saye for Christmas. By 28 December the Earl was again in Grosvenor Square.

Most of the journeyings of both the Earl of Verulam and the Earl of Wilton were probably made by road, few railways having yet been built by 1841. Verulam's real home was evidently at Gorhambury, and as this was little more than twenty miles from London he seems to have spent less time at his house in Grosvenor Square (around seventeen weeks) than did the Earl of Wilton. Wilton's country seat was much further away, and its proximity to Manchester was perhaps already reducing its residential attraction.* To cater for his two principal sporting interests of hunting and yachting he therefore had two subsidiary houses out of town, at Melton Mowbray and Ryde, plus a third, perhaps mainly for his wife and family, at Tunbridge Wells. But it may be conjectured that none of these gave him a social position out of town comparable with that of Gorhambury for the Earl of Verulam, who was Lord Lieutenant of Hertfordshire for over twenty years. Despite his more numerous residences Wilton therefore seems to have spent rather more time in Grosvenor Square—around twenty-one weeks—than Verulam.

Such influences of family heritage and of individual personal preference no doubt greatly affected the way of life of many other families moving about in the 'Fashionable World'. But it may be noted, firstly, that although neither of them was prominent in politics, the movements of both Verulam and Wilton conformed broadly with the general pattern of seasonal migration based on the parliamentary sessions; and, secondly, that even in out-of-season times of the year they (and particularly Wilton) were often in at least brief residence in Grosvenor Square.

The Censuses of 1841 and 1871

The vast amount of information about the demographic structure of the Grosvenor estate which is contained in the enumerators' books of the decennial censuses from 1841 onwards falls largely outside the scope of this volume, and only a brief analysis of those of 1841 and 1871 (the latter being the most recent for which the schedules are at present open to public inspection) can be attempted here.[32]

The results of this analysis are presented in the Table on page 94. At the outset it must be emphasised that the inter-censual comparisons made there should be treated with caution because the criteria upon which the censuses of 1841 and 1871 were taken differed in several important respects. But despite these differences, which are discussed below, some tentative evaluations can be made.

Firstly, the figures show that between 1841 and 1871 the total number of residents on the estate fell by 13 per cent. Almost all of this decline evidently occurred between 1841 and 1851, when the population of Mayfair as a whole, and of that other fashionable area, St. James's Square, also fell by a similar amount.[33] As will appear later, it seems that this decline was principally amongst the residents of independent means and their servants, rather than amongst those engaged in trade or non-domestic service; and it may be conjectured that some, at any rate, of this decline was due to the rival attractions of Belgravia, Kensington and Tyburnia.

Secondly, the figures show that only a very small proportion of the residents on the estate (some 5 to 10 per cent) belonged to the titled or leisured classes. The social *cachet* of a good address there might still, in Victorian times, be as highly prized as ever; but even in this citadel of the *beau monde* such residents were far outnumbered by the rest of the population.

The number of residents of title and leisure recorded in the census of 1841 is, however, more than double that recorded in the count of 1871, and this disparity requires examination. Some decline in their numbers evidently did take place, but it was probably not as great as the figures suggest, and the discrepancy can be largely explained by differences inherent in the two counts.

The first of these differences arose from the precise dates in 1841 and 1871 when the censuses were taken. That of 1841 was taken on 6–7 June, when Parliament was in session and the London Season was near its height, whereas that of 1871 was taken on 2–3 April, when both Houses had risen for the Easter recess, and many residents of wealth and fashion were therefore absent from their London homes: less than half the peers who are listed in *Boyle's Court Guide* as having addresses within the Grosvenor estate in Mayfair were actually resident there on the night of the census of 1871. In 1841 some eighty inhabited houses were not in substantially normal occupation (i.e. were occupied only by servants or caretakers), about forty of them in the principal streets, whereas in 1871 the number of such houses was 175, about one hundred of them being in streets where the titled and leisured classes generally lived. Furthermore, in 1841 the number of such occupants who may have been absent from their homes on the night of the census was in part counterbalanced by others who had taken houses for the Season, such as the Duke of Rutland, who was living at General Thomas Grosvenor's house, No. 50 Grosvenor Square, with two members of his family (and eleven servants).

A second important difference arises from the differing treatment of residents of independent means, which has resulted in a far larger number of such persons appearing in 1841 (906) than in 1871 (300). This divergence may be partly explained by the very catholic interpretation placed

* The house and park at Heaton were sold to Manchester Corporation in 1901.[27]

The Censuses of 1841 and 1871

	Census of 6–7 June 1841				*Census of 2–3 April 1871*			
Inhabited houses and mews dwellings	1,753				1,645 (containing 2,711 households)			
Blocks of model lodgings					3 (containing 75 households)			
Uninhabited houses and mews dwellings	85				125			
Total population	17,064				14,829			
			% of workers	% of total popn			% of workers	% of total popn
Residents of the titled and leisured classes	1,780			10.4	840			5.7
Peers		48				25		
Baronets		25				14		
Other persons of title		238				109		
Untitled independents		906				300		
Untitled landowners		*not available*				81		
Dependants of above		563				311		
Residents working for financial reward	9,213			54.0	8,422			56.8
Professional								
Army officers		83				50		
Naval officers		18				11		
Law		29				54		
Medicine		70				88		
Church		21				17		
Architects and engineers		11				6		
Total		232	2.5	1.3		226	2.7	1.5
Trade or service								
Servants		5,935	64.4	34.8		4,583	54.4	30.9
Transport		408	4.4	2.4		489	5.8	3.2
Dress and fashion		1,060	11.5	6.2		1,348	16.0	9.1
Food and drink		481	5.2	2.8		521	6.2	3.5
Building		270	2.9	1.6		202	2.4	1.4
Other trades		829	9.0	4.9		1,053	12.5	7.1

A 'household' (both as used in the above table under 1871 and in the text) comprises any distinct family group in which the head of the group is so described, or where an absent head is presumed by the designation of the first person within the group as wife, son, etc. Lodgers and boarders have not been counted as separate households. It has not been possible to determine the number of households in 1841 from the enumerators' books.

'Other persons of title' comprise peeresses; peers' widows, sons, daughters or daughters-in-law; wives or widows of baronets; knights and their wives or widows; and foreign nobles. In the 1841 census persons of independent means were generally classed simply as 'independent' and it has not been possible to determine the number of untitled landowners. In the figures derived from the 1871 census, in which more categories were used, 'Untitled independents' include fundholders, annuitants, gentlemen, and persons with 'income from dividends' or entered as of 'no occupation'. In both censuses M.P.'s who are described as such without any accompanying rank or profession are counted as independents. 'Dependants' include untitled relatives of the head of the household, and visitors, but governesses, servants, coachmen and grooms are excluded.

Soldiers' rank was not given in the 1841 census, and the 83 'Army officers' include eight residents whose addresses suggest that they may not have been commissioned.

In the 1841 census coachmen and grooms were generally entered as servants, but in 1871 they were classified separately. They then numbered 637, and for purposes of comparison have been included in the number of servants. Governesses, of whom there were 35 in 1841 and 48 in 1871, have also been classed as servants.

The parish workhouse on the south side of Mount Street was enumerated separately at each census and has not been included in the above table.

on the term 'independent' by the enumerators in 1841. They were instructed that 'Men, or widows, or single women having no profession or calling, but living on their means, may be inserted as *independent*',[34] but sometimes they extended this definition to embrace almost anyone with no occupation, including the wives and children of tradesmen. As far as possible the latter have been excluded in counting the number of 'independents' for the purposes of the Table, but some exaggeration in the total number of such persons is, nevertheless, probably inevitable. On the other hand there are numerous instances in both the 1841 and 1871 counts in which a householder's profession or occupation is not given, and, particularly in the latter year, many of the persons concerned are likely to have been untitled householders of leisure.

These differences in the time of year and in the methods of classification of the two counts point to the conclusion that in 1841 the number of titled and leisured residents was slightly overstated and in 1871 certainly understated. But despite these qualifications there is little doubt that there was indeed an overall decline between 1841 and 1871 in the number of such persons living on the estate. In Park Street, where many 'independents' lived in 1841, the number of residents occupying exactly the same number of inhabited houses dropped from 932 to 786 between the two censuses, and this pattern was repeated in other streets of 'middling' character. It is in such streets that persons living off moderate incomes, many of them women, would have lodged, and it may be that one of the factors in the general decrease in the population of the estate after 1841 was the migration of such people to the newly developing suburbs of Paddington and Kensington.

A similar decline in the number of M.P.'s listed in *Boyle's Court Guide* with addresses on the estate from 68 in 1840 to 49 in 1872 can no doubt be attributed to the same cause, but there was no corresponding diminution in the number of peers, who were perhaps more reluctant to leave such a long-established centre of fashion.

The residents who worked for financial reward comprised slightly over half the total population in both 1841 (53·99 per cent) and 1871 (56·8 per cent).* Very few of them were professional men, but the number of lawyers, physicians and surgeons had increased by 1871, while the number of army officers had fallen. 'City' men of business and commerce—bankers, stockbrokers and merchants—who at the turn of the century were to settle in the area in some numbers, were still very few.

In an area such as Mayfair most of the working population were engaged in supplying the wants of the relatively small number of wealthy residents, and by far the largest of these wants was, of course, for service, both domestic and out-door. In the census of 1841 grooms and coachmen (who were very numerous in this carriage-owning area) were generally classified as servants, and altogether servants amounted to over a third of the entire population (34 per cent) and to 64 per cent of all the working residents. Some 44 per cent of them were male.

By 1871 the total number of domestic servants, coachmen and grooms had fallen by nearly a quarter, but they still amounted to 30 per cent of the entire population and to 54 per cent of the working residents. Some 36 per cent of them were male. The domestic servants were now classified separately from the coachmen and grooms, and they alone numbered 3,898, equivalent to 26.3 per cent of the whole population and to 46.3 per cent of the working residents. Some 26 per cent of them were male.

Between 1841 and 1871 there was thus a substantial fall in the total number of servants, and in the proportion of male servants.

The census of 1871 demonstrates the extent to which the demand for domestic service was concentrated in a comparatively few very wealthy households. Some 63 per cent of all the households on the estate had no domestic servant, and thirteen per cent had one each; a further thirteen per cent had two or three servants, and only eleven per cent (303 households) had four or more. Expressed in a different way, some three hundred households with four or more servants employed almost 70 per cent of all the domestics on the estate in 1871.†

Comparable figures for 1841 cannot be calculated because of the difficulty of identifying separate households.

About three quarters of the three hundred houses with large domestic staffs in 1871 were in Grosvenor Square, Park Lane, Brook Street, Grosvenor Street, Upper Brook Street and Upper Grosvenor Street, and a similar concentration had no doubt existed in 1841. In Grosvenor Square in 1841 over 76 per cent of the residents listed in the census were domestic servants,‡ while in 1871 (when a greater proportion of householders and their families were absent on the night of the census) servants accounted for over 80 per cent of the inhabitants of the square. In those 43 houses which were in normal occupation at the time of the count in 1841, the average size of each household was 16.7, of whom 12.9 were servants. Twenty-six

* Excluding residents of the titled and leisured classes, the balance of the population consisted of the wives and children of the residents working in the professions, trade or service, students and all other untitled persons who left the 'occupation' column of the census schedule blank.

† These figures for servants may be compared with those for the Queen's Gate area of South Kensington in *Survey of London*, volume XXXVIII, 1975, p. 322.

‡ As has already been mentioned, the census of 1841 does not differentiate between domestic servants and coachmen and grooms, but the census of 1871, which does make this differentiation, contains hardly any coachmen or grooms resident in Grosvenor Square or other principal streets. It has therefore been assumed that in the census of 1841 the servants recorded at such addresses were indoor domestics and not stable staff, who were, of course, listed, also as 'servants', in large numbers in the nearby mews.

of these 43 houses had 12 or more servants, the largest number being at No. 44, where a staff of 23 attended to the Earl of Harrowby and four members of his family.

In 1871 the average size of household in the 29 houses in Grosvenor Square which were in normal occupation had declined to 13.8, of whom 10.8 were servants. The largest domestic establishment was at No. 41, the house of Sir Henry Meux, baronet, of the brewing family, where there were 21 servants. The largest complement of all, in either census, was at Dudley House, Park Lane, in 1871, where the Earl and Countess of Dudley, their infant son, a nephew and two nieces, were attended by 28 domestic servants, two coachmen and seven stable 'helpers'.

In 1841 domestic servants accounted for between 67 and 72 per cent of all the residents in Upper Brook Street, the western part of Grosvenor Street, and Upper Grosvenor Street. In the houses where normal occupancy existed on the night of the census the average size of each household was 10.9 in Upper Brook Street and 10.7 in Upper Grosvenor Street, and the average number of servants was 7.3. Households in the western part of Grosvenor Street averaged 12.8, of whom 9 were servants. In 1871 these figures had fallen only slightly, 66 per cent of the residents in these streets still being servants, and the average number of servants in each house being about seven. In the western half of Brook Street some 62 per cent of the residents were servants in both 1841 and 1871, but their numbers in the houses in normal occupation fell from an average of 7·0 to slightly below 5·7.

In addition to the domestic servants there were also the coachmen and grooms, of whom there were over six hundred living on the estate in 1871. Many of the great houses in Grosvenor Square and the streets leading off it had their own coach-houses and stables in the mews on to which they backed, but in the censuses the residents in the mews were almost always classified separately from their employers, and the precise number of stable staff belonging to any particular house cannot easily be found, even in the census of 1871, and in that of 1841 never: the previously mentioned case of Dudley House provides a rare exception, and the Marquess of Westminster's stables are known to have been near Grosvenor House in Reeves Mews, where in 1871 lived the head coachman and his family, an assistant coachman, a groom and two servants. The census of 1871 shows that in the yards and mews behind the principal streets, in such places as Adams Mews (now Row), Blackburne's Mews, Three Kings Yard and Wood's Mews, almost all the male working residents by then in fact worked with horses, the public-house keepers, of whom there were often one in each mews, being the most notable exceptions. A few farriers, jobmasters, ostlers, carmen, coachsmiths and such like could be found there, but by far the most numerous occupations were those of coachman and groom. In Three Kings Yard, for instance, ten of the twelve householders were coachmen or grooms, the other two being a female domestic servant and the keeper of the public house at the corner of Davies Street. The latter and one footman were the only men not working in the stables. The entire population of this busy little working community lurking inconspicuously behind the fashionable mansions of Brook Street, Grosvenor Street and Grosvenor Square upon which it was so totally dependent and yet from which it was socially so totally divided, amounted to sixty-five persons.

Apart from demand for personal service, both indoors and outdoors, wealthy residents' other great want, sufficiently extensive to reflect itself in the general pattern of employment on the estate, was in the field of dress and fashion. But while demand for domestic service declined between 1841 and 1871, demand for services providing for personal adornment was increasing. The Table above shows that whereas in 1841 1,060 residents had work dependent on dress and fashion, a figure equivalent to 11.5 per cent of the working population of the estate, by 1871 the corresponding figures were 1,348 residents, amounting to 16 per cent of the working population. During this period the number of dressmakers rose from 310 to 507, and of tailors from 205 to 269, but laundresses remained constant at 116 and 113. The remainder included such trades as milliner, draper, hosier, hatter, haberdasher, bootmaker, dyer, waistcoat-maker, hairdresser, lace merchant and lace cleaner. Apart from domestic service these trades provided *in toto* by far the largest source of local employment for women.

Unlike many of the servants, coachmen and grooms, the residents engaged in these trades were scattered over many parts of the estate, with particular concentrations in the poorer areas immediately to the south of Oxford Street and in what are now Grosvenor Hill and Bourdon Street. Many of the women were the wives or daughters of householders engaged in quite different trades, and the needlewomen and laundresses in particular probably often worked at home, the sooty grime of London and the absence as yet of a constant water supply providing the latter with continuous and arduous work. There were, however, half a dozen employers of large, generally resident, staffs of needlewomen or shop assistants. In 1871 three of these—a dressmaker (whose staff of eleven lived elsewhere), a lace merchant and a linen-draper—were in South Audley Street, and there was one each in Mount Street (court dressmaker) and the eastern parts of Brook Street (milliner) and Grosvenor Street (silk mercer). The biggest of these establishments was that of Smith, Durrant, Mayhew and Loder, at Nos. 58–60 (consec.) South Audley Street, where Francis Loder, living in 1871 with his wife and two infant sons, employed a male staff of six assistants, four porters, two clerks and two apprentices, and a female staff of sixteen assistants, plus a female domestic staff of seven—all living in.

The demands of wealthy residents on the estate may also have been at least partly responsible for the number of local workers engaged in the coachbuilding trades. This demand was of course very small in comparison

with those for personal service and the dress trades, the total number of workers in the trades of coachbuilder, painter, trimmer, smith, plater and springmaker being only 74 in 1841 and 81 in 1871. A large proportion of them lived in the area immediately south of Oxford Street, where they had been established for many years. This concentration may well, indeed, have originated in the low rents charged here at the time of the original development of the estate, for coachbuilding always required a considerable amount of space; but the close proximity of numerous wealthy customers was no doubt also an advantage, just as it is to-day for the motor-car dealers of Berkeley Square and Berkeley Street.

Few of the numerous other trades practised on the estate appear to have been notably directed towards the requirements of the rich residents upon which the occupations so far discussed did chiefly depend. Some of the firms (mainly shops) in which the 521 residents engaged in 1871 in the food and drink trades worked no doubt catered for expensive local tastes, and the poulterer John Baily, who employed sixteen men at his shop in Mount Street, was in later years known to the Duke of Westminster himself. But the relatively even distribution of the food and drink trade workers throughout all but the most exclusive residential parts of the estate suggests that most business was of a very local nature. In the High Victorian world of 1871 the 56 publicans living on the estate, at all events, are not likely to have been greatly dependent upon the custom of upper-class residents. Some of the 73 lodging-house keepers may, on the other hand, to judge from their numbers in such partly fashionable streets as Green Street, Park Street and Mount Street, have found much of their custom amongst persons of rank who had no town house of their own. It is a testimony to the accuracy of Anthony Trollope's observation that when, in *Framley Parsonage*, Archdeacon Grantly and his wife had occasion to come up to London they took lodgings in Mount Street, which in fact contained in 1871 the highest number of lodging houses of any street on the Grosvenor estate.

Although over half of all the residents on the estate worked in trade or service, there can have been little outward reflection of this in the streets, which were, of course, overwhelmingly residential in character except in such 'shopping' streets as Mount Street and Oxford Street. Dress and fashion, and domestic service, the two principal sources of employment in the area, were unobtrusive trades, and the noise made by the 'machinists' who are occasionally recorded in the census cannot have been so generally heard as in the industrialised quarters of London. Conditions in the two primarily labouring-class areas, immediately south of Oxford Street and in the south-eastern corner of the estate, must certainly have provided a striking contrast with those of the neighbouring Brook Street and Grosvenor Street, but even there the smell of horses must have been far more notable than the clatter of machinery.

The census of 1871 presents a detailed picture of the social composition of the estate as it existed about a decade before the commencement of widespread rebuilding in the early 1880's under the first Duke of Westminster's superintendence. This picture was made about a century after the completion of the original building development, and it shows very clearly how relatively little change had taken place during that period.

Aristocrats and gentlemen still lived mainly in Grosvenor Square and the four streets extending east and west from it. Norfolk (now Dunraven) Street, and the south ends of Park Street and South Audley Street were still fashionable, and Park Lane had come into its own in the early nineteenth century. Nor does the basic pattern of the seasonal movements of the fashionable world seem to have changed greatly since the mid eighteenth century, although November and December had probably become quieter because Parliament now seldom sat in those months.

The public houses in Upper Grosvenor Street and Upper Brook Street no longer existed, but such fashionable streets had become popular with physicians, of whom in 1871 there were three in the former and six in the latter. Rich businessmen were also beginning to appear in small numbers in the best streets—Joseph Baxendale, for instance, the senior partner in the firm of Pickford and Company, the carriers, which had some two thousand employees, lived at No. 78 Brook Street; and in addition to Sir Henry Meux in Grosvenor Square itself there were at least four brewers, those three of them (Sir Thomas Buxton, Sir Dudley Marjoribanks and Octavius Coope) who lived in Upper Brook Street each having a retinue of servants ranging between twelve and nineteen in number.

In both Grosvenor Street and Brook Street the number of tradesmen had declined since 1790, and members of the medical profession had settled there in large numbers. In Grosvenor Street in 1871 18 houses were occupied by physicians and surgeons and another five by four dentists and an oculist—equivalent to 31 per cent of all the houses in the street within the estate; and in Brook Street there were also 18 houses similarly occupied, plus another two by dentists, making 44 per cent of all the houses there within the estate. Another five houses in Brook Street were now occupied by two private hotels, Lillyman's at No. 43 and Claridge's at Nos. 49–55 (odd). Both these establishments had originated in the early nineteenth century, the former as Kirkham's, the latter as Wake's and Mivart's, and both belonged to that select class of hotel where 'no guests were received who were not known to the landlord either personally or through fit credentials ... An unknown and unaccredited stranger could, by the mere chance latch-key of wealth, no more obtain access to such hotels as these than he could make himself to-day [1920] a member of some exclusive club by placing the amount of the entrance fee in the hands of the hall porter.'[35] At Claridge's, on the night of the census in

1871, the thirty-nine visitors were attended by sixty-six living-in servants—a number that probably included both personal domestics and the hotel staff.

In Mount Street, despite the presence of one peer, two M.P.'s and two foreign nobles, the commercial element of the population may have increased slightly since the mid eighteenth century, some 75 per cent of the householders being engaged in trade or domestic service. In North Audley Street, too, there seems to have been a small increase, for here all but four of the householders in 1871 were in trade, the exceptions being two widows, a surgeon and a schoolmistress; but in South Audley Street no perceptible change had taken place, some 65 per cent of the householders being tradesmen, and most of the 'independents' being still at the south end. Most of the tradesmen in these streets kept few domestic servants, the average number in the commercial households of North Audley Street, for instance, being only slightly over one each. In Mount Street, it may be noted, the residence of several butlers (described as head of household) with their families shows that at any rate senior domestics did not always live at their place of employment; but elsewhere on the estate (in Davies Street and Binney Street) there are instances of households consisting of butlers' wives and children without a husband or father, who was presumably 'living in' at his employer's house.

The parts of the estate on which substantial social change first took place were in the poorer areas occupied by the labouring classes. The two main such areas were immediately south of Oxford Street chiefly east of North Audley Street, and in the south-eastern extremity of the estate in the mews now known as Grosvenor Hill, Bourdon Street and Place, Broadbent Street and Jones Street. Both these areas had been relatively poorly occupied since the time of the original building development, and both were greatly altered in the second half of the nineteenth century by the building of blocks of model lodging houses. But whereas in the area immediately south of Oxford Street the first such block (Clarendon Buildings in Balderton Street) was still in course of erection at the time of the census of 1871 and had not yet been occupied, in the south-eastern corner of the estate several blocks had already been completed; and the effect of this innovation can therefore be compared, at any rate for the years between 1841 and 1871.

The two censuses show that in the twenty-nine four-storey houses with basements in Robert Street (now Weighhouse Street), parallel with Oxford Street, there was no significant change in the total numbers of residents. In 1841 there were 526 and in 1871, 512, the latter figure being about ten per cent more than the population of the whole of Grosvenor Square. The average number of residents per house was thus 18.1 and 17.65 respectively. Many of the inhabitants were coachmen, tailors, porters, labourers, building tradesmen, needlewomen and charwomen. In 1871 each of the twenty-nine houses in this street contained an average of 4.9 separate households; and the average number of residents in each household was 3.6 (compared with 13.8 for the houses in Grosvenor Square in normal occupation on the night of the census). Comparable figures for households in 1841 are not available.

But in the south-eastern mews area the building of several blocks of model lodging houses in the 1850's and 1860's greatly increased the overall population of this little working-class territory. In 1841 there were 805 residents in the 76 dwellings there, and in 1871 857 in 81 dwellings, the average number per dwelling remaining constant at 10.6. But by 1871 the new model lodging houses contained 287 extra residents; the total population of this densely packed little enclave, only some two and a half acres in extent, was thus 1,144, equivalent to nearly eight per cent of the population of the entire hundred-acre estate.

Despite such wide variety of social circumstances, Grosvenor Square and the principal streets had to a notable extent retained for over a century the original social *cachet* of their first development. This was not always the case in originally fashionable areas. Covent Garden Piazza, built in the 1630's to attract 'Persons of the greatest Distinction' had lost much of its social prestige within two generations, the growth of the adjacent market being partly responsible.[36] Its later seventeenth-century successors, Golden Square, containing 'such houses as might accommodate Gentry', Soho Square, said in 1720 to be 'well inhabited by Nobility and Gentry', and Leicester Square, had all suffered a considerable social decline within two or at most three generations.[37] On the Earl of Burlington's estate (Cork Street and Savile Row area), where building had begun at about the same time as on the Grosvenor estate, the process took a little longer, but substantial change had nevertheless taken place by 1850.[38] On the other hand, Berkeley Square, Cavendish Square, Portman Square and above all St. James's Square (built as long ago as the 1660's and 70's) had retained their original social character largely unchanged. These varying fortunes suggest that favourable topographical situation and the absence of adverse social influences from surrounding areas were of more importance in preserving the original social quality of an estate than either the terms of land tenure at the time of first building or the watchful management of a ground landlord intent on maintaining the value of his property.

The Last Hundred Years

The census of 1871 was taken about a decade before the commencement of the period of greatest change in the whole history of the Grosvenor estate in Mayfair since its first development for building. The widespread rebuildings initiated by the first Duke in the 1880's and 1890's have already been described from the historical

viewpoint. Socially, they seem to have had two main effects—they increased the segregation both between class and class and between the private residents and the men of commerce; and they increased the proportion of private residents in a number of important streets on the estate, at least in part at the expense of the tradesmen.

These, at all events, are the impressions gained from such evidence—mainly the *Post Office Directories*—as is at present available. Sometimes they were the results of deliberate policies laid down by the Duke, and always they reflected the immiscibility of the numerous social gradations prevalent in the late Victorian and Edwardian world.

The provision of churches, schools, artisans' dwellings, a library and two public gardens, the removal of the workhouse and the drastic reduction in the number of public houses, were all as much a part of the first Duke's achievement as the replacement of hundreds of old and often dingy houses by solid expensive new ranges of shops and chambers and private dwellings. In many parts of the estate this tremendous tidying-up operation stamped Victorian social discipline and formality upon the more easy-going attitudes of earlier times, and even when it was not intentional, physical changes of this order of magnitude could not fail to produce correspondingly great social change as well.

The elimination of trade from certain streets or parts of them, and its concentration in others, were certainly intentional. This was done in Park Street, Green Street, Charles Street (now Carlos Place) and the western part of Mount Street which became exclusively residential, while shops were encouraged in South Audley Street.[39] Between 1871 and 1914 the number of both commercially and professionally occupied houses in the eastern part of Grosvenor Street was reduced, with a corresponding increase in private residence, and in Upper Grosvenor Street even the successful physicians and surgeons who had gained a foothold in the 1870's were eliminated. Only in the eastern part of Brook Street, where the proportion of commercial occupation increased between 1871 and 1914, did the Duke's separatist policies not prevail.[40]

Policies of this kind undoubtedly enjoyed the support of well-to-do residents, and after the first Duke's death in 1899 they were continued by his successor and his advisers. Some residents, indeed, notably those of Grosvenor Street and Park Street, were even successful in insisting that they should be adhered to in circumstances in which the Estate Board would have preferred to relax them.[41]

The new buildings erected in the 1880's and subsequent years also had a marked effect on the social composition of the residents. The houses built in Green Street, the western part of Mount Street and in South Street (Nos. 39–47 odd) always found ready buyers,[42] but their high price restricted the market to purchasers with substantial means. And so too, in somewhat lesser degree, did the price of the new flats built over shops in such streets as South Audley Street and the eastern part of Mount Street. Wealth was what counted in the recruitment of residents, and even though the first and second Dukes both wanted to have what they regarded as 'small private houses' such as those in South Street, no concession was made to slender pockets, as Miss Walpole was crushingly informed when she inquired in 1895 'if it is the intention of the Duke to build middle class dwellings in South Street. She wishes to live near Farm Street Roman Catholic Church and the flats in Mount Street are too expensive.'[43]

As early as 1880 H. T. Boodle had foreseen that 'flats should be encouraged for the upper classes as well as the working classes as they are found of great use'.[44] At first these had been built over shops in the commercial streets, one of the earliest examples being Audley Mansions in South Audley Street of 1884–6 (Plate 33d). This type of building was evidently extremely successful, for it provided a good address for both shopkeepers and private residents while keeping them quite apart from each other, the flats being approached by separate entrances. At corner sites, such as Audley Mansions, the private entrances could even be placed in a residential street (in this case the western part of Mount Street) while the commercial entrance could be at or round the corner in a shopping street.

By means of these large, carefully designed dual-purpose buildings the proportion of floor space in private use even in avowedly commercial streets could be substantially increased. Although there is no firm evidence on this point, the internal disposition of the buildings themselves suggests that the shopkeepers now generally lived elsewhere instead of generally upstairs, as the census of 1871 (made before rebuilding) shows to have been hitherto the usual practice. Taking the number of entries in the *Post Office Directories* as a rough guide (the only one available) the proportion of tradesmen fell substantially, and that of private residents rose correspondingly, between 1871 and 1914, in Mount Street, North and South Audley Streets and Duke Street. In Brook Street and Grosvenor Street (the whole of these streets on the estate being here considered) there were similar changes, though of lesser degree, and as we have already seen, trade was wholly excluded from Park Street, Green Street and the new Carlos Place. In about 1914, it may be hazarded, the private residents formed a larger proportion of the total population of the estate than ever before or since.

This increase finds indirect expression in the new social and financial origins of many rich residents willing and anxious to pay for a good address on the Grosvenor estate in late Victorian and Edwardian times—origins very different from those of the traditional landed aristocracy and gentry. Following the earlier example of the old-established brewers, it was now the turn of the new industrialists and capitalists, both native and foreign, to edge their way into even the innermost social sanctuary of Grosvenor Square itself, where at various times lived,

for instance, Sir John Kelk the building contractor, Baron Furness the Hartlepool shipping magnate, Sir Edward Mackay Edgar the Canadian company director, Samuel Lewis the moneylender, and the financiers John Pierpont Morgan junior and Sir Ernest Cassel. In Park Lane lived two Duveens, in Park Street (in houses looking out across the garden of Grosvenor House to Hyde Park), two Rothschilds; and so on.[40]

It was in the houses of such people as these, and in those of such old families as were still able to afford to compete at the highest level in the fashionable world, that in the years before the war of 1914–18 the traditional social round of the London Season reached its last opulent and glitteringly artificial climax. Entry to and status within even the innermost circles could now generally be bought, for the cost in itself provided the necessary degree of exclusiveness. In 1905 Sir Ernest Cassel paid a premium of £10,000 for the renewal of the leases of Brook House, Park Lane, and the adjoining house, and spent £20,000 on adapting them to provide an appropriately magnificent setting for his receptions there, the proposed approach to the dining-room being specially designed 'level with the ground floor...(for the convenience of the King)'.[45] A few years later Mrs. Keppel, before starting to spend some £15,000 on the renovation of No. 16 Grosvenor Street, submitted her plans to the King, 'who had approved of them', but who probably only visited the house on a single occasion before his death in May 1910.[46] And from such central points as these a succession of ever-widening ripples spread out all over both the fashionable and the would-be fashionable worlds, powerful enough to confer a rent 'for the season' of up to £1,000 on even a house in noisy dusty Hereford Gardens.[47]

Matching the increased private residential use of parts of the estate after the great rebuilding was the apparent decline in the proportion of commercial use. If there were fewer businesses after the first Duke's reconstructions, it was, evidently, because the weakest had gone to the wall. In his evidence before the Select Committee of the House of Commons on Town Holdings, H. T. Boodle had said that 'in many cases of rebuilding it is impossible to let the old tenants rebuild. The tenants would not be equal to it', and he had admitted that compulsory displacements had been made.[48] These casualties had been amongst the little men (and women) with a shop or business at home or round the corner, and whose numbers (attested in the census of 1871) must have made much shopping and petty commerce so local in character before the rebuildings. The survivors, on the other hand, were the strongest and fittest—men like W. J. Goode, the South Audley Street china-dealer, whose business expanded from a single house (where he lived with his family)[49] to take in the whole frontage between South Street and the Grosvenor Chapel; or James Purdey the gunsmith, who after building his own premises in South Audley Street, was only too anxious to speculate elsewhere on the estate; or T. B. Linscott, the confectioner, whose shop in Oxford Street flourished greatly after he had reluctantly rebuilt it.[50] These were the men able to stimulate and then cater for the demands of a wealthy clientèle, primarily in the luxury and semi-luxury trades in which many of the shops of the area were now engaged. And in its hotels—now the other commercial speciality of the estate—the change from the old-fashioned comforts provided by William Claridge and Auguste Scorrier in adapted private dwellings to the discreetly spacious splendours newly built by Claridge's Hotel Company Limited and the Coburg Hotel Company Limited must have been just as great.

For the working-class residents on the estate the principal result of the first Duke's rebuildings was a great improvement in the standard of their housing. The blocks of artisans' dwellings built immediately south of Oxford Street, mainly between 1886 and 1892, provided new accommodation for nearly two thousand people—equivalent almost to fourteen per cent of the total population of the estate in 1871—and in the early years of the twentieth century the flats there were in very great demand, often from locally employed servants (butlers and valets in particular) and policemen.[51] In addition an unknown but very substantial number of residents in the mews were rehoused by the widespread rebuilding of coach-houses and stables in such places as Adams Row, Balfour Mews, Bourdon Street, Mount Row and Three Kings Yard. Some of these premises were of considerable size, space for six or seven stalls and three or four carriages being sometimes provided,[52] and even when complete rebuilding did not take place, tenants were often required, as a condition for the renewal of their leases, to execute extensive works of modernisation.[53]

Much of this great surge of improvement in the mews took place in the years immediately preceding the gradual eclipse of the horse by the motor car. By 1910 tenants on the estate were said to have a 'general desire to get rid of horses',[54] and the second Duke and his Board were granting increasing numbers of licences for the use of coach-houses and stables as garages. At about this time this process was taken a stage further by the occasional conversion of stables into dwelling houses, the first known example being at No. 2 Aldford Street in 1908;[55] and in later years the size and quality of these equine palaces was such that many of them proved well suited for adaptation to domestic use for residents no longer able or willing to live in a great house in one of the fashionable streets.

The outbreak of war in 1914 marked the commencement of fundamental changes in the social character of the estate. Throughout Mayfair as a whole the population had been falling slowly since as early as 1851, and although the first Duke's rebuilding may have temporarily reversed this process on the Grosvenor estate, numbers in Mayfair as a whole were again falling in the early twentieth century. For the estate by itself no reliable figures can be calculated for some sixty years after 1871, but during that period the resident population fell from 14,829 in 1871 to some 8,775

in 1931.* By 1961 it had declined still further to an estimated 4,354.[56]

It has already been conjectured that in the years before 1914 the private residents formed a larger proportion of the total population of the estate than ever before or since. Whether this conjecture is correct or not, the steep decline in the aggregate resident population reflects the great increase in the number of non-resident business users which has transformed the social make-up of the estate since 1914.

At the very top of the social scale the evidence of the *Post Office Directories* suggests that in the 1920's and 1930's there was little change in the number of peers, baronets, knights and other persons of title resident on the estate, despite the numerous new creations made in those years. The ritual of the social Season still continued, and in the unfashionable months cruises to the Mediterranean or the West Indies, or forays to shoot big game in Africa replaced the visits of earlier days to the German spas. But cocktail parties ('by far the cheapest way of entertaining') and 'Cheap cabarets and *intime* night clubs' were replacing the lavish private receptions of Edwardian times; and the prevalence of jokes about income tax collectors showed that it was now becoming 'almost a social stigma to be rich. It is fashionable to pretend to be poorer, not richer, than you are.'[57]

The lack of change in the number of residents of title obscures important internal changes, however. Old families were giving place to new, and by 1947 the titles of approximately half the peers resident on the estate had been created since 1900. Between 1921 and 1939 the Dukes of Portland and Somerset and Earl Fitzwilliam and the Earl of Durham all left Grosvenor Square, whilst the newcomers included two new barons (Illingworth and Selsdon). By 1939 four of the eight peers resident in the square lived in the new flats there, and the fifteenth Earl of Pembroke, one of whose eighteenth-century ancestors had had a house in the square, now lived in Three Kings Yard. In 1933 the first Viscount Furness left Grosvenor Square for Lees Place, and by 1947 even such a traditional grandee as the Duke of Sutherland had moved from Hampden House in Green Street to a flat in Park Lane.[40]

In addition to the continuing decline in their absolute numbers, many residents were thus occupying less space individually. By 1939 only about a quarter of all the houses in Brook Street, for instance, were still in private occupation, and a diagram prepared for *The Grosvenor Estate Strategy for Mayfair and Belgravia*, published in 1971, shows not a single building in the whole of either Brook Street or Grosvenor Street still in solely residential use.[58] By that time a substantial proportion of the surviving residents lived either in modern blocks of flats or in the mews and the lesser streets—Adams Row, Reeves Mews, Balfour Mews and Culross Street are cases in point—and Grosvenor Square itself could only be considered to be still predominantly residential by virtue of the two large hotels recently built there. The fall in the number of residents had, indeed, gone so far that throughout the whole estate only about one third of all the floor space was still, in 1960, in residential occupation[59]—a remarkable reversal of the traditional character of the area.

Some of the buildings hitherto in private use are now occupied by foreign diplomatic missions, for which imposing mansions provide an appropriate setting. In the eighteenth and nineteenth centuries embassies and legations had from time to time alighted for a while on different parts of the estate, but in 1910 there was only one—the Italian Embassy, then at No. 20 Grosvenor Square—and the permanent presence of a foreign diplomatic community here dates only from the 1920's. In 1921 there were seven embassies and legations (four of them in Grosvenor Square), but to-day there are nine, plus five high commissions and two consulates; and some of them are very large—notably the embassies of Egypt and the United States and the Canadian High Commission—and with their ancillary premises occupy more than one building.

A much greater proportion of the accommodation previously in private residential use had, however, been converted into offices, which in 1960 occupied about one third of all the floor space on the estate.[59] As early as 1929 *The Evening News* reported that 'Ancient families are leaving Mayfair and modern dressmakers or beauty or health specialists are arriving'; and 'a West End property expert' declared that Mayfair 'is going over to business as fast as it can...Not so long ago a large house... remained to let for a year without a single inquiry. At last a condition against the use of any part of it for business was withdrawn. It was snapped up then within the next 48 hours.'[60]

In the 1920's and 30's the Grosvenor Estate itself was 'strongly opposed'[61] to the spread of offices, but in 1934 the second Duke's advisers acknowledged that trade and business had for many years been moving westward, and in streets such as Brook Street and Grosvenor Street they had conducted a slow rearguard action, here and there permitting first a professional occupation (usually by a doctor or dentist), then an inconspicuous business (usually dressmaking) and finally, perhaps, a shop window. By 1939, however, this process had advanced a little further, for some of the doctors and dentists in their turn were beginning to move out of Brook Street and Grosvenor Street. Those that remained, instead of living there in individual houses as at first had been the practice, were congregating together in houses evidently

*The figure for 1931 is obtained by counting the number of resident voters contained in the electoral register and multiplying this figure by the factor of 1.505, provided by the Population Studies Section of the Greater London Council's Policy Studies and Intelligence Branch. The electoral registers cannot be satisfactorily used for this purpose prior to 1928, when women under thirty years of age were given the vote.

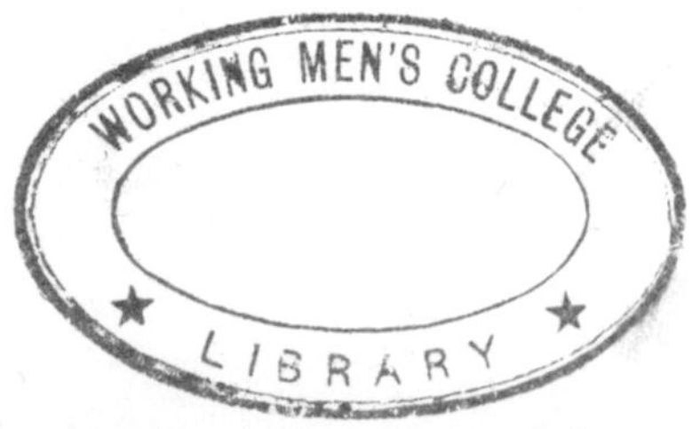

used only as non-resident consulting rooms, of which No. 86 Brook Street, for instance, contained some twenty sets. Even in Upper Grosvenor Street, where a few physicians and surgeons had again settled in the 1870's (only to be subsequently eased out again in favour of private residents), clubs, couturiers and other businesses began to appear in the late 1920's, soon after the building of the new Grosvenor House on the south side.

It was at this time of delicate transition that the impact of the war of 1939–45 tilted the balance heavily towards office use. During the war a number of buildings were requisitioned for this purpose, and after the destruction of large parts of the City of London by bombing, many businesses moved into the mansions of Mayfair, then often vacant through the departure of the residents to the country, and in rapidly changing social conditions no longer suitable for private occupation.[62] The Grosvenor Estate itself reversed its previous opposition to the growth of offices on its Mayfair properties, leaving Belgravia unchallenged as London's principal fashionable residential quarter. On the Mayfair estate the professions—no longer dominated by the doctors and dentists, who did not return in large numbers after the war of 1939–45—and the diplomats were joined by businessmen with either relatively small staffs or small headquarters staffs, all of whom required a prestigious address and often a sumptuous 'Board Room' office suite in an adapted Georgian or Victorian town house. Advertising and public relations firms (of which there were some thirty in 1965) found a natural milieu here; expensive restaurants did well, and many of the shops dealt in the fields of fashion or luxury. Despite this new emphasis on business and commerce the estate has thus maintained its traditional prestige; but in 1970 the *Post Office Directory* listed only one solitary duke as still resident there; and even the Duke of Westminster himself now lived in Belgravia.

CHAPTER VI

The Architecture of the Estate

The Early Buildings

A glance at the map or a short walk through the district will show that the Grosvenors' Mayfair estate, with its regular grid of broad streets and narrow mews, conforms in layout and structure to the characteristic development patterns of early-Georgian London. But though some few surviving buildings still remain from that period, an equally casual inspection will reveal how much of the original basic stratum has been concealed, overlaid or obliterated. Nineteenth- and twentieth-century flats, shops, office blocks and hotels have taken over upon the peripheries of the estate, while its very centre of Grosvenor Square has been so thoroughly rebuilt that only the merest traces survive from the initial development there. The four main sides of the square, to follow this example further, are now nearly all given over to modern flats, hotels, and diplomatic buildings, with the exception of two embassies that occupy the only surviving 'houses'; and even these houses (Nos. 4 and 38) are rebuildings or recastings of differing date, hardly related except in plot to the predecessors on their sites. Only along the four chief residential thoroughfares, Grosvenor, Upper Grosvenor, Brook and Upper Brook Streets and towards the bottom of South Audley Street, an outlying but always fashionable district of the estate, can the original Georgian fabric and character of the whole area be readily appreciated today.

Even here, as with the surviving houses of the square, qualifications have immediately to be made. Anywhere in these streets, what looks like a Georgian house may be only a Georgian façade; and, *vice versa*, what appears to be a Victorian or Edwardian rebuilding may just be a Victorian or Edwardian refronting. For throughout the smarter parts of the estate, one rich inhabitant has continually replaced another over the years; succeeding estate managers have, since the early nineteenth century, enforced a strict but variable set of demands for improvements (especially to fronts); and, latterly, there has occurred a near-universal change from single-family occupation to offices or flats. As a result, each and every house has been incessantly liable to refacing, internal alterations small and large, or complete rebuilding.

All this is a common pattern on London's older and larger leasehold estates, but it is particularly marked on the Grosvenor estate in Mayfair, for two perhaps connected reasons. One is that the district has never lost its high property values, nor since its construction fallen out of fashion; the other, that its acme of repute as an upper-class residential district was reached only quite recently, at the end of the last century and the beginning of this one. Viewed in this light, the older areas of the estate are a palimpsest, of no vast antiquity perhaps, yet subject to continual rewritings. What is remarkable is not so much that parts of the original are still decipherable, but that these should have so vividly affected, shaped and often fixed the labours of those that came after.

The method, organisation and chronology of the initial development on 'The Hundred Acres' have already been discussed in Chapter II. Something, too, has been said of the rationale of its plain and grid-like layout (Plate 1), evidently the work of the estate's first surveyor, Thomas Barlow. Ambitious in scale but aesthetically unadventurous, its chief debts were to its immediate predecessors and neighbours, Lord Scarbrough's Hanover Square development and the Cavendish-Harley estate north of Oxford Street, both of which schemes were initiated a little before development on the Grosvenor estate began in 1720.[1] The one obvious dramatic feature of Barlow's layout was, of course, Grosvenor Square—at 680 by 530 feet larger than any previous square laid out in London. In plan it had resemblances to Cavendish Square (*c.* 1719–24), the first London square to incorporate two roads at precise right-angles to each other running into the corners, thus making each side of the square in some degree a continuation of the grid of streets around it.[2] But in Cavendish Square this occurred in only the north-west and north-east corners, for on the south side the only road running out of the square did so from the middle, crossing Oxford Street and debouching into the north side of Hanover Square. Grosvenor Square takes the Cavendish Square principle to its logical conclusion, with two streets running into each corner, making eight altogether. But though the long north and south sides might naturally have been bisected by further streets running into the centre of the square, this was not done. The line of George Street (present-day Balderton Street) together with the passage known to have been projected from Providence Court into the middle of the north side of the square gives a hint that such a street may have been considered but abandoned.[3] If it had been cut through, the shorter frontages thus created would have lent themselves to expansive sites for individual noblemen's houses such as were encouraged in Cavendish Square. That some such scheme may seriously have been mooted is hinted at by the survival in the Grosvenor Office of a drawing (Plate 4a) showing neat plans and elevations for a large house on a corner site, bigger than anything ever built in

Grosvenor Square, with a 'front to ye square' of some seventy-five feet. Though there is nothing but its provenance to connect it with Grosvenor Square and it fails to fit any of the sites as actually developed, it may well be an early scheme for the west end of the north side, made at a time when palatial houses were possibly being contemplated. In style, this drawing with its distinctive pilasters and its aprons under the windows is much more consciously attuned to the English Baroque than anything actually built in the square, and has a flavour of the work of Thomas Archer (who did indeed have an interest on the north side of the square, though at the east end, on a site with which the drawing can have no connexion).

However, if this kind of scheme was ever seriously considered, it came to nothing. It may have been the difficulties encountered with individual noble lessees in Cavendish Square that helped to persuade Barlow and the Grosvenors to stick on all four frontages to the kind of terrace housing familiar from St. James's Square and Hanover Square, and now rising along Grosvenor and Brook Streets. This decision, together with the arrangement of streets at the corners, meant that Grosvenor Square was more integrated into the surrounding estate layout than any previous square in London. But to dispel just a little the insistent rectilinearity of the scheme, the building line on all four sides of the square was set back thirty feet from that of each of the incoming streets, as on the short sides of Hanover Square. This led to extra spaciousness in the square itself, and to the creation of four distinctive L-shaped corner sites; on one of these (Nos. 9 Grosvenor Square and 88 Brook Street in the north-east corner) something of the original fabric survives. Though the square was doubtless less easy to take in as a whole than is suggested by early engravings (Plate 5a), these corner sites must have helped to give to its peripheries some much-needed solidity, and thus contributed to its 'squareness'. In the centre, the oval garden probably had some slight softening effect upon the contours of the square, though the paths were strictly formal, the planting was minimal, and the whole scheme centred upon John Nost's gilded equestrian statue of George I in the middle. The garden layout (1725) was the work of the little-known John Alston; the traditional attribution to William Kent appears to have no basis.

One other obvious feature in the planning of the estate, also shared by the Hanover Square and Cavendish-Harley schemes, was the exclusion of its main public place of worship from the square. In any comparable French or Italian town-planning project of this date, a church or other public institution would have been the natural point of focus, but in England this was not the custom, despite the early precedent of St. Paul's, Covent Garden. St. George's, Hanover Square (1720–5), the parish church for the Grosvenor estate and a building with which Thomas Barlow was involved, had despite its importance been sited outside Hanover Square itself, rather as St. James's, Piccadilly, had been related to St. James's Square some fifty years before. On the Cavendish-Harley estate, James Gibbs's Oxford Chapel (the modern St. Peter's, Vere Street) was situated well away from Cavendish Square and in no way emphasized. So too the Grosvenor Chapel was allotted an equally inconspicuous position in South Audley Street, though it did at least have the advantage of a vista along Chapel (now Aldford) Street. Nor can it have been deemed essential to the early success of development, for though it was projected from the start it was not built until 1730–2. At one stage indeed, Edward Shepherd thought of erecting a chapel in North Audley Street, again on a relatively modest site, but this came to nothing;[4] the Grosvenor Chapel, when built, became the estate's only place of established worship. Likewise, other special buildings, whether public or private, were equally slow to develop and tended to occupy peripheral sites. The layout, in fact, was designed with terrace housing alone specifically in mind, and it is the nature of this that must now be examined.

In the 1720's and 1730's it was not as yet feasible for a landlord to impose absolutely regular frontages upon the London speculative building lessees of the day. But if only because the Grosvenor estate was by far the biggest single area of high-class domestic building at the time, attempts were made here and there, notably in the square, to combine individual house fronts into the kind of disciplined architectural composition beloved of the Palladians. This has to be seen in perspective. Palladian ideals being as yet new in the 1720's, Barlow and the master builders who dominated the estate development still practised an architecture in the tradition of speculative building going back to the era of Nicholas Barbon fifty years before, but tempered by modest innovations from the school of Wren. Further, in conjunction with the short-lived period of the English Baroque, there appears to have been a reaction against uniformity of town-house fronts, especially for houses of the larger sort, and this was still reflected in the estate development. In Grosvenor Square, the only part of the area for which there is good evidence as to the original appearance of the houses, the variations were considerable. Some of them were due to the leasing history of the various plots, some to stylistic uncertainty following the onslaught of Palladianism, but some may have been the outcome of a conscious desire for variety. Almost certainly, the surrounding streets looked more uniform and more disciplined, but this would have been in the interests of economy rather than classicism. Nevertheless, the Palladian movement did have much influence on the estate. Colen Campbell, Roger Morris, William Benson, Thomas Ripley and Edward Shepherd, five important figures in the implementation of Palladian ideals, all had a hand in the development. Their precise involvement is specified elsewhere (see pages 20–2), but here something must be said of its nature and results.

It was upon Grosvenor Square that the new movement naturally concentrated its powers. Here Colen Campbell contributed in 1725 an intriguing but unexecuted design

for the east side, known only from an engraving showing a front elevation and ground-floor plan of the whole composition (Plate 4b). The elevation presents a striking antithesis to speculative building traditions of the time: an absolutely even and symmetrical range dressed in the whole Palladian finery, with stone arches to the ground floor, first-floor balconies, an engaged order to the upper storeys, elaborate window dressings and balustrading with crowning statues masking the roof. The backs of the houses are shown on the plan as very curtailed but absolutely regular, while no allowance is made for the corner sites, so this was probably something of an ideal solution. Nevertheless John Simmons, the developer of the square's east side (Plates 5, 8a), did manage within the limits of a plain brick architecture to maintain the symmetry and regularity suggested by Campbell; he raised a central pediment and emphasized the ends, thus distinguishing the range from the rest of the square and other parts of the estate, and setting an important precedent for London street architecture.

Campbell was very likely involved in the two long sides of Grosvenor Square as well. A similar design of his for a block of three houses, perhaps for the south side, was again not followed, but on the north side the story is more intriguing. Though lavish in the scale of its houses, this side as built ended up as an irregular and frankly clumsy range because of the inclusion among its façades of two Palladian compositions with attached orders and pediments and, between them, a third less 'correct' interloper adorned with pilasters (Plate 5). Had these buildings balanced each other, all would have been well, but this they failed to do, thereby exciting the derision of acerbic critics such as James Ralph.[5] Close to the west end of the side Edward Shepherd's massive composition occupied three houses (Nos. 18–20, to follow modern numbering); near the middle, the pilastered part extended over two (Nos. 15 and 16), while to the right of centre there was just John Aislabie's elegantly pedimented house at No. 12 (fig. 2a), conspicuous amidst a run of otherwise orthodox fronts. Individually, Shepherd's development and the Aislabie house were of high merit, and since Colen Campbell had been patronised by Aislabie at Waverley Abbey and Studley Royal and was an associate of Shepherd's, he could have had some hand in either of these ambitious buildings. That a 'regular range' had at first been designed by Shepherd for the whole of the north side is claimed by Robert Morris,[6] and it would have been natural for Shepherd, though clearly the architect for his development, at least to consult Campbell. It may be no coincidence that the window surrounds on Campbell's surviving own house, the modest No. 76 Brook Street (fig. 2e), on a plot made available to him by Shepherd, appear to be similar in shape, character and material to the 'plaister' ones specified for Shepherd's Grosvenor Square houses.

So despite the participation of two experienced undertakers, Simmons and Shepherd, and the enthusiasm of Campbell, the pioneering Palladian, the attempt to build uniform classical frontages in the square met with very limited success. It was even harder where plots were parcelled out among different builders in smaller divisions. Outside the square, one such effort to impose a uniform frontage on a number of builders in Upper Brook Street as late as 1742 soon met with opposition and failed (see page 31). Normally, the different lessees and sub-lessees were building on plots of limited frontage with little or no restriction as to proportion and style, and so there was naturally opportunity for plenty of variation from house to house. Width of plot, height and number of storeys, proportions of windows, quality and type of brickwork on the front: all these features varied according to the position and status of the house in question (Plate 8b, c, e). The simple overall layout meant that these small tendencies to indiscipline were enlivening rather than disruptive, whereas an elaborate composition in town planning might have been wrecked by them.

Along the estate's chief streets and in most of the square, the effect was quite different from the monotonous regularity of later Georgian thoroughfares like Baker Street or Gower Street. Instead, the finished appearance must have consisted of variations upon the well-tried but ever fertile theme of flat, stock-brick fronts, of unpredictable width and slightly irregular height (fig. 2). Where two or more houses were undertaken together, there was sometimes no architectural break between them; more frequently, it was the practice to draw attention to the division by means of projecting brick piers or 'pilaster strips', a favourite device along the estate's main streets and one probably borrowed from the Hanover Square development. These curious strips, which can still be seen in places in Grosvenor Street, gave definition to the individual houses. Where adjacent plots were developed by a single builder, the strips would usually span the party wall. Elsewhere they were less formally organized, belonging sometimes to one house, sometimes to another (Plate 8c), and a few of the widest plots included two strips, to the deprivation of their narrower neighbours. Sometimes these strips were plain, sometimes rusticated like quoins. In the square itself, proper stone quoins were common (Plate 8a), but this seems to have been infrequent elsewhere, though there are surviving examples at No. 16 Grosvenor Street and Nos. 35–36 Upper Brook Street (Plate 6b; fig. 2f). At the ends of these unevenly divided but otherwise flat-fronted ranges, it became a charming habit to give the return frontages to some of the corner houses delightful bay windows or other features to the upper storeys, carried out on piers or pillars and sometimes projecting right over the pavement. Though the only examples that survive are those at Nos. 9 and 71 South Audley Street (Plate 6d), these upper-storey projections (which may frequently have been early additions) were not uncommon, and were also to sprout here and there along the main frontages.

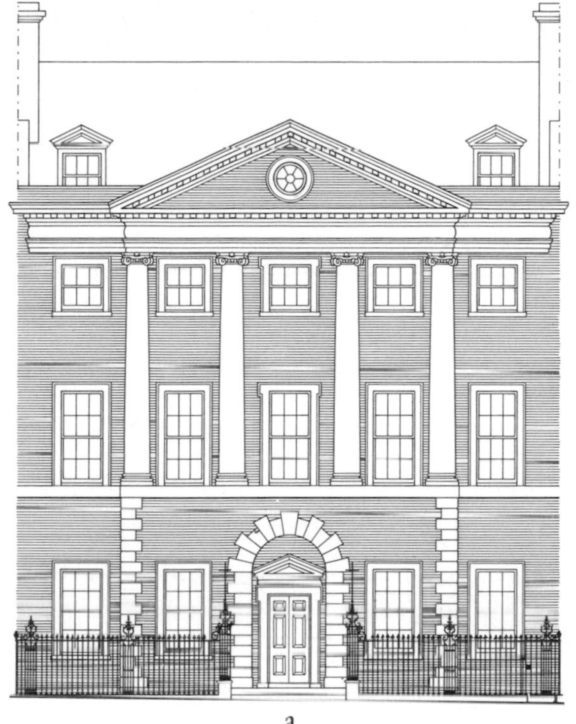

a

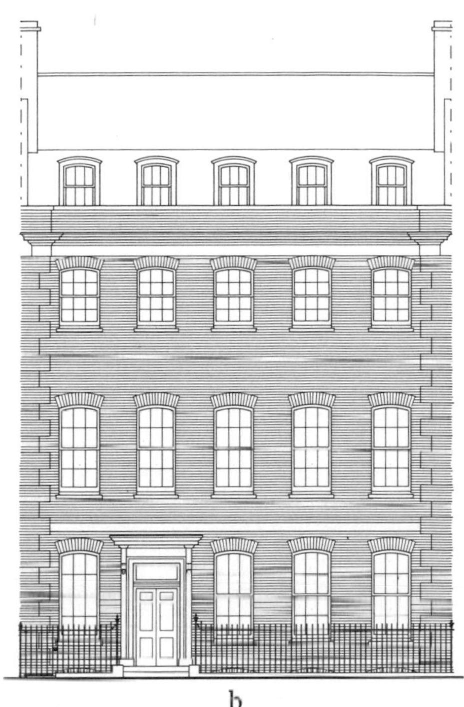

b

a. No. 12 Grosvenor Square. *Lessee*, John Kitchingman (timber merchant), 1727; *architect*, possibly Colen Campbell for John Aislabie, the first occupant. *Demolished*

b. No. 51 Grosvenor Street. *Lessee*, Israel Russell (painter), by direction of Benjamin Timbrell (carpenter), 1724

Fig. 2. EARLY-GEORGIAN ELEVATIONS

As for the fronts themselves, these were of anything between two and five windows' width. The windows generally were still segment-headed, with their wooden frames set well back in accordance with the Building Act of 1709, and their surrounds dressed liberally with red cutters and rubbers to set off the grey-brown of the stock bricks. Indeed many of the original fronts were probably quite colourful, to make up for the lack of stonework. Stone dressings were common only in the square and other special places; elsewhere, bold plaster cornices and wooden doorcases ruled the day. In height, there was rough uniformity along the main streets, but little attempt to make storey levels coincide. Three storeys above ground sufficed for Georgian wants, with a further one in the attic, usually with dormers perching over the cornice and set within a roof of double pitch, or more rarely treated as a fourth full storey flush with the front. The whole house would be raised upon a basement storey, its front area protected by stout iron railings (a feature often specified in the building agreements) and frequently containing an ornamental lead cistern.

Though none of these terrace fronts along the main streets remains absolutely unscathed, two sets of houses designed as pairs, Nos. 44 and 45 Upper Grosvenor Street and Nos. 35 and 36 Upper Brook Street, are good but rather different types of survivors (Plate 6a, b; fig. 2f). Both pairs were built in two tones of brickwork; but in Upper Grosvenor Street the houses (*c*. 1727–31) have the segmental window heads and wooden doorcases typical of early development, whereas the later Upper Brook Street houses (*c*. 1737–42) adopt the embellishments by then familiar from the square, of string courses between the storeys, stone quoins, keystones, and rusticated door surrounds. All four of these houses have had balconies added and windows lengthened at first-floor level, and the Upper Grosvenor Street houses have been heightened. Similar changes have been made at Nos. 70 and 76 Brook Street, 51 Grosvenor Street, 10 and 13 South Audley Street, and 48 Upper Grosvenor Street, all terrace houses whose fronts still have much of their old character, without more than the most superficial admixture of stucco (fig. 2b–f).

Photographs of the lost Grosvenor Square houses confirm the slightly different picture there already suggested. The houses whose fronts survived best until the square's recent rebuilding were No. 1 on the east, Nos. 12, 14 and 17 on the north, No. 25 on the west, and Nos. 37, 44 and 46 on the south. But of this group, if those on the north

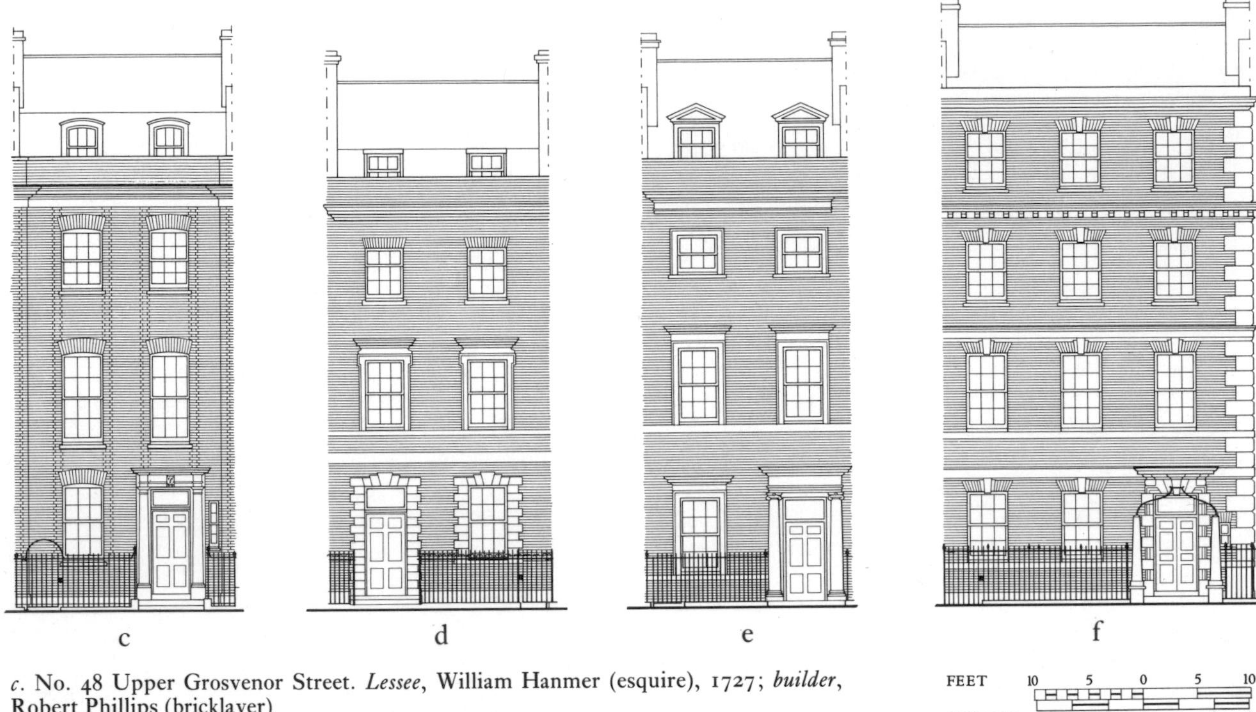

c. No. 48 Upper Grosvenor Street. *Lessee*, William Hanmer (esquire), 1727; *builder*, Robert Phillips (bricklayer)
d. No. 13 South Audley Street. *Lessee*, William Singleton (plasterer), 1736
e. No. 76 Brook Street. *Lessee*, Colen Campbell (architect), 1726
f. No. 35 Upper Brook Street. *Sub-lessee*, Anthony Cross (mason), 1737

and east side bear out the greater formality intimated in early engravings, the south side ones show the extent to which a pre-Palladian brick architecture continued even in the square. No. 44, one of a row of similar houses here, was particularly attractively organised, with the red dressings flanking the windows carried up without break between the floors to cornice level; this emphasized the pilaster strips at either end and gave the whole building a strong vertical accent, augmented by treating the attic as a full storey flush with the front (Plate 7).

The smaller residential houses of the estate have nearly all been demolished (Plate 8e). But the survivors show that they differed in scale and plan rather than in front from their superiors. A well-preserved group at Nos. 70–78 (even) Park Street, originally quite a respectable row of small houses and including an almost untouched façade at No. 72, gives an idea of the appearance of some of the secondary streets, a sequence of modest fronts in two tones of brick (Plate 8b). Further down the social scale, the disappearance has been total. Simplicity must have been the rule, since in many districts tenements with only a single room per floor were crammed into a riddle of back alleys, as in Brown's Court, Green Street, one of the few places of this kind for which we have a reliable plan (see fig. 1 on page 32).

In general, most of the lesser houses on the estate followed the common London terrace plan. It is well known that in the late seventeenth century there evolved a standard arrangement for the smaller London terrace house, consisting of two rooms per floor, a dog-leg staircase rising alongside the back room and, often enough, an additional small rear parlour or closet facing the yard. This plan appears, for instance, throughout Nos. 70–78 (even) Park Street and in many places along the main streets where frontages were narrow (fig. 3a), but it could also be used outside a strictly residential context. At this period there were no special plans for shops, taverns or even small manufactories, and this established arrangement quickly proved itself both adaptable and economic. As a result the standard plan became the norm in streets of mixed character like Mount Street and Duke Street, where for over a century it steadily continued to perform the varied functions laid upon it.

But though this plan suited small houses, it would not do for the smarter parts of the estate, which abounded in generous frontages and deep plots leading right through to stables some 150 feet or more away. A separate servants'

staircase was hard to include in the standard arrangement, and the areas of circulation and main stairs themselves tended to be cramped. Alternatives of several kinds were evolving for larger houses at the time the estate was being developed; consequently the individuality of the first-class Grosvenor estate house was more strikingly expressed in its plan than in its elevation (fig. 3).

Where a secondary staircase was felt to be *de rigueur*, the most fashionable plan, much employed on the recently built Burlington estate,[7] was to have a 'great stair' starting from the front compartment of the house inside the entrance hall and turning back towards the street, from which it was lit (fig. 3f). This staircase rose only to the first-floor reception rooms; the upper storeys were served by separate stairs (usually with a toplight high above) which was situated behind the great stair in the central or back compartment of the house and climbed most or all of the way from basement to attic. Houses of this kind were built throughout the square and surrounding streets where the plots were of thirty-foot frontage or over, allowing at least four windows towards the street, sometimes five, and therefore giving enough space for ample front rooms on ground and first floors beside the great stair. Examples with parts or more of the main stairs surviving can still be seen at Nos. 67 Brook Street, 34 and 59 Grosvenor Street (Plate 9b, d), and 14 and 74 South Audley Street, and plans remain of many other lost ones, e.g. at No. 43 Grosvenor Street (fig. 3f). It must have been a particularly common type in the square, but there documentation of the original plans is sadly scant.

Although this was the most distinctive and fully evolved type of plan for the larger terrace house, there were plenty of other options available. One was the central toplit staircase arrangement, whereby the entrance hall was left clear and the great stair, lit by a skylight high above, rose immediately behind to first-floor level, with the secondary staircase again behind that and sometimes relegated right to the very back of the house beyond a large reception room. The advantage of this disposition, which survives at No. 33 Grosvenor Street and can be clearly seen on plans of various demolished houses, for instance Nos. 43 and 45 Brook Street (fig. 3g, h), was to allow a large room facing the front at first-floor level, which compensated for loss of living space on the ground floor below. This plan was relatively novel when it first appeared on the Grosvenor estate, but was to grow in popularity throughout the eighteenth century; the lengthy rear wings often incorporated in such arrangements were commonly used as private suites, for the master of the house on the ground floor, for the mistress on the floor above. In its full form, the central toplit plan was again at its best for houses of four or five windows' width, but it could also be used in a curtailed version for those of three windows' width; in houses of this kind the need for a separate servants' staircase was beginning to be increasingly felt. A remarkable variant survives at No. 44 and originally existed also at No. 45 Upper Grosvenor Street (fig. 3d), both three-bay houses, where the back stairs are in parallel to the main staircase, which is toplit from a low dome in the centre; this creates a fine effect but necessarily curtails the size of the rooms at front and back. In other houses of three windows' width, for instance No. 16 Upper Grosvenor Street (fig. 3b), the presence of a conventional dog-leg staircase did not inhibit the inclusion of a secondary one, placed behind the rear wing closet and accessible only through the back room on each floor. For houses on the estate without back stairs, a central staircase was also a common variant from the conventional type of plan, as it long had been. In various houses of lesser width of frontage like Nos. 10 and 73 South Audley Street and No. 38 Upper Brook Street (before alteration) the toplit stairs were thrust between front and back rooms with small closets or passages behind (fig. 3c). This was basically an old-fashioned arrangement, especially when the staircase was of the dog-leg variety, but it survived well into the 1730's and beyond.

Happily, there is good proof to show how heterogeneous the plans of the houses along the main streets really were. There survives at the Grosvenor Office a large body of ground-floor plans of individual houses, showing their state round about the beginning of the nineteenth century; these were made by William Porden and his assistants for the purposes of leasing, at the time that the estate management was being put upon a more professional footing. By this date many of the houses had already been altered, and as the drawings were done at different times they vary in detail and accuracy. But when used judiciously together with a survey made by Robert Taylor and George Shakespear in 1778–9 showing in detail the triangle within Davies Street, Grosvenor Street, and South Molton Lane/Avery Row (fig. 4), they demonstrate the variety of possible arrangement. For instance, the relative frequency of the three main plan types is given by the crude statistic that of some 120 fully enclosed terrace houses along Brook, Upper Brook, Grosvenor and Upper Grosvenor Streets for which the arrangement is known, 51 were of the conventional staircase type, 35 had their chief staircase in the front compartment, and 33 had some form of main central stairs. More sense can be made of these figures in terms of plot widths and the presence of secondary stairs. In Grosvenor Square, where frontages habitually exceeded thirty-five feet in breadth and had more than three windows, few if any houses had the conventional staircase arrangement, and none is known to have been without back stairs. In the surrounding streets, the houses of three windows' width and approximately twenty-five feet in frontage are the unpredictable ones. If they had back stairs, usually they adopted some form of main central staircase, but if they omitted back stairs, either the conventional type or a central staircase was possible. To sum up, a central staircase could be found in all kinds of houses, while a front compartment staircase tended to be reserved for those of

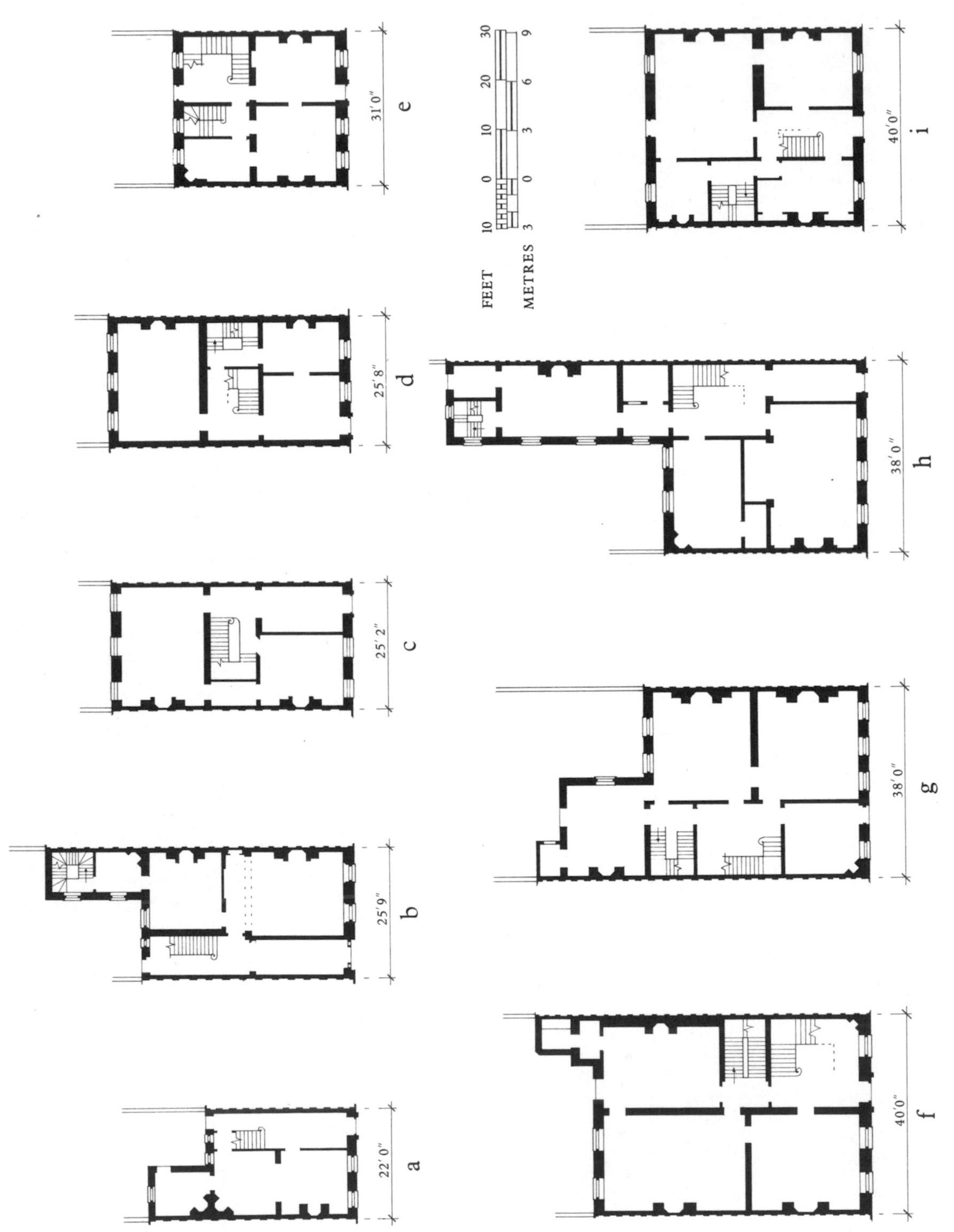

Fig. 3. EARLY-GEORGIAN GROUND-FLOOR PLANS

The dates are of building leases or sub-leases

a. No. 13 Upper Brook Street, 1728. *Demolished*. *b*. No. 16 Upper Grosvenor Street, 1730. *c*. No. 38 Upper Brook Street, 1736. *d*. No. 45 Upper Grosvenor Street, 1727. *e*. No. 36 Grosvenor Street, 1726. *Demolished*. *f*. No. 43 Grosvenor Street, 1726. *g*. No. 45 Brook Street, 1723. *Demolished*. *h*. No. 43 Brook Street, 1725. *Demolished*. *i*. No. 47 Brook Street, 1723. *Demolished*

wide frontage and a conventional dog-leg staircase for narrow ones of three bays or less.

In houses of the largest size, the characteristics of the terrace house plan might be virtually lost and much of the spaciousness of the nobleman's free-standing town house could be obtained, despite enclosure. In examples like No. 47 Brook Street (with a frontage of forty feet but, curiously, only three windows towards the street) or No. 19 Grosvenor Square (five windows wide with a sixty-foot frontage), the entrance was in the centre of the façade, and the plan resolved itself into a series of separate but equal compartments *en suite*, with toplit stairs where required (fig. 3i). Despite the efforts of Simmons and Shepherd to create symmetrical compositions, this grandest of all the house types was the distinct exception, even in Grosvenor Square. Thus Isaac Ware, propagandizing in his *Complete Body of Architecture* on behalf of a Palladian programme for symmetrically planned town houses, found cause to complain of 'one very striking instance of placing the door out of the centre. This errs both in proportion and situation, and must be named as a caution to the young builder. The house is in Grosvenor Square; the edifice is large and conspicuous, but one is puzzled to find which is the way into it. It appears a house without a door, and when the eye is cast upon the little entrance at one side, one scarce knows how to suppose it is the door to that house; it seems to belong to the next.'[8]

An analysis of the plan types and plot widths offers no logical answer to the question of why small and large houses were so closely intermingled along the four main streets. In Grosvenor Street there was some tendency for the grander houses to be sited nearer the square, and there were few plots in Upper Brook Street and Upper Grosvenor Street with the width of frontage sometimes found in Brook and Grosvenor Streets, but to both these rules there are exceptions. The size of houses erected in any one area depended upon the inclinations, capacities and ambitions of the developers, especially when they were taking large plots, and not upon any clear conception on the part of Thomas Barlow or any other officer of the estate. To take one instance visible on the 1778–9 survey plan mentioned above (fig. 4), the north side of Brook Street between Davies Street and South Molton Lane was taken in 1720 by Henry Avery and Robert Pollard as one lot. Fifteen small houses, nearly all of conventional plan and probably of quite uniform appearance, were built here, though scarcely anything of them survives today. Yet immediately opposite on a strip of similar length along the south side of Brook Street, the land was divided between several undertakers; here only eleven houses were built, but these were of greater size and varying plan The rich and the not-so-rich were therefore staring each other in the face, a situation which had polarized by the 1780's, when the majority of the houses on the north side

Fig. 4. Plan of area east of Davies Street and north of Grosvenor Street, showing ground-plan of buildings. *From a survey of 1778–9 by Robert Taylor and George Shakespear. Original torn in places as indicated. The vacant house plots were not surveyed*

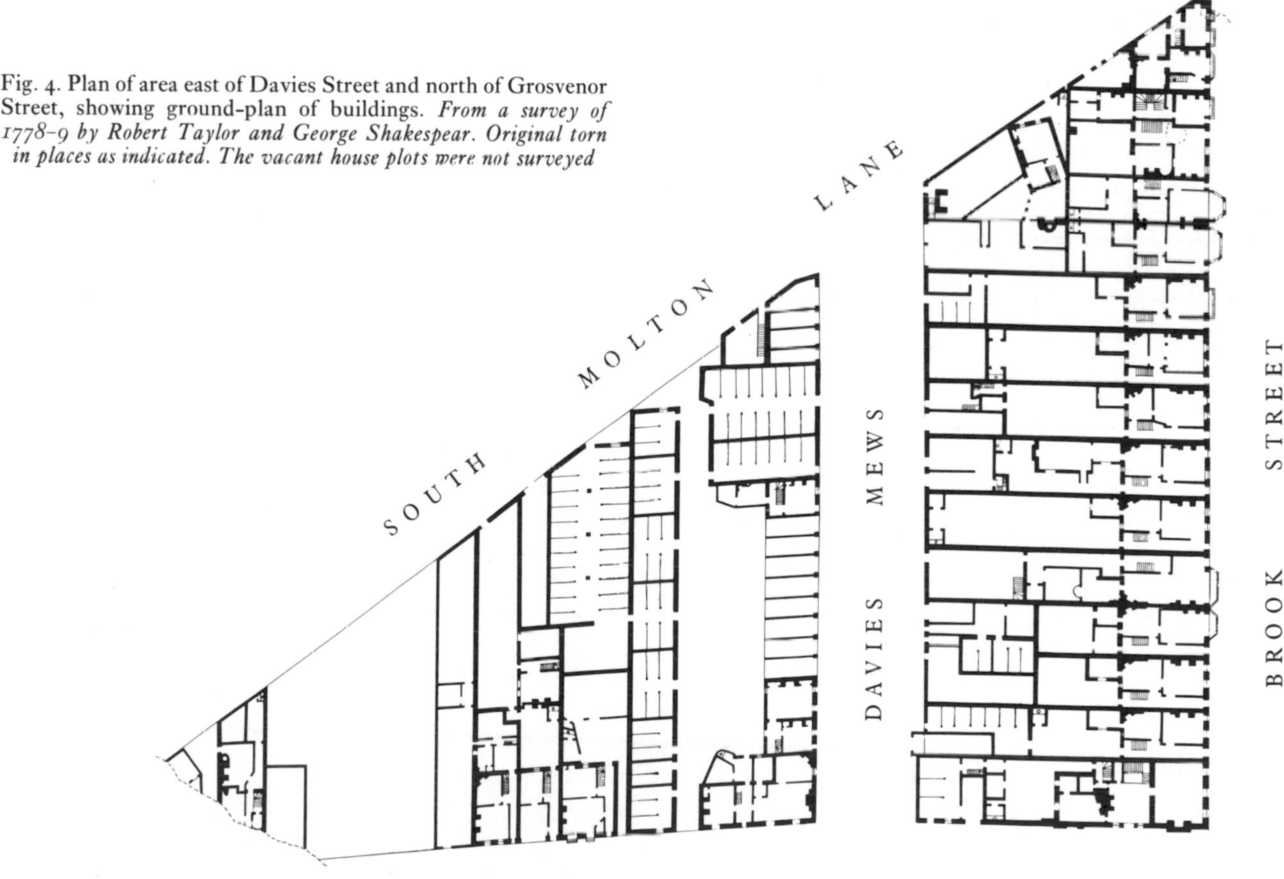

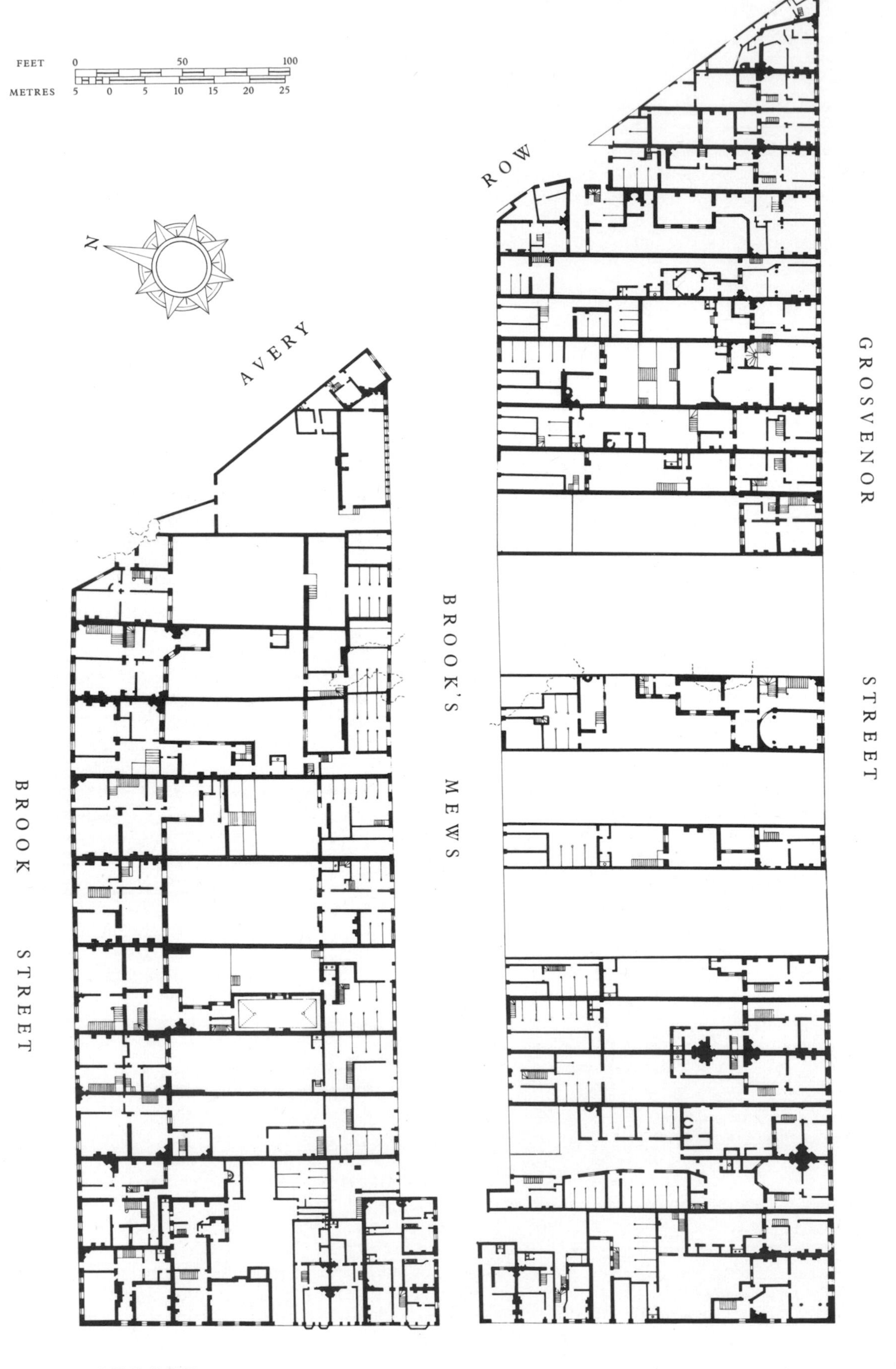
FEET 0 50 100
METRES 5 0 5 10 15 20 25
N
AVERY ROW
BROOK'S MEWS
GROSVENOR STREET
BROOK STREET
STREET

were occupied by tradesmen. In 1805, when William Porden was asked to consider the conversion of one of the south side houses into a hotel, he reported that the good houses here were neither so fashionable nor so profitable as they ought to have been, because of the proximity of lesser ones.[9] There was a similar contrast (though less sharp) in Grosvenor Street east of Davies Street, where most of the houses on the north side were smaller than those on the south. Why the better class of house in the eastern parts of both these streets occupied the south sides we do not know. In Upper Brook and Upper Grosvenor Streets, nearly all the houses had frontages of between twenty and thirty-five feet and there was much less unevenness between the sides.

Despite the remains of much original work here and there, a clear idea of how the interiors of these houses first appeared or how they functioned is hard to come by. In view of later attempts, often successful, to convey a 'period' authenticity in their redecoration, the nature of the original schemes cannot easily be seen objectively. The evidence of memoirs and correspondence is scanty, building accounts rarely survive and are even less frequently helpful; early inventories, however, are not so uncommon, and have been much depended upon for what follows.

From our review of its planning, it is plain that the early Georgian first-class terrace house on the Grosvenor estate was rarely a composition of great formality. One reflection of this is the nomenclature of rooms, which were most often designated not by their function but by their position or sometimes by their embellishment. On the ground floor were the parlours, usually 'fore parlour' and 'back parlour', the normal focus of private family activity. At first-floor level the front room, especially if it was at the head of a 'great stair', might be the grandest room of the house in which guests were received and entertained. More remarkably, the 'eating room' was often also at this level. It was certainly so at Handel's house, just off the estate at No. 25 Brook Street;[10] inventories of 1757 and 1772 show dining-rooms at first-floor level at Nos. 9 and 6 Grosvenor Square respectively;[11] and in 1756 Isaac Ware takes it for granted that the dining-room of an ordinary house would naturally come over the hall.[12] Still, by the mid century, dining-rooms were sometimes at ground level, more often at the front. Thus at No. 29 Grosvenor Square, a schedule of 1746 mentions one on the first floor, but by 1757 it has descended to ground level.[13] In the best houses, this change meant the re-organization of the ground-floor parlour so as to make a capacious room with a recess or sometimes a screen of pillars marking off the serving area, thus often curtailing the back room behind (figs. 3h, 4). By 1800 many of the houses on the estate had been altered in this way, but it is a moot point whether in some the change did not take place shortly after completion; at No. 50 Grosvenor Square, a surviving set of what appear to be very early plans already shows this arrangement.[14]

A dining-room on the first floor must have meant a long trek from the kitchen; this was most frequently in the basement along with the other 'offices' and normally faced the front area. But in at least one of the larger Grosvenor Street houses (on the site of the present Nos. 71–72), it had already been relegated from the start to a position 'away from the house',[15] and a similar arrangement, found at No. 16 Grosvenor Street in about 1763, was probably also original.[16] Such a long separation of kitchen and dining-room was inconvenient to gentry as well as to servants, who must have had to cross some of the important public spaces with hot dishes and dirty plates. But it seems not to have troubled the Georgian builders, or the inhabitants of their houses, still content to live at close quarters and without complete privacy.

The houses were certainly very fully occupied at certain seasons. In 1763 Lady Molesworth's reputedly 'small' house at No. 49 Upper Brook Street burnt down one night (a peril to which early Georgian town houses, with their stud partition walls, their wooden stairs, and their stretches of panelling, were prone). Horace Walpole says that seven inhabitants perished, another account claims ten, but certainly several escaped. This means that there were probably some fifteen people in the main house, though admittedly at a time when there were visitors, since Lady Molesworth 'to make room had taken her eldest daughter, of 17, to lie with her' in the front room on the second floor (a casual, crowded arrangement which would have been avoided at a later period).[17] Again, when in 1726 Sir Thomas Hanmer moved into his new house at No. 52 Grosvenor Street, one of the district's largest, it appears that he had at least fourteen servants (mostly male) in and around the house, besides his wife and family. But if these houses were intensively used, that was not the case all the year round. Hanmer's accounts show him, with fair regularity, living in Grosvenor Street between November and May and moving to the country-side for the rest of the year.[18] From the architectural point of view this seasonal migration meant that for some five months of the year the houses were merely looked after by servants, and therefore there was ample time and scope for the decorative improvements that were so frequently demanded, right from the early days of the estate's history.

There must always have been a wide variety in the degree and elaboration of internal finishing in these early houses. One useful hint for interpreting their original quality is the mix of panelling and plaster. The basic material was of course panelling, and on moving into her new house in Grosvenor Street (on the site of Nos. 71–72) in the early 1720's Lady Hertford was pleased to report 'that (except the garrets) there is not a corner unwainscotted'.[15] But though panelled interiors were practical, they were not in any way special. Many quite modest houses, for instance Nos. 7 and 8 Upper Brook Street or Nos. 70 and 74 Park Street, retain much panelling, while some of the more luxuriously appointed ones such as Nos. 71, 73 and 74 South Audley Street have, and probably always had, little (Plate 10a): prosaically

enough, an early inventory of No. 45 Grosvenor Square records in the garden a wainscotted 'Boghouse'.[19] In fact deal panelling without any mouldings ('square work') could be cheaply run up and was regularly used in attics and up to dado level in basements. It could be framed directly on to internal brickwork, or be attached to studs to make thin partition walls not bearing any load. On the main floors, it would be more or less elaborated, with at the simplest a 'quarter-round' or 'ovolo' moulding (often carved with egg and dart) framing the panels, which were set back from the stiles and characteristically rose high in proportion to their breadth. One better than this was the raised and fielded panelling that formed the wainscotting of the parlours in the best houses. These were the two basic types of good panelling, which though subject to variation are nevertheless distinguishable from later imitations. The cornices in panelled rooms of high quality would include a run of egg and dart or of modillions; on bedroom floors, wooden box cornices seem to have been the norm.

However this wainscotting was originally treated, it is clear that at least in the best houses it was primarily regarded as a background to other things. Most of it was made from imported deal, which was very nearly always painted, and sometimes grained to look like oak. The tone of the painting remains a difficulty but light colours seem to have been the commoner. Ware must have been thinking of white or cream when he spoke in 1756 of panelling 'painted in the usual way' as lighter than stucco,[20] and in 1769 the building agreement for Lord Bateman's house in Park Lane (later Somerset House) specified that the main rooms should be left a dead white but the bedroom floor and attics a stone colour, presumably as a basis before the upholsterer moved in.[21] Later in the century, shades of green were popular for panelling and by 1800 stronger tones were frequent. But whatever its tone, the panelling served chiefly as a background for broad, brightly coloured areas of fabric, with mirrors ('pier glasses') frequently interspersed in between. Thus Sarah, Duchess of Marlborough, in 1732 tells her grand-daughter, then about to move into No. 51 Grosvenor Street: 'Though several people have larger rooms, what you have is as much as is of any real use to anybody, and the white painting with so much red damask looks mighty handsome. All the hangings are up in the four rooms above stairs except some pieces that are to be where the glass don't cover all the wainscott, and I think that will look very well.'[22] Thus too in an inventory of 1767 for No. 18 Grosvenor Square the bedrooms, which were probably panelled from head to foot, were called after their hangings and soft furnishings in general: 'green silk damask bedchamber', 'printed cotton bedchamber', 'green harrateen bedchamber' and 'blue mohair bedchamber'.[23] Such names reveal the crucial, sometimes tyrannical, part played by the upholsterer in finishing these houses. Little is known of the men who originally furnished the great Grosvenor estate houses, but of their successors there will be much to say.

Panelling apart, the joiner was of course responsible for doors, which on the main floors might have pediments and friezes, and occasionally for chimneypieces. But fireplaces were basically part of the mason's job, a point on which the early inventories are surprisingly unanimous. The good houses usually had marble fireplaces, often of no great pretension, right through to bedroom level, with Portland stone equivalents in the basement and the 'garrets'; the lesser houses were content with ordinary stone chimneypieces throughout. Perhaps because of their simplicity, few of these remain in either marble or stone; later accounts for Grosvenor Square mention the replacement of fireplaces with particular frequency. The characteristic early Georgian high chimneypieces have also rarely survived in their entirety, though there are wooden examples at No. 71 South Audley Street (Plate 10a) and a more elaborate one of marble below and plaster above on the first floor at No. 66 Brook Street (Frontispiece). This type of fireplace must have meant calling in a skilled carver or statuary specially for this task; thus Hanmer employed Rysbrack for a lost fireplace at No. 52 Grosvenor Street.[18]

Some elaborate survivals suggest that the plasterers were particularly active on the Grosvenor estate. To a degree their trade overlapped with that of the carpenters, since cornices could be of wood and walls could be panelled but either feature could be plastered instead. They may even in places have encroached upon the traditional spheres of other tradesmen. Because the houses were built by a mutual system of sharing jobs and bartering in labour, there had to be co-operation between the trades, but the actual lessee presumably had the final say as to the permanent finishings of his house and would naturally bias them in favour of his own craft. Certainly stucco was already gaining ground on the fronts of houses, especially where plasterers like Edward Shepherd were involved. For his group of houses at Nos. 18–20 Grosvenor Square (Plate 5), Shepherd agreed in 1728 to execute all the 'Plaistering worke of the front...(Vizt) The Intableture Rustick Story Cellar Story and ornaments to Windows',[24] and though exterior stuccowork remained unreliable in quality for fifty years and more after this, it is likely that several other houses on the estate took advantage of the material. Similarly, quite a few surviving interiors of quality can with fair certainty be ascribed to Shepherd, one of the most prolific and individual of the original developers, or to craftsmen close to him. These are Nos. 66 Brook Street, 72 Brook Street (for a time Shepherd's own house), 12 North Audley Street, and 71, 73 and 74 South Audley Street, all in a block taken by Shepherd and let to him and his associates. On the other side of South Audley Street five further houses, Nos. 9, 10, 12, 13 and 14, retain interesting ornamental plasterwork; here the plasterer William Singleton, of whom little is known, was one of the lessees.

What all these houses have in common is a series of entertaining decorative ceilings (fig. 5). More unusually,

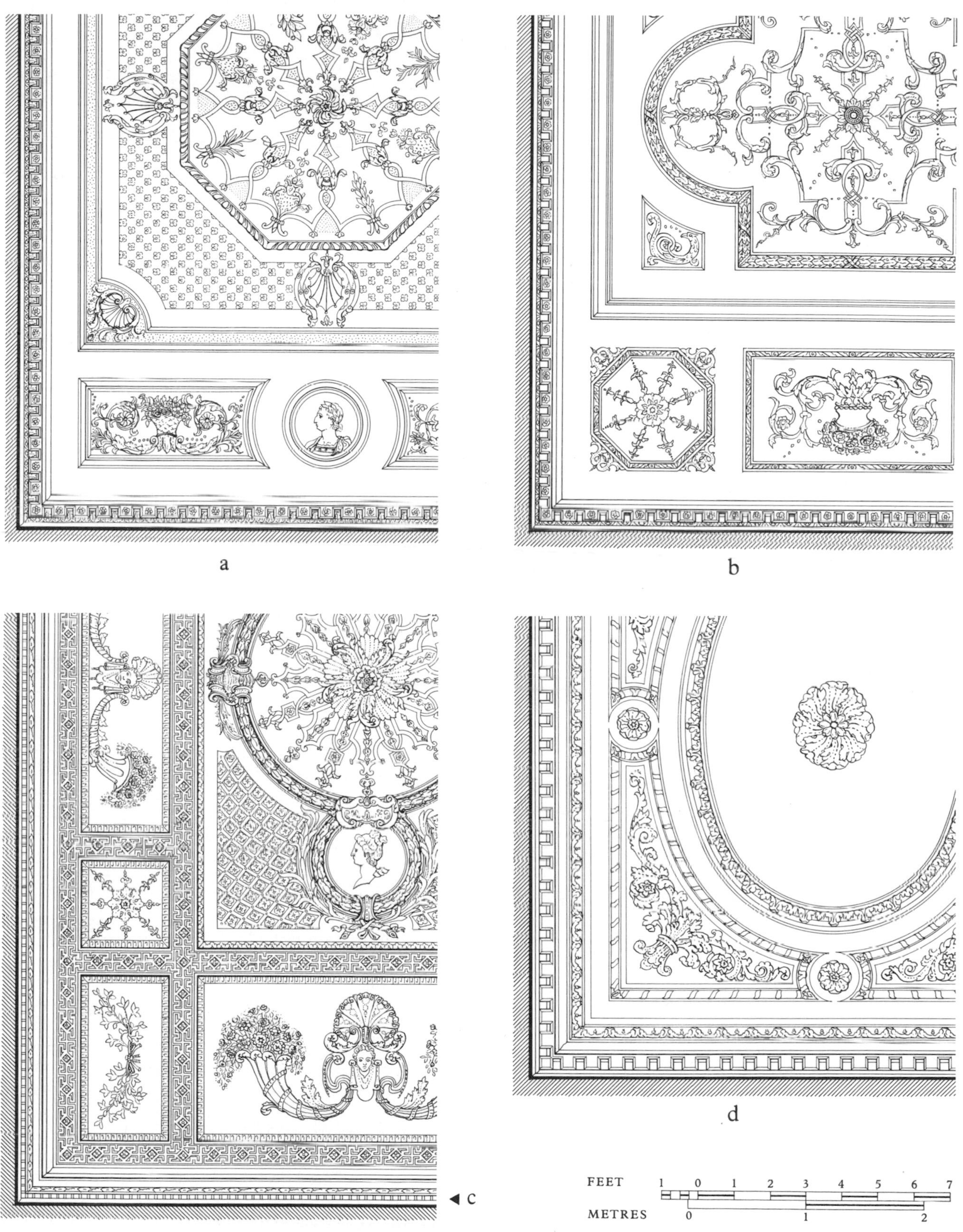

Fig. 5. EARLY-GEORGIAN PLASTER CEILINGS

a. No. 12 South Audley Street, ground-floor front room. *Lessee*, William Singleton (plasterer), 1737. *b*. No. 73 South Audley Street, ground-floor back room. *Lessee*, John Shepherd (plasterer), 1736. *c*. No. 74 South Audley Street, ground floor, main back room. *Lessee*, Edward Shepherd (esquire, formerly plasterer), 1736. *d*. No. 34 Grosvenor Street, over main staircase. *Lessee*, Richard Lissiman (mason), 1725

many of them also have interesting plasterwork to the walls as well. Nos. 12, 71 and 73 South Audley Street share in many of the principal rooms the characteristic of eccentric sunk plaster wall panels with shouldered heads (Plate 10a). These, clearly the plasterer's equivalent to wainscotting, were meant to receive pictures and hangings. Sunk plaster panels occur again at No. 66 Brook Street on the walls and ceilings of the ground-floor front room, as part of a more elaborate composition including pilasters, flowerpieces, and ornamental cartouches destined for 'pier glasses'. This house undoubtedly contains the finest of all Shepherd's surviving interiors on the estate, for besides this room there is a plaster-vaulted staircase (Plate 9a) leading on the first floor to a splendid and festive apartment, long recognized as one of the best Baroque interiors in London. It boasts elaborate doorcases, engaged Corinthian columns on all sides and, as a climax, an exuberant double-storey chimneypiece, marble below and plaster above, with a standing *putto* set in relief in the upper part (Frontispiece).

The surviving ceilings and staircase decorations of Shepherd and his circle show that, left to their own devices, they expressed themselves with an almost rustic floridity. This was not uncommon at the time, even with quite Palladian houses. William Kent was a fertile and frequently unclassical designer of ornament, and even true Italian *stuccadori* like Bagutti (who is known to have worked on the lost staircase at No. 52 Grosvenor Street[18]) could produce ceilings bordering on the quaint. This rampant style of plasterwork is well shown in four fine surviving ceilings at No. 73 South Audley Street, where Shepherd's brother John, also a plasterer, was the lessee (fig. 5b). They are highly compartmentalized compositions, relatively flat in relief; but within its borders each compartment breaks out into a rash of arabesques and strapwork patterns, with the occasional naturalistic flowerpiece or portrait medallion reserved for the sides or corners. The manner is too stiff to be connected with the real Rococo that was shortly afterwards to triumph in the great London *palazzi* of Chesterfield House or Norfolk House, and it may in part reflect surviving plasterers' traditions from an earlier period. This is not to say that Edward Shepherd could not turn out disciplined, dignified plasterwork when required to. The vaulting over the stairs at No. 66 Brook Street (Plate 9a), perhaps done specially for Sir Nathaniel Curzon, and the ceilings at No. 74 South Audley Street, originally the Portuguese ambassador's house (fig. 5c), are at once deeper in relief, severer in conception, and more gracious than his average production. Still more 'correct' is the plasterwork in the long gallery at No. 12 North Audley Street, the house that Shepherd probably built for Lord Ligonier and one of the outstanding survivals on the estate (Plate 11). Here Ligonier had a tripartite single-storey gallery built for himself at the back, very possibly designed by the Irish architect Edward Pearce; but though its proportions, plaster vaulting and engaged columns show a restraining hand at work, there are still traces of Shepherd's florid manner. At No. 72 Brook Street, his own house, some hint of his idiosyncrasies also survives, despite much alteration. It should be added that Shepherd can have had no monopoly of high-class plasterwork. The two houses leased to William Singleton at Nos. 12 and 13 South Audley Street included accomplished plaster decorations (Plate 9c; fig. 5a), while much elaborate work of which we now know nothing must originally have been executed for houses in Grosvenor Square.

The last feature of these early Mayfair interiors that remains to be singled out is the treatment of the 'great stair'. As the most formal part of the house, the staircase had to be handled with fitting pomp. Up to this time, main staircases in enclosed town houses had usually been of wood, but the Grosvenor estate shows the joiner beginning to give ground to the mason and the smith. Here they were often built of stone, the steps cantilevered out from the wall and cut away on their undersides, with hand-wrought iron balustrades in simple, attractive patterns (fig. 6). There are good surviving examples in each of the three traditional staircase positions at Nos. 33 and 34 Grosvenor Street (Plate 9b; fig. 6c, f) and No. 16 Upper Grosvenor Street (fig. 6d). With a front compartment staircase, this might make part of a considerable architectural composition. Over the stairs would come an ornamental plaster ceiling (Nos. 14 and 74 South Audley Street, 34 and 59 Grosvenor Street, 20 Upper Brook Street), or even a plaster vault (No. 66 Brook Street). Sometimes this plasterwork was extended to the walls, as at No. 13 South Audley Street, where the decoration has been comparatively recently destroyed (Plate 9c). An inventory records similar treatment at No. 6 Grosvenor Square, and at No. 34 Grosvenor Street the lessee Richard Lissiman agreed in 1728 with Sir Paul Methuen, the intending occupant, 'to wainscoat the Staircase with Oak, in the same manner as the Staircase is wainscoated, in the house where Sir Thomas Hanmer now lives [No. 52 Grosvenor Street]. And...to cover all that part of the Staircase and Sealing above it, that is plaisterd, with Ornaments of Stucco, to the Satisfaction of Sir Paul.'[25] However this was evidently not done in exact accord with the agreement, for the surviving staircase at No. 34 Grosvenor Street, a fine and authentic example, is wainscotted from head to toe in elegantly elongated panels, with the plasterwork confined to the ceiling (fig. 5d).

Another and more dramatic alternative was to fresco the stairs. How common this was we do not know, but it was probably fairly regular in the 1720's and 1730's, having been done often enough in country houses since 1660, and having acquired a new impetus in London after William Kent painted the great stair at Kensington Palace. It certainly required craftsmen of ability, but they are usually anonymous. Israel Russell, a 'painter-stainer' who was one of the original lessees of some of the houses, may have specialized in this direction; another

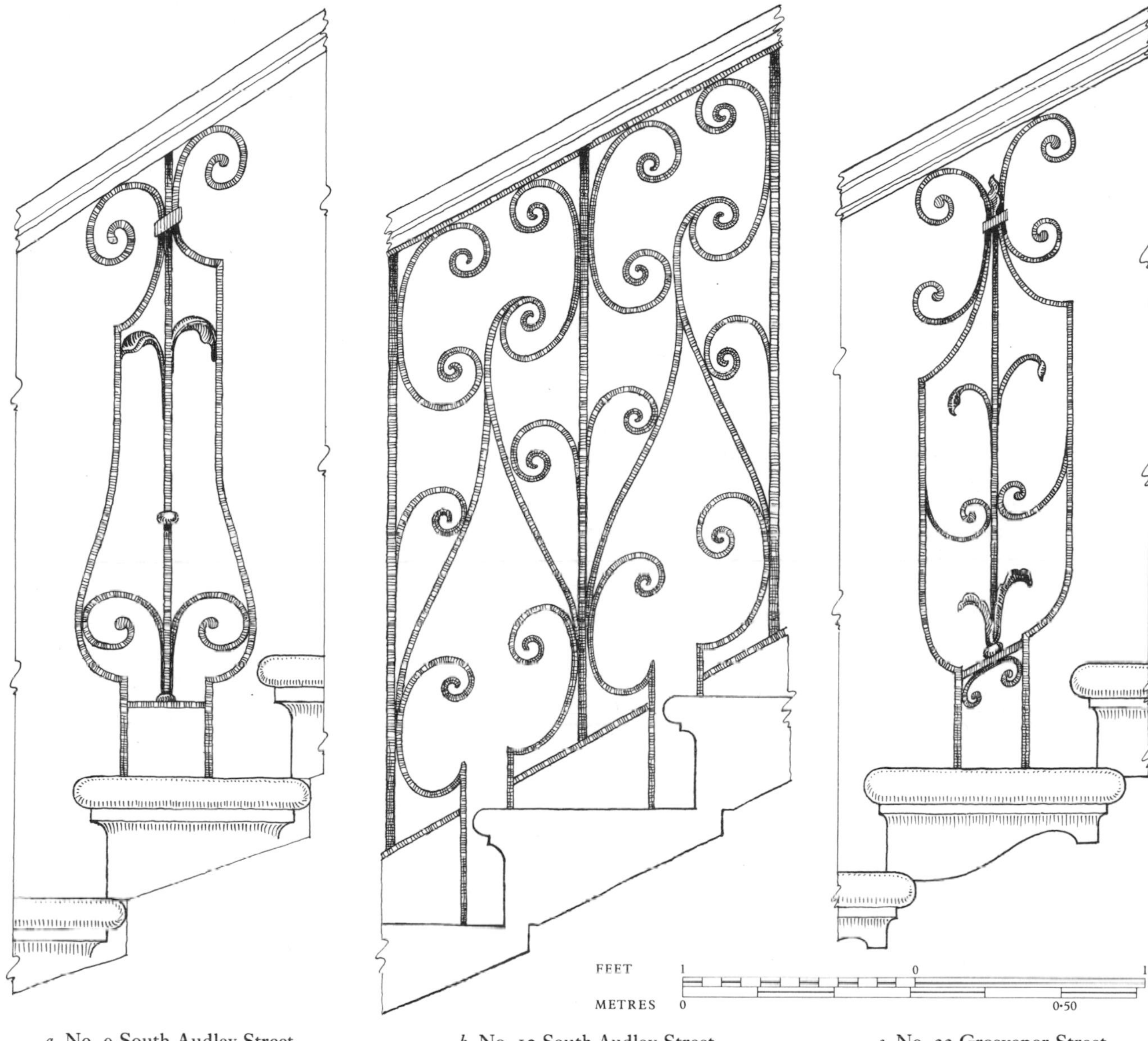

a. No. 9 South Audley Street *b*. No. 10 South Audley Street *c*. No. 33 Grosvenor Street

Fig. 6. WROUGHT-IRON BALUSTRADES FROM EARLY-GEORGIAN STAIRCASES

possibility is Mark Antony Hauduroy, who had worked with Shepherd at Chandos House and lived in one of his houses at No. 11 North Audley Street. A charming figurative staircase mural, found at No. 44 Grosvenor Square, was removed to the Victoria and Albert Museum before the destruction of that house. An attribution of this fresco has been made to John Laguerre, son of Louis Laguerre, and seems the more convincing in so far as an inventory of 1750 for No. 48 Grosvenor Street informs us that the 'Great Stair Case' was 'Wainscotted Rail'd high with Oak and the rest painted in a Composed Order with figures and Trophies done by John Legare'. Several of the other houses, especially in the square, must have had painted staircases, though none survives; besides those mentioned, inventories allude to long-lost examples at Nos. 45 Grosvenor Square and 29 Grosvenor Square, the latter 'painted in Architecture and History'.[26]

To round off this discussion of the interiors of the great Grosvenor estate houses, the reader is referred to Appendix II, where he will find the full text of one of the several inventories mentioned above, that of 1733 for No. 45 Grosvenor Square. This will provide some idea of the typical positions, names and uses of the smaller rooms, as well as of the basic fixtures and fittings of such a house.

A few general comments can be added about the gardens

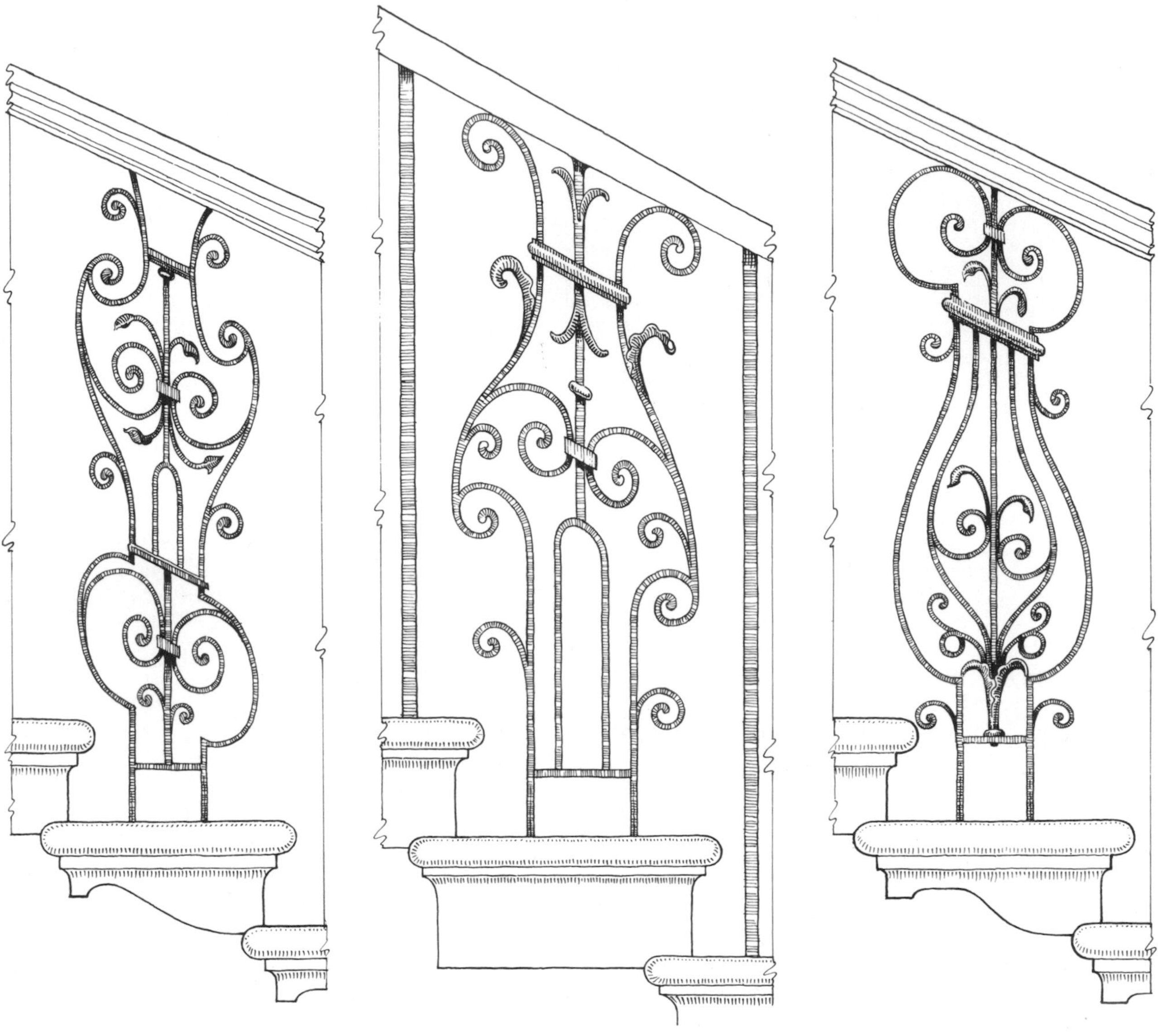

d. No. 16 Upper Grosvenor Street

e. Dudley House, Park Lane (basement stairs, from older house)

f. No. 34 Grosvenor Street

of these large houses. Sutton Nicholls's engraving of Grosvenor Square (Plate 5a) gives an idealized representation, showing in each back garden numerous straight gravel walks enclosing small grass plots or flower beds, with espaliered fruit trees against the walls, a few minor shrubs here and there, and the occasional architectural feature at the back to disguise a stable block. Though this picture of seventeenth-century formality may be misleading in many respects, it demonstrates that these town-house gardens were no mere plain and functional backyards. Even where a basement extended behind the main house, a proper garden could from early on be had, as an inventory of 1799 for No. 16 Grosvenor Street shows; here the yard is described as 'covered with Lead Clayed and Gravelled for Garden'.[27] Yet another inventory, this time of 1742 for a house on the south side of Grosvenor Street, shows that the 'features' too were no mere figment of the imagination, for here there could be found 'an Alcove at the end of Garden after the dorick order covered with lead, the alcove back and sides wainscotted quarter round and raised pannells with a seat, Portland pavement before ditto'.[28]

Flowers in abundance were certainly common and, as time went on, so were fair-sized trees. Sir Thomas Hanmer's accounts of 1726–9 for No. 52 Grosvenor Street itemize several payments for tending flowers to gardeners

(one of whom was French), and include a note to pay one man more 'when the flowers appear to be right in number and kinds'.[18] So too in 1734 Mrs. Delany, keeping her provincial sister up to date with details about her modest (but surviving) house at No. 48 Upper Brook Street, could write: 'You think, madam, that I have no garden, perhaps? but that's a mistake; I *have one* as big as your parlour in Gloucester, and in it groweth *damask-roses*, *stocks* variegated and plain, some purple, some red, *pinks*, *Philaria*, some dead some alive; and *honeysuckles* that never blow'.[29] And in 1748 Fanny Boscawen of No. 14 South Audley Street was boasting that 'my garden is in the best order imaginable, and planted with 100 shrubs and flowers'. Half a century later, still living in the same house, Mrs. Boscawen could in the more picturesque spirit of the age go further: ''tis well I have some trees, whose leaves wave close by me, and that about me I behold purple lilacs, white lilacs, and yellow laburnums in my own or my neighbours' gardens, and no bricks or tiles'.[30] How mature Mrs. Boscawen's trees were is hard to say, but they were probably bigger than the trees which in 1763 William Chambers was advising his client at No. 25 Grosvenor Square to trim and nail up against the wind, in a garden which contained wooden 'lattice work', that is presumably trellises for espaliers against the walls.[31] So from quite early days, there was a fair amount of variety, colour and greenery in all these gardens and by the end of the eighteenth century precious little austerity, if the Boscawen case is at all typical.

Finally, something must be said of the few larger buildings that interrupted the estate's original pattern of regular terrace housing. Here and there, especially west of Grosvenor Square, a few individual houses of size did spring up. Among these, pride of place must go to the freestanding house built in about 1730 for Lord Chetwynd in Upper Grosvenor Street near its west end. Though it was to become the future Grosvenor House little is known of its original appearance, except that Porden characterized the interiors as being in 'a heavy, antiquated, but respectable stile'.[32] This was written in 1805, just before the Grosvenors began their transformation of the house; at that time it was a sizeable, symmetrical villa in plan, set back some ninety feet from the south side of the street at the rear of a court with a narrow street entrance. In this respect it was like some of the large noblemen's houses that still in part survive on the north side of Piccadilly, but instead of having office wings flanking the court, the side plots were let off, so that the house must have been inconspicuous from the street. In the later eighteenth century other big houses were to be built close to the park in this western sector, but for nearly thirty years Lord Chetwynd's house stood alone.

For the largest surviving individual house of early date on the estate one must look further north, to No. 61 Green Street, later known as Hampden House. This was the home of the Palladian architect Roger Morris. Of the Palladians who were involved in the estate development, Colen Campbell has already been discussed; Thomas Ripley built a very large house that survives in altered form at No. 16 Grosvenor Street but does not seem to have varied greatly in elevation from the estate norm; and William Benson may have been responsible for two small lost houses in Grosvenor Street of which, however, little is known. But Morris was evidently more ambitious on his own behalf. The result was the big brick house and spacious garden, dating from 1730, that survive at the east end of Green Street. This was then a relatively open position, with a few sizeable houses nearby in North Audley Street, some smaller but seemingly detached houses mainly belonging to other builders on either side of Morris's plot, and empty land close by on the north and west. It is now a gaunt and much altered building on both elevation and plan, but the slightly recessed wings and high central rooms of this seven-bay house still bear witness to Morris's ambition and wealth. By contrast, at the south end of Davies Street stands a much quainter survival, Bourdon House (Plate 12a). Built in about 1721–3 and therefore one of the earliest of houses on the estate, it still despite alterations and an added top storey keeps its modest brick character, with a south-facing pediment looking down on what must once have been the main approach, through a rather deeper front garden than now exists. Within, the interior has retained an early Georgian flavour almost better than any other house on the estate, and there is some excellent original woodwork in the 'ante-dining room' (Plate 10b).

These are the main early houses independent of any terrace arrangement of which something is known. There is little to add about the estate's few public buildings. Since there was originally no market, these really comprise only two, the parish workhouse that stood until 1886 on the south side of Mount Street, and the Grosvenor Chapel in South Audley Street. The workhouse, erected by Benjamin Timbrell and Thomas Phillips in 1725–6, was a functional and capacious building which could accommodate 160 persons and ran to no elaboration except a central cupola. The chapel (Plate 12b; fig. 7), erected in 1730–1, also involved Timbrell (with Robert Scott as fellow carpenter and William Barlow senior as bricklayer), and this is the more interesting since it bears distinct resemblances to James Gibbs's Oxford Chapel (St. Peter's, Vere Street) on which Timbrell had worked a few years before. Both are simple auditoria of similar length having galleries on three sides, with groined plaster vaults over the aisles and a curved ceiling to the nave, and on the outside two tiers of windows along the sides, and pedimented and turretted western features. A comparison is instructive, as it shows the difference in fluency between the work of the specialist architect and that of the master builder; but though the Grosvenor Chapel is second best in most respects and has been more altered than St. Peter's, its quaint steeple at the termination of Aldford Street provides one of the few minor features of town planning in the estate layout. Of original interior

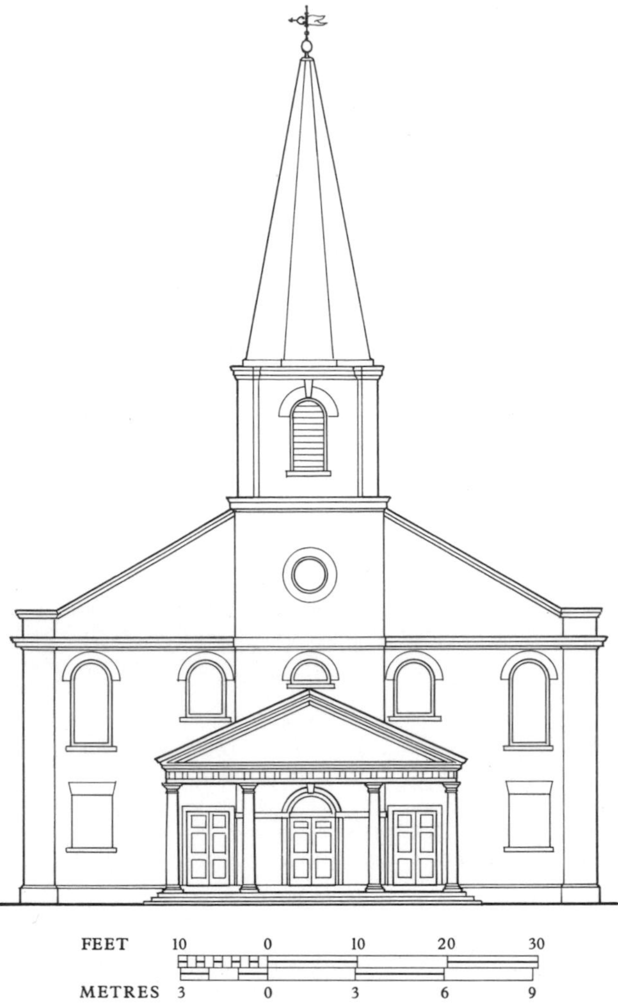

Fig. 7. Grosvenor Chapel, west front as originally built in 1730–1

fittings it still retains its old stairs to the gallery, some pleasant panelling and plasterwork, an organ and a pulpit, but much else has been changed in subsequent restorations.

First Changes

Since the plots at the western end of the Mayfair estate were slow to let, a date at which the original development was finished is hard to pinpoint. Beyond Park Street building proceeded very spasmodically, especially in the north-west. Though little of the old fabric in this sector survives in recognizable form, one or two characteristics can be determined. Where rows of houses were built, they deviated little from the norm. Park Lane, then an unimpressive thoroughfare with a high wall on the park side, was reached at one point by the early 1730's, when King's Row, an ordinary set of small houses, was built at the end of Upper Grosvenor Street on the site of the present Nos. 93–99 (consec.) Park Lane. The lane in fact presented a considerable problem to would-be developers, since the original estate grid had taken no account of its irregular course; plots west of Park Street, therefore, were of very variable size. Towards the south end of the estate, between Mount Street and South Street, the houses on the west side of Park Street occupied deep plots running right through to Park Lane, so the inhabitants certainly, and the houses probably, were of quality, but none of the fabric here remains.

Further north in Green Street, there is equally scant record of the appearance of the terrace houses; surviving lease plans show the usual variety of plan-type here, which suggests irregularities too in the elevations. A chapel was built at the south-east corner of Green Street and Park Street (1762), but it also was of small architectural significance. In Norfolk Street (now Dunraven Street), developed in the late 1750's with a good class of house, especially on the west side, there was again little or no uniformity. The survivors here, though much altered, do provide some idea of the original scale and quality. The houses on the west side are not deep, since Park Lane is close behind, but they are reasonably wide, often with a frontage of thirty feet or more; Nos. 21 and 22 Dunraven Street, the only ones for which old plans are known but probably reasonable guides for several others, had front compartment staircases and canted bays at the back. It must be emphasized that because Park Lane was at this date so inconsiderable, these rear bays facing towards the park were quite simple and cannot have been thought of as alternative fronts. King's Row, the only terrace actually entered from the lane itself, had completely flat fronts at this date, sheltered behind a screen of trees (Plate 13a, b). In the 1750's and '60's very little new development occurred on the estate, except in Norfolk Street, already mentioned, and Portugal Street, a short thoroughfare between Mount Street and Chapel (now Aldford) Street, on the line of what is now Balfour Place, where a few modest but well-inhabited houses were erected. Then in 1773 began the construction of Hereford Street, marking the completion of the ordinary estate development. This street, running west from close to the northern end of Park Street beyond North Row, has been entirely obliterated; it occupied a large part of the site of the present Hereford House, but was quite distinct from development along the south side of the Oxford Road. Even at this late date, the old pattern of individuality was scarcely disrupted, with a number of houses on the north side of different extent and, presumably, appearance. But for the south side of Hereford Street the architect and speculator was John Crunden (1740–1835), a capable designer in the Adam manner, and responsible for Boodle's Club in St. James's Street at just about this date. Along the main frontage Crunden erected a series of high-class houses with what were probably quite conventional façades except at No. 13, which boasted a pediment, perhaps because it was the only house visible from Oxford Street. But on the return frontage to Park Street,

illustrated in one of Soane's lecture diagrams (Plate 13c), he attempted something more ambitious, a group of three houses with fronts of stucco or stone, the central one having touches of attenuated classical detail and a pediment. Crunden lived in the corner house with Hereford Street, and the centre house was Mrs. Fitzherbert's.

It was on this western part of the estate that there also arose a number of big houses distinct from any terrace arrangement, which were to be the precursors of the later Park Lane palaces. The first of these, Lord Chetwynd's house in Upper Grosvenor Street, has already been mentioned (page 118). Close by were the Park Lane mansions of Lord Petre (later Breadalbane House) and of Lord Dudley, the latter on the northern half of the site occupied by the present Dudley House. Both were five-bay houses, with high but plain brick façades, as befitted what was still a modest right of way of little pretension. Breadalbane House, designed in 1769 by James Paine with a complicated plan because of its restricted site, had the advantage over Dudley House of a pair of brief recessed wings (Plate 13b). Abutting Dudley House to the south, at the corner with modern Culross Street, stood another substantial house in an up-to-date Palladian style, shown on an aquatint of 1801 (Plate 13a). This engraving well conveys the ragged but not unattractive medley of backs and fronts which made up this part of Park Lane at that date.

Higher up and closer to Oxford Street, there was space for more large houses, but they took longer to get under way: Sir Thomas Robinson advised Lord Bute in 1762 against building a house here or on the Portland estate north of Oxford Street on the grounds that it was 'too farr either from publick business or publick pleasure'.[33] John Phillips the master carpenter eventually took a large area here, and was responsible for Lord Bateman's house, later Somerset House, erected in 1769–70 on a site now covered by part of Nos. 139–140 Park Lane, and probably for the building of Thomas Pitt's Camelford House (1773–4) on a site squeezed in between this and the Hereford Street development. Despite their proximity, they were dissimilar houses. Somerset House (Plate 14b) was very much a builder's house, always asymmetrical and probably never distinguished in elevation, without a particularly grand front even towards the park. But the owner of Camelford House, Thomas Pitt, was an amateur architect of accomplishment and an intimate of the young John Soane; so his house was of some moment, though inconspicuous from Oxford Street or Park Lane. A self-conscious late-Palladian villa (Plate 14a), it boasted a courtyard before it like that at Lord Chetwynd's house, canted bays at front and back, a strictly symmetrical plan, and able neo-classical interiors.

With these houses of the western sector, the names of well-known architects begin at last to crop up. But before Paine, Crunden or others had been active here, the houses in and around Grosvenor Square were already undergoing alteration. Hardly a noble family would change its London abode in the eighteenth century without manifold rearrangements and re-upholsterings, and these often involved architects. As early as 1743 Henry Flitcroft was undertaking works at No. 4 Grosvenor Square for the Earl of Malton, who had just moved in; this was to be followed by a series of improvements up to 1764, when the ageing architect superintended the stuccoing of the back of the house. This was the kind of job that one might expect to have been undertaken by an architect of the younger generation, William Chambers or his great rival Robert Adam. In fact in 1763 Chambers, just then building his fine early villa for the Earl of Abercorn at Duddingston, did also renovate the Earl's town house at No. 25 Grosvenor Square. This was often how high-class architects came to be involved in houses on the Grosvenor estate, altering them in sometimes quite trifling respects following more important country house work for the same client. Adam was in the field straight after Chambers in 1764–5 with a larger job, the internal updating for the Earl of Thanet of the stately No. 19 Grosvenor Square, the pedimented house by Edward Shepherd on the north side (Plates 15b, 17a, b). Each architect went on to cap the other's work with further commissions in the square, Chambers by redecorating No. 20 in 1767 for the Duke of Buccleuch, Adam with what amounted to a rebuilding of No. 26 for Lord Stanley (later the Earl of Derby) in 1773–4: this was the famous Derby House. Chambers also worked at No. 28 Grosvenor Street, while the Adam brothers were involved in one capacity or another at Nos. 5, 12 and 28 Grosvenor Square, at No. 16 Grosvenor Street (Plate 16b), at Claudius Amyand's house on the corner of Berkeley Square and Mount Street (Plate 15c), and perhaps too at No. 75 South Audley Street, the town house of Robert's great Scottish patron Lord Bute. The Adams' list is the longer not just because of their popularity or their better documentation but also because they were well placed to cultivate their contacts; from 1758 to 1771 they lived at No. 76 Grosvenor Street, a house which they appear to have altered but which is now long demolished.

By the turn of the century, plenty of well-known architects had acted in alterations of one kind or another. Thus John Vardy spent lavishly at No. 37 Grosvenor Square for the Duke of Bolton (1761); Robert Taylor appears to have rebuilt No. 33 Upper Brook Street (fig. 8b) in about 1768; the shadowy Kenton Couse made alterations at two houses in Grosvenor Square, in 1774–5 at No. 2 and in both 1764–5 and 1774–5 at No. 29; Henry Holland worked with his early partner Capability Brown at No. 75 South Audley Street (*c.* 1775) and, it seems, alone at Bourdon House (*c.* 1783); the less-known George Shakespear made changes at No. 41 Upper Brook Street in 1776–7; James Playfair added a gallery at No. 34 Grosvenor Square for Sir George Beaumont (1790); John Nash was supervising work at No. 34 Grosvenor Street (1798); and John Soane was in almost constant employment on major or minor estate works, the chief of them being the gradual internal reconstruction of No. 49 Grosvenor Square (1797

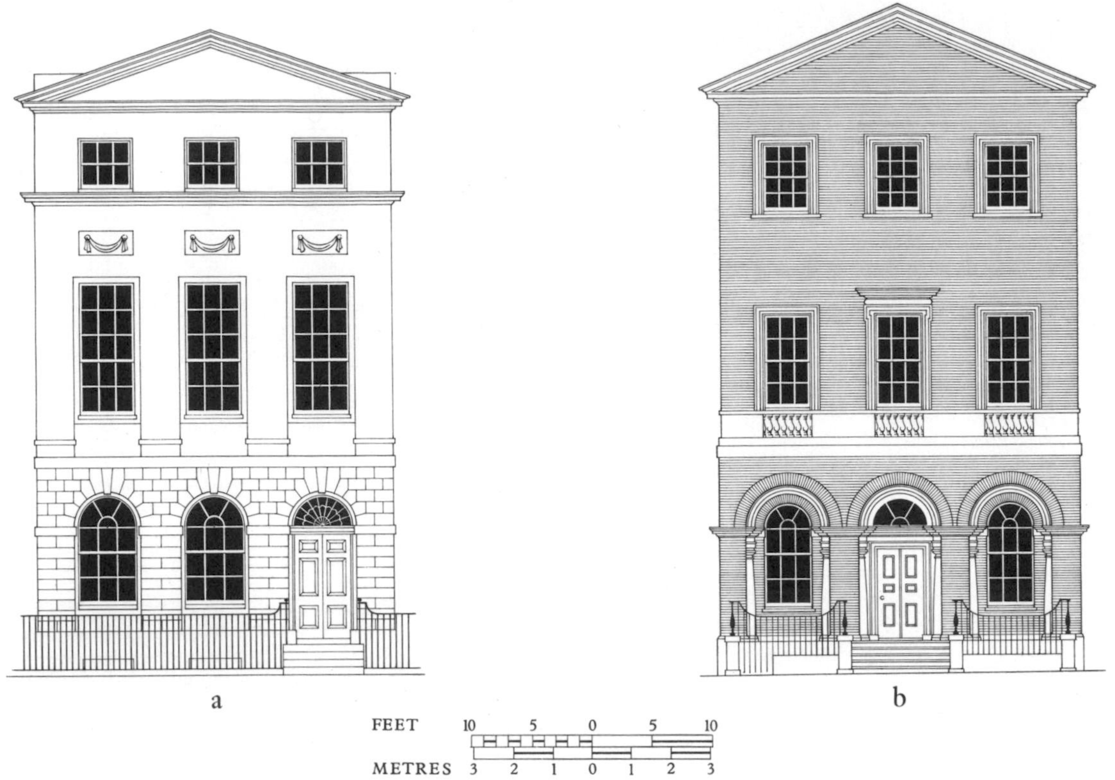

Fig. 8. MID-GEORGIAN ELEVATIONS

a. No. 6 Upper Brook Street. *Architect*, Samuel Wyatt, 1787–9. *Demolished*
b. No. 33 Upper Brook Street. *Architect*, probably Robert Taylor, *c*. 1768. *Now without pediment*

onwards). Soane, the best documented of these architects, had dealings with at least seventeen different houses on the estate in the course of his long career, and a similar intensity of practice hereabouts may be presumed for others. Frequently they were working simply as surveyors, valuing properties, bargaining on behalf of their clients, or acting as estate agents. A document of the 1740's at the Drawings Collection of the Royal Institute of British Architects in the hand of the architect John Sanderson describes and gives rough plans of a number of town houses, several of them on the Grosvenor estate, which he had evidently looked over on behalf of an intending purchaser;[34] rather later, Robert Mylne's illuminating diary is full of little entries mentioning visits to houses in a similar capacity,[35] while some letters of P. F. Robinson show that as late as the 1800's it was still common for eminent architects to find town houses for their customers.[36] Holland, Soane, S. P. Cockerell and Wyatville are all also recorded as 'acting' for clients in negotiations with the Grosvenor Office, no doubt usually in hope of rather than in connexion with more remunerative work.

One architect whose work on the estate is worth more than passing attention is Samuel Wyatt, who until recently has lived in the shadow of his brother James's greater reputation. In the earlier and more thorough period of his career James Wyatt did indeed work on two major houses in Grosvenor Square, No. 16 for William Drake of Shardeloes (1773–4) and the larger No. 41 for the dissolute Peter Delmé (1778), and made minor alterations at a third, the Grosvenors' own No. 45 (1783–4). Both No. 16 and No. 41 had ornamental ceilings of the new Adam type, and No. 41 was one of the first houses to have its front stuccoed in Higgins's patent cement. Having been his brother's reliable assistant and principal contractor in these two houses and in several other jobs, Samuel Wyatt struck out on his own in the late 1770's, with great success. Thus on the Grosvenor estate he is found in 1778 stuccoing the basement of No. 66 Brook Street with Higgins's cement for Assheton Curzon, the brother of Wyatt's first patron under Adam at Kedleston Hall.[37] In the ensuing period he acted in at least three lease renewals, altered one house (the western of the two on the site of No. 10 Grosvenor Square, in 1801–3), and virtually reconstructed two others (No. 6 Upper Brook Street for William Weddell in 1787–9 and No. 45 Grosvenor Square for Lord Petre in 1803–6). Weddell's house was of the greatest interest; having employed Adam to remodel his country seat at Newby Hall, for his town

house he opted for the versatility and practicality of Samuel Wyatt. Wyatt seems to have excelled himself, achieving some ingenious interiors behind a stone pedimented front of only three bays (fig. 8a). He even earned himself the hyperbolic title of the 'wonder-working Chip' from a friend of Weddell's, whose surviving letters enthuse, as work proceeds, over 'the fine curve of the Trunk Cieling in the sky light', 'the light and airy look of the Eating room with the new circular end behind the columns', and finally, 'the Chip's new invented design for lighting the staircase, a fanciful *Machine*, that pours forth such a blaze of glory, that the Sun in it's meridian splendor will shew to it but as a *rush light*'.[38] Of all this interior work there is now no record except a few photographs of detail (Plate 17d), but they are enough to show that No. 6 Upper Brook Street was exceptional, even within Wyatt's *oeuvre*.

Like that house, nearly all the results of this first epoch of alterations have been swept away today. There is nothing recognizably by the Adams left on the estate, nothing by Chambers, just one room with characteristics of Holland's touch at Bourdon House, a few presumed fragments of the work of Brown and Holland at No. 75 South Audley Street, and little by the assiduous Soane except for a balcony and parts of a porch at No. 22 Dunraven Street (Plate 19c). However there are two major mid-Georgian survivals, No. 33 Upper Brook Street, a rebuilding of *c.* 1768 almost certainly by Robert Taylor for John Boyd of Danson Park, and No. 38 Grosvenor Square, a reconstruction of *c.* 1780 done so much in Samuel Wyatt's manner that an attribution to him is hard to resist. These houses are very different but equally important. No. 33 Upper Brook Street shows what could occur when updated Palladianism was applied to a modest three-bay house of little depth. Taylor reorganized the façade (fig. 8b) by putting the door in the centre, setting it and its flanking windows between small engaged columns carrying semi-circular heads, emphasizing the first floor with a sparing use of ornamental dressings, and topping the house with a neat pediment (now obliterated). Inside, the ground floor had to be limited to just two units, a spacious plaster-vaulted entrance hall and stairs, and a large octagonal room behind. Because this kind of arrangement left little compass for manoeuvre, mid-Georgian architects more frequently adhered to the basic lopsidedness of the town-house plans that they inherited. That is what occurred at No. 38 Grosvenor Square, where a front compartment staircase may have been removed, and a deep back wing with windows to the side was certainly added, stretching right through to the stable block and ending with a private stair between the suites of the master and mistress of the house (fig. 9c). This wing was plastered over, and so also in all probability was the front to the square, since rebuilt. At the same time the interior was gutted throughout and refashioned with features of greater delicacy and lightness: a stone staircase with a lively iron balustrade and oval toplight, drawing-rooms with voluptuous marble chimneypieces (Plate 17c), and plasterwork ceilings incorporating inset allegories painted in the fashionable manner of the Carracci (Plate 16c).

Such also, to judge from plans, was the character of Samuel Wyatt's No. 45 Grosvenor Square, and also of Derby House, Robert Adam's great masterpiece at No. 26 Grosvenor Square. Here again in both houses was a main central staircase generously toplit, and a long rear wing with a bow culminating in a private stair (fig. 9a, b). All three of these houses, in fact, betray the new preference for central stairs; the days of the front compartment staircase were over by 1770 and would not return. But at Derby House, with that extra conviction and fertility that separate him from his followers, Adam transformed the resulting sequence of straightforward rooms, each in itself symmetrical, into an eventful suite, by introducing circular and oval apartments and by blurring the contours of the other rooms with bowed ends, niches, vaults and pillared screens, so producing the effects of light and shade dramatized in Pastorini's famous perspective of the third drawing-room (Plate 15a). The intention to create such a suite even within the confines of a terrace house of fifty-foot frontage, despite attendant difficulties, is confirmed by the commentary on Adam's published plans, which refers to Derby House as 'an attempt to arrange the apartments in the French style, which... is best calculated for the convenience and elegance of life...The smallness of the scites upon which most London houses are built, obliges the artists of this country to arrange the apartments of the ladies and gentlemen upon two floors. Accordingly Lord Derby's are placed on the parlour story: the French, in their great *hôtels*, with their usual attention to what is agreeable and commodious, would introduce both these apartments upon the principal floor; but this we can only do in our country-houses, where our space is unconfined.'[39] So by 1773 French influence was already beginning to invade the London terrace house.

Adam's published plans of Derby House (fig. 9a) show also that the function of rooms was becoming more specified. As in some earlier houses, the kitchen was to be found here in the basement of the stable block facing inwards towards the paved court; because of smells, noise, and the danger of fire, such a position or one actually under the garden was to become standard in all subsequent rearrangements. In the main block of Derby House the reception rooms consisted of a 'great eating room' and library downstairs, and three drawing-rooms above, with appropriate antechambers on each floor. The private suites in the rear part of the wing referred to above, were a survival from the days of the 'great apartment', a concept ably explained in Fowler and Cornforth's *English Decoration in the 18th Century* (1974); they are a reminder that intimate friends would be received as a matter of course in these more sequestered parts of the house. One further point about Derby House,

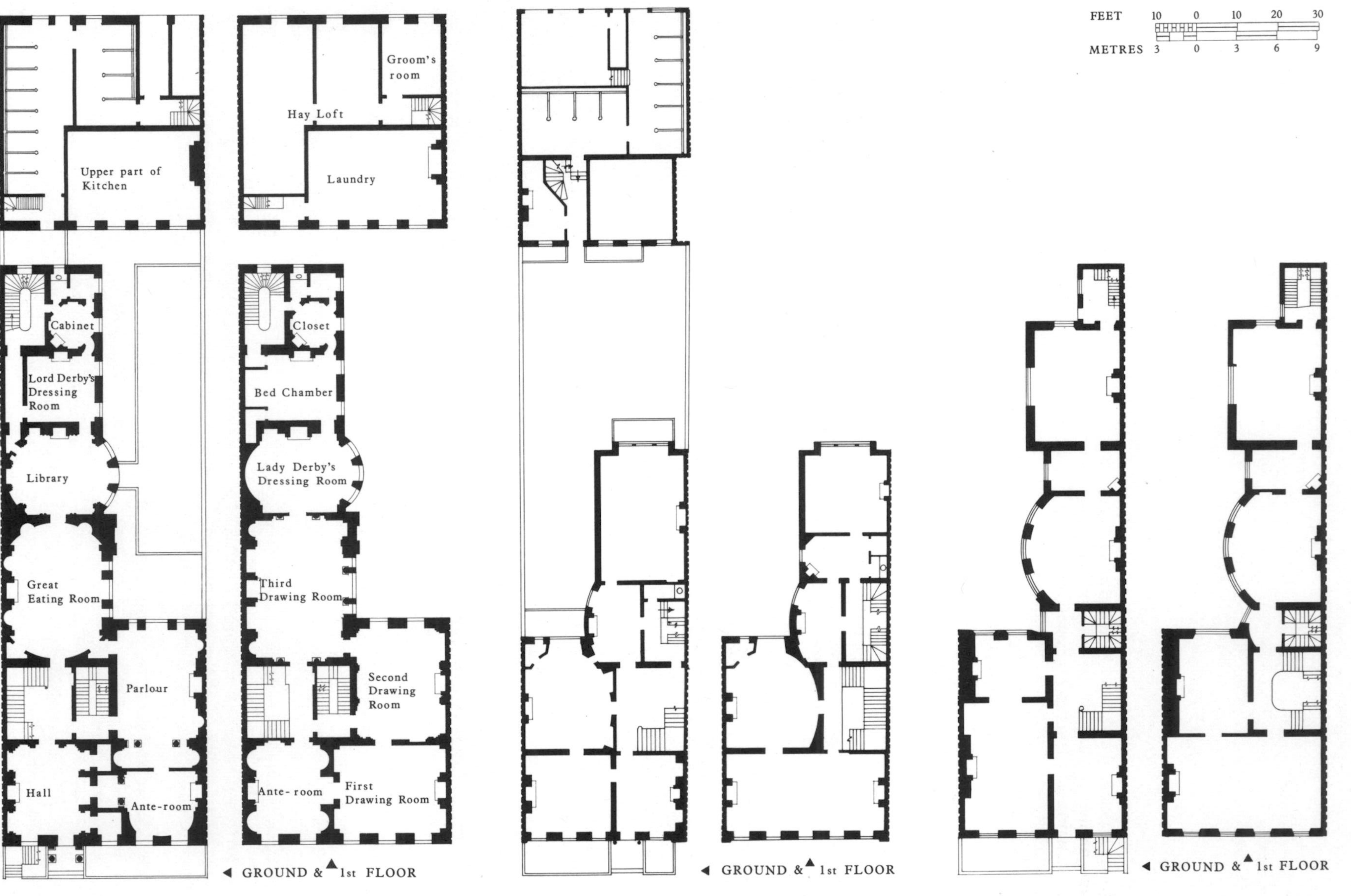

a. No. 26 Grosvenor Square. *Architect for reconstruction*, Robert Adam, 1773–4. *Demolished*

b. No. 45 Grosvenor Square. *Architect for reconstruction*, Samuel Wyatt, 1803–6. *Demolished*

c. No. 38 Grosvenor Square. *Architect for reconstruction unknown*, *c*. 1780

Fig. 9. MID- AND LATE-GEORGIAN GROUND- AND FIRST-FLOOR PLANS

originally made by Soane in his Royal Academy lectures, is worth repeating; the front elevation was scarcely altered by Adam and retained its modest brick early-Georgian character, in token of the proud 'disregard to external appearance' of which English noblemen liked to boast.[40]

The 'Adam' style of interior decoration, exemplified by Derby House, looks radically new when compared with the efforts of Shepherd and his contemporaries. But there had certainly been a transition. Paine's ceiling design for the drawing-room of Lord Petre's Park Lane house (Plate 16a), published in the second volume of his *Plans, Elevations and Sections of Noblemen and Gentlemen's Houses*, combines the old deep compartments with a single painted roundel of the new type in the centre, and there is still a certain floridity to Adam's early ceiling designs such as that for Lord Hertford's drawing-room at No. 16 Grosvenor Street (Plate 16b). Nevertheless, the new style embodied archaeological sophistication of a kind that had been rare in earlier town houses. Not all designers could pick up its every resonance, but they were at least aware that a novel self-consciousness and unity were expected of their decorative schemes. This entailed the ousting of the heavy panelling that had been the hallmark of the original houses and a new supremacy for the more delicate skills of plasterer, painter, gilder, paperhanger, and last but not least, upholsterer.

Apart from a few master builders like Benjamin Timbrell and Edward Shepherd, the craftsmen responsible for the estate's original development remain shadowy figures. For the later Georgian period we are rather better informed. High-class architects like the Adams or the Wyatts brought with them experienced men whose practice was by no means exclusively metropolitan and who were no mere tradesmen. A few of them indeed appear to have enjoyed something of a monopoly within their trade. Thus the name of John Deval, mason (both father and son), appears in connexion with alterations at no less than five houses in Grosvenor Square (Nos. 2, 4, 16, 18 and 29) between 1736 and 1775, that is to say for almost all the houses in the square for which we have full records of work during the period. Sometimes this family firm was acting as mason-contractors, sometimes as specialized sculptors.

Another equally well-known name that constantly crops up is that of the great plastering concern of the two Joseph Roses. In 1764 Flitcroft was enthusing over the care taken by the elder Joseph Rose in stuccoing the back of No. 4 Grosvenor Square, which he thought would be 'an Example worthy of Imitation Mr Rose having taken great care in Chusing and mixing the materialls for it'.[41] Rose and his nephew went on to work in the 1760's and '70's at Nos. 16, 26, and 29 Grosvenor Square under James Wyatt, Robert Adam and Kenton Couse respectively, and doubtless did jobs at other houses of which we know nothing. By the turn of the century, plasterwork was in general becoming less elaborate, and the Roses had been superseded by men like the William Rothwells, Soane's favourite plasterers, and Francis Bernasconi, who executed large contracts for Samuel Wyatt at No. 45 Grosvenor Square (1803–6) and for William Porden at Grosvenor House (1806–8).

One or two other special craftsmen are worth particular mention. Sefferin Alken was the carver in three of the mid-century jobs in Grosvenor Square already mentioned; Thomas Carter the younger worked as sculptor at No. 16 Grosvenor Square under James Wyatt and also elsewhere; Richard Westmacott the elder sculpted a chimneypiece at No. 41 Upper Brook Street; and John Mackell occurs constantly as a smith in contracts towards the end of the century. The early nineteenth-century bills for No. 45 Grosvenor Square and Grosvenor House include two names which were to become increasingly familiar in the years to come, those of Bramah for water closets and other ironwork at both houses, and of Skidmore for cast iron at Grosvenor House. Men like these were laying the foundation of firms of industrialized craftsmen in the modern sense at about this time. At the opposite end of the scale were the decorative artists, who held a particularly high status and operated more or less on their own; such were Antonio Zucchi who painted door panels at Derby House, and Biagio Rebecca, James Wyatt's choice for ceilings at No. 16 Grosvenor Square.

As elusive as any of these craftsmen but far more important for the history of the estate were the cabinet-makers and upholsterers, ancestors of the modern interior decorator. For obvious reasons, their work hardly survives in town houses at all. Yet because of their concern with the finishings of houses, they dealt directly with clients and frequently wielded much authority. Furnishings in the latest taste might be destined to last perhaps only a very few years before they were supplanted by something more up-to-date. But the lure of a spick-and-span interior was compelling, and certainly more powerful in London, where the proximity of neighbours encouraged rivalries, than in the country. Thus in 1748 we find Mrs. Boscawen rattling on to her absent admiral husband about their new house at No. 14 South Audley Street. 'This afternoon I saw company in my dressing-room for the first time since its being furnished...and everyone admired my apartment, which is indeed a very pretty one and wants nothing but the approbation of its Lord.' Then a little later: 'My house is an hourly expense to me, as you may imagine...My furniture, which is now pretty complete, costs many a penny. So elegant am I, that my fender is a Chinese rail. *Je connais des gens qui portent tellement envie à ma maison et à mes meubles qu'ils en sont presque malades*, and worry their husbands night and day to go out of that odious, beastly house.'[42]

Though Mrs. Boscawen's letters mention papers, hangings, chintzes, muslins, carpets and mattings galore, she includes only one craftsman's name, that of the famous early paperhanger Thomas Bromwich. In its later forms,

firstly Bromwich, Isherwood and Bradley, later Isherwood and Company, this firm also made papers for No. 29 Grosvenor Square (1777), No. 45 Grosvenor Square (1784) and for Grosvenor House (1807–8). In the later eighteenth century, wallpaper, as a cheaper and daintier background material, was increasing in popularity against hangings, and was available for quite humble houses. Surviving records of Joseph Trollope of Westminster reveal his firm at about the turn of the century papering houses of varying status, from Nos. 49 and 34 Grosvenor Street (the latter under Nash's guidance) to an evidently small house in South Audley Street, where Trollope was asked to 'take coals in return'.[43]

While very little is known of the earliest upholsterers who worked on the estate, the bills for alterations in houses in Grosvenor Square are soon full of the names of the most eminent concerns of the day: Vile and Cobb at No. 4 Grosvenor Square (1775 and later); William France, at No. 29 Grosvenor Square (1764); John Bradburn, paid £2576 for work at the Marquis of Carmarthen's house, No. 2 Grosvenor Square, in 1774–5; and Chippendale, for whom posthumous works by his firm are recorded at No. 29 Grosvenor Square (1781–2) and No. 16 Grosvenor Square (1789).

For the display of their wares, cabinet-makers and upholsterers such as these required a proper shop, which tended to be strategically sited, close to fashionable society: Soho, Oxford Street, Bond Street, or increasingly the Grosvenor estate itself. A modicum of high-class trade has always flourished at the east end of Grosvenor Street, and here the firm of William Campbell (later George Campbell), advertised as 'upholders', had premises between 1727 and 1785, the first of several such enterprises in the street. Not far away, on the north side of Berkeley Square (the only side on the Grosvenor estate), John Linnell, in succession to his father William Linnell, ran his famous workshops from 1763 until 1796. From here he was excellently placed to supply furniture to the local houses of the great, for example No. 16 Grosvenor Square in 1773–4, and No. 4 Grosvenor Square in 1776 and 1782–3. As a subcontracting carver to the building concern of John Phillips and George Shakespear, Linnell is likely to have done much other work on the estate. Then in Mount Street nearby was the establishment of William Marsh (Elward and Marsh), another celebrated upholsterer who from about 1795 was in partnership with Thomas Tatham, a close associate and legatee of Linnell. Marsh and Tatham may possibly have inherited the goodwill of Linnell's business. In the firm's later incarnations as Tatham and Bailey, later Tatham, Bailey and Saunders, it became one of the dominating forces in the world of decoration, and included in its orbit two architects, C. H. Tatham, Thomas's brother, who lived for several years on the estate but is not known to have done substantial work hereabouts, and John Linnell Bond, who altered the Tatham and Bailey shop in Mount Street.[44]

By the early nineteenth century, to digress further into the obscure but influential world of these upholsterers, the commercial parts of the Grosvenor estate together with Bond Street had become virtually their most important centre of activity. From *c.* 1795 to 1814 Gillows, the well-known cabinet-makers who decorated the interiors of Grosvenor House and Eaton Hall under William Porden, held a lease of the grand house at Nos. 11–12 North Audley Street, and they retained the yards and workshops behind; these were premises additional to their main Oxford Street shops not far away, on part of the present site of Selfridges. In the next generation Thomas Dowbiggin had by 1816 started his very successful and high-ranking business in Mount Street, not far from Tatham and Bailey. For the following thirty-five years Dowbiggin was to work widely on the estate, sometimes as a speculator, before being absorbed into Holland and Sons, a firm which has only recently disappeared. Lastly, Thomas and George Seddon of Aldersgate Street took and probably greatly altered the large No. 16 Grosvenor Street in 1824 as their West End branch. Houses like this and Nos. 11–12 North Audley Street must have been fitted up not as mere places of work, but as elaborate showrooms. Into such centres these firms could entice the local gentry and nobility and tempt them to extravagance in their own homes.

The extent of upholsterers' work at this time is rarely known except when short-term speculation was involved. The seasonal occupation of fashionable Mayfair houses encouraged firms to buy up leases, refurnish the premises and let them at exorbitant rents for short periods, especially near the end of leasehold terms, a practice which could lead to serious problems (see Appendix III). In 1792 when the parish vestry of St. George's, Hanover Square, debated a rating question, they noted that 'when Gentlemen go into the Country leaving Furniture and a Person in their House (which generally wants more or less Repair every Year) such Gentlemen pay Rates for the whole Year; also that Upholsterers and others who lett Houses ready furnished pay Rates for the whole Year though the Houses may be unlett for a great part of the Time'.[45] One example of such a house was No. 74 Grosvenor Street, for which the reputable cabinet-making concern of Mayhew and Ince are entered in the ratebooks 'for tenants' during the whole of the period 1778–1801; another may be No. 65 Grosvenor Street, where Taprell and Holland, ancestors of the firm of Holland and Sons, are entered between 1833 and 1847. It was a short step from this kind of practice, a perfectly normal one for upholsterers and house agents, to that of early hotels like Mivart's (later Claridge's) in Brook Street, by which an entrepreneur took on contiguous houses and let them to different clients for short periods, not just fully furnished but fully staffed as well.

After the Regency period, the advent of the professional builder began to scale down the broader activities of upholsterers, but in their heyday they are found acting

on the Grosvenor estate as house agents and speculators far more often than architects, and quite frequently also as surveyors. In 1819 when the lease of No. 16 Grosvenor Street (the house eventually taken by the Seddons) came up for renewal, it was reported that 'three upholsterers have applied for the terms, viz Mr Key, Mr Rainy and Mr Johnston'.[46] No more is known of Rainy, but George Key was associated with a good cabinet-maker, Charles Smith, who had a house on the opposite side of Grosvenor Street, while John Johnstone of New Bond Street acted both as a major speculator (he took four houses in Grosvenor Street and one in Upper Brook Street between 1819 and 1824[47]) and also as agent and surveyor for the Duke of Newcastle in 1811, when the Duke was thinking of purchasing No. 75 South Audley Street.[48] Possibly the most ambitious speculator of this type was Charles Elliott, yet another well-known Bond Street upholsterer of high quality. Of the several large houses that Elliott took on, at least three radically altered or rebuilt by him between 1790 and 1810 survive: No. 66 Grosvenor Street, No. 18 Upper Grosvenor Street, and No. 65 Brook Street. One of them, No. 18 Upper Grosvenor Street, still has the appearance of a high-class speculative house of the 1790's, with its stucco façade (Plate 44d), neat central stone staircase, and Adam-style marble fireplaces; to these the original finishings would doubtless have added a spick-and-span flavour.

Of course upholsterers were not alone in such speculations. Since the start of estate development, builders or other tradesmen had often been the holders of head leases, merely subletting to gentry. Now others bought up the ends of leases, especially of houses that were dilapidated. In the period 1797–1819, for instance, a speculator called Bartholomew bought up at least six houses at the Bond Street end of Grosvenor Street in this way, radically improved and relet them.[49] The system frequently provoked dissatisfaction among their clients, who were not too happy to be so dependent upon 'tradesmen'. Thus in 1811 the economist David Ricardo bought No. 56 Upper Brook Street, a small new house built as 'infill' behind Nos. 24 and 25 Grosvenor Square, from the builder Charles Mayor, the original lessee of Nash's Park Crescent and very soon a spectacular bankrupt.[50] Ricardo, ironically disregarding the laws of the market at the whim of his wife and children, paid Mayor what he considered an 'enormous' price and was soon lamenting his decision: 'that Mayor of whom I bought the house was a complete knave, and from the holes in the chimnies, and the communication between them and the beams, he perhaps intended that it should be destroyed by fire, so that no one might ever find out the total insufficiency of the materials to support the house.'[51]

One might think that these were the kinds of difficulty that led to Lord Grosvenor's appointment of an estate surveyor in about 1784. But the evidence is clear that the main brief was financial, to compile an accurate record of property values and to make satisfactory terms when leases were renewed. When in 1778–9 Robert Taylor and George Shakespear were employed by the Estate to survey the area north of Grosvenor Street and east of Davies Street in detail, the purpose cannot have been to see where estate improvements could be effected but to get adequate information about this part of the estate in case of lease-renewals. William Porden, Lord Grosvenor's eventual choice as surveyor, was a relatively unknown architect at the time of his appointment. His selection is possibly a little surprising, since John Jenkins, a local surveyor, had recently been employed in some small family jobs for the Grosvenors; Jenkins had also designed the Grosvenor Market (1784–5), a modest group of houses and shops with a covered way behind, on the triangular stretch of ground at the top of Davies Street and South Molton Lane (the present Boldings site). Porden may have been chosen because he had been a pupil of James Wyatt, who had also been working for Earl Grosvenor, if only in a minor capacity, at his main town house, No. 45 Grosvenor Square. In any case Porden soon proved his worth and his individuality and was to handle estate matters with a stout and hearty independence for thirty-five years and more. A number of large architectural jobs away from the estate showed that he could design too, and that with talent and idiosyncratic taste. From 1804 he was working for the Prince of Wales at Brighton, and had started reconstructing Eaton Hall for Lord Grosvenor on the most lavish scale, in the Gothic style that he made no bones about favouring. Then in 1806–8 he became equally busy with his one major work on the Mayfair estate, Grosvenor House. This was the reconditioning of Lord Chetwynd's old house in Upper Grosvenor Street, which had passed to the Duke of Gloucester and was acquired by Lord Grosvenor in 1806 for use as the family's London seat.

There is no reliable record of the appearance of Grosvenor House when Porden had finished with it in 1808. Though well over £16,000 was spent, the only major change to the outside of the house was the addition of a bow towards the garden (Plate 18a). Most of the work, in fact, was interior and decorative, since the house was intended to show off Lord Grosvenor's collection of pictures to best advantage, and Porden prided himself on his particular taste and care in such matters. There was inevitable (and instructive) friction with the upholsterer, Gillow, who was often consulted by Lord Grosvenor, doubtless because he was less independent-minded than Porden. Disagreeing with Gillow about the colour of a dado, which he wanted 'sattin wood' in tone and Gillow a more dashing pink and white, Porden could damningly say of his opponent, 'in his own province, he is only governed by fashion'.[52] In the end, all turned out for the best; when Grosvenor House was thrown open in 1808, the results earned for Porden society's accolade. *The Times* was at its most orotund: 'Never do we recollect to have seen a more judicious and pleasing application of classical enrichments to domiciliary character and accom-

modation.'[53] There was, however, an argument about Porden's fee. Still, in 1817 Porden was again chosen as architect to add a gallery to accommodate Lord Grosvenor's growing picture collection.

The places where Porden significantly influenced the appearance of the rest of the Mayfair estate were few. Unlike later surveyors, he does not seem to have required plans for new houses or alterations to old ones to be submitted to him, nor did he solicit employment on the estate as a private architect. In the early years of his tenure relatively few leases were falling in, so his opportunities to assert himself architecturally or to promote a coherent policy for improvements were small. But one example of a notion of Porden's eventually bearing fruit was the reconstruction of King's Row (Nos. 93–99 consec. Park Lane), by the Grosvenor Gate into Hyde Park. As early as 1791 he saw that the jumbled appearance of Park Lane could be improved in places. He therefore persuaded Lord Grosvenor not to renew leases in King's Row so that in due course better houses could be built there. In 1808 Porden once more counselled against premature renewals, but it was not until 1823–8, after his death, that most of the range was rebuilt. Though the designs adopted were not uniform, Nos. 93–99 Park Lane remain one of the estate's most charming and individual ranges (Plate 19a). The only architect known to have been involved, John Goldicutt at Nos. 98 and 99, certainly did not have overall control. Yet somehow, since the plots were very shallow, the promoters all took up the idea suggested by the backs of houses fronting Norfolk (now Dunraven) Street higher up and Park Street lower down the lane, and canted out the new façades with a delightful set of bays, bows, iron balconies and verandas (Plate 19; fig. 10). This conception of backs turning into fronts was the vital factor in transforming Park Lane into a thoroughly fashionable address. Up and down the park frontage, bigger and better bays started to sprout on existing houses, while beyond the estate the reverberations reached Tyburnia.

In his last years as surveyor, Porden was sometimes represented at the Grosvenor Board by his son-in-law, Joseph Kay.[54] He retired in 1821, shortly before his death. By then the emphasis of Grosvenor estate development had shifted to Belgravia, the main sphere of activity of his successors, the Cundys. From their tenure of the surveyorship, a new phase in the character of the Mayfair estate may be dated.

The Reign of the Cundys

In September 1821 Thomas Cundy of Pimlico, architect and builder, succeeded Porden as the second Earl Grosvenor's surveyor. Cundy may have been recommended by his predecessor, as like Porden and Kay he had been a protégé of S. P. Cockerell, the district surveyor of St. George's, Hanover Square. He was certainly conversant with the Mayfair estate already, having altered two houses in Grosvenor Square, No. 7 (1808) and No. 30 (1815–16), acted in lease-renewals for two others (Nos. 11 and 29), and applied for the lease of at least one property close to Grosvenor House. His brother, the engineer Nicholas Wilcox Cundy, had also lived briefly first in Brook Street just off the estate, then in Norfolk (now Dunraven) Street.[55] But the decisive factor must have been Thomas Cundy's connexion with the 'Five Fields' area of Pimlico, towards which all eyes were now turning as the next logical place for expansion on the Grosvenor estates. By 1811 serious plans had already been laid for the development of Belgravia;[56] there were at least two false starts, but by the time that Cundy became estate surveyor development was about to take off, and since he operated from Ranelagh Street (now Beeston Place and the eastern end of Ebury Street) he was well placed to superintend affairs. For the next forty years Mayfair was to take a back seat, as a style both of development and of architecture was evolved for Belgravia and Pimlico, and then reflected back upon the older estate. The principal early figures in this evolution were the speculative builders, the great Thomas Cubitt, Seth Smith, and to a lesser degree Joseph, James and Thomas Cundy II, the sons of the estate surveyor.[57] But though Thomas Cundy I must have matured the layout of Belgravia, and certainly had a hand at the start of his sons' speculations there, he died in 1825 before matters were at all advanced. Thomas Cundy II, his eldest son, now took over the surveyorship to Lord Grosvenor, an appointment he was to hold for over forty years and then pass on in turn to his third son Thomas Cundy III, who retained the post until 1890. Day-to-day architectural control of the London estates was thus in the hands of the same family for nearly seventy years.

Officially the briefs of Thomas Cundy I and II seem to have exceeded Porden's in one important respect only. This was that the Cundys began to consider and approve plans for any new buildings or rebuildings undertaken by tenants. This duty, obviously evolved with Belgravia in mind, was to become vital on the Mayfair estate as well. Here a new era of general rebuilding, small perhaps compared to the volume of development further south, but still significant, was ushered in with the retirement of Porden. If the falling-in of Mayfair leases was partly the cause, the Cundys must also have encouraged this distinctly new policy, as it offered them greater opportunities as well as more responsibilities. The family certainly took their early chances in Belgravia while Thomas Cundy I still lived, and though Thomas Cundy II relinquished his interest in his brother Joseph's 'take' of land round Chester Square on becoming surveyor,[58] he probably continued designing for the family speculations, as his father had done.

How much Thomas Cundy II designed on the estates during the first twenty years of his surveyorship, before the accession of the second Marquess in 1845, is hard to

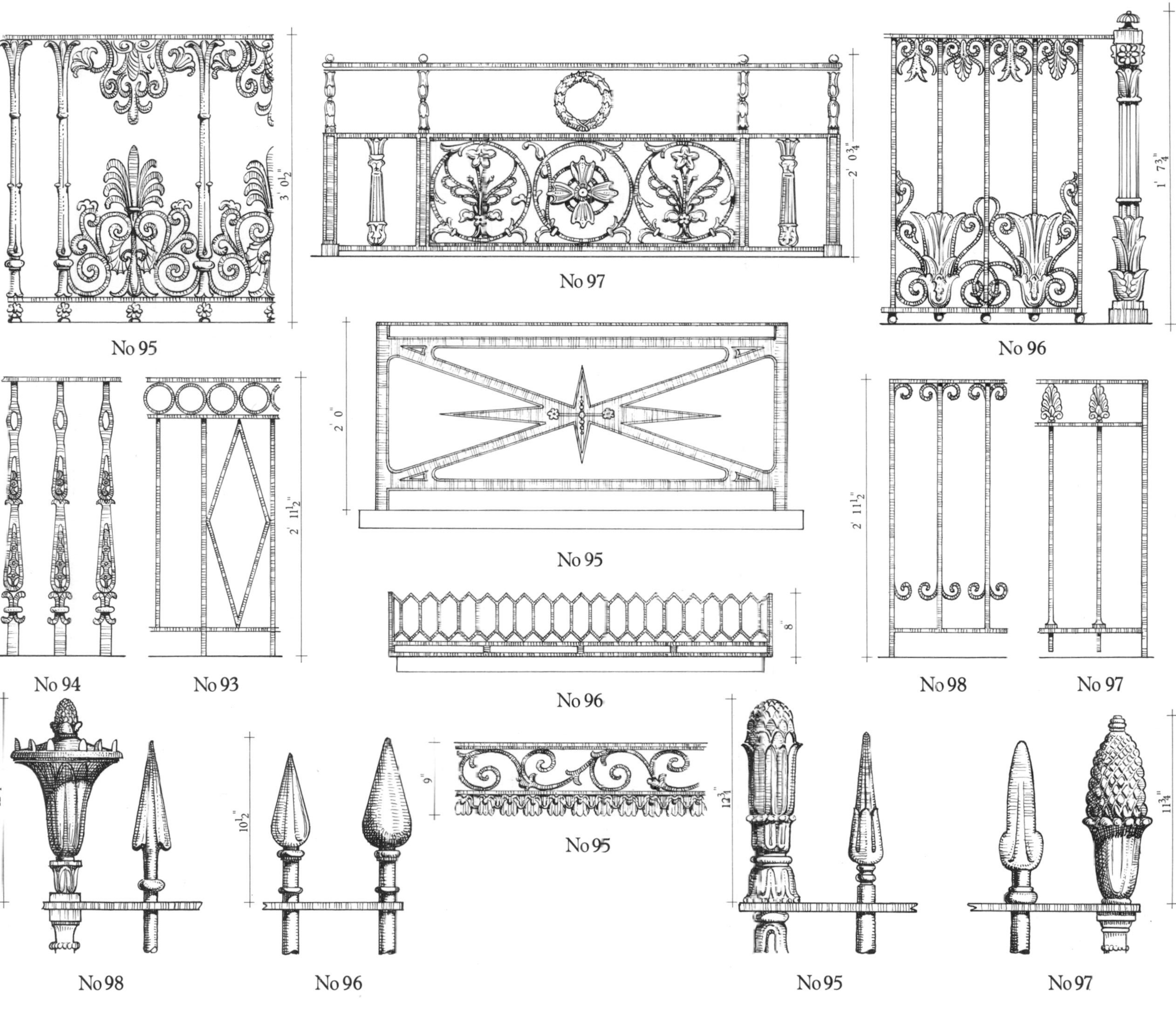

Fig. 10. Nos. 93–98 (consec.) Park Lane, details of decorative ironwork, mainly of 1823–8

say. Well before his father's death he had been engaged in the architectural side of the practice, and for works of the mid 1820's their hands are indistinguishable. What is undoubtedly true is that their most lucrative Mayfair commissions of this period were undertaken for the Grosvenors themselves. The first one, the reconstruction of Nos. 15 and 16 Grosvenor Square as Belgrave House, has hitherto escaped notice, but was a large business. In 1819 the second Earl Grosvenor's heir, Viscount Belgrave, had married Lady Elizabeth Leveson-Gower; the wealthy couple soon had children and wanted for a substantial London house. The answer was the pair of houses in the middle of the north side of the square, which between 1822 and 1824 were transformed by the Cundys into a regular palace, at a cost of over £12,000. They acquired a new stucco front some seventy-five feet in length, with four giant engaged columns running through first- and second-storey levels (Plate 20a). This illustrious mid-terrace composition must have been an influence on the façades of Belgrave Square, which were being evolved shortly after this date. The interior of Belgrave House, though modest on plan, can scarcely have been less magnificent, as John Davis, a Brook Street cabinet-maker, presented a bill for £3829 for work done here.

Immediately afterwards, in 1824, Earl Grosvenor initiated an even more massive rebuilding scheme for Grosvenor House itself. Porden had reconditioned the house but had scarcely enlarged it, and this was what the Cundys now prepared to do. Thomas Cundy I must have been a party to the scheme's inception, but all extant drawings date from after his death. The only major addition actually erected, the great picture gallery of 1826–7, was certainly in the hands of Thomas Cundy II, assisted in the execution of the work by his brothers, the short-lived mason James and the soon-bankrupted carpenter Joseph. As architects, the first two Cundys had neither the sophistication nor the individuality of a Porden: their Grosvenor House scheme, therefore, though lavish and imposing, was essentially pedestrian, relying much upon engaged columns for exterior effect (Plate 18a, b). In contrast to this heavy Roman effort, a chaster scheme submitted (without invitation) by Smirke makes one sigh for more imaginative patronage on the part of the second Earl Grosvenor (Plate 18c). Later, in 1842–3, Thomas Cundy II added a noble screen equipped with florid iron gates to front the courtyard towards Upper Grosvenor Street. Though modelled on Holland's Carlton House screen, it has been translated into the same sober Roman idiom (Plate 20c).

Still, the second Cundy does appear to have had a lighter side at times, if the façade of the Grosvenor Office at No. 53 Davies Street, a fresh and cheerful essay of the 1830's in the stucco of Belgravia, can be taken as his (Plate 20b). There is no evidence for the authorship of this engaging composition, enlivened by touches of Greek detail, but Cundy is the obvious candidate, and stylistic parallels

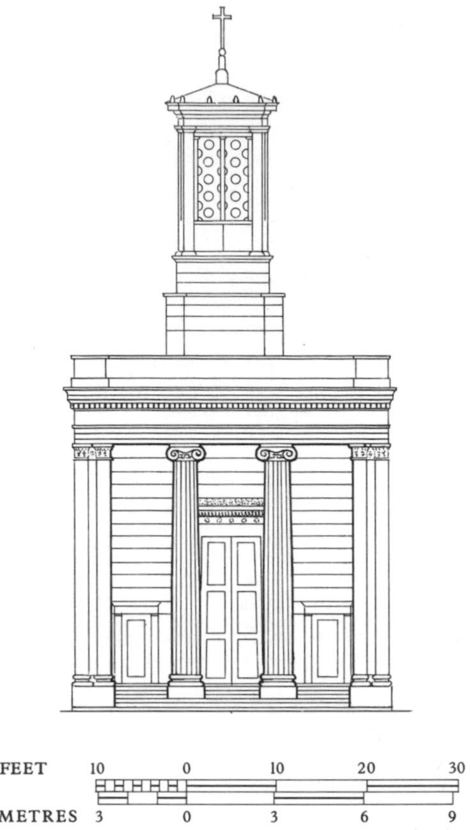

Fig. 11. St. Mark's Church, North Audley Street, west front. *Architect*, J. P. Gandy-Deering, 1825–8

with the demolished Belgrave House, also fronted in stucco, seem to suggest his hand. Meanwhile, he was also well supplied with out-of-town work for the Grosvenors, for instance at Moor Park in Hertfordshire, where over £15,000 was spent by Earl Grosvenor between 1828 and 1831.[59]

With the Cundys at the helm, the Greek Revival scarcely got an airing on the Mayfair estate. The chief exception is the work of that rare architect, J. P. Gandy-Deering. He was the winner in 1824 of a competition for the new church of St. Mark's, North Audley Street. The surviving portico and pronaos of his church (fig. 11) display able scholarship and exceptional purity of detail, and go some way to explain why the extant designs of another competitor, John Goldicutt, were not chosen. Goldicutt also participated in the redevelopment at Nos. 93–99 (consec.) Park Lane, but there was nothing very Greek in the outline of this range (Plate 19a). Here and elsewhere, lessees were mostly content to display the new fashion, as far as exteriors were concerned, in pretty cast-iron balconies and verandas on the fronts and backs of their houses (figs. 10, 12b). Again, Gandy-Deering was the exception. A unique and highly fashionable terrace of

houses designed by him in *c.* 1825–35 at Nos. 14–24 (even) South Street (Lord Melbourne lived in one of them) manifested the same careful discipline and sense for proportions as his St. Mark's designs (Plate 24c; fig. 12c). So it is lamentable that only two forlorn houses in this row remain, while of other work by Gandy-Deering in the South Street area virtually nothing survives.

Another architect employed on the western half of the estate was William Atkinson. His rebuilt Dudley House (1827–8) is the most important house of this period to remain. Its stucco façade follows the lead of some of the simpler Regent's Park terraces, whilst some handsome passages of its interior decoration mark the point of transition from a chaste Greek style to the more fulsome manner associated with the Italianate of Charles Barry (Plate 21).

In the 1820's one or two interesting architects had their homes upon the estate, a circumstance which easily led to their employment here and there. One such was George Stanley Repton, son of the landscape gardener, who in 1821 was encouraged by his banking friends the Loyds to come and live close to them in Norfolk (now Dunraven) Street. His house, overlooking the park, has been demolished, but in the early 1820's he designed stabling in Wood's Mews for Samuel Jones Loyd, the future Lord Overstone (Plate 22c), and is likely to have done more work, either for Loyd or for himself. P. F. Robinson, an affable and ingenious ex-assistant of Porden's who is best known for his books of picturesque cottage designs, lived and worked for many years at a house on the site of the present No. 80 Brook Street; he altered Somerset House, Park Lane, in 1819 and on various occasions acted for his regular clients, the Osbaldestons, in their search for a Mayfair house;[36] an instructive account of one such episode, in connexion with No. 51 Brook Street, will be found in Appendix III. Though the houses of Repton and Robinson have disappeared, the more original residence of Jeffry Wyatt (Sir Jeffry Wyatville) still survives at No. 39 Brook Street (Plate 22a). Wyatt moved into this pleasant and unusually planned early Georgian house in about 1802, at which time he was partner in a building business with premises behind in Avery Row and Brook's Mews. As his architectural practice expanded he seems to have relinquished the building side, and shortly after 1821 he smartened up the old house substantially by remodelling several rooms, constructing a small circular entrance hall, and adding a large and long toplit gallery at first-floor level behind on the Avery Row side. The character of this work is classic in the manner of Soane, but far more subdued. Wyatt also acted in lease-renewals and altered several houses in Grosvenor Square, principally No. 6 in 1809 for the Marquess of Bath, his patron at Longleat, and he may also, like Robinson, have made a small addition at Somerset House, Park Lane (1811).

Other leading architects of the period are less well represented on the estate. Smirke's scheme for Grosvenor House was never seriously considered and his only other known design, a small addition at Camelford House, does not seem to have been built. The substantial works done by C. R. Cockerell at No. 88 Brook Street in 1824 have been swept away, and the house he altered for his brother at No. 1 Upper Grosvenor Street has been demolished. In Grosvenor Street there are few traces of the internal alterations made by Decimus Burton at No. 18 (1835–6), but rather more of those by Lewis Vulliamy at No. 51 (1836). Anthony Salvin is said to have worked at Grosvenor House in 1835, but the nature and extent of his employment remain a mystery. As for Charles Barry, he appears to have been employed on the estate only in his later career, and again his two known works, both refrontings, have disappeared. That at No. 41 Brook Street (1852–3) was not particularly significant, but his recasing of No. 2 South Street in 1852 was a lavish affair. This house, which had been enlarged by the Duke of Orleans, the famous Philippe Egalité, during his English exile (1789–90), had a return front to Park Lane, by then a highly fashionable address. Barry therefore dressed the building in a noble outfit of Italianate stucco façades with a festive and ornamental frieze, rather in the manner of some of the houses in Kensington Palace Gardens (Plate 22b).

In general, the reign of the second Earl Grosvenor and first Marquess of Westminster (1802–45) brought few drastic changes to the fabric in the smartest parts of the Mayfair estate. Since leases were often renewed without particular conditions, rebuilding occurred only as and when the lessees desired and was rarely prompted by the estate. Apart from the recasting of Belgrave House, only one house along the main sides of Grosvenor Square is known to have been completely rebuilt between 1804 and 1854, and that was No. 47, reconstructed in 1814–15 because of its poor state to the designs and under the superintendence of a little-known builder, Thomas Martin.

Yet elsewhere there was no shortage of building activity, a fact which is partly obscured by the spate of subsequent reconstruction in the first Duke's day. To take the clearest instance, a good deal of Davies Street and of the small streets south of Grosvenor Street and north of Brook Street was transformed in the 1820's and 1830's. The main operators were Seth Smith and, to a lesser extent, Thomas Cubitt, famed as developers in Belgravia. But both had built on the Mayfair estate before turning to Belgravia, Smith on the west side of Davies Street between Brook Street and Three Kings Yard (1818–20), Cubitt at the north end of Berkeley Square, next to the corner with Davies Street (1821–2). Cubitt was of course to outstrip Smith in Belgravia, but in Mayfair Smith was the bigger speculator. Yet of the sixty-three small but decent houses he put up between 1822 and 1833 in the Gilbert Street, Binney Street and Weighhouse Street area, possibly to the designs of William Maberley (Plate 23a), only a single one, No. 27 Gilbert Street, survives (fig. 12a); even his dissenters' chapel has disappeared. Cubitt's slightly later developments have fared no better. In 1837–40 he rebuilt

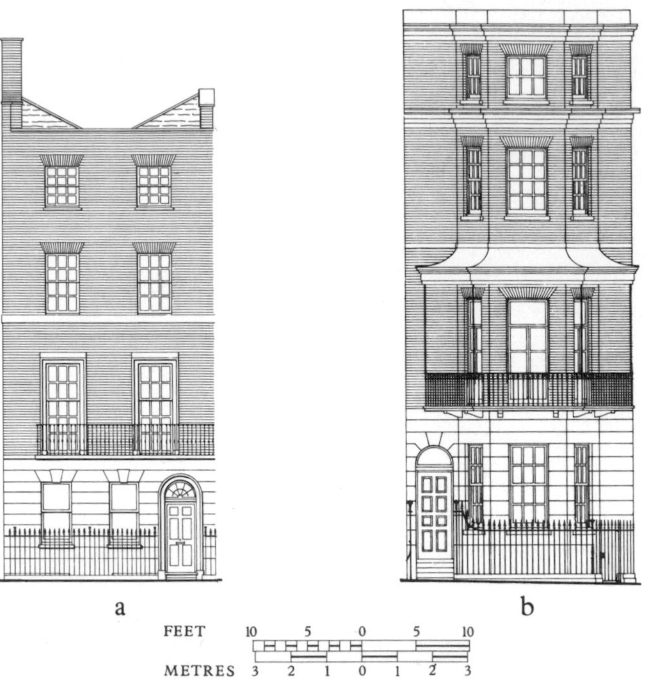

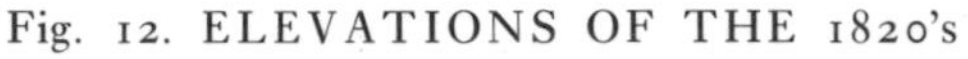

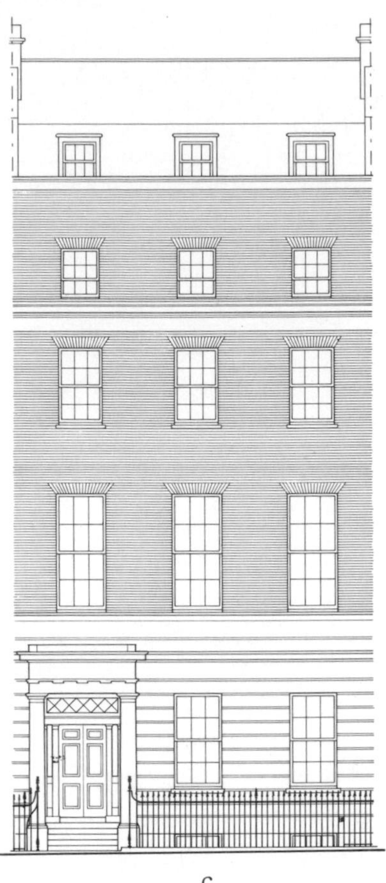

Fig. 12. ELEVATIONS OF THE 1820's

a. No. 27 Gilbert Street. *Builder*, Seth Smith, 1828–9. *Now extended*

b. No. 98 Park Lane. *Architect*, John Goldicutt, 1823–5

c. No. 16 South Street. *Architect*, J. P. Gandy-Deering, *c*. 1825–30. *Demolished*

much in the Grosvenor Hill–Bourdon Street area, a group of houses on the west side of Davies Street, and three substantial houses in Grosvenor Street. None of these remains. In Cubitt's case these enterprises may have been intended to take up the slack from his undertakings elsewhere, but Seth Smith's smaller workforce was more probably stretched by his Mayfair developments.

A third, much smaller improvement in this area that happily survives is the Running Horse public house together with Nos. 52–54 (even) Davies Street of 1839–40 (Plate 24b). This originally comprised the pub, a pair of houses, and building workshops behind, erected by the small contracting firm of Joshua Higgs and Company as their headquarters. Though the business here never seems to have grown to great proportions, a nephew of Joshua Higgs apprenticed here was to become co-founder of the much bigger Higgs and Hill.[60] Also, in the year of the firm's establishment at this address, 1839, a son, Joshua Higgs junior, submitted to the Select Committee on Metropolis Improvements an elaborate scheme for improving the north end of Davies Street with shops and a chapel in the Grecian style of Regent Street (Plate 24a). But the scheme came to nothing, and the top of Davies Street had to wait another fifty years for its improvement.

Two other districts underwent major change at this time. One was the Green Street area, where the presence of several minor architects and surveyors such as Samuel Erlam, Edward Lapidge and Daniel Robertson was a stimulus to rebuilding activity in the 1820's. A principal builder-speculator here was John Elger (Plate 23c), a native of Bedford who from about 1825 had a yard on the estate in South Street, east of South Audley Street. Over the following twenty years he took a substantial number of good sites in different parts of the West End, and he was also the builder of Thomas Cundy II's screen at Grosvenor House (1842–3). Elger's niece was to marry Thomas Cundy III, and in the 1840's his South Street premises were passed on to John Kelk, who in his turn relinquished them in about 1862 to George Smith and Company.[61] All these are highly reputable names in the London building world of the time, and all are frequently met with on the Mayfair estate. The connexions between these figures, though often unclear to us, were evidently crucial to their operations. Yet despite Elger's importance, the only estate work of his to survive in any recognizable form is No. 138 Park Lane (Plate 19c), a house at the corner with North Row, originally two premises but united by him in 1831–2.

The last district to be substantially redeveloped at this time, South Street, Chapel Street (now Aldford Street)

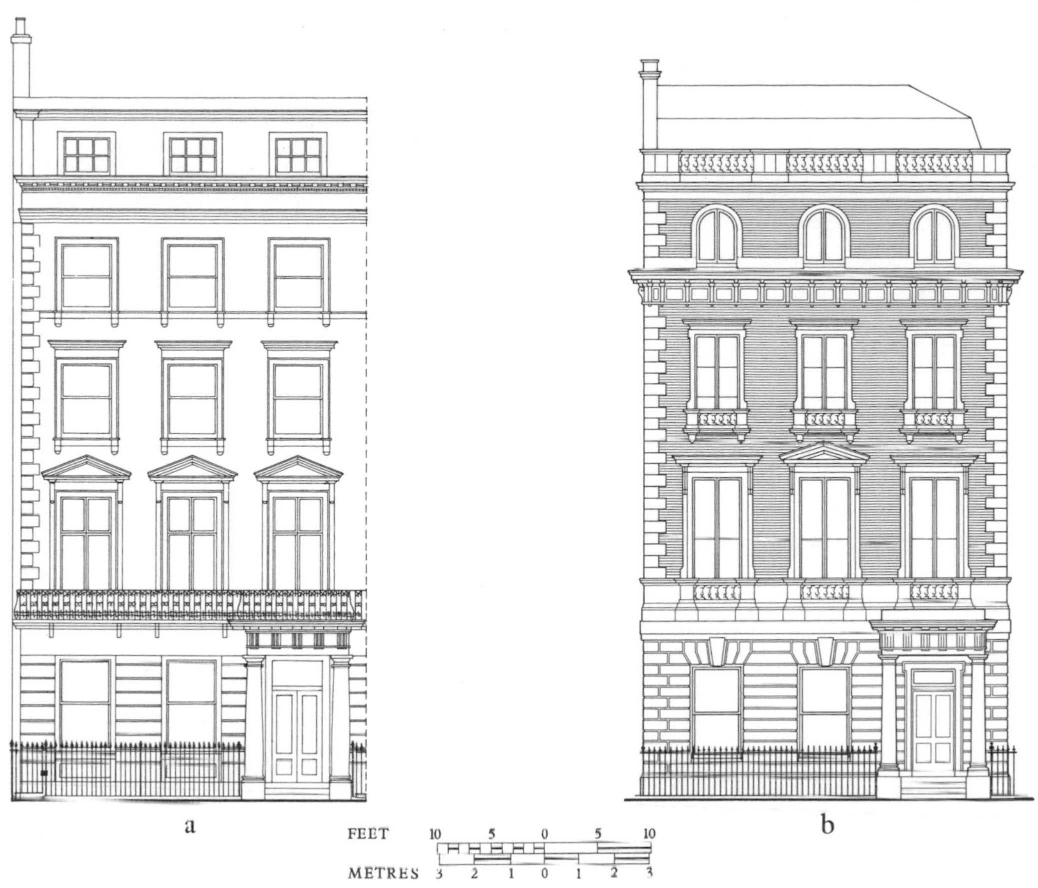

Fig. 13. EARLY-VICTORIAN ELEVATIONS

a. No. 11 Upper Grosvenor Street. *Architect*, Henry Harrison, *builder*, James Ponsford, 1842–3
b. No. 50 Grosvenor Square, elevation as submitted in 1849; altered in execution. *Builder*, Sir Matthew Wyatt. *Demolished*

and Portugal Street (now Balfour Place), also brings up its individuals, but by and large they are more obscure. The Gandy-Deering developments in the western part of South Street have already been mentioned. One of his associates here was James Gallier, who soon became bankrupt and departed to America, where he won some fame and fortune as an architect in New Orleans.[62] Gallier's chief backer was John Robson, who had a large coach manufactory behind the north side of South Street and the west side of South Audley Street and built houses hereabouts. In the late 1820's Robson, a Mr. Arber and Thomas Oliver divided a good deal of the ground round here for redevelopment, but there were other figures too such as William Skeat on the south side of Mount Street close to Park Lane (Plate 23b). Oliver and his successor John Feetham appear to have been the largest operators; they did much work in Portugal Street and Chapel Street and among the larger houses which Feetham took was No. 74 South Audley Street, where he altered the main house, pulled down the old Portuguese Embassy chapel behind, and erected stables on the site, which survive as the present No. 26 South Street (1833). It was probably also at this time that the Grosvenor Chapel acquired its present external dressings of stucco; major works were undertaken by William Skeat in 1829–30, after the chapel had become the property of the parish.

The developments in this district also mark the first appearance of Wright Ingle, for nearly forty years a speculator upon the Mayfair estate. In the 1820's his activities were modest in scope, but they gradually enlarged. Between 1841 and 1851 he was absent from the estate scene, but in the following eleven years he was constantly at work altering or reconstructing one house or another, his largest single task being the rebuilding of No. 42 Grosvenor Square (1853–5). He eventually died in 1865, full of years and riches, and was buried in his native town of St. Ives, Huntingdonshire.[63] The two survivors from Ingle's speculations are Nos. 11 Upper Brook Street and 20 Grosvenor Street, a pair of similar small houses both of 1852–3. It is significant that though Ingle is sometimes described as a builder, he was not one in the ordinary sense of the word at least in his later years, nor so far as is known was he an architect. His enterprises of the 1850's were invariably erected by other building firms and usually, it appears, designed by Henry Harrison, an architect who lived for some years in Park Street and had experience of designing for speculative builders. In about 1843 James Ponsford, a major speculator in

Tyburnia, now developing apace on the other side of Hyde Park, called in Harrison to design a pair of large houses at Nos. 10 and 11 Upper Grosvenor Street (fig. 13a) and a smaller one behind at No. 62 Park Street. Those in Upper Grosvenor Street are among the few remaining examples on the Mayfair estate to adopt the full Belgravia manner: completely stuccoed with Italian porches, pedimented first-floor windows and iron balconies, and spaciously planned so as to include ample public space and internal light-wells. Harrison may also have designed a set of houses erected by Ponsford in North Audley Street (all now demolished), and he certainly altered Hampden House, No. 61 Green Street, and Derby House, No. 26 Grosvenor Square. Under Ingle's aegis he was responsible for Nos. 11 Upper Brook Street, 20 Grosvenor Street, and 42 Grosvenor Square, except for the façades. These, in accordance with a policy that must now be discussed, were the work of Thomas Cundy II (figs. 14, 15, 17).

The death of the first Marquess of Westminster in 1845 marked the start of a twenty-two-year heyday for Thomas Cundy II. Just like his father before him and his son after him, the second Marquess celebrated his accession with an outburst of building. In the country, his principal architects were William Burn, who altered Eaton once again and designed a new house on the family's Fonthill estate in Wiltshire, and T. H. Wyatt, who scattered a handful of Grosvenor-financed churches across the Salisbury diocese, churches being the enthusiasm of the age.

But in London the Cundys still ruled supreme. Thomas Cundy II had already been laying his plans, for in 1844 he obtained the consent of the first Marquess to a proposition for adding stuccowork, porticos, window dressings, cornices and balustrades in Grosvenor Square to 'such of the houses as may be thought to require it. The terms for renewal in all houses to contain stipulations to this effect and a drawing to be submitted by the parties applying.'[64] This was more than a vague idea, it was a proposal for refronting on a vast scale. In May 1845 measurements were being taken from the façades of the south-side houses, the new Marquess telling inhabitants 'I am anxious to obtain a correct design for some proposed improvements';[65] four years later, Cundy produced to the Grosvenor Board 'a drawing showing his suggested alterations' for all the houses along this side.[66] There is also more than a suspicion that Cundy prepared a uniform elevation for the north side of the square. In 1855, at the time that substantial reconstruction on this side first became a practical proposition, an elevation of the whole frontage as existing was drawn; moreover, the houses eventually rebuilt here, No. 10 at the east end (fig. 15) and Nos. 20 and 21 at the west (Plate 25b), were allotted unusual and matching pilastered fronts, as though they were to form flanking wings to Nos. 15–16, formerly Belgrave House. (Soon after the Marquess had moved into Grosvenor House in 1845 this house became free. It had then been taken by a speculative businessman, Kensington Lewis, and divided back into two in 1848–9, with some alterations to the front.) It appears therefore as if the Marquess and Cundy now conceived their old Belgrave House as the centre of a splendid composition embracing the whole north side of the square.

Whether, as all this implies, there was serious thought of refronting the whole square over a long period so as to make the houses 'range uniform' in the Belgravia manner is not clear. But it soon became apparent that the new policy had no prospects of quick advancement. The first practical opportunity to refront a house in the square did not come until 1851. By chance it was the famous Derby House, No. 26; Henry Harrison was the lessee's architect, and not unnaturally wanted a slightly different front from the type prescribed by Cundy. In the event Cundy designed the new façade, but probably with some concessions. A similar compromise with the new estate rule must have been reached at the next house to be refronted, the surviving No. 38 Grosvenor Square (1854–5); unlike most of the square it already had a completely stuccoed front, and therefore Cundy had to provide different detailing (Plate 25a).

Soon, Cundy and the second Marquess, knowing there was no chance of a quick, clean sweep in the square, were also soberly applying themselves by means of compulsory clauses in terms for new leases to refronting almost every house in the main streets as it came up for renewal. The first house that appears to have fallen under this fiat was No. 18 Grosvenor Street (since refronted again), for which Cundy provided an elevation in February 1846. At first the policy was slow to get off the mark, but by the mid 1850's it was well under way, and between 1850 and Thomas Cundy II's death in 1867 almost fifty separate refrontings can be traced as having been carried out in the major streets, nearly all in conjunction with lease renewals.

Although these refrontings had to be proceeded with piecemeal, it is not improbable that a coherent design existed for the frontages in each major street, to which Cundy turned when an individual house was being renewed. In 1848 he produced a general design for the north side of Brook Street east of Davies Street, and the wording of the original terms of renewal for Nos. 41 and 43 on the south side suggests that he may have proposed another one for this side. There is indirect evidence too for such a design on the north side of Grosvenor Street, where a large number of houses between Avery Row and Davies Street, some of them contiguous, were rebuilt or refronted with similar façades of a uniform height and with a distinctive frieze (fig. 14c). In Grosvenor Square nearly all the fronts rebuilt on the south and west sides had common characteristics, with stone dressings instead of the cement used in the side streets, harder and lighter bricks for the walling, and stone balustrades to the areas rather than iron railings (Plate 25). Even in South Audley Street, where little refronting took place in the Cundy era, the one block to be rebuilt, Nos. 53–55 (consec.) of

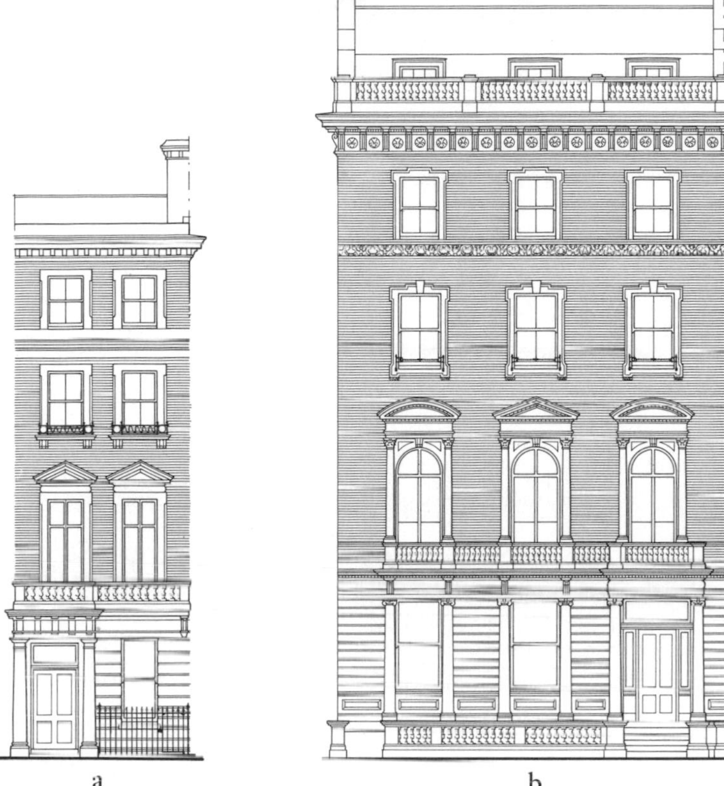

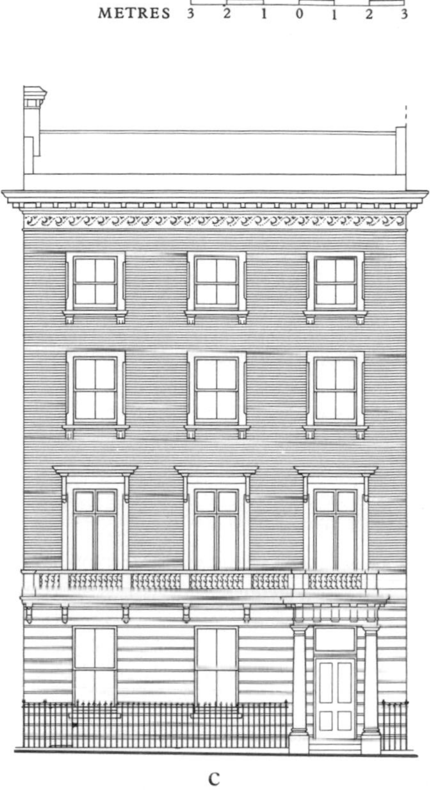

Fig. 14. ELEVATIONS BY THOMAS CUNDY II

a. No. 11 Upper Brook Street. *Builder*, Wright Ingle, 1852–3
b. No. 55 South Audley Street. *Builders*, Reading and William Watts, 1858–9
c. No. 17 Grosvenor Street. *Builder*, John Newson, 1855–6

1858–60, had its special, markedly ornamental design, though only No. 55 (fig. 14b) has survived to tell the tale.

Inevitably there were exceptions to the policy, especially early on, as the cases of Nos. 26 and 38 Grosvenor Square have already shown. Some few lessees escaped the condition of refronting or successfully rejected Cundy's elevations. At No. 2 South Street his design was supplanted by that of the lessee's own architect, Charles Barry, no doubt because of the latter's superior prestige; at No. 41 Brook Street Barry again had his own way. At No. 50 Grosvenor Square, the home of the aged General Grosvenor, Lord Robert Grosvenor (the brother of the Marquess) took charge of the rebuilding deemed urgently necessary in 1847. He brought in (Sir) Matthew Wyatt, the developer of Victoria Square and of much of Tyburnia, who was allowed to build the whole house, and the Marquess was reduced to twice requesting Wyatt to simplify and tone down his elevation, presumably because the originals (fig. 13b) were too brash for the estate norm. Generally, however, the Marquess supported Cundy to the hilt. At No. 41 Upper Brook Street, Sir Henry Meux and his architect Samuel Beazley had to submit to the stone balcony insisted upon; and even so eminent a domestic architect as Burn, who had twice worked for the Marquess, had to employ an elevation by Cundy when he rebuilt No. 18 Grosvenor Square for Earl Fortescue in 1864–7 (Plate 54a).

The refronting policy raises several issues. What were the precedents? Were the Estate's motives primarily commercial or aesthetic? And was it the fruit of Thomas Cundy II's ambitions, or did it in the main reflect the desires of the tenants? Though the answers must in part be guessed, it is plain that Belgravia and its newer outliers westward, beyond Grosvenor land, lay at the root of Estate thinking. There, uniformity and the stucco style had proved an asset, not a liability, and there must have been some anxiety that Mayfair might go into decline unless something of the kind were tried there. Rebuilding, though frequently undertaken in the main streets and square during the period of the second Marquess, was often unrealistic, wasteful and unnecessary, and could deprive the estate of valued tenants; as there was no way of influencing internal alterations, refronting was the only other option. Nevertheless, the whole operation was to

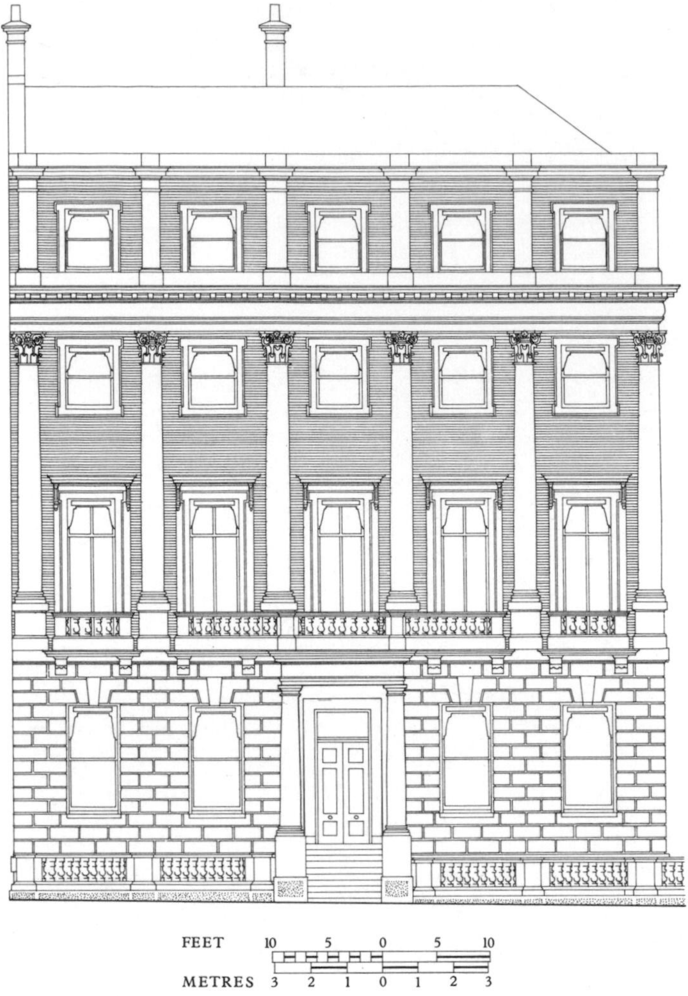

Fig. 15. No. 10 Grosvenor Square, elevation to the square. *Architect*, Thomas Cundy II, *builder*, C. J. Freake, 1864–6. *Demolished*

a degree eccentric. There was no obvious precedent, and the few successors, like the Bedford Estate's refronting of Russell Square at the turn of the century, were not strictly parallel. It was also a destructive policy. Thomas Cundy II and the second Marquess were not sensitive souls when it came to the architecture of the past, and in their anxiety to promote a revitalized Mayfair estate in good repair, not only did much of the Georgian appearance of the streets and square vanish, but many fine houses, including Derby House, were entirely destroyed. If the epochs of the second Marquess and the first Duke are compared, it cannot seriously be questioned that the first Duke built more that was of permanent merit and destroyed less of real value than his father had done.

Still, many of Cundy's fronts (Plate 25; figs. 14, 15, 17) were able compositions in their own right, especially where plots were broad enough to allow him adequate space. One fine surviving example, at No. 52 Grosvenor Street, involved Lord Radnor in large expenditure in 1854–5. This front (fig. 17) is still in the strict Italian style, with a deep cornice upon consoles, individual balconettes to the first-floor windows, and the cement rustication running evenly up the sides of the building. Later on, these elements begin to change. Another big surviving elevation is that to No. 4 Grosvenor Square, in fact a complete rebuilding of 1865–8 (Plate 25d). Here the basic material is the hard, unyielding white Suffolk brick so fashionable during this period; upon this have been fitted the conventional appendages of refronting policy, i.e. deep cornice and roof balustrade, window dressings, rusticated quoins, pediments to the first-floor windows (here supported on columns), first-floor balconies, stuccoed ground storey, and projecting open portico. But by this time the various details have something of a French flavour, consistent with the appearance of Thomas Cundy III as an important power under his father. Thomas Cundy III, who was, as will be seen, a designer of distinctive Francophile tendencies, was in fact paid for drawings for No. 4 Grosvenor Square. His first recorded appearance on the Grosvenor estate was in 1854–6, when the very large job of rebuilding Nos. 20 and 21 Grosvenor Square, ascribed in *The Builder* to 'the firm of T. and T. Cundy', was in fact almost entirely the work of the younger man.[67] From then on he played an increasing part

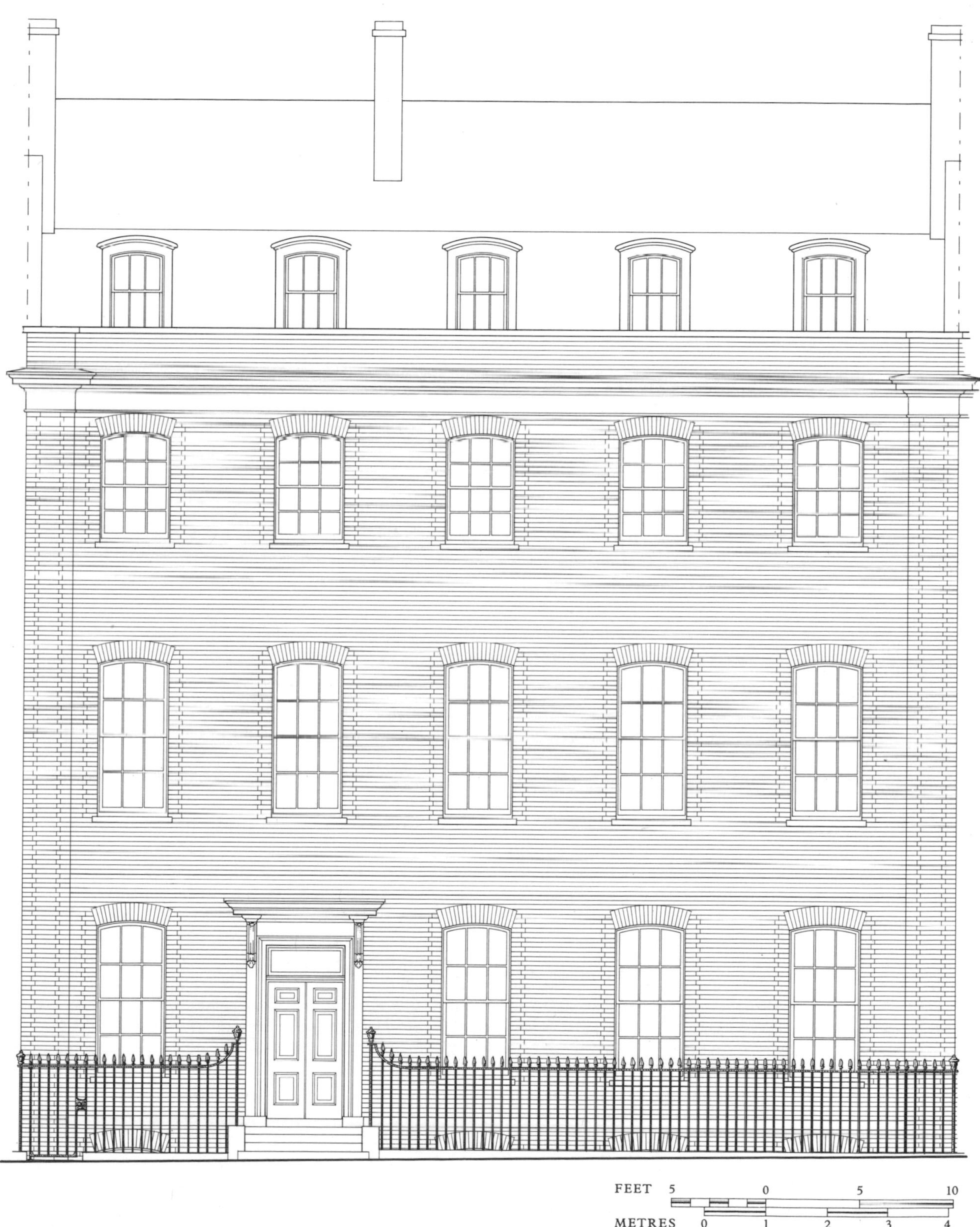

Fig. 16. No. 52 Grosvenor Street, elevation as originally built. *Lessee*, Benjamin Timbrell (carpenter), 1724

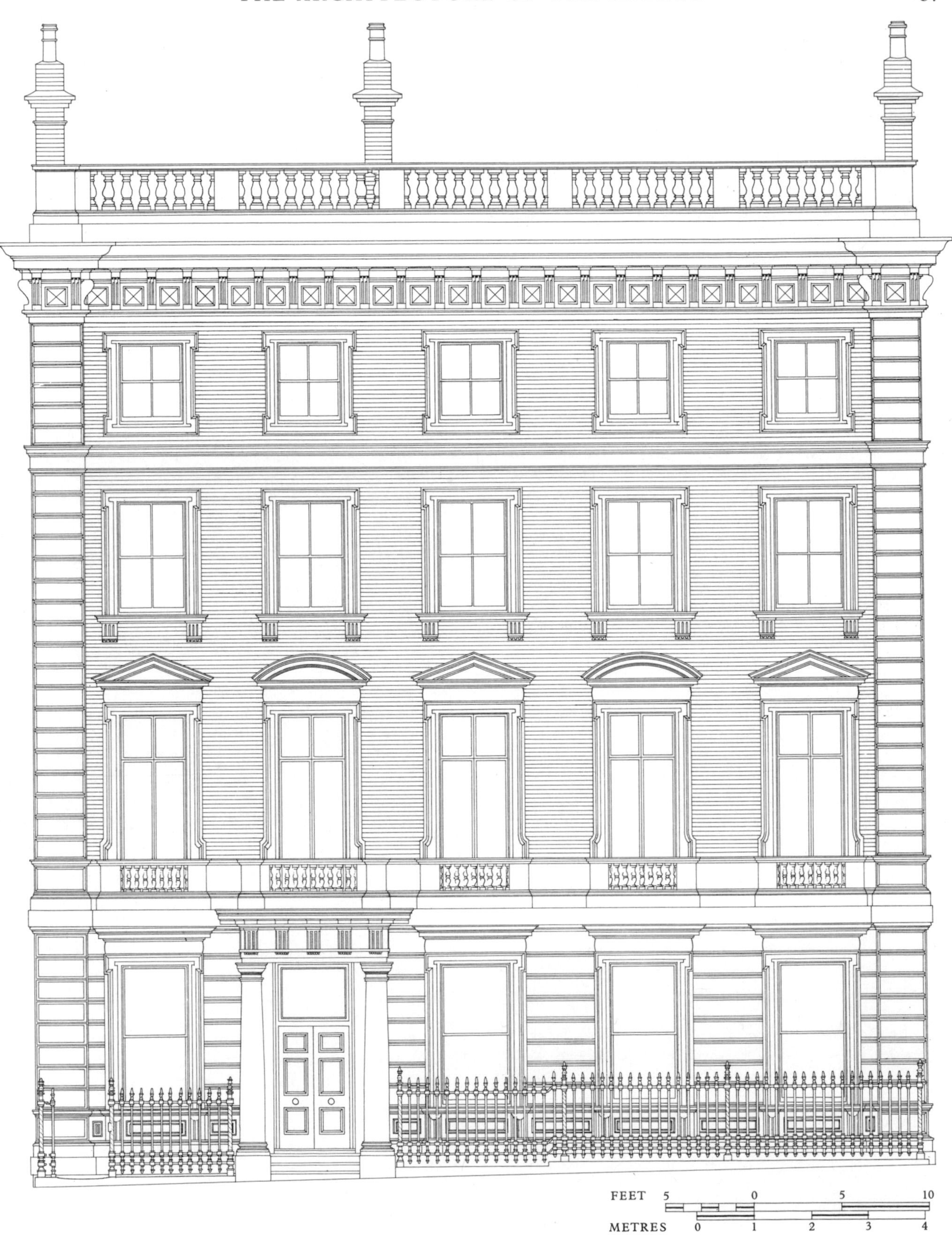

Fig. 17. No. 52 Grosvenor Street, elevation after refronting. *Architect*, Thomas Cundy II, 1854–5

in matters of design on the estate, and from 1864 until he replaced his father as estate surveyor in 1867 it is likely that a good proportion of 'Cundy' designs were his.

In the large majority of cases involving the Cundys, their role was confined to refronting, even where there was a complete rebuilding. Lessees and speculators acquiesced in this arrangement because they knew that Cundy designs would generally pass the increasingly stiff hurdle of acceptability for façades at the Grosvenor Office, while behind the fronts they could proceed much as they did elsewhere. As usual, we are best informed for Grosvenor Square (Plate 25). Here, out of ten reconstructions with Cundy fronts between 1853 and 1867, two actually were planned by the Cundys. These were Nos. 20 and 21, where they were employed directly by the tenants, no doubt through the mediation of the Grosvenor Office, and the successful builder, John Kelk, got the contract as the result of tendering for their already formulated plans. Only one other of these ten houses is known to have been planned by an independent architect acting directly for a client. This was No. 18, the house rebuilt by William Burn for Earl Fortescue. The remaining seven were probably all planned by large builders with experience in speculation, or more correctly by architects working under them according to an arrangement already common: No. 42 by Henry Harrison for Ingle, Nos. 10, 26 (the 1861–2 rebuilding), and possibly also Nos. 4 and 40 by William Tasker for Freake, and the other two by unknown designers, No. 2 under Kelk, No. 30 under George Trollope and Sons. Varying degrees of speculation were involved in these houses. Sometimes there was technically no speculation at all on the builders' part, as at No. 30 where it was the tenant who stood to gain, bringing in Trollopes and then selling on his own behalf the house that they built for him. In some other cases a client was found at an early stage, and not only was the lease granted to him but the finishings of the house and on occasions even the planning were determined by his requirements. Thus at No. 10 Grosvenor Square, Freake built a single house instead of the two he had originally contemplated for the site to meet the wishes of his client Lord Lindsay, who paid £35,000 for the privilege. At this house no less than four architects were involved in one way or another: Lewis Vulliamy, the Lindsay family's old architect, who was consulted over the planning at an early stage; Freake's architect Tasker, who actually provided the plans and was probably responsible for most of the interior; Cundy, who designed the fronts (fig. 15) on behalf of the Estate; and lastly a Mr. Young, a surveyor who was called in at the insistence of Lord Lindsay's solicitor to look over the specifications and proposed one major alteration.[68]

Nevertheless the critical role in most of these Grosvenor Square houses was that of the independent speculative builders, whose repute and reliability were vital to the successful carrying out of the refronting policy. Of Wright Ingle something has already been said. C. J. Freake was principally a Kensington figure, not widely active in Mayfair, but whose high status and respectability were affirmed by houses like those in Grosvenor Square: with Lord Lindsay, for instance, Freake could conduct his correspondence on a level almost of social equality. John Kelk too had broken through from the level of mere tradesman or entrepreneur to that of public benefactor and (eventually) baronet; his commitments on the estate were wider than Freake's. Trollopes on the other hand were an up-and-coming if somewhat faceless firm: they were to be incomparably the most important builders on the Grosvenor estate at the turn of the century.

But for the period of the second Marquess, the most significant and typical estate builder was none of these, but John Newson of Grosvenor Mews. According to tradition, Newson came to London in the 1830's from Woodbridge in Suffolk, took a contract for roadsweeping in Berkeley Square, and graduated via the making of trunks for maidservants into the building industry. Whatever the truth, he was big enough by 1835 to make a sizeable speculation in the Ebury Street district of Pimlico, where he built the delightful houses of Bloomfield Terrace in one of which he made his home.[69] He also had a Mayfair base and began here with a series of rebuildings near his workshops, in those parts of modern Grosvenor Hill and Bourdon Street that Cubitt had not touched. He then proceeded to larger works in the main streets, especially Grosvenor Street, where he rebuilt or worked on nine of the minor houses (Nos. 13, 14, 17, 23, 24, 25, 65, 79 and 80) between 1851 and 1857. Newson was small enough to employ outside architects. In the 1840's he had an association with the Mount Street cabinet-maker Thomas Dowbiggin,[70] while for the surviving No. 25 Grosvenor Street the recorded architect is F. W. Bushill, and for Nos. 79–80 Sydney Smirke (who had his office here). But Newson appears to have had a good understanding with Thomas Cundy II, and participated whole-heartedly in the refronting policy. Yet frequently, many of the surviving Newson houses with Cundy fronts turn out to be less than complete rebuildings and retain a few older features.

Though by no means an operator on the scale of Thomas Cubitt, and perfectly content to do contract as well as speculative work, Newson did well enough to build himself a country house, Haskerton Manor near Woodbridge, and buy other Suffolk property. On his retirement, one son took over his Mayfair interests, another his property and yards in Pimlico, and the latter side survives as W. H. Newson and Sons, timber merchants of Pimlico Road.[71] But what separates John Newson from the speculative builders of the previous generation is his interest in working-class housing. In the 1850's he built in Grosvenor Hill and Bourdon Street the first two blocks of an important series of 'model lodging houses' erected on the Mayfair estate: St. George's Buildings (1852–3) and Bloomfield Flats (1854–6), as well as the smaller Oxford House, Grosvenor Market (1860), now

demolished. St. George's Buildings was for the newly formed St. George's Parochial Association, but Bloomfield Flats was Newson's own enterprise, and in both the initiative appears to have been his, at least according to Henry Roberts, who reports similar ventures by Newson elsewhere in London.[72] Roberts, the best-known of the early architects to specialize in working-class housing, was brought in to plan St. George's Buildings, an austere, galleried block of workman-like appearance (Plate 30a).

For the time the estate did not manifest much interest, but the second Marquess must have been impressed by the success of the experiment. In the 1860's he began to encourage much larger developments of working-class flats on his estates, at first with the Metropolitan Association for Improving the Dwellings of the Industrious Classes, later with the Improved Industrial Dwellings Company. Before the Marquess died in 1869 this campaign was mainly confined to Pimlico, so there are no I.I.D.C. blocks in northern Mayfair prior to Clarendon Flats in Balderton Street (1871–2). But in 1868–9 the St. George's Parochial Association did add to their previous ventures with a further block in Bourdon Street, Grosvenor Buildings, this time designed by R. H. Burden and built in two tones of brick to cheer up its essentially sober elevations (Plate 30b).

The last years of the second Marquess were ones of stylistic restlessness. Gothic had scarcely yet been seen on the estate, nor was it ever to secure more than a toehold. However when it did appear its teeth could be sharp, as was manifested in a chemist's shop at No. 26 South Audley Street, an eccentric and controversial creation of 1858 by Thomas ('Victorian') Harris demolished in the first Duke's rebuildings. Some of this kind of assertiveness percolated through to other styles deemed more suitable to town houses. In this context a number of significant schemes on the northern part of the estate, now almost entirely lost, must be mentioned. One was a single house. In 1866–9 Sir Dudley Marjoribanks rebuilt his residence at the corner of Upper Brook Street and Park Lane. The new Brook House was on the grand scale (Plate 27a); its architect was T. H. Wyatt, a choice possibly prompted by the Grosvenors (who had long patronized him in the country), and the style was rebarbatively French. It proclaimed for all Park Lane to see that the fustian classic of Thomas Cundy II had had its day upon the estate. But a little further north, larger developments were in the mid-1860's already springing up in confirmation of this message. These were the reconstructions of the whole of Hereford Street (soon to be called Hereford Gardens) and of a range nearby at Nos. 489–497 (odd) Oxford Street (Plate 27b), while further east at Nos. 411–413 (odd) rebuilding of a similar kind was contemplated but could not yet be undertaken.

Hereford Gardens and the Oxford Street ranges are inseparable from the Grosvenor Place improvements, that is to say the rebuilding of properties along Grosvenor Place and the laying out of Grosvenor Gardens on the eastern edge of the Belgravia estate. All of these works as built betray the hand of Thomas Cundy III working untrammelled by the restrictions of previous estate policy. Grosvenor Place itself had a complicated history and was the last of these improvements to be undertaken, but for Grosvenor Gardens, initiated in 1863, Thomas Cundy III provided designs for the street fronts; behind these, high-class builders were allowed to proceed much as they pleased. Cundy's elevations here were of a French-style Second Empire character and of an elaboration and colourfulness hitherto unknown in London terrace architecture, with tall mansards and pavilion roofs, lavish stone dressings, and plenty of red brick, terracotta and polychrome slatework. Though his inspiration was no doubt the New Louvre, mediated through such recent buildings as Burn's Montagu House and Knowles's Grosvenor Hotel, Cundy showed that he had learned something too from the proponents of Advanced Gothic.

The Mayfair schemes matured at the same time as Grosvenor Gardens and by the same methods, with Thomas Cundy III as architect for the elevations once again, but because the developments were smaller and the neighbourhood of Oxford Street was less fashionable, the façades were somewhat more sober, but with a similarly animated roof-line (Plate 14b). Hereford Gardens, the only strictly residential development of the three, was originally to comprise nine houses, which were to be set back from Oxford Street with an open space in front. The terms for its development were taken by Trollopes, but at a high price just before a big building slump, and they were soon in trouble with the venture. To make them easier to sell, twelve houses instead of nine were built and the elevations of six of these were simplified, so that the final result as built between 1866 and 1876 had little of the *brio* of Grosvenor Gardens. By contrast Nos. 489–497 (odd) Oxford Street, a block of shops with accommodation over, proceeded without a hitch in 1865–6, Mark Patrick and Son being the builders for all the lessees. The appearance of this handsome range (Plate 27b), with an unanswered pavilion at the Park Street corner, suggests that it may have been the Estate's hope to rebuild the remainder of the block up to North Audley Street when leases fell in. Further east, Cundy also in 1864–5 provided modest French-style elevations (with proposed terracotta dressings) destined for a rebuilding at Nos. 411–413 (odd) Oxford Street; these were eventually extended to Nos. 407–409, and the block was carried out in 1870–4. This rather forlorn range is now the only survivor of French-style elevations in Mayfair, but it testifies to what may have been the start of a systematic attempt by the second Marquess to smarten up the bedraggled appearance of Oxford Street, a policy frustrated by difficulties with leases and by his own death.

If the French-style developments of the Oxford Street area and of Grosvenor Place marked the end of the long sway of Thomas Cundy II, they were also in their way a turning point for his son. For though Thomas Cundy III

succeeded as surveyor to the second Marquess on his father's death in 1867 and held this post under the first Duke right up until 1890, he was never again so largely employed as an architect on the Mayfair estate. He certainly did some smaller designing jobs under the first Duke, but his role was mainly confined to that of a surveyor. In fact the Duke seems firmly to have shut Cundy out from the architectural aspects of the great rebuilding undertakings he was to initiate from the 1880's. With his accession in 1869 (at first as third Marquess) the whole refronting policy finally collapsed, and yet another distinctive epoch in the estate's architecture was ushered in.

Ducal Heyday

The first Duke of Westminster was one of English architecture's great private patrons. Bodley, Clutton, Devey, Douglas, Edis, Lutyens, Robson, Wade and Waterhouse were among the different distinguished Victorian architects whom he employed in a personal capacity. But the range of talents engaged through him on estate work was far wider. On his estates, the notable architectural achievements of the Duke and his servants were twofold. Round Eaton Hall, the Cheshire countryside was studded with a series of internationally acclaimed cottages and model farms from the picturesque pencil of John Douglas, while in London, many of the more down-at heel streets of the Mayfair estate were taken by the scruff of the neck, and then scrubbed, polished and outfitted anew. From this latter transformation there emerged a remarkable batch of buildings, almost invariably in the fresh red brick personally insisted upon by the Duke, and usually approximating in style to the 'Queen Anne', that undogmatic town-house manner initiated in the 1870's. Individually, these buildings are a mixed bag, some brilliant, some worthy, and some poor; together, they then offered and still offer a sharp, invigorating contrast with the character of the rest of the estate, and please in accordance with the old canon of variety within uniformity. Duke Street and Green Street both have a share in these virtues, but the great success of the first Duke's rebuildings was undoubtedly Mount Street, a thoroughfare whose *élan* and cheerful homogeneity are unique not just on the estate but in the whole of the West End (Plate 34a, b).

In contrast to his father, the first Duke felt a special affinity with and concern for questions of architecture, as the detailed comments and suggestions he made on Douglas's drawings for estate buildings round Eaton show.[73] For his London estates the second Marquess had continued to prefer the Italianate fashionable in his youth, though we have seen a more lavish French manner beginning to creep in under architects like T. H. Wyatt and Thomas Cundy III. But his son was keen to explore new possibilities; his tastes were in fact broad and eclectic. In 1863, several years before his father's death, he had sauntered down from his home in Princes Gate to see the new brickwork of what is now the west side of the quadrangle of the Victoria and Albert Museum.[74] This visit may have fuelled his enthusiasm for red brick and terracotta. In 1875 the Duke was to ask for the use of these materials in connexion with the rebuilding of W. J. Goode's shop in South Audley Street, and to recommend Goode to view a certain house in South Kensington, no doubt one of the very recently erected ones by J. J. Stevenson or Norman Shaw. This suggests a partisanship for the idioms of 'South Kensington' and the Queen Anne revival, and certainly Mount Street and other developments testify to the sway that these styles were to enjoy upon the Duke's estates.

But he was no architectural dogmatist, except in this matter of brickwork being red. In the countryside, for instance, he was an avid enthusiast for half-timbering, a feature which he was sensible enough not to try and force upon his London estates. There is a suspicion, too, that it was he as Earl Grosvenor rather than his father who in 1864, as part of the improvements of the time in Belgravia and Pimlico, promoted an abortive limited competition for two blocks in Grosvenor Place, where it was his definite intention to live in a specially designed house.[75] The participants for the blocks were G. E. Street (Gothic), H. B. Garling (Gothic), Robert Kerr (French Renaissance with significant terracotta detailing) and Thomas Cundy III (designs lost, but presumably also French Renaissance), while E. M. Barry contributed an ornate villa design for a corner site, again in a French Renaissance style with terracotta details and presumably destined for the son and heir to the estates himself. Gothic designers like Street and Garling were not the sort of architects whom the second Marquess normally patronized, nor was competition his natural method of selection. Although the designs were set aside, the records show that Earl Grosvenor was involved before his succession in decision-making for all the big blocks actually erected by Cundy during this period, in Grosvenor Gardens (1864–9), Hereford Gardens (1866–76) and Grosvenor Place (1867–71).[76] No. 5 Grosvenor Place (now demolished), at the corner with Halkin Street, was indeed specially built in 1867–9 to Cundy's designs for the Earl,[77] though because of his father's death he appears never to have lived there. The French style of all these buildings, therefore, though not normally associated with his preferences, was probably one of the several facets of his catholic architectural taste, at a period when town-house styles were in a state of uncertainty and flux. At the least, the Earl was well versed in all questions of design upon the Grosvenor estates before his succession in 1869. His later patronage was to show that he was always more concerned to get the right architect for the right job, and to experiment accordingly, than to adhere to any one single man or style.

However, it is vital not to attribute too much to the personality of the first Duke. For a start, his important rebuildings in Mayfair belong only to the second half of

his reign, from about 1885 to 1899, and were of course dependent upon the falling-in of leases, not upon personal initiative. Except in Oxford Street the years 1869 to 1885 were a reasonably quiet period on the Mayfair estate, during which the Duke had merely to maintain the smooth-running management machine perfected by the second Marquess, the Cundys and the Boodles. The only drastic change he made was to drop the refronting of houses, a policy which had already become something of a dead letter since the demise of Thomas Cundy II in 1867. He did indeed involve himself specially in the charitable projects inherited from his father, principally the campaign for better working-class housing in both Pimlico and Mayfair. But otherwise he was at first content to let the estate jog on much as before under the professionals.

Indeed as a dynast, a Liberal and a Balliol man, the first Duke was as much bound up with fulfilling the duties of family, politics, social life and conscience as with the artistic aspects of architecture. His patronage reflected these concerns and prejudices; Alfred Waterhouse, who rebuilt Eaton, was most likely the choice of the Liberal politician in him, while the very different Henry Clutton, architect for the Grosvenor House alterations, was probably the notion of the family man, as Clutton had worked for the Duke's father-in-law at Cliveden. Eaton and Grosvenor House were in fact set in train shortly after he had succeeded as third Marquess in 1869, the latter perhaps in compensation for the unoccupied mansion in Grosvenor Place. The Grosvenor House job, though modest in comparison with Eaton and hardly affecting the exterior at first, was certainly lavish. The whole of the Cundy wing and most of the reception rooms in the old house were being redecorated from top to toe in 1870–2, and were certainly finished before the third Marquess was created first Duke in 1874. Clutton's outstanding features were the ceilings, magnificently painted, gilded, and in part designed by J. G. Crace. They varied between dainty neo-classicism in the saloon, dining- and drawing-rooms, and exceptional muscularity and depth in the Rubens room and the gallery (Plate 28b). The awesome 'chain-link' ribs of the gallery ceiling were of *cinquecento* inspiration, but the handsome painted frieze beneath was by a Frenchman, F. J. Barrias, and the Rubens room and many of the fittings throughout were in a candidly Empire style.

It is instructive thus to see Clutton, a Goth by instinct though certainly a Francophile one, and the Duke, an Englishman to his marrow and client for the most confident Gothic Revival house of its day at Eaton, turning automatically to French classicism, in however imaginative a rendering, as the natural answer for the grand town-house interior. The gallery ceiling was constructed under a special fireproof iron framework and could if it became necessary be hoisted to a higher position, proof not so much of the Duke's delight in prudent ingenuity as of his plans for the future extension of Grosvenor House. But as with his grandfather this was not to be. In 1880–1 Clutton did add on a semicircular open loggia with Ionic columns at the newly conspicuous Park Lane end of the gallery wing, matching Cundy's exterior in general style and materials but once again using markedly French details (Plate 28a). Yet the fuller reconstruction of Grosvenor House forecast in 1871 never materialized, so that the interior, right up to demolition in 1927, remained much as Clutton had left it fifty years before.

Though the Duke's first thoughts were of rehousing himself, the claims of conscience and religion were being settled simultaneously. His uncle Lord Ebury had been instrumental in securing a favourable hearing for the Association in Aid of the Deaf and Dumb, when they brought their request for a chapel site before the Grosvenor Board in 1868. Earl Grosvenor, as the Duke then was, promised virtually for nothing a site in Oxford Street, upon which St. Saviour's Church was erected in 1870–3. The architect was Arthur Blomfield, brother-in-law to one of the Association's trustees. It was a valuable commission to him, for he went on to design the reconstructions of St. Peter's, Eaton Square, St. Mark's, North Audley Street and the new church of St. Mary's, Bourdon Street, all on the Grosvenor estates. St. Peter's, in Belgravia, does not concern us here, but Blomfield's three Mayfair churches (Plate 29) all showed the resourcefulness that this frequently humdrum architect could muster when faced with a special brief. St. Saviour's, Oxford Street, though conventionally 'second-pointed' in style, was given a centralized plan to ensure maximum visibility for the deaf and dumb, and a wooden octagonal vault above. On the other hand St. Mark's (1878), where since 1851 the Reverend J. W. Ayre had pursued an industrious ministry directed particularly towards the poor of his parish, was a prestigious reconstruction job. Here, Blomfield kept Gandy-Deering's portico and pronaos, but rebuilt the body of the church in the Romanesque style that was one of his occasional specialities. The result is a fine high-roofed vessel of considerable dignity, with internal walling of coloured brickwork and some fittings and glass of merit, though there have been several alterations since Blomfield's time. The third church, St. Mary's, Bourdon Street, was a less ambitious venture, built for the poor of the Grosvenor Mews district and entirely paid for by the Duke. It was a simple church in a Gothic rather old-fashioned for its date (1880–1), but it had two distinctive features, passage aisles and concrete piers, concrete being an expedient Blomfield sometimes used for cheapness. Some of the same craftsmen worked at the three churches. Maceys were the builders of St. Saviour's and St. Mary's, in both of which there were windows by Blomfield's favourite firm of Heaton, Butler and Bayne; while Thomas Earp did carving and Burke and Company mosaic work at St. Mark's and St. Mary's. Blomfield also provided clergy houses for St. Saviour's (1876–8) and St. Mark's (1887–8), next to the respective churches. The St. Mark's vicarage survives at No. 13 North Audley Street, an unexceptional brick house

unusual only as a rare essay by Blomfield in the full Queen Anne manner and because of its fine position at the head of Green Street. Later again in the Duke's reign, the estate was to become even better 'churched'. In Duke Street, the King's Weigh House Chapel replaced Seth Smith's Robert Street Congregational Chapel, while in Davies Street there rose the unusual church of St. Anselm's; both of these important designs will be discussed later.

Behind St. Mark's, two further buildings still to be seen in Balderton Street (Plate 30c) highlight the concern of both vicar and landlord for the lot of the local working classes. One is St. Mark's Mansions (1872–3), an unusual institution for the Church of England at that date, combining a club, kitchen, mission room, classrooms and apartments in the same functional brick building by R. J. Withers. Adjacent is Clarendon Flats, originally Clarendon Buildings (1871–2), the first of the Improved Industrial Dwellings Company's blocks upon the Mayfair estate, complementing several others erected in Pimlico in this period in accordance with a policy worked out in the late years of the second Marquess.

But though his son approved and carried out this block, as he did with the others in Pimlico, he was when Clarendon Flats were finished to express 'his dissatisfaction at the elevation as built'.[78] Consequently, when fifteen years later the I.I.D.C. came to construct the large series of tenement blocks round the present Brown Hart Gardens and east of Duke Street (1886–92), their habitual type of elevation was dropped in favour of something more cheerful in the red-brick idiom of which the Duke was so fond, with a modicum of gables and decoration (Plates 30d, 31a, b). However, with working-class housing the plans were what mattered. The later I.I.D.C. blocks (fig. 18) adhere to the complete self-containment for each

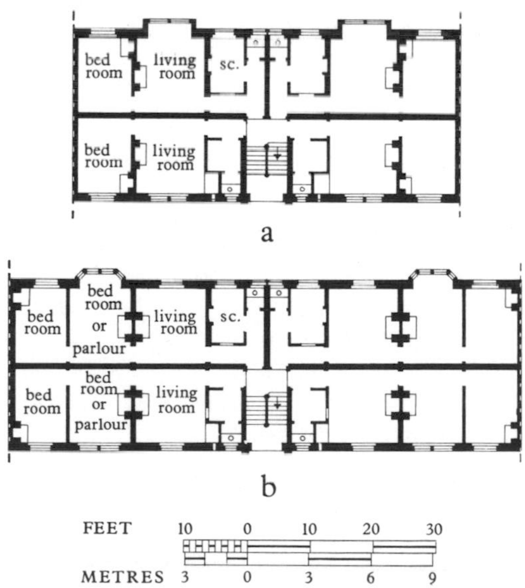

Fig. 18. Standard plans for flats, Improved Industrial Dwellings Company's estate, 1885. *a*. Three- and two-room flats. *b*. Four- and three-room flats (sc = scullery)

flat that was a hallmark of this company, but drop the awkward contours of Clarendon Buildings and their similar early ventures elsewhere and go instead for greater linearity of plan, more even ventilation, and better light. Who designed these flats we do not know, but the principal throughout their construction was the I.I.D.C. secretary, James Moore. Though the 'coffee tavern' that was to accompany them never materialized, they did enjoy the unusual amenity of communal gardens. The 'Italian Garden' in the centre of what is now Brown Hart Gardens was soon replaced by the Duke Street Electricity Sub-station, but the quiet little garden dividing the two parts of Moore Flats survives as a pleasant urban oasis between Binney Street and Gilbert Street.

Meanwhile, there was further expansion of working-class housing by other bodies. In 1883–4 a small parish institute was erected in Bourdon Street in combination with model dwellings, designed by Joseph Peacock and now demolished; between 1887 and 1890 the Artizans Labourers and General Dwellings Company tucked in two small blocks by F. T. Pilkington, one at Nos. 20 and 22 Lees Place, still surviving, the other in Mount Row, now gone, and for the St. George's Parochial Association, a body distinct from the vestry itself, their secretary and architect R. H. Burden designed a substantial block in North Row (1887–9) and extended Grosvenor Buildings in Bourdon Street (1891–2). As Thomas Cundy III and the Estate were behind the Association's initiative, Burden's North Row Buildings, though peppered with a few more Queen Anne touches, keep to a basic idiom compatible with the I.I.D.C.'s Brown Hart Gardens blocks.

Returning now to the early period of the Duke's reign, only a few houses along the four major streets were rebuilt in his first years. One such was No. 78 Brook Street, destroyed by fire in December 1872. Its replacement by C. F. Hayward, a tall, gaunt affair (1873–5), shows the Estate's predilections of the time: minimally Gothic elevations of the 'prescribed' red brick and stone, with 'numerous projections' for light and air (Plate 33c).[79] The biggest single block along these streets to undergo major change in the 1870's was Nos. 37–40 (consec.) Upper Grosvenor Street (now demolished), the leases of which had been planned to fall in so that the Duke's stables in Reeves Mews could be improved. Yet significantly in the event only Nos. 39 and 40 were completely rebuilt (1875–7). Though both houses have gone, they were a landmark in the return of individualism for terrace houses. Both had porticos, but their elevations were by no means uniform; No. 39, by Clutton, had a stone front, while No. 40, the home of John Walter, proprietor of *The Times*, was in brick. When Walter had dabbled in architecture before, at his country house, Bear Wood, he had employed the 'gentleman's architect' Robert Kerr and had had his fingers burnt for his pains, so for Upper Grosvenor Street he relied upon his surveyor, one S. Deacon, perhaps supplemented by his own efforts.

The only other big house to be rebuilt in these years was No. 3 Grosvenor Square (1875–7) by John Johnson for Sir John Kelk, with a rather restless front elevation again of stone, which the Duke was plainly prepared to allow if a tenant would run to it. Clearly it was drab stucco which he could not stomach, as he showed when he had the exterior of the Grosvenor Office painted orange in 1883.

If complete rebuildings of individual first-class houses were for the time rarer, the pace of internal reconstruction and redecoration never slackened. This was an age of large households and specialized servants, and Georgian town-house accommodation could not hope to meet Victorian requirements. Many tenants had long since begun adding extra storeys to answer this problem, and in 1874, when one of several attempts was being made to rationalize building regulations, a proposed height limit of sixty-five feet to the cornice was canvassed for London houses. E. M. Barry, giving evidence before the Select Committee on the eventually abortive Metropolitan Buildings and Management Bill, took as an example No. 66 Grosvenor Street, a house which he had just altered internally. This house then had a height to the cornice of 41 feet 6 inches, and Barry demonstrated how two good extra floors could be added and the main storeys raised behind a suitably embellished front, without exceeding the proposed limit. He also pointed out that the recently built Brook House, which actually exceeded the limits slightly, boasted merely two bedroom storeys below the cornice, whereas if pressed he could get in three at No. 66 within the limit, apart from the attics.[80]

If Brook House shows what spacious storey heights were then in vogue, the Grosvenor Street house is a typical instance of the predicament in which fashionable tenants found themselves. There was little they could do to alter the proportions of their reception rooms unless they undertook total reconstruction. Usually they had to content themselves with palliatives: building on at the back (though space here was at an increasing premium as more and more additions were made), putting on extra storeys, or rearranging the main rooms. Adding on servants' rooms was a rather anonymous sort of work, radically different from the great Grosvenor Square reconstructions of a hundred years before, in which leading architects had vied with each other. But occasionally distinguished men were still employed in additions or alterations; No. 49 Grosvenor Street was set about by Alfred Waterhouse in 1868–71, and in 1878–9 that rare architect Eden Nesfield is found engaged on one of his even rarer London works, the partial refurbishing of No. 26 Grosvenor Square. One development of these years was the more sensitive treatment, in some cases, of Georgian interiors, as at No. 19 Grosvenor Square, where Frederick Arthur presided in 1880 over a full restoration of the Adam work.

The coming of 'Queen Anne' in the mid 1870's gave a fillip to the staid progress of the Mayfair estate and

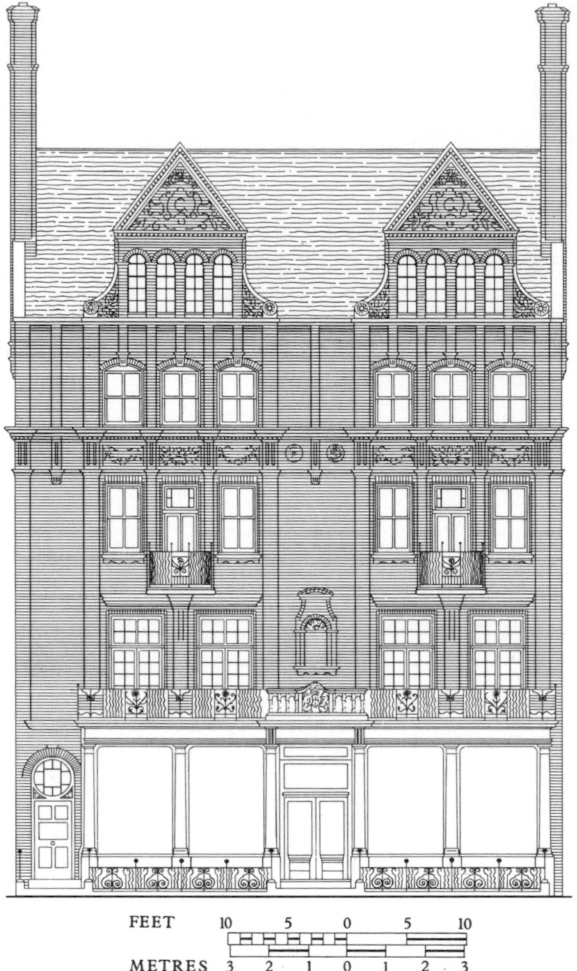

Fig. 19. Nos. 18 and 19 South Audley Street (Goode's), elevation. *Architects*, Ernest George and Peto, 1875–6

heralded the estate revolution of the 1880's and 1890's. Its indubitable harbinger was W. J. Goode's china and glass shop at Nos. 17–21 (consec.) South Audley Street (Plates 32, 33a, b). Goode's is a powerful and picturesque if slightly ungainly building by Ernest George and Peto, in the reddest of red brickwork and tricked out with the complete panoply of the new domestic revival: carved and moulded brick dressings and panels of great elaboration, mighty chimneys, touches of half-concealed tile-hanging, blue and white pots in the Oriental taste to enhance the façade, and within, dapper aesthetic interiors mingling stained glass, ceramic tiles and leather paper. Two points need to be emphasized about Goode's. Firstly, it is not a single composition; Goode began rebuilding on the enclosed sites of Nos. 18 and 19 in 1875, added No. 17 on the corner shortly after, and only extended his premises to Nos. 20 and 21 together with the houses in Chapel Place in 1889–91. The original design, therefore, though short-lived as an independent composition, seems to have

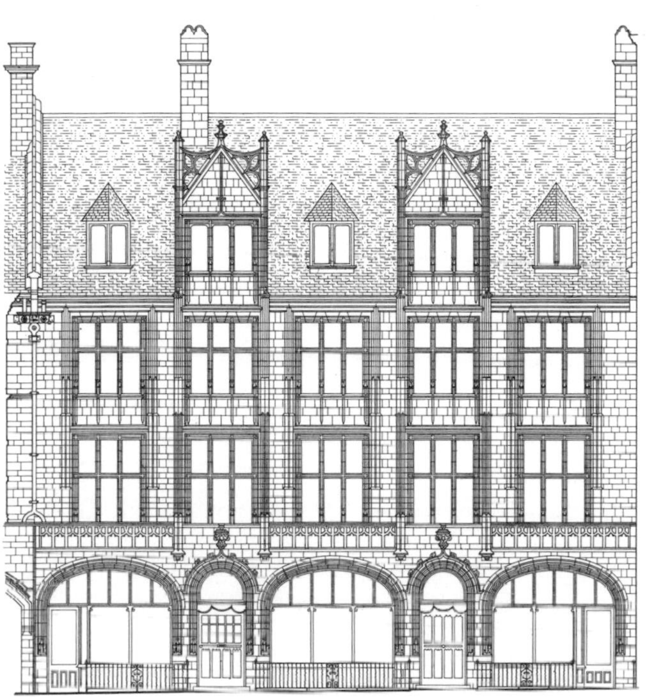

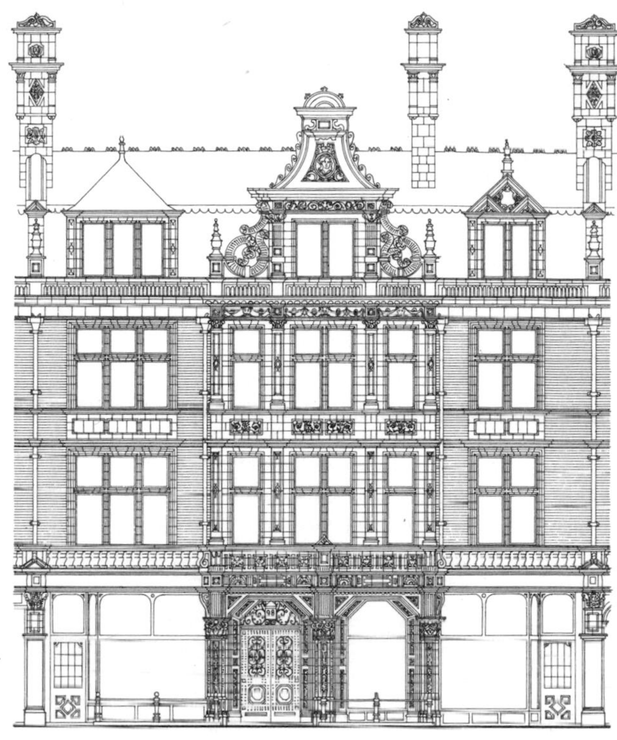

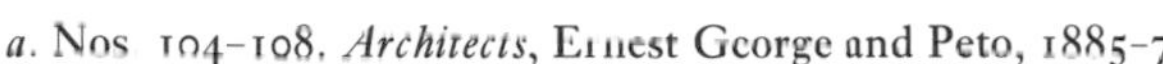

a. Nos 104–108. *Architects*, Ernest George and Peto, 1885–7

b. Nos. 97–99. *Architect*, Albert J. Bolton, 1889–91

Fig. 20. MOUNT STREET REBUILDING: ELEVATIONS

involved only a pair of terrace houses, and in this context one can make sense of the Duke's advice that Goode's architect should look at a particular house in South Kensington (probably No. 8 Palace Gate by J. J. Stevenson, less likely No. 196 Queen's Gate or Lowther Lodge by Norman Shaw), and of the designs then produced by George (fig. 19), slightly asymmetrical but kept in order by two regular gables. Secondly, if the Duke's advice was helpful, it fell on receptive ears, for Goode himself was an enlightened 'artistic' tradesman, eager to reflect the latest taste. To him must be credited the employment of Ernest George and the consequent architectural panache of the building. Goode's in fact was a double precedent; besides being the Grosvenor estate's first Queen Anne building, it was apparently George's own first full essay in a style that was to be the medium of many of his happiest inventions. From two more of these Mount Street was to profit, while in the 1890's George went on to rebuild Motcombe in Dorset for the Duke's brother, Lord Stalbridge.

The street where the new manner was most quickly taken up was Oxford Street, where a systematic policy of rebuilding when the time was ripe appears to have been decided in the mid 1860's. The first rebuildings here had been in the French style favoured in the late days of the second Marquess, and Thomas Cundy III's Nos. 407–413 (odd) Oxford Street (1870–4) still survives as a reminder of the type. Under the first Duke, Queen Anne was soon to prevail, but if Goode's shows how well the new style could be applied to commerce, in Oxford Street it was often watered down and degenerated into banality. The most prolific architect here was T. Chatfeild Clarke, who designed a number of shops of variable style and merit, the best being the extant Nos. 385–397 (odd) of 1887–9 and the demolished Nos. 475–477 (odd) of 1887–8. But the first Queen Anne range appears to have been Nos. 443–451 (odd) of 1876–8, a perfunctory design by J. T. Wimperis notable only as an attempt at stylistic compromise between the French elevations provided for Oxford Street by Thomas Cundy III and the new preferences of the Duke. Wimperis, a prolific West End architect, was known to Cundy, and his later partner, W. H. Arber, came from a family of local surveyors equally established with the Grosvenor Board. Wimperis built quite widely on the estate, and a cousin of his was later to become its surveyor. He is a representative Queen Anne designer of varying accomplishment. His other surviving buildings include Nos. 130 Mount Street and 34 Berkeley Square (1880–2); Nos. 51–54 (consec.) Green Street (1882–3); Audley Mansions at the north-west corner of South Audley Street and Mount Street (1884–6); Duke Street Mansions, a block of shops and flats that straggles along the west side of that thoroughfare (1887–8); and the premises of John Bolding and Sons, the plumbers and sanitary engineers, in Davies Street (1890–1). The Berkeley Square house has a stylish interior; Audley

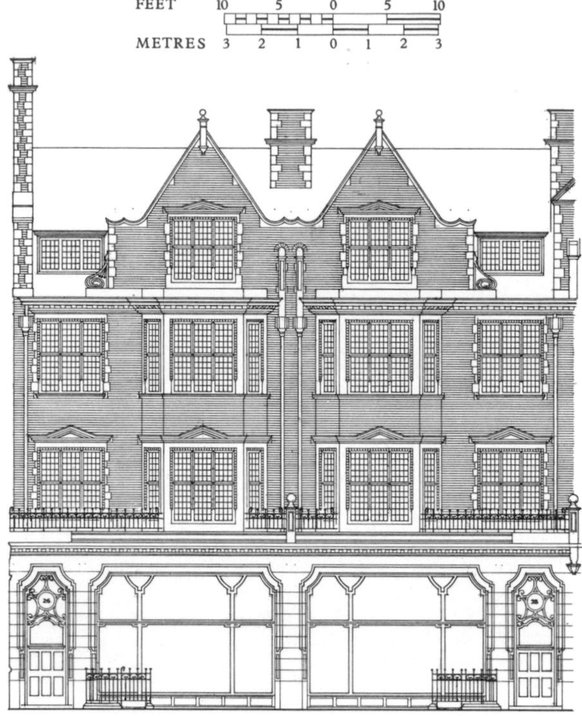

c. Nos. 23–26. *Architects*, Read and Macdonald, *builders*, Holloways, 1896–8

Mansions (Plate 33d) is one of the earliest and not the least satisfying set of high-class flats on the estate; and at Boldings, Wimperis's chunky pink blocks of terracotta make up a dignified elevation for yet another corner site, and skilfully conceal the nature of the only major surviving factory building on the whole estate. Though J. T. Wimperis was often a speculating architect he could ascend the social scale too, making alterations at No. 23 Grosvenor Square in 1876 and 1879, and completely rebuilding No. 27 Grosvenor Square in 1886–8. In several of these works, lowly as well as high class, he found room for a little stained glass, as if to validate his claims to just a touch of aestheticism.

The work of J. T. Wimperis offers a preview of the building types and styles soon to dominate in the great reconstructions of 1885–99. At much the same time rebuilding began in three separate areas, centred upon Mount Street, Duke Street and Green Street. By the turn of the century the first two districts were substantially complete, but in Green Street west of Park Street building activity was to recommence just before the war of 1914–18. The methods by which these rebuildings were organized and architects chosen are explained on pages 54–60; here it remains to consider the results, beginning with Mount Street.

To understand the genesis of present-day Mount Street (Plate 34), the most representative and best sector to take is the range on the south side between South Audley Street and the cul-de-sac opposite Carlos Place. Ignoring J. T. Wimperis's two corner blocks mentioned above, one may say that the reconstruction of the street began when Albert J. Bolton won a limited competition of 1884–5 for a Vestry Hall on the site of No. 103 (in the centre of this block), the freehold of which had been recently bought by St. George's Vestry. Of the Vestry Hall, one of only two losses in Mount Street, we know little except that the Duke preferred a rival design. Nevertheless in 1889–95 Bolton was allowed to build the adjacent Nos. 87–102 (consec.) to the west, together with the deep return plot to South Audley Street and the library in Chapel Place North. For the first part of this long frontage, the Duke had hoped but failed to get Bolton to follow the lines of Ernest George and Peto's designs at Nos. 104–111 (consec.) Mount Street (1885–7), the Vestry Hall's neighbour on the other side and the first block to be reconstructed in the body of the street at the Estate's initiative. These two ranges (Plate 34a, b) are archetypal for Mount Street. Both consist of shops with chambers over; both, so far as overall uniformity of design permits, are divided into distinguishable units, to suit the wants of different parties among the consortia that built them; and both boast street fronts spectacularly decked out in bluff pink terracotta. The differences are almost more illuminating. Bolton contents himself with a straightforward elevational division between shops and upper floors, arranges his flats in an orthodox manner, and where necessary leaves out a little of his normally riotous façade ornament (fig. 20b). But Ernest George boldly chooses two different styles for his lessees, a simple late French or Flemish Gothic for W. H. Warner (fig. 20a), a gentle Jacobean for Jonathan Andrews. He then binds his block together with a continuous roof, corresponding storey heights, and a line of firm arches over the shops. He also experiments with the planning of the chambers, providing conventional bachelor apartments for Warner's tenants over Nos. 104–108, but a brilliant split-level arrangement of larger flats over Andrews's portion, Nos. 109–111. Then, when Andrews decides to take the corner site with the cul-de-sac in 1891–2, George is able to extend his design two bays eastwards to cover Nos. 112–113 without a visible break, and to vary his plan again, this time with another arrangement of bachelors' flats.

The problems raised by this collective method of architecture were formidable. On the whole the Mount Street designers solved them most creditably. Of the two big blocks that followed in 1886–7 hard upon Ernest George's brilliant lead, J. T. Smith's Nos. 116–121 (consec.) appears overloaded in comparison with W. H. Powell's Nos. 125–129 (consec.), a disciplined range in orthodox Queen Anne taste (Plate 34c), with good touches in the planning of the flats. A capable architect, Powell designed a pair of corner houses which the Duke admired at Nos. 33–34 Grosvenor Square (now demolished) at the same time, but disappeared from the metropolitan scene shortly afterwards. The other building to be noted on this part

of the south side of Mount Street is No. 114 by the Catholic architect A. E. Purdie (1885–8), which includes, behind its somewhat lumpy terracotta façade, presbytery accommodation, a hall and a chapel, all for the Church of the Immaculate Conception in Farm Street.

In 1888–9 work began on the north side of the street, with George and Peto again in the forefront of affairs. There was to be less terracotta along this side, so the high façades that George devised here (to the plans of others) between Davies Street and Carpenter Street at Nos. 1–5 (consec.) were of brick, with neat cut and moulded brick dressings in his whimsical early Flemish or French Renaissance manner. The western half only of this range survives. Progressing further west, the opening out of Carlos Place, formerly Charles Street, was one of the major Estate undertakings of the early 1890's. The pleasant houses around the eastern curve here (Plate 34d) are to the designs of John Evelyn Trollope, working for his brother George Haward Trollope's building firm (1891–3); the same combination was busy simultaneously on houses at Nos. 45–52 (consec.) Mount Street, in the sector west of South Audley Street where the Duke had decided that trade should be barred, and a little later at the adjacent No. 53 Mount Street and Nos. 34–42 (even) Park Street. On the western side of Carlos Place rose in 1894–6 the rebuilt Coburg (now Connaught) Hotel. It was designed by Isaacs and Florence, and much of its rich, original interior survives behind a somewhat banal façade. Further along the north side of Mount Street, at the east corner with South Audley Street, Thomas Verity's Audley Hotel (1888–9) was a very different animal from the Coburg; a 'public house bar' was at first prohibited in the Coburg, but the Audley, as one of the few pubs that escaped the scythe of ducal temperance, was frankly a drinking establishment. This truth is reflected in the block's popularly beefy two-tone appearance, albeit moderated from Verity's first elevations, which the Duke had rejected as too 'gin-palace-y'.[81] Between these two havens is the latest and possibly the most charming of the Mount Street ranges, Nos. 14–26 (consec.) by Read and Macdonald (1896–8), in a Tudor style handled with a convincing flair for overall composition and with effective Arts and Crafts touches in the stone dressings, ironwork and shop fronts (Plate 34a; fig. 20c).

Both Verity and Read and Macdonald were to work again on the west side of North Audley Street, another thoroughfare much rebuilt in the first Duke's time. Verity's Nos. 24–29 (consec.) North Audley Street (1891–3) is a big block of flats much like the Audley Hotel and again incorporating a pub; while Read and Macdonald designed another pretty block in their Mount Street idiom, unfortunately now demolished, at the corner with Oxford Street (Nos. 453–459 odd Oxford Street and 22–23 North Audley Street, 1900–2), and the stone mansion at No. 22 Grosvenor Square stretching up North Audley Street as far as Lees Mews, a not altogether happy speculation of 1906–7 by Holloways the builders.

Duke Street is more easily dealt with. On the west side the dominant feature, J. T. Wimperis's Duke Street Mansions (1887–8), evidently sited so as to enclose the Improved Industrial Dwellings Company's new blocks built round Brown Hart Gardens, looks like a coarser and bigger version of one of the Mount Street ranges. Then, before the present Electricity Sub-station was built, came the Duke's 'Italian Garden', a welcome open space, and to the south of this, a pair of undistinguished rebuildings at Nos. 78–82 (even) flanking Chesham Flats, the biggest of the I.I.D.C. blocks.

Opposite, however, are three notable buildings. At the north end Nos. 55–73 (odd), a long range of shops stretching through to Binney Street, has a large central Dutch gable, refined brick detailing, and very picturesque roof treatment. Reminiscent of Ernest George at his most flamboyant, it is in fact an early work by W. D. Caröe (1890–2), who went on to design the more remarkable Nos. 75–83 (odd) Duke Street, south of Weighhouse Street (1893–5). This is one of the estate's most original buildings, a compact, asymmetrical composition whose square profile and chimneys, clipped roof line, well-organized windows and graceful shop arches are all features eloquent of the Arts and Crafts spirit (Plate 35b). The handling of materials on both blocks is delicate and careful. Caröe had doubtless been given these jobs by the Duke on the strength of another design of his a little further east, the Hanover Schools in Gilbert Street (1888–9). This now-demolished building was a more orthodox composition in the School Board manner, but with an idiosyncratic outline and touches of adventurous detailing.

Between Caröe's two Duke Street ranges rises one of Mayfair's chief landmarks, Alfred Waterhouse's King's Weigh House Chapel (now the Ukrainian Catholic Cathedral), built in 1889–91 and serving as a replacement for both Seth Smith's Robert Street Chapel and the old Weigh House Chapel, which had been displaced from the City. The Weigh House congregation was independent and, on the whole, wealthy; originality, therefore, was to be anticipated. Waterhouse, in one of his few ecclesiastical ventures, complied, with an elliptical galleried auditorium candidly expressed outside as well as in, and a Romanesque street front of brick and terracotta designed with his customary rigour and culminating in a tall, cleverly balanced tower at the street corner (Plate 35b; fig. 21). Round into Binney Street the composition continues with a presbytery and associated buildings, of which not the least interesting feature is a meeting room in the attics with a fine open-timber roof. Though a late work, the King's Weigh House Chapel conveys in both conception and detail the energy and compulsiveness so characteristic of Waterhouse throughout his career.

Where ranges of houses were built, rather than the shops with flats over that make up the bulk of Mount and

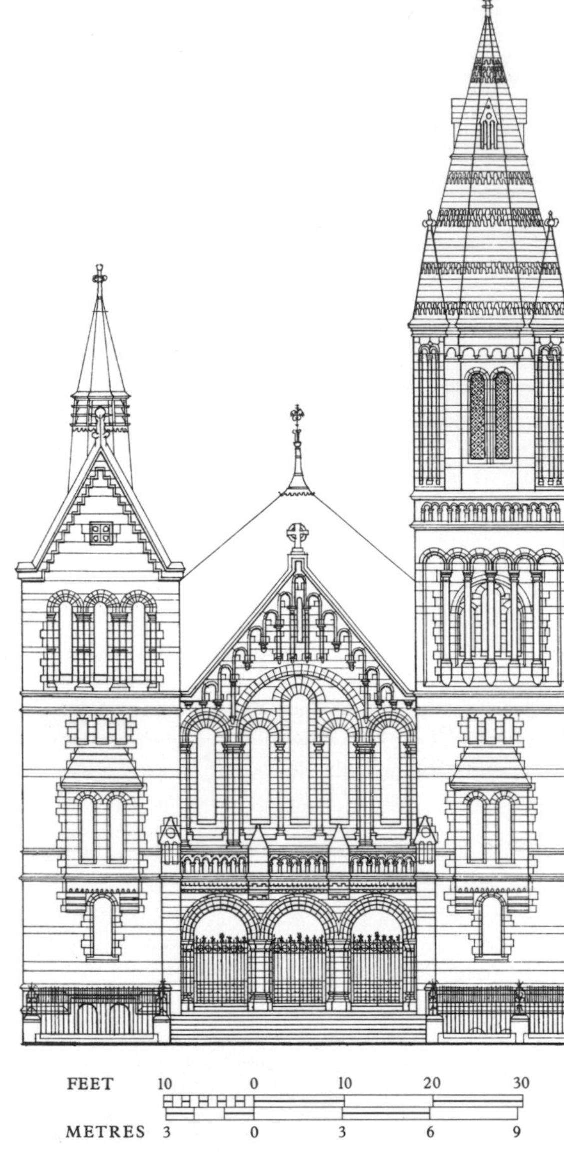

Fig. 21. King's Weigh House Chapel, Duke Street, west front. *Architect*, Alfred Waterhouse, 1889–91

Duke Streets, the results were by and large inferior, because the Grosvenor Board let direct to speculative builders and exercised less control over their designs. In any case, Queen Anne was a style evolved for individual houses, and rarely looked as well when strung out unrelieved along a domestic terrace. These are the reasons why Green Street is a duller and less distinguished thoroughfare than its commercial counterparts. As before, J. T. Wimperis was the Queen Anne standard-bearer here, with Nos. 51–54 (consec.) for Charles Fish the builder on the site of the Park Street chapel (1882–3). Most of the succeeding development of 1887–94 was opposite, on the north side, and neither the promoters nor the designers need to be individually mentioned here; the blocks uniformly consist of houses rather than 'chambers' or 'mansions', and are scarcely distinguishable from similar work elsewhere in London. The only prominent name is that of R. W. Edis, architect and speculator for Nos. 25–31 (consec.) Green Street and 105–115 (odd) Park Street (1891–4). Edis had been in high favour earlier on, having been employed by the Duke himself both at Eaton and at Cliveden and having rebuilt the prominent Nos. 59–61 (odd) Brook Street, opposite the Grosvenor Office, together with the long return to Davies Street in 1883–6. But as a result of his activities in Green Street he fell from grace, for by the 1890's the Grosvenor Board had decided against allowing independent architects to speculate on their own behalf.[82]

The fate of Edis raises anew the question of the choice of architects who worked on the estate at this period. With Thomas Cundy III firmly in his place as surveyor and no more, the Duke and his estate managers could often select architects themselves. From 1887, shortly after large-scale rebuilding began, a list of 'approved architects' was inaugurated, a practice which may have been shared by other contemporary estates. This list was made up in the main of architects who had already built on the estate and conducted themselves without signal incompetence. The original seven of 1887 comprised the two doyens of contemporary domestic architecture, Norman Shaw and Ernest George, four middle-ranking names, T. Chatfeild Clarke, R. W. Edis, Thomas Verity and J. T. Wimperis, and the rather dim figure of James Trant Smith, altogether an odd assortment.[83] Shaw's name was doubtless included out of pious hope; he never built anything on the Grosvenor estates, though he did at one stage sketch out a scheme for houses on the future Aldford House site.

Obviously the list was an amalgam of the Duke's suggestions, mainly aesthetic, and his advisers' business-oriented ideas. It was never exclusive, always haphazard and inconsistent, with names being inserted or dropped in an *ad hoc* manner. In 1891 Aston Webb and Ingress Bell were added, evidently at their own request and on the strength of their Victoria Law Courts at Birmingham, which the Duke 'highly approved of',[84] but they never worked on the estate. Basil Champneys, on the other hand, a leading Queen Anne architect, was never added to the list, although he applied for work on the estate and was championed by his friend and ex-pupil Eustace Balfour, the Duke's new estate surveyor.[85] At one stage Champneys prepared plans for reconstructing the Grosvenor Chapel, but these came to nothing, as did the suggestion that he should undertake part of Carlos Place.

In 1894 the revised list looked like this: J. Macvicar Anderson, Ingress Bell and Aston Webb, A. J. Bolton, H. C. Boyes, W. D. Caröe, T. Chatfeild Clarke, T. E. Collcutt, R. W. Edis, Ernest George and Peto, Isaacs and Florence, C. E. Sayer, J. J. Stevenson, and J. T. Wimperis.[86] Apart from Sayer, Webb and Bell, all these men had already worked on the Mayfair estate or were to do so in the future. Of those not already mentioned, Anderson and Collcutt seem only to have been involved in minor private house-alterations in Mayfair, but may have had work in Belgravia or Pimlico; Boyes designed

a small and respectable block at Nos. 10–12 (consec.) Mount Street; and Chatfeild Clarke was active in Oxford Street, designing, besides his creditable Nos. 385–397 (odd), a long run of shops, all now demolished, between North Audley Street and Park Street: Nos. 461–463 (1886), 465 (1885), 467–473 (1885–6), 475–477 (1887–8), 479–483 (1883–4), and 485–487 (1883–4). He and (later) his son Howard also designed the large and ornate block at Nos. 64–70 (consec.) South Audley Street (1891–1900). J. J. Stevenson was responsible in 1896–8, by which time he had largely abandoned his early austere Queen Anne manner, for a small, select and ornamental little block of speculative houses for William Willett the builder, tucked away at Nos. 39–47 (odd) South Street.

Four men (H. Huntly-Gordon, E. W. Mountford, E. P. Warren and Howard Ince) were subsequently added to the list of 1894, most of them at their own request, but none of them is known to have worked on the Mayfair estate.[87] In fact the list was always something of a fiction. The real estate 'discoveries' such as the young W. D. Caröe owed their opportunities to the Duke's seeing something good by them and giving them a run for their money. Indeed the estate's appearance benefited more from the Duke's obsession with architecture and from his almost capricious desire to put a new architect or two through his paces every so often, than from the sound but staid advice of H. T. Boodle and the luminaries of the Grosvenor Office. Sometimes, of course, it was a lessee who came up with a good and previously unknown designer, as at Nos. 52–54 (even) Brook Street, where the young Percy Morley Horder displaced an incompetent architect and produced what must have been virtually his first work (1896–7), a neat brick design with mullioned windows in the manner of Voysey.

But a crucial contributor to the changing tone of the estate in the last years of the century was the new estate surveyor, Eustace James Anthony Balfour, who took over when the Cundy era finally came to a close with the retirement of Thomas Cundy III in 1890. Though a short list appears to have been made of candidates for the job, it was characteristic of the Duke that social and dynastic considerations in the end swayed his choice and led to his appointment of a man not on the final list. Eustace Balfour (1854–1911) was impeccably connected; his mother was a Cecil, his brother was A. J. Balfour the politician and future Prime Minister, his father-in-law was the eighth Duke of Argyll, and most critically of all his uncle by marriage was the Duke of Westminster himself. Balfour in fact was on terms almost of social equality with the Duke, and rather as in the case of Cecil Parker, the Duke's agent at Eaton and another of his nephews, this entitled him to a position of special eminence, since the estate, to quote Balfour's wife writing much later, 'was run, not as today on commercial lines, but more as a Principality'.[88] Balfour however was not an autocrat in the Parker mould, but a fastidious and to some extent withdrawn individual, with a strong feeling of class loyalty, an interest in shooting, and, at least in later life, a sense of commitment about his work with the army volunteer corps, in which he served as a colonel. Yet as a pupil of Basil Champneys he was also a conscientious and well-trained architect, he knew Burne-Jones, De Morgan, and others in early Arts and Crafts circles, and, having a horror of modern Gothic, he had been involved in some of the early work of the Society for the Protection of Ancient Buildings, a body with which his friend and partner since 1885, Hugh Thackeray Turner, had a lifelong association.

Thackeray Turner (1853–1937), a man of a reticence and modesty equal to Balfour's, had been brought up in Sir Gilbert Scott's office and then became his son George Gilbert Scott junior's trusted assistant. Deeply versed in English mediaeval churches, Turner ardently admired the principles of William Morris and the work of Philip Webb, and was a close companion of W. R. Lethaby, loyalties all discernible in his architecture, and most notably in the beautiful house he built himself at Westbrook outside Godalming in his beloved Surrey. Turner appears as the more active and abler architect of the two, and while Balfour was clearly in ultimate control of all the work they did on the Grosvenor estates, Turner seems to have been the busier at the drawing board.

Of designing the partnership had much to do, since the first Duke was disposed to give them the chances he had denied to Thomas Cundy III. The main area of their Mayfair activity was between Mount Street and Aldford Street. Here, and especially round the eponymous Balfour Place, they showed that Green Street was not an inevitability, in fact that one could combine with the speculative builder to get lively but disciplined street fronts in the brick style of the day. The first range by Balfour and Turner, Nos. 1–6 (consec.) Balfour Place (1891–4), is still tentative and unsatisfactory despite some imaginative planning. But the block bounded by Mount Street, Rex Place, Aldford Street and Balfour Place (1891–7), together with the stables on the east side of Balfour Mews (1898–1900), shows late Queen Anne elevations at their best, with delightfully shaped gables and individual touches of Arts and Crafts detailing and carving upon each house (Plate 35a). Further west, the firm designed another good range of houses fronting Park Street at Nos. 14–22 (even), which with A. H. Kersey's Nos. 2–12 (even) Park Street and Balfour and Turner's demolished Aldford House in Park Lane virtually completed the Duke's transformation of this sector. Elsewhere, they built Nos. 21–22 Grosvenor Street (1898–9) in brick with gay stone banding and a prominent pair of gables, the long range at Nos. 40–46 (even) Brook Street of 1898–9 (fig. 26a), the beautiful Webb-influenced stabling on the south side of Duke's Yard of 1900–2 (Plate 35c), and one odd house in the Green Street development, No. 10 of 1893–5, with delightful carving round the door probably by Thackeray Turner's sculptor brother, Laurence Turner, who worked on other of the firm's buildings on the estate. There were further works by Balfour and Turner under the second

Duke, but none so characteristic as these. All convey an originality passing at times into self-conscious eccentricity, a mood particularly marked in their two major demolished buildings on the estate, St. Anselm's Church in Davies Street (1894–6) and Aldford House (1894–7).

St. Anselm's, a building which by repute was largely or wholly the work of Thackeray Turner, was a typical Arts and Crafts attempt at style-blending (or style-bending). The interior (Plate 38b) was basilican, with more than a hint of *quattrocento* Florence in the texture of grey stone coupled pillars against white-plastered walls, and a few bald and massive fittings; but the tracery was Gothic and the exterior uncompromisingly plain except for some big buttresses and a vicarage building squeezed on to the site at the corner between St. Anselm's Place and Davies Street. In fact for all its originality it was a little-loved church, and when its demolition was being canvassed in 1938 even H. S. Goodhart-Rendel had to admit that 'St. Anselm's has always seemed to me a purely personal record of Thackeray Turner's particular tastes'.[89] And so it disappeared, to be replaced by the far less worthy British Council building.

Aldford House, the diamond magnate Alfred Beit's grand free-standing stone mansion in Park Lane, was also far from an unqualified success, partly because of difficulties over the site, partly because Balfour and Turner insisted on deploying the elements of classicism borrowed from nearby Dorchester House so casually and eccentrically. The result (Plate 38a), an ornate but stunted affair, earned a muted reception, soon dated like St. Anselm's, and therefore was the more easily demolished. There is no doubt that brick domestic buildings were the firm's *forte* on the Grosvenor estate, and these have happily nearly all survived.

Aldford House was one of the last-built of the Park Lane palaces, those ebullient mansions of the super-rich that adorned the park frontage from Marble Arch to Hyde Park Corner, interspersed among the more modest stucco houses. Though many were old, their halcyon days date from after the improvement of Park Lane as a thoroughfare about 1870. At the turn of the century those on the Grosvenor estate were as follows, from north to south: Somerset House, with Camelford House behind in its shadow (Plate 14); Brook House, which was to be transformed internally for the financier Sir Ernest Cassel in 1905–7; Dudley House, with its façade appearing by 1900 much as it does today (Plate 21a); Grosvenor House, whose westward aspect towards the park was opened out shortly before Clutton added his loggia in 1880–1; and finally Beit's Aldford House, below which Dorchester and Londonderry Houses raised their massive bulks.

Though Dudley House is the sole survivor from this galaxy, two grand houses of the 1890's still remain in 'also-ran' positions close behind the park frontage, to testify to its lure at that date. One is No. 32 Green Street, a corner house close to Park Lane, built for Lord Ribblesdale in 1897–9 to the designs of Sidney R. J. Smith. Though a large, conventional edifice (Plate 36b), it is a valuable precursor of the subdued brick neo-Georgian soon to be so fashionable, and contrasts distinctly with the neighbouring Nos. 16–19 (consec.) Dunraven Street, where Smith allowed himself rein with some beefily detailed terrace housing. Much more spectacular is No. 54 Mount Street, on a similar corner site, but originally with an open view towards the park over the garden of Grosvenor House. This was the town house, built in 1896–9, of Lord Windsor, an affluent but discriminating client, whose profuse patronage fell on this occasion upon Fairfax B. Wade, never a prolific but, in his later practice, always an interesting architect. Wade's design (Plates 36a, 37) makes both Aldford House and No. 32 Green Street appear lacking in assurance. It has a festive pair of pedimented brick and stone elevations mixing French and English late seventeenth-century motifs, and a unique and forceful plan combining upper and lower vaulted halls, ample reception rooms, and unusually spacious office and sleeping quarters, all marked by many little originalities of conception and detail. Happily these palatial interiors still remain and must be counted one of the estate's surviving glories. They are possibly the only place on the Grosvenor estate where the true flavour of the late Victorian aristocracy at home still lingers on in Mayfair.

The other great survivor from this palmy period is Claridge's. This splendid and always exclusive hotel had long been operating in a handful of spacious houses stretching along Brook Street from the south-east corner with Davies Street when rebuilding was first contemplated in 1889. The Estate willingly fell in with the idea, for though commerce was at best tolerated along the main streets, this had to be an exception. The classes for whom Claridge's catered were precisely those whose good opinion mattered to the Estate; and, in a period of already shrinking rented accommodation, the hotel fulfilled the specific needs of the many gentlemen, noblemen, magnates and potentates, British and foreign, who wished to stay in town for a limited season and would in former years have hired a house on the estate for the purpose. Caröe was appointed architect and devised a comprehensive scheme with a courtyard, but after the promoters had got into financial difficulties and were bought out by the Savoy Hotel Company in 1893, he was replaced by C. W. Stephens. The main part of the hotel as rebuilt in 1894–8 is the work of Stephens, whose tall and ruddy brick elevations (Plate 39a) call for no great notice. But the lavish decorations of the main reception areas (Plate 39b) were given to Ernest George and Yeates, and although these were drastically altered in the 1930's, in these august apartments, something of the gracious, unhurried life-style of that late Victorian golden age also still obtains.

If such sumptuous edifices are symptomatic of the imperial spirit of the 1890's, that epoch's luxurious but formal way of life can be traced, too, in the vast extent and

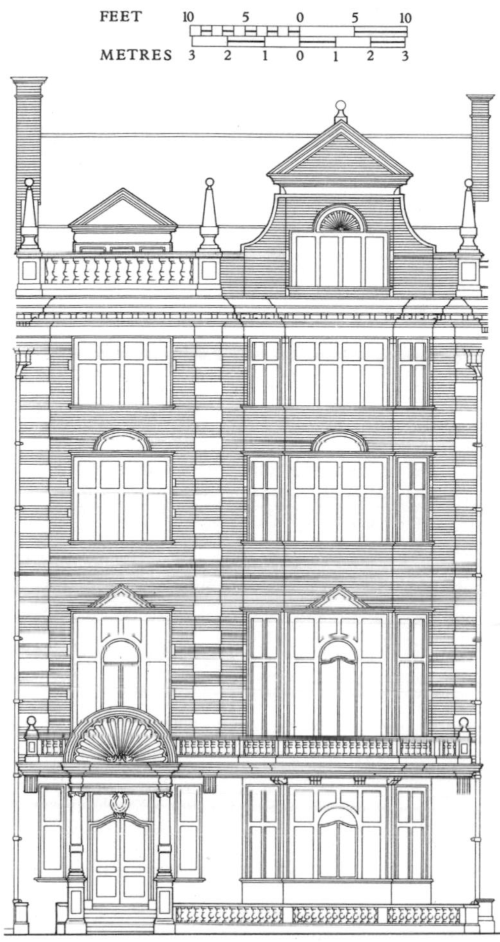

a. No. 41 Grosvenor Square. *Architect*, George Devey, 1883–6. *Demolished*

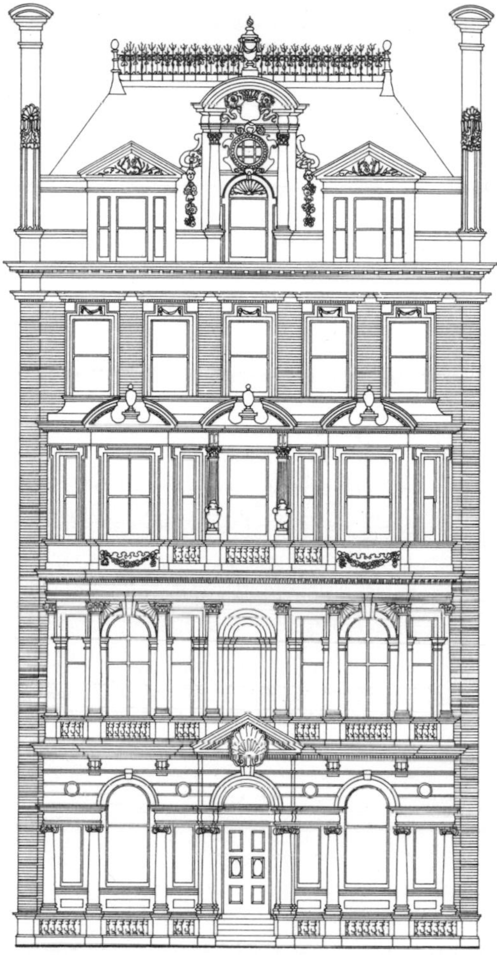

b. No. 27 Grosvenor Square. *Architect*, J. T. Wimperis, 1886–8. *Demolished*

Fig. 22. ELEVATIONS OF THE 1880's

expense of works privately undertaken between 1890 and 1914 in Grosvenor Square and the surrounding streets. This era saw the undoubted climax of the great houses of the estate, after which they were soon to decline and, nearly every one, fall victim to demolition or conversion. While the first Duke lived, there were indeed few entirely new terrace houses rebuilt along the main streets, but in the latter half of his reign, yet another tide of replanning and redecoration had begun to carry his smarter tenants along, until from the second Duke's accession in 1899 up to the war of 1914–18, the Mayfair estate was immersed in wave after frenetic wave of internal reconstructions and redecorations, sometimes engulfing the same house twice. For this period, records of many of these (to modern eyes) almost incredibly lavish conversions remain in photographs taken by the firm of Bedford Lemere after the work was done. From these a coherent picture of this part of Mayfair at the apogee of its fashion emerges.

The lead-up to this great splash was tentative. Possibly because of the prevalent tone of existing houses, 'Queen Anne' never somehow caught on on the estate as a style for the houses of rich individuals, as it did in Kensington and Chelsea. There are really only three candidates, all rebuildings in Grosvenor Square between 1883 and 1888. George Devey's No. 41 for C. H. Wilson, later Lord Nunburnholme, (1883–6) and J. T. Wimperis's No. 27 for the Earl and Countess of Aberdeen (1886–8) were both political gathering points for prominent Liberals. Neither was as typical a Queen Anne composition as Nos. 33 and 34, a busy pair of houses by W. H. Powell in the south-west corner (1886–8), which sported ample terracotta dressings, and bay windows and gables. In contrast to this, Devey, nearing the end of his career as a progressive country-house architect, still believed, even in town, in an irregular Jacobean front with a prominent multi-storey bay and casement lights, while Wimperis

invested in equal protuberance coupled with a more cautious symmetry and some distinctly French detail (fig. 22). Both houses had newly specialized plans, Devey in particular showing ingenuity in getting natural light to the stairs and securing a storey-and-a-half ballroom (though Cundy, noticing his poor arrangement of the offices, could surprisingly inform the Grosvenor Board that 'he does not think that Mr Devey can have had any experience in planning a large house').[90] Wimperis, on the other hand, who had been brought in when the Duke insisted that the Aberdeens must have an architect, was well under the thumb of his employers, for whom an exotic 'Indian room' decorated by the firm of Liberty was devised at first-floor level next to the mews and accessible by a separate entrance, since it was destined mainly for meetings (fig. 24a). This is a token of how stable blocks were beginning to be squeezed out by expanding families at this period. By another late-Victorian innovation, dinner guests in the Aberdeens' 'Indian room' were accommodated at separate small tables, a change in fashion which opened up the possibility of new types of reception-room planning.[91] Yet by 1912 Wimperis's arrangements were sufficiently old-fashioned for No. 27 Grosvenor Square to require radical updating in both plan and décor.

Bedford Lemere's surviving photographs of No. 41 Grosvenor Square show this house at two dates, 1909 and 1926 (Plate 41). The opulence of interior finishing that they reveal is matched only by its transitoriness, and in this they may be taken as paradigms of the kind of continual renewal that so many of the houses in the square underwent in this era. Devey had indicated the lines that the decoration would have to follow, having designed the staircase details, fireplaces and panelling for at least some of the main rooms, and probably also the ceilings. But by a division of labour typical of the time, the main onus of the finishings must have been left to the professional 'interior decorator', as the old upholsterer was now beginning to call himself. His work, even more than that of the architect, was naturally subject to dramatic shifts in fashion. Thus by 1909 the Nunburnholmes' ballroom was given over to a riotous Viennese Rococo quite out of character with anything known about Devey; yet this in 1926 had in turn been ousted and the room redecorated in the cooler eclectic classicism of the years immediately after the war of 1914–18. By contrast the dining-room, an apartment still treated much in Devey's manner in 1909, with light-painted panelling up to dado level and framed tapestries above, had been enlivened seventeen years later by marbling parts of the panelling and fireplace, and by covering the whole of the upper walls with an old pictorial wallpaper.

Decorators' schemes such as these, characterized by their almost reckless extravagance and panache, were amazingly common on the estate during this era. Before 1914, however, they were invariably derivative in style, the common stylistic factor nearly always being France. The French taste lurks behind so many stages of the history of interior decoration in Britain since the seventeenth century, cropping up even in English architecture's most chauvinist periods, and its importance in Mayfair is so great that it calls for a short excursus.

French-derived interiors were always far commoner in London than in the country. Chesterfield House and Norfolk House were decorated in a French Rococo taste at the height of English Palladianism; Carlton House revealed the Prince Regent as a regular Francophile; and York (now Lancaster) House and Apsley House show the conquerors of Bonaparte transformed into enthusiasts for 'Empire'. For all these jobs the upholsterers and other decorators were of equal or greater importance compared with the architects, and the numerous French immigrants among them naturally passed on their skills to Englishmen. So by the 1820's at the latest all the big Mayfair cabinet-making firms such as Tatham and Bailey, Dowbiggin (the decorator of Apsley House) and Seddon, had a good grasp of the French style of interior. But at this time it connoted an exclusive style reserved for the court or the nobility, which the ordinary Mayfair resident either did not want or could not afford. Earl Grosvenor, for instance, might well have chosen such a manner for Cundy's picture gallery at Grosvenor House, or his heir for the refashioned Belgrave House (Nos. 15–16 Grosvenor Square), though what evidence we have suggests that they did not do so. In fact the first French scheme of decoration on the Grosvenor estate of which there is reliable record was at Samuel Daukes's ballroom for the first Earl of Dudley at Dudley House, finished off in a dazzling Empire splendour of glass and gilding in 1858, by the Paris firms of Laurent and Haber (Plate 40a). Though the ballroom has gone, many passages of French craftsmanship survive in the fabric of Dudley House and presumably date from this time.

From this epoch on, the French manner was to grow in popularity and make more of a specifically architectural impact. Many mid-Victorian country houses espoused one French style or another, but in London, under the influence of Haussmann's Paris and especially after the building of a number of grand mansarded hotels, the impulse to go French was particularly strong. Under Thomas Cundy III at Grosvenor Gardens, Grosvenor Place and Hereford Gardens, and in great mansions like T. H. Wyatt's Brook House (Plate 27a), there emerged briefly in the 1860's a fully fledged French architectural style for the high-class London town house. Though the Queen Anne revival succeeded in putting a stop to this kind of street architecture, it did not establish itself widely as an aristocratic style for interiors, and here the French manner was never seriously challenged, instead gradually and imperceptibly broadening its own appeal, particularly for the mercantile bourgeoisie. As an international style, equally idiomatic in Paris, New York, Vienna or London, it became particularly popular with the foreigners who in increasing numbers made their homes in Mayfair. Not

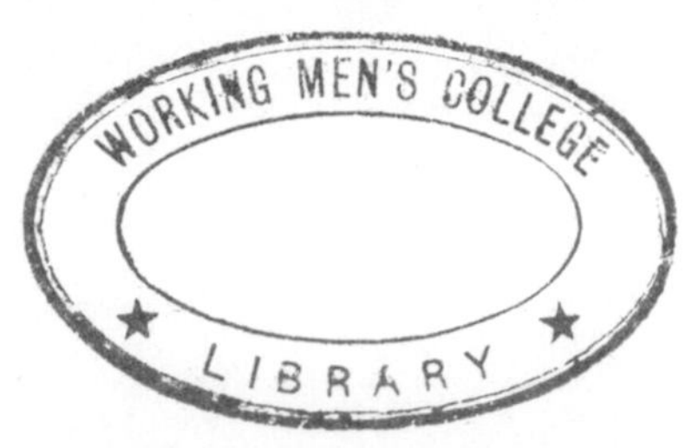

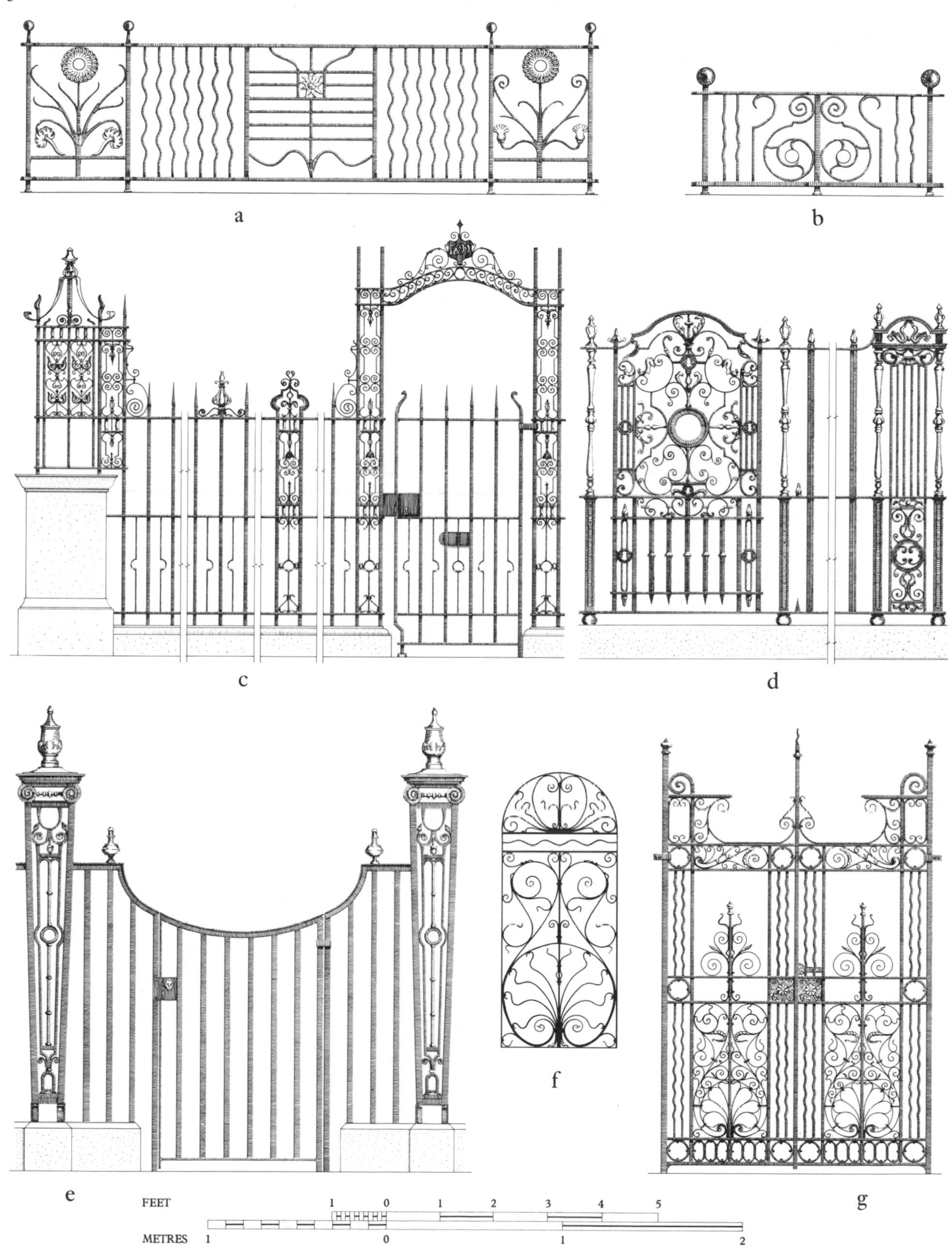

Fig. 23. VICTORIAN AND EDWARDIAN EXTERIOR IRONWORK

a, *b*. Goode's, South Audley Street. *c*. No. 10 Park Street. *d*. No. 54 Mount Street. *e*. No. 28 South Street. *f*, *g*. No. 13 North Audley Street

just the peerage, but financiers, diplomats, industrialists and entrepreneurs of every variety were now crowding on to the estate, and lavishing more money than ever before on their town houses, in the attempt to make their mark on society. No longer was it merely tiresome tradesmen who were predictably uncivil to Boodle and the rest of the Duke's minions; magnates when making their whimsical alterations might also fret at estate restrictions, and more reverence had to be shown to them. Thus F. W. Isaacson, millionaire colliery owner, who in 1886 spent some £7,000 on improvements and decorations at No. 18 Upper Grosvenor Street, coupled a cheque for the renewal of his lease eleven years later 'with some expressions of a very offensive nature'.[92] What such persons in increasing numbers wanted and could now command was the French interior, which by 1890 was well on the way to becoming not just the natural idiom of the great Mayfair house, but a symptom of the conspicuous consumption of the day. Architects had either to learn how to manage the style or leave the job to the real professionals. Mostly they chose the latter course, and from this time dates the heyday of the interior decorator.

Two quite early but typical Grosvenor estate clients for the French interior were H. L. Bischoffsheim of Bute House, No. 75 South Audley Street, and Walter H. Burns of Nos. 69–71 (odd) Brook Street. Neither of them spared any expense. Bischoffsheim was a millionaire banker originally from Amsterdam, with close ties in Paris. Some time between 1873 and 1902, he transformed Bute House into a suite of immaculate *dixhuitième* rooms as a showcase for his famous collection of pictures and furniture (including the G. B. Tiepolo ceiling painting which found its way to the National Gallery in 1969). These interiors were to be supplanted in yet another French-style campaign of 1926–7; but Burns' palatial house in Brook Street survives behind a pair of unpromising exteriors as the Savile Club. Burns, an American who had married a sister of Pierpont Morgan and whose City job involved looking after the great financier's British interests, bought himself a country estate at North Mimms, Hertfordshire, where he employed Ernest George as his architect. Yet significantly for his town house Burns appears (in about 1890) to have put himself in the hands of a Parisian architect, the Dutch-born W. O. W. Bouwens van der Boijen,[93] who for the very extensive structural works relied heavily upon Trollopes the builders. The results (Plate 42b) were ornate, imposing, but haphazard, the climax being an enormous Louis XV ballroom now shorn of its once liberally frescoed ceiling.

There were various smart ways to procure a French interior. One was to buy original *boiseries* and other fittings—no problem for the big dealers like Duveen who now regularly dealt in 'period' rooms. Much panelling from decaying Parisian *hôtels* must have been shipped to England, cleaned, regilded, and neatly made up for the fashionable drawing-rooms of the period. One such beneficiary was No. 66 Grosvenor Street, fitted out in 1913–14 for Robert Emmett (after alterations by W. H. Romaine-Walker) with Louis XV panelling from the Hôtel Cambacères in the boudoir, and Louis XVI panelling from the Hôtel Prunellé in the drawing-room.[94] This is just one case for which the evidence survives; in many other houses on the estate, imported originals cannot be reliably distinguished from modern copywork, such was the stylishness and craftsmanship of the crack interior decorating firms of the day.

The old upholstering concerns were now fading into the background or changing their complexion. Several of the new firms founded in this period still survive today. Among these, pride of place must go to Turner Lord and Company of Mount Street, who have been involved in works on the Mayfair estate, many major, ever since the early 1890's, when they were busy redecorating the Aberdeens' ballroom at No. 27 Grosvenor Square and enlarging the veranda on the front of Dudley House. A typical example of their high standards is No. 33 Grosvenor Street, thoroughly recast by Turner Lord in 1912 for Princess Hatzfeldt with a new stone front and delicate interiors, part French and part English. At this date and just after the war of 1914–18, this firm boasted full-time architects (W. Ernest Lord and Sidney Parvin) on their staff, and could design, build and decorate complete houses, for instance Nos. 41–43 (consec.) Upper Grosvenor Street (1912–14) and Nos. 42–44 Hill Street (1919), though in each case the Grosvenor Board insisted on the involvement of independent architects as well. Some other familiar firms like Maples, White Allom, Green and Abbott, and Lenygon and Morant came to prominence during this era. White Allom and Company in particular were as prolific in this period as Turner Lord. Their largest job, the recasting of the interior of Brook House, will be mentioned a little later, but work by them at No. 128 Park Lane (1905), No. 17 Upper Grosvenor Street (1906–7) and No. 59 Grosvenor Street (1910) should also be recorded here. Another firm of comparable status which does not survive today was the cabinet-making concern of Charles Mellier and Company, by whom several big schemes of decoration, apparently all in the French style, are known: Nos. 45 Grosvenor Square (1897, Plate 42d), 14 Grosvenor Square (1901–2), 19 Upper Brook Street (1903–4), 58 Grosvenor Street (1908–9) and 27 Grosvenor Square (1912).

No. 19 Upper Brook Street, one of the more extravagant of these works, was undertaken by Mellier under the supervision of W. H. Romaine-Walker, one of the few English-trained architects to take a real interest in French interior work and therefore a popular choice among plutocrats; besides this house and No. 66 Grosvenor Street, Romaine-Walker altered No. 128 Park Lane for Henry Duveen (brother and partner of the famous dealer Sir Joseph Joel Duveen), two houses in Park Street (Nos. 34 and 46) for members of the Rothschild clan, and No. 1 Upper Brook Street for C. F. Garland. After some

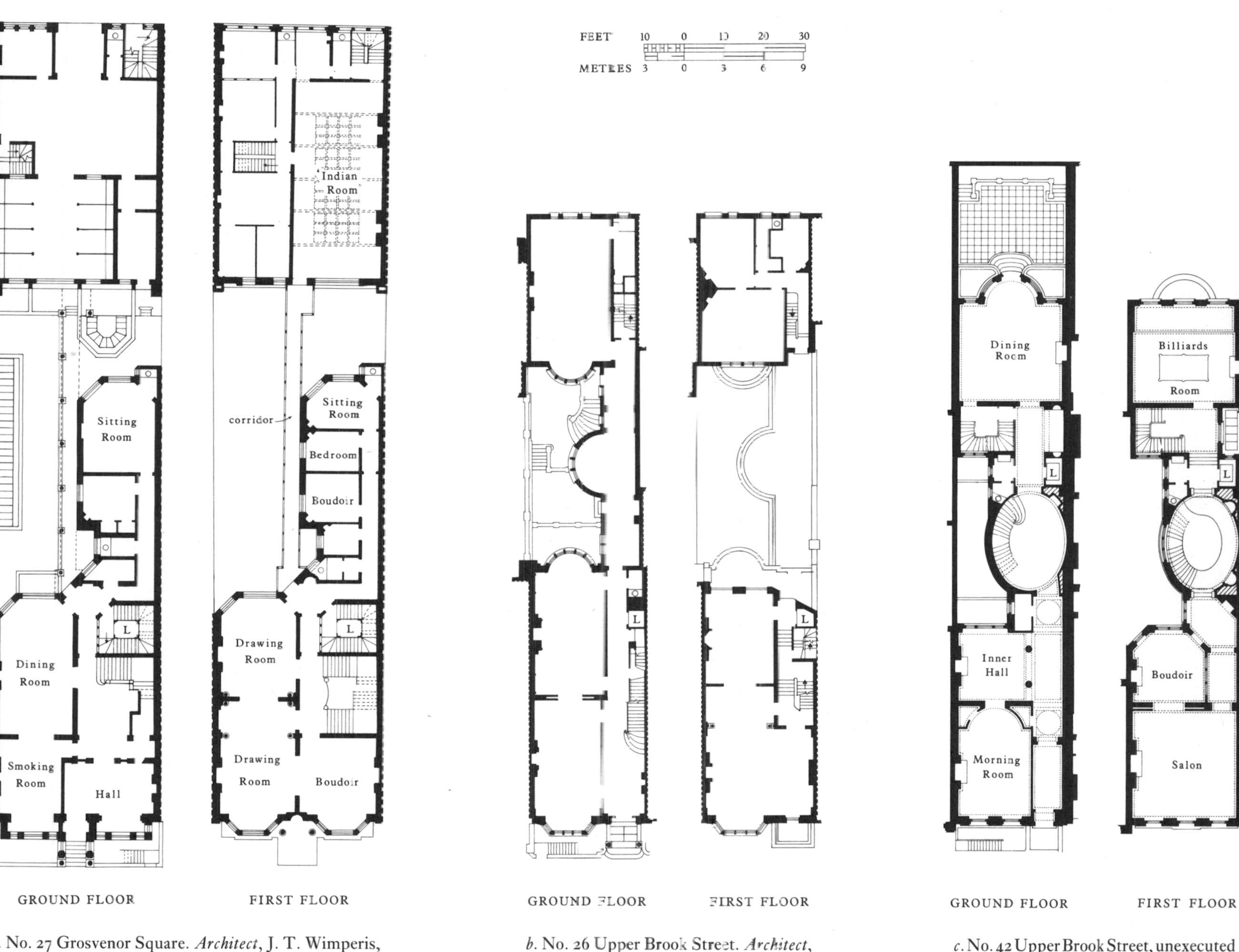

a. No. 27 Grosvenor Square. *Architect*, J. T. Wimperis, 1886–8. *Demolished*

b. No. 26 Upper Brook Street. *Architect*, Arnold Mitchell, 1908–9

c. No. 42 Upper Brook Street, unexecuted plans. *Architects*, Mewès and Davis, *c*. 1914

Fig. 24. GROUND- AND FIRST-FLOOR PLANS, 1880–1914 (L = lift)

£20,000 had been lavished upon No. 19 Upper Brook Street, the Grosvenor Board felt obliged, not uniquely for this period, to warn the tenant that such reckless expenditure would not guarantee for him the renewal of his (very short) lease. The Board also noted that 'French workmen had decorated the house to fit and display his works of art', presumably under Mellier.[95] This was an old and by no means unusual tradition, dating back to Georgian times and beyond. On the estate, we have seen Parisian firms working at Dudley House, and by the Edwardian period this was a frequent occurrence. Thus Marcel Boulanger of Paris was commissioned in 1910 by Lady Essex (one of the many Americans who married into the English aristocracy at this period) for decorations at Bourdon House; he also carried out some decorations at Claridge's under the French architect René Sergent (1910), and worked at No. 27 Grosvenor Square (1912). The smartest thing, in fact, for a client to do if he could not command old French work was to command modern French craftsmen.

But a specifically late-Victorian and Edwardian development was the introduction of Beaux-Arts-trained architects as well as craftsmen. One such was Sergent at Claridge's, another Bouwens van der Boijen, mentioned earlier in connexion with Nos. 69–71 (odd) Brook Street. A third was Arthur J. Davis, English partner in the international firm controlled from Paris by Charles Mewès. Mewès and Davis, though best known for their great commercial successes like the Ritz Hotel, were also busy and capable domestic architects. From a number of estate jobs that fell to them, the remodelling of No. 27 Grosvenor Square in 1912 and an unbuilt speculative house design for Trollope and Colls at No. 42 Upper Brook Street (fig. 24c) excel in elegance and amplitude of plan.[96] But the outstanding survival is their complete rebuilding of No. 88 Brook Street, tactfully carried out behind the existing façade in 1909–10, and culminating in an architectural garden at the rear, small, sculptural, and tastefully *chic*. Such gardens, conservatories and verandas were now constantly being jammed into the few awkward remaining spaces between houses and mews, in an effort to instil yet more lushness into the tone of life in this palmiest of periods.

The most significant Beaux-Arts architect to appear on the Grosvenor estate scene was in fact a Frenchman, Fernand Billerey (1878–1951). Billerey came to England in about 1902 and joined up with Detmar Blow, an architect who, like his friend Lutyens, had struck out a line in very English small country houses and cottages, designed and constructed along fervent Arts and Crafts principles. Blow and Billerey were to feature largely in the twentieth-century history of the estate, and a fuller account of their careers will be found on pages 73–4. But at the time they went into partnership, Blow's only substantial independent job on the Mayfair estate was (and still remains) No. 28 South Street, the rebuilding of a stable as a private house, done in 1902–3 for a stockbroker, Sir W. Cuthbert Quilter of No. 74 South Audley Street. The best feature of this house is its neat front elevation (Plate 45a), executed in a reticent neo-Georgian notable for its date but quite characteristic of Blow's beliefs and previous practice. A few years later Blow secured the job of designing the second Duke's French hunting lodge at Mimizan, and by 1911 the established team of Blow and Billerey was working on the gardens at Eaton, had started designing a big block of houses for the building firm of William Willett looking into the garden of Grosvenor House at the corner of Upper Grosvenor Street (Nos. 37 and 38) and Park Street (Nos. 44–50 even), and was engaged on a large new house on the site of two old ones at No. 46 Grosvenor Street, for the ostentatious financier Sir Edgar Speyer.

Stylistic and documentary evidence alike point to Billerey as the design partner for these and other of the firm's London works. The contrast between Blow's quaint and almost pugnaciously English manner in the country, and Billerey's sumptuous Beaux-Arts urban confections, reflects the schizoid state of Edwardian architecture and, indeed, society. In his elevations for both the Willett block and Speyer's house, Billerey insisted upon rigidly disciplined classical elevations in stone, with refined though sometimes overscaled French detailing (Plate 46a; fig. 25). As so often with this type of architecture, this could only be achieved in each case at the expense of true logic of plan; the elevations had constantly to be juggled to make them fit, often at the last moment, which failed to endear the architects to either the London County Council or the Grosvenor Board. To achieve the 'easy certainty of grouping' that impressed Professor Goodhart-Rendel at the Willett speculation (1911–12), one bay of the main façade covering Nos. 44–50 (even) Park Street fronts no more than a light-well.

But this is nothing compared with what occurs at No. 46 Grosvenor Street (1910–11). Here, since Speyer was obliged by the Board to arrange his house so that it could be converted back into two houses at some future date, Billerey's heroic three-bay elevation conceals many an oddity of plan. Not only do two asymmetrical staircases start from opposite ends of the entrance hall, but they are clothed in two styles, with a riot of flamboyant Gothic woodwork such as might be found in the Musée de Cluny clambering up one side (Plate 42a), and more modest Italian Renaissance detailing on the other. Indeed the whole of Speyer's house passes from exoticism to exoticism with dazzling rapidity, mixing features genuine and antique upon its path, until the comparative calm and familiarity of Louis XV are reached in the first-floor music room. The astonishing woodwork of No. 46 Grosvenor Street appears to have been put in by a Paris firm, L. Buscaylet, and though some of the craftsmen were British, such as W. Bainbridge Reynolds for metalwork (he designed a silver bath for Speyer) and George P. Bankart for plasterwork, the frescoes in the music room must have been painted by a Frenchman, most likely

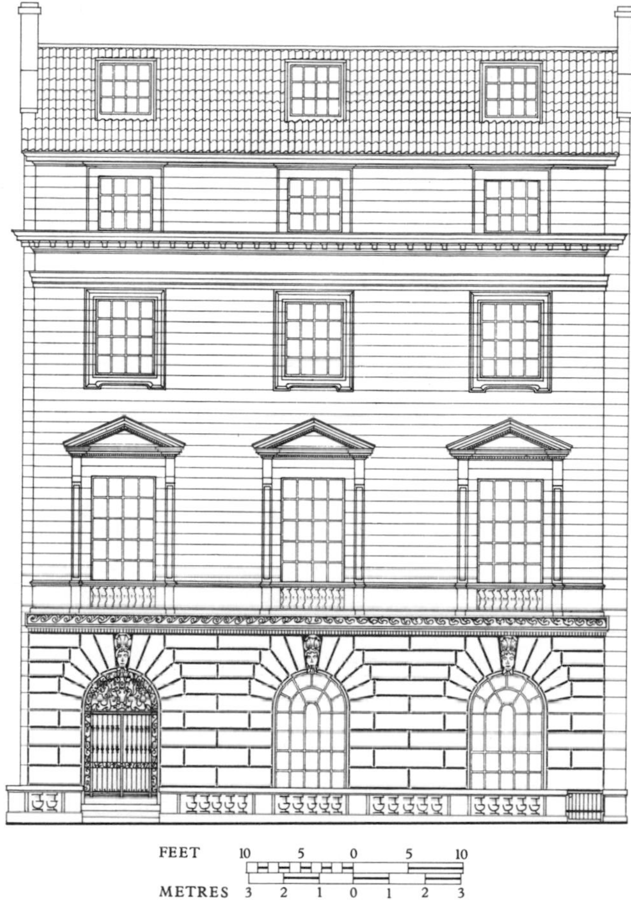

Fig. 25. No. 46 Grosvenor Street, elevation. *Architects*, Blow and Billerey, 1910–11

Billerey's close friend Henri Tastemain. Other members of Billerey's regular team of French craftsmen may have worked on the architect's most satisfying later job on the estate, the final and complete internal remodelling of Bute House, No. 75 South Audley Street, as the Egyptian Embassy, done in *c.* 1926–7 after Blow and he had parted company (Plate 43a). The decorous Louis XVI and Empire interiors on the first floor here were far removed from the flamboyance of No. 46 Grosvenor Street, and happily they remain to this day appositely furnished and kept up in the old style. As for Billerey's other post-war role on the estate, in connexion with the rebuilding of Grosvenor Square, this must be deferred till later.

If the interior embellishment of Speyer's house is the *ne plus ultra* of the exotic vulgarian, it is also a reminder that other styles besides French ones were common currency in the Edwardian years. Often, inhabitants stuck to something discreetly English for ground-floor rooms and went French only up at drawing-room level. Such a house is No. 26 Upper Brook Street, rebuilt in 1908–9 by Arnold Mitchell (fig. 24b); on the ground floor the front room is in the Adam style, the dining-room behind and the room right at the back are panelled in Old English taste and allotted pretty plasterwork in the manner of the Bromsgrove Guild, but upstairs the inevitable French drawing-rooms appear. The decorators here may have been White Allom, who had in 1905–7 certainly done the lion's share of the work in transforming Brook House next door under Mitchell into yet another up-to-date magnate's palace, this time for Sir Ernest Cassel, financial confidante of Edward VII. Royal connexions with the estate were closer than ever at this time; indeed right at the end of the reign No. 16 Grosvenor Street became the home of Mrs. Keppel, after the typical fashionable renovation under F. W. Foster (1909–10). 'Adam' (often still termed 'Adams') such as Mrs. Keppel had here was the commonest rival to French, but there were plenty of other options. Beneath its French drawing-rooms, No. 24 Upper Brook Street boasted a series of rich ground-floor rooms (including a 'museum') hallowed by liberal helpings of polished and carved oak, half Jacobean and half Loire Valley in character, and no doubt the speciality of some interior decorator who held Ernest George in high regard (Plate 42c). Again, No. 33 Grosvenor

Street was briefly fitted up in 1910 for Auguste Lichtenstadt, a stockbroker, with drawing-rooms 'in the German medieval style',[97] but these were expeditiously removed only a year later when Princess Hatzfeldt took the house. Best of all, perhaps, Mr. J. Bland-Sutton, surgeon, of No. 47 Brook Street, doubtless hoping to outdo his many medical neighbours, in about 1904–5 introduced as his dining-room a reproduction ('of course to a smaller scale') of the Palace of Artaxerxes at Susa.[98]

Turning from these interiors to the development of street architecture during the early years of the second Duke's reign, it has first to be remembered that there was a marked downturn in the volume of total rebuildings promoted between 1899, the year of his accession, and 1906. This hiatus, together with the fact that Eustace Balfour was less closely attuned to the second Duke's taste and to his casual and sporadic way of dealing with architectural questions, led to some uncertainty as to design policy. One sure trend, however, was the decline of red brick along the main streets in favour of stone. The first instance of this seems to have been at No. 18 Grosvenor Street, where the builder John Garlick in 1901–2 provided a new stone front. In Grosvenor Square, No. 45 was refronted in Portland stone on the tenant's initiative by Edmund Wimperis and Hubert East in 1902 (Plate 44a); and when in 1906–7 Nos. 22 and 32 were both rebuilt speculatively, the fronts were again of this material. Sir Edgar Speyer and Princess Hatzfeldt both adopted stone at Nos. 46 and 33 Grosvenor Street respectively, and in Upper Brook Street practically all the many rebuildings of 1905–16 were stonefronted: Nos. 1, 2, 16–18 (Plate 44b), 25, 26, 37, 39, 41, 49–50 and 51. There was one exception, the now demolished No. 54 (1912–13). This was Ernest George's swansong on the estate (fig. 26b), a delightful brick house handled in the seventeenth-century manner to which he had always inclined, but with a gentleness and understatement far removed from the exuberance of his earlier work at Goode's in South Audley Street.

The new liking for stonework is of particular significance in two places. One is in the ranges facing Grosvenor House, where the Duke naturally took an interest and the estate managers therefore exercised special prudence. Hence the appearance of a now seemingly purposeless full order and pediment on the prestigious stone block at Nos. 37–38 Upper Grosvenor Street and 44–50 (even) Park Street by Blow and Billerey of 1911–12 (Plate 46a). Across the road from the Grosvenor House screen, too, reconstruction of individual houses with stone fronts was proceeding apace from 1906 onwards (Plate 44d). Balfour and Turner acquired the first job here, the rebuilding of No. 17 Upper Grosvenor Street, and a typically interesting and idiosyncratic job they made of it, with large expanses of small-paned windows and plenty of naturalistic carving. No. 19 by Maurice C. Hulbert has an able individual elevation (fig. 27a) and plan in the French manner, while for No. 21 another considerable talent, Ralph Knott of County Hall fame (in partnership with E. Stone Collins), produced an attractively florid front with oval windows beneath the cornice (fig. 27b). Both Knott and the architects of the less interesting No. 20, probably Boehmer and Gibbs, came up against Balfour's opposition, for he plainly wanted small window panes throughout this range to match his own No. 17; but the pressures of the fashionable French style and of the social influences brought to bear upon his pliable master the Duke forced him to concede big plate-glass windows.

A little further east, at the north-west corner site between Park Street and Upper Grosvenor Street, comes an interesting illustration of the status by now attached to a stone front (Plate 46b). Here Caröe was chosen architect for a big speculative block at Nos. 37–43 (odd) Park Street, after the Estate had applied some pressure upon its undertakers, Higgs and Hill. Abandoning most of the stylistic mannerisms of his Nos. 75–83 (odd) Duke Street but retaining some similarities of outline, Caröe produced a design articulated in two separate parts. Both are in a wholehearted seventeenth-century French idiom, but with the ornate stone façades significantly confined to the corner site (No. 37 Park Street), while the northern portion, invisible from Grosvenor House, drops back quickly into a cheery red brick with stone dressings.

The other important set of stone fronts occurs in South Audley Street, near the southern boundary of the estate. Drastic reform in this area was contemplated in 1907, when a proposal to demolish the best houses on the east side, Nos. 9–16 (consec.), was after some indecision deflected by the Duke's innate conservatism. Opposite, on the west side, something like a Cundy refronting policy was followed, apparently for no more substantial reasons than fashion (Plate 44c). In 1906 H. L. Bischoffsheim, forced thus to set about the great No. 75, chose an obscure architect called Cyrille J. Corblet for the lushly classical façade which this house still presents (though the door has been moved); in 1908 Balfour and Turner refronted No. 74 in their idiosyncratic style; and in 1909 Paul Waterhouse followed with a new elevation to No. 73. But the policy went no further. Edwardian fronts of these years normally imply Edwardian houses behind. The rest of South Audley Street remained as it was, excepting for some major and controversial alterations to the interior of the Grosvenor Chapel by J. N. Comper in 1913.

By 1909 Balfour's constitution was breaking down, and a change in the surveyorship again became imminent. What Thackeray Turner and he had designed since the second Duke's accession, besides No. 17 Upper Grosvenor Street and the refronting of No. 74 South Audley Street, did not amount to much: an inconspicuous but pleasant building at Nos. 439–441 (odd) Oxford Street (1906–8) and a new wing at Bourdon House (1910), the latter on the personal initiative of the Duke. Balfour had, however, been instrumental in improving various designs which came before him in the course of estate work, notably

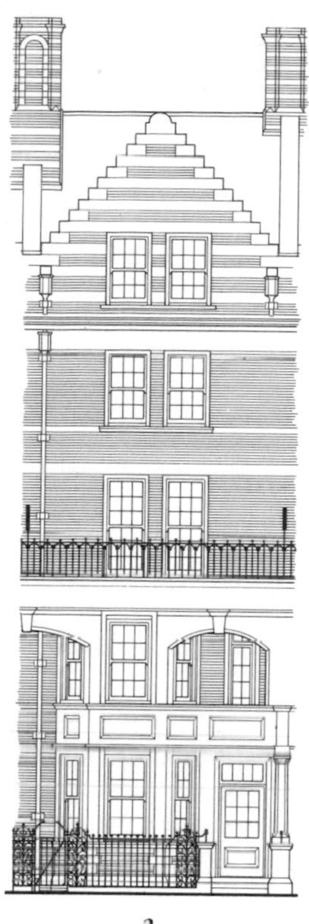

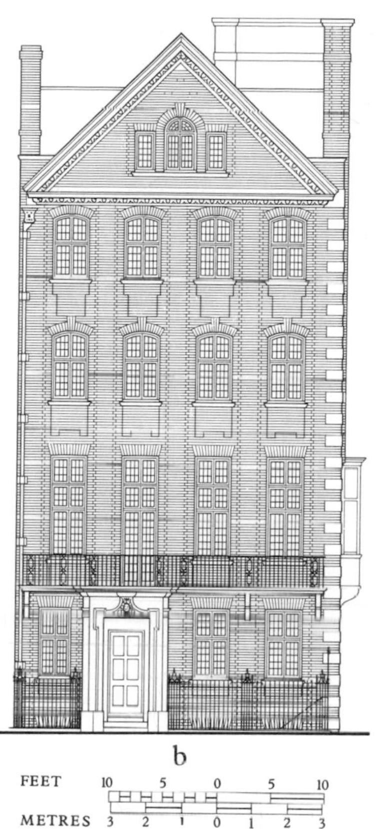

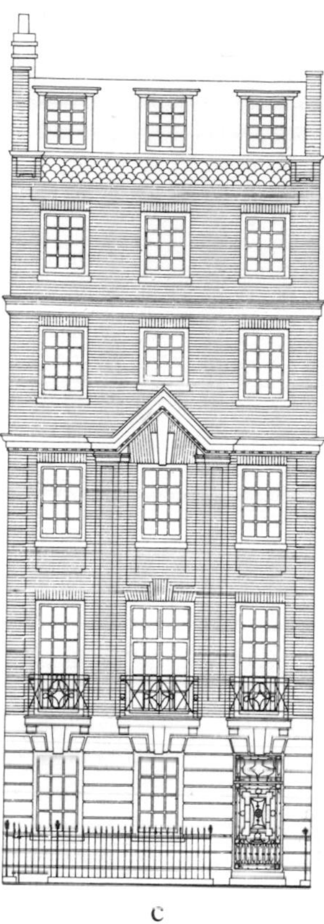

Fig. 26. BRICK ELEVATIONS, 1890–1914
a. No. 44 Brook Street. *Architects*, Balfour and Turner, *builders*, Holloways, 1898–9
b. No. 54 Upper Brook Street. *Architects*, Ernest George and Yeates, 1912–13. *Demolished*
c. No. 26 Grosvenor Street. *Architects*, Wimperis and Simpson, 1913–16

C. Stanley Peach's Duke Street Electricity Sub-station (1903–4). This heroic replacement for the Italian Garden is the Mayfair estate's fullest flight in Edwardian Baroque. Peach was a practical architect of much ingenuity and a pioneer in the planning and design of electricity stations; in 1890–2 he had already erected a generating station and some not uninteresting flats on the estate (now demolished) at the corner of Davies Street and Weighhouse Street. But his more ambitious elevations for the Duke Street Sub-station (possibly in part designed by C. H. Reilly, who worked briefly for Peach at this time) did not satisfy Balfour until he had expended much effort on them.

Balfour's successor as surveyor in 1910 was perhaps surprisingly not Detmar Blow, who had by now worked personally for the Duke, but Edmund Wimperis (1865–1946), son of E. M. Wimperis the painter, brother of Arthur Wimperis the playwright, and a cousin-once-removed and pupil of that J. T. Wimperis who had designed so much in Mayfair in the first Duke's day. At this date he was in partnership with J. R. Best at No. 61 South Molton Street and had already carried out a few substantial works on the estate: the refronting (with Hubert East) of No. 45 Grosvenor Square (1902, Plate 44a), a rebuilding at No. 1 Upper Brook Street (1907–8) and the first part of what was to be an attractive run of three stone elevations further west at Nos. 16–18 (consec.) Upper Brook Street (1907–16, Plate 44b). He it was who was to carry out the rebuildings now planned for the Green Street and Davies Street areas, and with his later partners W. Begg Simpson and L. Rome Guthrie to preside over the estate's gradual change of style to neo-Georgian.

No doubt because of their expense, the Edwardian liking for Portland stone façades was not shared by developers building on more than one plot. Therefore the only two ranges built on the estate in the period 1899–1906, Nos. 6–9 and 61–63 (consec.) Grosvenor Street (1900–1 and 1904–6), both adopt a rather dull late Queen-Anne brick style. Even in the square Joseph Sawyer's new No. 51 (1908–11), entered from Grosvenor Street, adhered to brick with stone dressings, out of loyalty to its neighbours. Edmund Wimperis's own first big undertaking is again in brick; it fronts Grosvenor Street at Nos. 55–57 (consec.), and Davies Street at Nos. 4–26

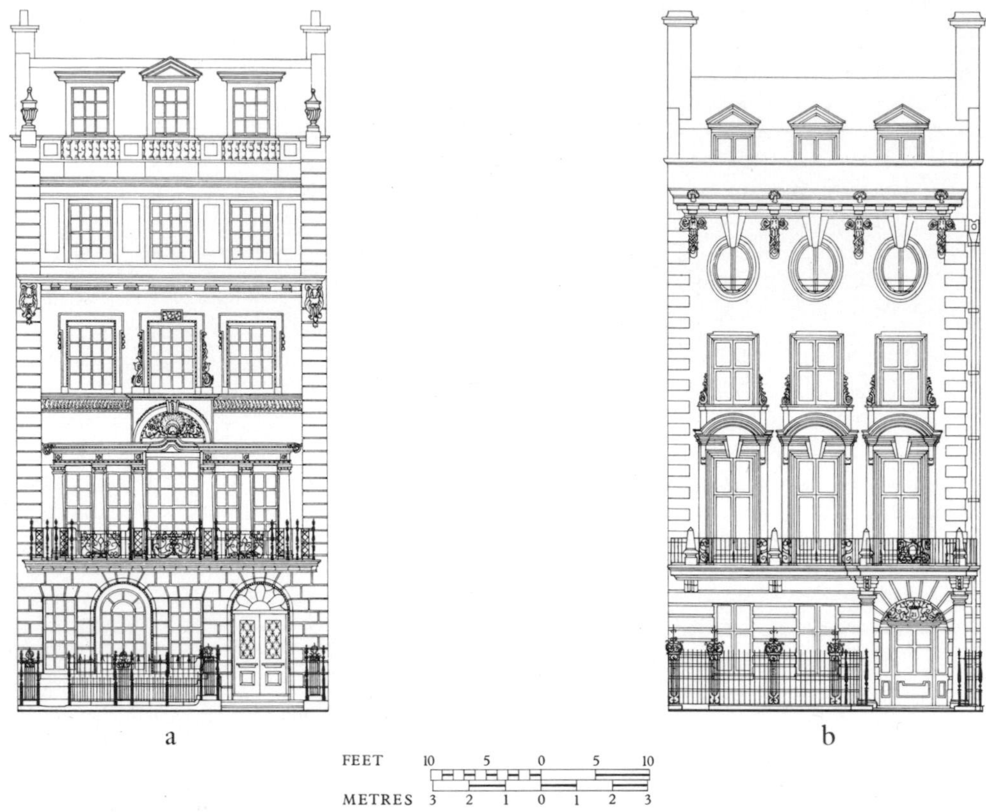

Fig. 27. EDWARDIAN STONE ELEVATIONS
a. No. 19 Upper Grosvenor Street. *Architect*, Maurice C. Hulbert, *builders*, Matthews, Rogers and Company, 1909–10
b. No. 21 Upper Grosvenor Street. *Architects*, Ralph Knott and E. Stone Collins, 1908

(even), where it stretches all the way back to Bourdon House. Though already architect (with J. R. Best) for this development before becoming estate surveyor, Wimperis was at the helm by the time it was actually built (1910–12). It is not an elegant or entirely coherent building (Plate 47a), but, foreshadowing as it does the bulky blocks soon to multiply upon the estate, it is an important one. The incoherence is due only partially to the division of the range between three separate developers, for it exhibits a measure of stylistic uncertainty as well. Minimally French or neo-Grec still in some of the details at the Grosvenor Street corner, along Davies Street the building shows study of Lutyens and a hankering for the flatter, suaver possibilities of elevation offered by neo-Georgian. With the arrival of W. Begg Simpson in 1913 as a partner, the neo-Georgian contribution begins to outweigh the subdued half-French, half-Greek detailing that seems to have been the urban idiom natural to Edmund Wimperis, and the firm's work quickly improves. Nos. 75 Grosvenor Street of 1912–14 and 26 Grosvenor Street of 1913–16 (fig. 26c) are indications of the ample scope that neo-Georgian was to offer for individual houses. Both façades are founded upon an entirely orthodox Georgian manner, but though they come closer than anything yet built on the estate to the original house-style of the area, their different proportions, subtle red-brick textures, and wooden window frames flush with the surrounds (a feature only legalized since 1894) make them distinctive. Yet if asked to design a front in stone, as at No. 39 Upper Brook Street (1913–15), elements of a more sober, less inventive classicism recurred in the work of Wimperis and Simpson.

To trace the evolution of neo-Georgian on the Mayfair estate a stage further one must look at Green Street. Here Edmund Wimperis was the agent of a policy agreed upon under Balfour to rebuild, on the south side between Park Street and Norfolk (now Dunraven) Street together with the deep return along those streets, 'small or moderate sized houses, of much the same frontage as those now standing, with a large common garden in the centre, and a motor house or motor houses towards Woods Mews'.[99] A similar decision was made for the short section of Waverton Street on the estate together with the return frontages to South Street and Hill Street. Though the

houses here were to be fewer and bigger, the principle of completely rebuilding a range with some allowance for individualism of plan and elevation but with a communal garden behind was again followed. These policies, interrupted by the outbreak of war, remained pre-war in conception. Wimperis's firm was to design both the pleasant South Street and the Green Street gardens together with most of the houses, that is to say Nos. 38–39, 41–44, 46 and 48 (consec.) Green Street, 91–103A (odd) Park Street, 40A and 40B Hill Street and, after the war, the mighty No. 38 South Street. Despite some variety in elevation, most of these houses are generically similar (Plate 47b), with bow windows towards the gardens and decent neo-Georgian façades, most of them in two tones of carefully textured brick. Where the level of design, exterior or interior, rises higher, it is usually, like No. 46 Green Street, the largest house in this section of the street, a design to meet an individual's requirements by W. Begg Simpson (Plate 45b). But most of the houses were undertaken directly for big speculative builders, and are therefore merely decent and simple.

Well before this time, indeed shortly after the great rebuildings began in the 1880's, the procedure by which large and respectable firms of builders could speculate upon the estate had been formalized, and it remains to look at the character and achievements of some of the principal contractors. Compared to earlier developers, their power was more limited because the Grosvenor Board took a more stringent line towards design and would often prescribe architects for them. But on the other hand it was now easier for good builders to get hold of large rebuilding plots and work out, in co-operation with the Board, a unified design for a whole range, or even an area. This could secure them a better return. The frequency with which builders were offered 'takes' by the Estate naturally depended upon their efficiency, their quality of work, and, because of the social tone of the area, upon their speed and discretion.

For the period 1890 to 1914, there is no doubt that of the builders regularly working on the estate George Trollope and Sons were foremost in all these virtues. Trollopes had long been connected with the Grosvenor estates, having been house agents for Cubitt in Belgravia before they entered into block contracting.[100] In the 1860's they had taken plots in Grosvenor Gardens and were responsible for the whole of Hereford Gardens, but the latter undertaking was nearly disastrous for them and made them unpopular in the Grosvenor Office. However, by 1890, under George Haward Trollope, they had recovered their credit completely. In the Mount Street rebuildings they secured on their own account the whole of the block fronted by the eastern curve of Carlos Place and, further west, Nos. 45–52 (consec.) and 53 Mount Street and 34–42 (even) Park Street. These were all erected to the very respectable designs of their own architect, John Evelyn Trollope (of Giles, Gough and Trollope), brother to G. H. Trollope, but the firm was just as ready to build to the designs of others. Fairfax Wade's No. 54 Mount Street, Balfour and Turner's Aldford House, W. D. Caröe's Nos. 75–83 (odd) Duke Street and C. W. Stephens's rebuilding of Claridge's were all works of the first importance carried out by them in the 1890's, while at Nos. 69–71 (odd) Brook Street Trollopes did the reconstruction for W. H. Burns under Bouwens of Paris. After the lull of 1899 to 1906 the firm took up their chances more selectively in the following new period of activity, here recasting a house direct for an aristocratic client (No. 20 Upper Grosvenor Street for the Countess of Wilton, or No. 44 Grosvenor Square for the Duchess of Devonshire), there going for designs to Edmund Wimperis (Nos. 2 Upper Brook Street, 75 Grosvenor Street) and even Mewès and Davis (No. 42 Upper Brook Street, unbuilt, fig. 24c), or, with greater orthodoxy, taking part of the block at Nos. 91–103A (odd) Park Street under Wimperis on lease from the estate. After the war of 1914–18 Trollope and Colls (as they had been since 1903) indulged little if at all in speculation but continued to do a lot of high-class private work. The reasons for their special reputation are not far to seek. They were a well-capitalized firm, relatively secure against fluctuations in building activity and therefore liable to be prompt in taking on, executing and completing contracts; they were diversified, including under their umbrella an estate agent's business which must have been the means of bringing them a proportion of their private work; they were staunch conservative builders with a tradition of opposition to the unions, which doubtless endeared them to much of their clientèle; and lastly, as specialists in high-class work, especially in superior joinery, they could always provide the elaborate materials and workmanship constantly specified in Mayfair but sometimes hard to obtain from lesser firms.

Other great concerns of comparable size to Trollopes did not on the whole work widely on the Mayfair estate at this time, though Higgs and Hill were the developers of A. H. Kersey's Nos. 2–12 (even) Park Street, W. D. Caröe's Nos. 37–43 (odd) Park Street and Joseph Sawyer's No. 51 Grosvenor Square, and William Willett of J. J. Stevenson's Nos. 39–47 (odd) South Street and the large Blow and Billerey block on the opposite corner to Caröe's in Park Street (Nos. 44–50 even) and Upper Grosvenor Street (Nos. 37 and 38), while Holloways promoted three separate major developments with Read and Macdonald as architects, Nos. 14–26 (consec.) Mount Street, 22 Grosvenor Square, and 453–459 (odd) Oxford Street together with 22 and 23 North Audley Street. Three smaller firms, however, deserve a special mention: Matthews, Rogers and Company, John Garlick and Sons, and F. Foxley and Company.

Matthews, Rogers had been building in Egerton Gardens, Kensington (under the name of Matthews Brothers), when in 1891 they took on their first Mayfair speculation at Nos. 25–29 (consec.) North Audley Street and 1–11 (consec.) Green Street. Thomas Verity was the

architect appointed by the Estate for the North Audley Street elevation, but in Green Street the company was allowed to stick (except at No. 10) to its own architect, Maurice Charles Hulbert. Architecturally undistinguished, this range was very profitable and led Matthews, Rogers on to further developments fifteen years later, at Nos. 37 and 49–50 Upper Brook Street (1907–8), 19 Upper Grosvenor Street (1909–10) and 80–84 (even) Brook Street with 22–26 (consec.) Gilbert Street (1910–13). The surprise about these later houses is that they show the obscure Hulbert transformed from a dull builder's architect into a free and spirited interpreter of the Mayfair French Renaissance manner. Outstanding is the Brook Street range, which unites three large houses in a single composition built of judiciously picked orange-red bricks and creamy stone, with a row of smaller dwellings of equal quality running back into Gilbert Street (Plate 45d). Here and at No. 19 Upper Grosvenor Street the plans are as well and individually conceived as the elevations, while at Nos. 49–50 Upper Brook Street Hulbert showed what he could make of a pair of elaborate stone fronts in a more English style, Balfour having recommended that he 'take for a model the Adams house in St James Square formerly Sir Williams-Wynn's'.[101] Was Hulbert 'ghosted' for these excellent houses, as so many architects of the time reputedly were? The question, now virtually impossible to answer, should at least be raised.

John Garlick was a more prolific operator but visually his output is less striking. Garlick started out as a large-scale public-works contractor based on Birmingham, but according to an obituary in 1910, 'in later years he had given special attention to West-end mansions, in connexion with which his name was well known on the Portman, Grosvenor, and Cadogan estates'.[102] His first known appearance on the estate was in 1897 when, already over sixty years of age, he took a lease of No. 35 Grosvenor Square. Between then and 1910 his activity, usually but not invariably speculative, was incessant, and it unusually bridged the gap of 1899 to 1906 when few other speculative developments were proceeding. Sometimes Garlick went to outside architects, for example Edward I'Anson III for Nos. 6–9 Grosvenor Street (1900–1), R. Stephen Ayling and Lionel Littlewood at No. 32 Grosvenor Square (1906–7) or Edmund Wimperis at No. 1 Upper Brook Street (1907–8), but R. G. Hammond was his regular man. Several of the plainer surviving fronts of these years are due to Hammond, not a designer of particular talent: Nos. 61–63 (consec.) Grosvenor Street (1904–6), 51 Upper Brook Street (1905–6), and 47 Upper Grosvenor Street (1905), while No. 25 Upper Brook Street (1907–8) is his work in association with another builder. On the other hand the façade of No. 18 Grosvenor Street (1901–2), evidently the first case of an Edwardian stone 'refronting' on the estate, looks less like Hammond, more like Ayling and Littlewood. When Garlick died in 1910 (worth £88,863) he had headquarters at No. 43 Sloane Street, Knightsbridge, a furniture shop at No. 40 North Audley Street, and substantial steam-joinery works in Manresa Road, Chelsea, for like other builders of this area he was a specialist in joinery. His son William J. Garlick continued the family's involvement in the area, building part of the big Wimperis block at Nos. 4–26 (even) Davies Street in 1910–12 and No. 26 Grosvenor Street in 1913–16, but after the war the firm faded from the Mayfair scene, though they still exist in Wandsworth today.

The third and last building firm of note begins to appear only late in the period. This is F. Foxley and Company, who from 1909 make frequent showings in the district surveyor's returns, mostly in the Green Street area and often in conjunction with F. W. Foster, architect and speculator. Foxleys built most of the Green Street houses designed by the Wimperis firm in the period 1913–16, together with much of the east side of Dunraven Street south of Green Street, but this apparently did not include the vast but not very accomplished Norwich House, No. 4 Dunraven Street (1913–16), a design by Foster based loosely upon Lutyens's No. 7 St. James's Square. The Foxleys–Foster relationship is unclear, but in 1914 Foster seems to have been using a firm of architects called H. H. Fraser and H. R. Peerless, suggesting that he himself was more of an entrepreneur than a designer. Foster was very busy in both Belgravia and Mayfair at this date and was responsible for No. 47 Grosvenor Square (1913–15), the last private house in the square to be completely rebuilt. He was badly hit by the housing slump when the war came, and disappears quickly from the scene. But the houses built by Foxleys are perfectly worthy, and Wimperis must have found the firm satisfactory, for they continued like Trollope and Colls to be trusted builders in the years after the war and to work often on the estate.

But along with much else, the war of 1914–18 spelt an end to the activities of the great self-capitalizing speculative builder. Soon the bottomless purse of the old Mayfair client began to close and as his servants slipped away one by one, the services of his town-house architect were in less and less demand. Though the interior decorator was to enjoy an Indian summer in the 1920's and '30's, the Mayfair house had started upon its inexorable decline.

Modern Times

Twentieth-century development upon the London estates of the Grosvenors, as previously, has kept in general respects of pattern and style to the ordinary progress of English architecture. Thus a conservative vein, gradually shorn of its classical attributes in response to the dictates of function and cost, has long persisted, giving way only very recently to the more forthright modes of the present day. But because of its homogeneity and its special blend

of domestic and commercial occupation, the Mayfair estate is a good area in which to focus upon the conflicts and trials that have beset modern urban architecture. Here, more particularly, one may ponder upon the achievements and the failures of neo-Georgianism as a style not just for our houses but also for our city centres. The contrasts are struck most starkly in Grosvenor Square, scene of one of London's most ambitious and comprehensive rebuilding projects of modern times, yet with Eero Saarinen's American Embassy at flagrant stylistic odds with its three other sides. Elsewhere, in a less dramatic instance of the same seemingly contradictory tendencies, bulky blocks of flats and offices invaded the main streets, while 'bijou' Georgian-style houses sprang up in the refurbished mews behind. Complete uniformity in so large a compass could of course be neither expected nor applauded. Yet there can be no doubt that over the last fifty years the architectural personality of the estate has been continually in question.

After the war of 1914–18, it at first looked as though the Mayfair estate might quickly resume its old role as the doyen of high-class residential areas. Despite post-war shortages and high costs of building materials, the Green Street–Park Street and South Street–Waverton Street redevelopments were soon completed and two large individual houses erected, No. 38 South Street for Henry McLaren (later Lord Aberconway) by Wimperis and Simpson (1919–21), and No. 15 Aldford Street for Cuthbert Heath by George Crawley (1919–21). No. 38 South Street, 'the last private house of great size to be built in London' (as *The Times* was to call it),[103] was a sophisticated essay in the mature brick manner of Lutyens for a client who knew the great architect but did not choose to employ him, possibly fearing his expense. As if to compensate for the vast, pre-war scale of the rooms, its polished interiors, partly designed by Harold Peto, were in a restrained, up-to-date style (Plate 43b). Heath's house was more old-fashioned, a staid stone mansion with a garden frontage towards Park Lane and some elaborate ironwork; its architect, George Crawley, was an amateur of some standing, who seems equally to have enjoyed designing palatial edifices in the United States and stockbroker manors in Surrey.[104] Crawley also altered Aldford House close by, and at one stage produced a complex scheme of flats for the Grosvenor House site, so his connexions with this part of Park Lane were strong. But his epoch was over; no work of Crawley's survives on the estate, which began reaping the whirlwind of change soon after these two big houses were finished.

Park Lane is the most graphic illustration of the sudden change of tack. After five years of prevarication, Grosvenor House was torn down in 1927. Aldford House followed in *c.* 1930, Charles Barry's No. 2 South Street and its neighbours at much the same time, and in 1936, after only fifteen or so years of existence, No. 15 Aldford Street disappeared together with all its neighbours on the present Fountain House site. So by the war of 1939–45, the whole of the Park Lane frontage of the estate south of Upper Grosvenor Street had been dramatically redeveloped and replaced by the high buildings familiar today. Further north, the rebuilding of Brook House and of Nos. 105–108 meant that only Nos. 93–99, No. 100 (Dudley House), and the two ranges between Nos. 117 and 138 including the backs of the houses in Norfolk (now Dunraven) Street (Plates 19, 21) survived as reminders of the old scale and dignity of this once charming thoroughfare. As brutally as the age of the great town house was over, the age of the high-rise block had begun.

In terms of mere extent, these big inter-war buildings were no novelty to Mayfair. Many of the ranges built during the first Duke's campaigns and, more recently, the block erected by Wimperis and Best at Nos. 55–57 (consec.) Grosvenor Street and Nos. 4–26 (even) Davies Street had been as ambitious. But (with the significant exception of Claridge's) they had been humanized by frequent subdivision, moderate height, and much plasticity, whereas now the revolution of steel-framing had unleashed a new scale of overall design. The first important example of steel-framing on the estate is the group of flats situated on the corner with Oxford Street at Nos. 139–140 Park Lane, and characterized by Goodhart-Rendel as 'much the best architecture that can be found in that thoroughfare'.[105] Erected in *c.* 1913–18 to the designs of Frank Verity, who had built a similar, smaller block of flats at No. 25 Berkeley Square some years earlier, the prominent Park Lane project attracted much attention and even made the favourably-inclined Grosvenor Board 'somewhat nervous as to the effect on the residents and public' (not least because the estate's only cinema was included behind).[106] Their apprehension cannot have diminished as building dragged on through the war years, but the various changes and delays did allow the capable and reliable Verity to mature an admirable set of neo-Grec elevations in stone to clothe his steel frame (Plate 48a).

For a few years it looked as though Verity's kind of idiom, with its capacity for easy translation into the smart Egyptian, Assyrian and Aztec modes of the 1920's, might have a future in Mayfair. But the only building overtly of this nature was the reinforced concrete garage in Balderton Street (1925–6, surprisingly by Wimperis and Simpson with strong support from structural engineers). Bolder and more conspicuous ventures of the Selfridges type do not seem to have been welcome on the estate. Nevertheless, one or two large stone-faced and steel-framed buildings did appear in the immediate post-war years. One, Brookfield House at Nos. 62–64 (even) Brook Street on the corner with Davies Street, was among the first purpose-built office buildings on the estate, with a bank on the ground floor. It had been projected in 1917, but when it was built in 1922–3 its architect Delissa Joseph was asked to make its elevation, at least towards Brook Street, 'as much as possible bear the appearance of a private residence'.[107]

Another and more meritorious example of steel-framing on the estate is the range of shops and offices at Nos. 415–419 (odd) Oxford Street, between Duke Street and Lumley Street (Plate 48b). This composite free-standing block, begun in 1923–4 with No. 419 designed by G. Thrale Jell (architect of the Piccadilly Arcade), was completed as one range in the same style by Wimperis, Simpson and Guthrie (No. 415 in 1926–7, No. 417 in 1935), but the overall design is probably Jell's. Because of its location on a candidly commercial street he was able to adopt the principles of Chicago, with plenty of window space for shops below and showrooms and offices above. America henceforward was to be an important factor in Grosvenor estate buildings. Just a little further east, another hint of changes to come occurred when in 1924 Charles Holden (of Adams, Holden and Pearson) did one of his earliest jobs for London's transport, the modest but prototypical remodelling of the exterior of Bond Street Tube Station with a neat stone frame, a canopy, and illuminated signs. It should be added that the station was no longer on the estate, as the site had been conveyed to the Central London Railway in 1897, so the Duke was in no way responsible for Holden's employment here.

For the core of the estate, still a distinctly domestic neighbourhood, those in architectural control had other ideas. Whatever frictions arose between Edmund Wimperis as estate surveyor and the second Duke's secretary Detmar Blow, they and their allies (Wimperis's partners W. Begg Simpson and L. Rome Guthrie, and Blow's old associate Fernand Billerey) were agreed in their adherence to a more or less classic style for future developments, and specifically to the type of reduced neo-Georgianism of 'Wrenaissance' embraced by Lutyens and his school for London buildings. These men, with the possible exception of Billerey, were broadly speaking architects of texture rather than structure. In the early 1920's their feeling was still primarily for domestic work, and they were firm believers in a refined neo-Georgian brick architecture as the right treatment for both private houses and flats. And by now, more flats were an inevitability. The too-great size of many of the old houses on the estate may have been just one of several factors contributing to a southward movement of the epicentre of fashionable Mayfair, to the more resilient areas of Hill Street and Charles Street. Something had to be done to keep the Grosvenor estate up to date, and flats and smaller dwellings were the most obvious answer. Thus for instance No. 7 Grosvenor Square was converted from one house into four in 1925, and in Upper Brook Street, where a grand house had been destined for the site of No. 42 before the war, what eventually went up in 1928–9 was a small luxury block of flats by T. P. Bennett. In a somewhat different vein of multi-occupation, No. 86 Brook Street was virtually rebuilt in 1922 to the discreet designs of C. H. Biddulph-Pinchard, becoming the headquarters of a team of consulting physicians and surgeons and gaining an elegant new front to Binney Street. There were still a few optimists, notably in the square, who were keen to expand their houses. One was Major Stephen Courtauld of No. 47 Grosvenor Square, for whom Vincent Harris added a music room (1926) and, further behind the house, a 'racquets court' (1924). Several such private courts appeared on the estate during these years, but this is the only one to survive conspicuously; its cheerful brick-and-pantiled façade can still be seen on the west side of Carlos Place, sandwiched between two large blocks. Again, as late as 1936 Collcutt and Hamp added bedrooms and radically altered the interior at No. 25 Grosvenor Square for Lady Cecilia Baillie. But subdivision and conversion were the commoner trends.

Still, conversion and infilling could by no means satisfy the demand. Therefore the firm of Wimperis, Simpson and Guthrie, who took the lion's share of major commissions on the estate in the mid 1920's, had like so many architects of the period to change the tenor of their work. A few words on the character of this firm are worth including. By this time Wimperis, Simpson and Guthrie were developing into one of the busiest and most respected practices in London, specializing in large commercial commissions throughout the West End, though the Grosvenor estate was their stronghold. The partners were Edmund Wimperis, still until 1928 the estate surveyor and ever the dignified and courteous Edwardian gentleman; W. Begg Simpson ('Simmy'), always dapper with a carnation in his buttonhole, and increasingly occupied by the business work of the firm; and L. Rome Guthrie, a Scot, son-in-law of William Flockhart, and established as a well-known architect before he joined the practice in 1925. At their office (just off the estate in South Molton Street) this trio presided benignly over an assiduous body of underlings. New jobs were normally assigned to one particular partner or another, though it is rarely possible to say which job went to whom. But it does appear that from the time of Guthrie's arrival he gradually took on more of the most important designing work, while Wimperis especially began to reduce his commitments.[108]

On the Grosvenor estate, the crucial buildings erected by the firm in the 1920's were not the occasional private houses like No. 38 South Street or the pert No. 64 Park Street, but their big new blocks of flats. These, like the houses, were designed with elevations of the elegantly textured red bricks (mainly from Daneshill) that were then fashionable, and for a time still sported ample classical details in stone. The first of these blocks was the justly admired Mayfair House, Carlos Place (1920–2). It was followed by three at the corner of Upper Brook Street and Park Street: Upper Feilde (1922–4), Upper Brook Feilde (1926–7), and No. 80 Park Street (1929–30). Also in the group is the important Nos. 49–50 Grosvenor Square (1925–7) in the south-east corner, precursor of much that was to follow in the square. Of these blocks of flats, Upper Feilde (at No. 71 Park Street) is worth singling out as an instructive early attempt to enliven an essentially plain six-storey elevation (Plate 49a); it

embodies cleverly contrived bonding patterns, delicate diapers in the brickwork, and even a small gable or two. Close by, on Upper Brook Feilde (at No. 47 Park Street), the architects fought back against monotony by means of a giant order on the main front and, to get extra accommodation, crammed two storeys instead of one into the roof, above the line of the 'architecture' (Plate 49b). But here and in their big corner block at Nos. 49–50 Grosvenor Square, stretching back along the east side of Carlos Place, they came up against the problem then exercising half London's architects. How could a style that was domestic in scale be articulated to fit the height and density required in the new, large city buildings equipped for modern living? This was the real, practical crisis for neo-Georgianism: not the challenge of Corbusier, but its own ultimate lack of elasticity for urban buildings of scale. What so often occurred was that the style was gradually deprived of its most obvious appurtenances so as to minimize two quite distinct problems, those of cost and those of proportion. Divested of its stylistic features, it easily sank into monotony and fell prey to critics of new persuasions.

However, on the Grosvenor estates this steady tendency towards simplification was to be stoutly, if briefly, resisted at the behest of Detmar Blow, now in the ascendant at the Grosvenor Office. In an unusual step, two independent architects, Edwin Lutyens and Fernand Billerey, were called in to help on different Estate schemes of redevelopment, while a third, Frederick Etchells, was entrusted with a variety of minor employments. More than anything, it seems to have been the question of Grosvenor House, uninhabited by the Duke since the first World War and temporarily under Government occupation, that precipitated this move. As early as 1923, Billerey and Etchells had been involved by the Estate in proposals for the site, and several abortive schemes followed, notably one worked out by the New York architect Whitney Warren, and another by George Crawley and Gervase Bailey. But it was not until 1926, when proposals for a new building on the site of the old house were finally agreed upon, that Lutyens was called in.

From this time the short but vital era of architectural consultation begins. Its peak coincides in fact with Blow's heyday between 1928, when Wimperis relinquished the estate surveyorship, and his own abrupt retirement in 1933. In this period, loose but distinct spheres of interest speedily emerged. Lutyens took the big blocks ripe for redevelopment, principally Grosvenor House and Hereford House; Billerey was called in over the proposed rebuilding of Grosvenor Square; and Etchells quietly diverted himself with private commissions in the mews. At first sight the emergence of these particular individuals appears arbitrary: Lutyens, acclaimed first architect of the day and prince of English traditions of design; Billerey, reclusive and meticulous Beaux-Arts designer; and Etchells, young Vorticist painter, translator of Le Corbusier, Anglo-Catholic enthusiast, and clever amateur in all the arts. Doubtless, the heterodoxy and informality of their characters appealed to Blow, weary of the steady efficiency of the Wimperis firm. Strong individualism was a particularly necessary quality for Lutyens and Billerey, since their job was to bestow grace and style upon the exteriors of a new set of buildings, most of which had a more mundane character and function than those of earlier epochs. What is remarkable is the extent to which their answers to the problems which Blow presented to them coincided uniformly in a reinforcement of that brick-classic tradition that was now gradually vanishing from so much of urban architecture.

The most graphic example of this is Grosvenor House. In 1926 A. O. Edwards, a speculator who had gained experience on part of the site of Devonshire House, came forward with a comprehensive scheme to include a hotel and flats, his architect being L. Rome Guthrie. It is said that Guthrie brought the job with him into the office of Wimperis and Simpson, whose ranks he joined as a partner at just this time. But by the time that Guthrie's drawings were complete, Blow had brought in Lutyens and made various suggestions to him. The deliberate plainness of Guthrie's submitted elevations evidently did not appeal to the Duke's advisers, and this gave Lutyens the chance to take over, alter and dramatize the façade-composition; and also to add some extra height. So Grosvenor House, as built in 1926–30, is in its plan basically Guthrie's and in its dress mainly Lutyens's: the hand of the latter is easily betrayed by the special brand of classicism employed on the ground storeys and on the high stone pavilions, so reminiscent of his work at Delhi (Plate 48c).

But there were other influences at work as well. Grosvenor House was intended by Edwards to cater 'specifically for the American market',[109] so in the layout good note was taken of American models and the complex was broken up into several separate blocks with deep set-backs from the street between them, instead of the internal light-wells traditional to Britain. Lutyens, who in 1925 had visited the United States for the first time, discovering much to admire in contemporary architecture there, had thought the skyscrapers 'growing from monstrosities to emotions of real beauty'.[110] Ever quick to adopt and perfect an idea, Grosvenor House shows him refining the American innovation of a crowning classical storey, as in his contemporary Midland Bank, Poultry, and Britannic House, Finsbury Circus.

At Grosvenor House, Lutyens was closely confined. His attic pavilions had to be limited to the ends of the four blocks, the linking bridges he had wanted between the two main portions were omitted, and the upward recession in mass for which he constantly strove in his later civic works could hardly be realized. The result was in fact a compromise and because of its great bulk inevitably controversial. It has never been thought wholly successful. Lutyens's official chronicler A. S. G. Butler believed that the criticism really stemmed from the fact

that new Grosvenor House spelt the knell of one-time fashionable Park Lane as a residential street.[111] But a shrewd contemporary article in *The Times* sums up the real problem: 'what is the matter with Grosvenor House is precisely that it is not designed as a big building. It is an overgrown small building, stretching a familiar and endearing style of domestic architecture beyond its capacity to please. Every architectural style has its proper scale, and it is a fairly safe general rule that, if you greatly enlarge—or diminish—scale, you must change style.'[112]

Nevertheless Lutyens had furnished the estate with a spectacular building, and was to do so again, at Hereford House in Oxford Street. Here the whole of the Victorian development of Hereford Gardens together with the open space in front was destined to disappear in favour of a grand store for Gamages with flats above, to plans by C. S. and E. M. Joseph. Lutyens provided elevations in September 1928 and building took place in 1929–30. This time, though the site was more enclosed, the design problems were not so great and Lutyens could respond to the scale with the high recessed classical features that he loved on all four sides. Towards Oxford Street he also introduced a small engaged colonnade, thus restoring to the Grosvenor estate side of the street a little of the swagger stolen by Selfridges across the way. On the whole Hereford House, though a ruinous enterprise for Gamages, turned out more satisfactorily than Grosvenor House. It was beyond even Lutyens's power entirely to redeem the problems of scale. But in each case he had given a touch of distinction to what might otherwise have been just another pair of massive rebuildings.

The smaller rebuildings in which Lutyens was involved need briefer comment. One was Audley House, Nos. 8–10 North Audley Street, where he provided a sketch elevation for the block of shops and residential flats planned by J. Stanley Beard and erected in 1927–9. Like Grosvenor House and Hereford House, Audley House is of red brick with some distinguishing stone dressings. But at No. 8 Upper Grosvenor Street, also in 1927–8, Lutyens surprisingly was asked to improve a single stone house-elevation. For this and two other advisory jobs on further sizeable rebuildings along Park Lane, Aldford House (1930–2) and Brook House (1933–5), he was paid a standard fee of fifty guineas each time. It must have been an *ad hoc* consultative procedure, for he played no known part in either the decent Nos. 105–108 Park Lane of 1930–2 (Plate 49c), designed like the new Brook House by Wimperis, Simpson and Guthrie, or the inferior Nos. 56–62 Park Lane (1933–4), by Trehearne and Norman, Preston and Company. Billerey, too, was consulted on some of these sites, particularly Brook House, but there is good circumstantial evidence that neither he nor Lutyens had any substantial hand in the design of this interestingly planned block, where Guthrie once again was the principal architect. The best of all these buildings is the new Aldford House (Plate 49d), for which the architects were George Val Myer and F. J. Watson-Hart, designers of Broadcasting House. As usual, it is divided between banks and shops below and flats above, but the flats have continuous, canted balconies that form a horizontal banding to the block and contribute to a more lively and up-to-date treatment than any of its neighbours received. The receding top storeys, culminating in the surprise of end pediments and a gabled roof, suggest the possibility of a more extensive and specially constructive piece of intervention by Lutyens here, but this is not known for certain.

After Blow's eclipse, however, Lutyens was no longer used by the Grosvenor Estate as a consultant. He was briefly superseded by Sir Giles Gilbert Scott, who was well paid for advice on Fountain House, Park Lane (1935–8, also by Myer and Watson-Hart), but this appears to have been the single instance of his consultation. In a personal capacity, Lutyens also made a number of minor domestic alterations on the estate, from those at No. 12 Grosvenor Square, probably of 1895, to those at No. 5 Balfour Place in 1934, but none was of consequence.

It is surprising, possibly even disappointing, that the job of rebuilding Grosvenor Square did not fall to Lutyens, the only designer of the period who had the stature, temperament, and needful mixture of charm and aggression to force such a bold concept through to fulfilment. Fernand Billerey had no such natural advantages. Neither his French background nor his self-effacing modesty was calculated to work to his benefit in a situation where the support and co-operation of estate managers, speculators and fellow-architects had to be secured for the elevations that he was commissioned to impose upon them. Many of the difficulties Billerey did manage to overcome, but others turned out to be insuperable.

The chronology of the long-drawn-out Grosvenor Square rebuilding has already been given (see page 77), but it remains to consider the architectural character and assess the outcome of this great scheme. Today there is no longer any need to challenge on doctrinaire grounds Billerey's choice of style for Grosvenor Square as old fashioned, since the fashion which it represents has now passed into history. His neo-Georgian, in textured brick with ample stone dressings, tested, formalized and refined through contact with the Beaux-Arts disciplines that were his own particular strength, corresponded precisely with that partial view of eighteenth-century tradition that the guardians of the estate's image cherished most dearly. Nor can Billerey be blamed in any way for the failure to complete the square. Given the leasehold system of tenure, the rupture between his ally Blow and the Duke in 1933, and the depressed economic situation that persisted through the decade, a quick completion to unified designs was impossible. But one pertinent question, having little to do with style but much to do with the history of Grosvenor Square, has to be asked. Was the

conception of a unified, composed rebuilding of the square in itself a wise one?

In the eighteenth century, attempts to sustain a single composition along individual sectors of the square had succeeded on the east but failed on the north. Then in the Cundy era, though Blow and his associates probably did not know it, what appears to have been an attempt to secure uniformity by refrontings had also died the death. So a composed, classical Grosvenor Square was a recurrent theme, and because of modern leasing policies it stood real chances of success in the twentieth century. But the British, traditionally respectful of the rights of property, have been equally often rebels against formality in aesthetics and dictatorship in design, even when initiated by the very same landlords. So much the estate managers might have learned from the painful recent histories of Regent Street and Kingsway. In Grosvenor Square they were to get nearer to success, but a major factor in their frustration was to be the old conception of the London square in terms of individual, private plots. In this conception there was much aesthetic sense as well as practicality. The Grosvenor Square which the twentieth century demolished was not meant to be 'read' as one, but as a set of variations upon the domestic theme, to which the amenity of the garden gave relief. Though the old houses of that square could hardly all survive into the age of the apartment block, the case for judicious variety and gradual replacement was a strong one. Since modern developers press both for height and for breadth of frontage, the variations would certainly have been difficult to control; arguably indeed, uniform development has meant that Grosvenor Square has escaped the fate of, say, modern Golden Square or Hanover Square. But this has been at a cost. The long sides of today's square, however well composed, cannot comfortably be taken in at a glance. The thinning of trees and opening out of the central garden, though intended to pull the square together, actually draws attention to this problem. As a result, the modern visitor scurries through Grosvenor Square, absorbing little of the refined architecture that is about him, or at best fixing on the comparatively brash but finite bulk of the American Embassy upon its western side.

Billerey was in some measure alive to the dangers of an over-extended composition on the two long sides. Evidently the Place de la Concorde, most obvious of models for a large open square, was much before his Gallic consciousness. Indeed in a design of 1936 for the south side he actually divided the range into two, with a wide gateway in the centre. This was doubtless not feasible because of the sacrifice of space involved, but it was visually a good principle and makes the loss of his overall design for this side the sadder. It is only on the north, the one side completed recognizably to his design (except for the roof), that Billerey's grasp of an architecture of scale and texture, with its refinements of sculptural detail and brickwork and its small breaks and recessions to avoid monotony, can be readily appreciated (Plate 54b).

Even on this side, and much more visibly on the others, variations of detail in parts of different date can naturally be found. These variations are more dramatically apparent on the return flanks and backs of the new Grosvenor Square, some of which have an interest of their own. The return flank along North Audley Street of No. 21, part of the first block to be rebuilt (1933–4), adopts the then fashionable light-well set back from the street, whereas at the other end of the north side, Lewis Solomon, Kaye and Partners' Europa Hotel (1961–4) has an expansive façade towards Duke Street incorporating a small drive-in. Brutally different again are the rear elevations of the square's other hotel, the Britannia by Richard Seifert and Partners (1967–9) at Nos. 39–44 in the middle of the south side; here, in compensation for the loss of a modern façade or entrance to the square, the design breaks with redoubled vigour towards Adams Row into the blocky pre-cast concrete idiom so characteristic of this firm. One of the minor entertainments of modern Grosvenor Square is to stroll around the neighbouring streets and mews and note how many disparate bedfellows in the way of embassies, hotels and flats can be found snuggling together under Billerey's all-enveloping classical counterpane.

Of the architects regularly employed to advise the Estate during this period, the third, Frederick Etchells, is something of an elusive figure, and his direct work for the Estate was much less far-reaching than that of Lutyens or Billerey. A dilettante of the best and most capable kind and an associate of Blow as far back as 1911,[113] Etchells liked small jobs with which to keep himself amused, and of these the Grosvenor estate had plenty. In 1923 he had a model prepared in connexion with one of the Grosvenor House proposals, a task he again undertook for Lutyens in 1929. By 1925 he was also being paid in connexion with a variety of small commissions, sometimes matters like lettering on signboards. But by the time that Wimperis retired in 1928, Etchells was privately establishing himself as monarch of the mews, with all that this now implied.

The 'bijou' mews house in Mayfair had, perhaps surprisingly, a short pre-war history. Possibly motors took up less space than horses, for as early as 1908 the Grosvenor Board agreed to the conversion of some of the stables in Balfour Mews and Streets Mews (now Rex Place) which were letting badly, and duly in that year No. 1 Streets Mews was turned into a private house (now No. 2 Aldford Street). Then after a gap of about five years, the architects Gilbert and Constanduros added a storey at No. 1 Balfour Mews (now No. 3 Aldford Street) for Monty Mendelssohn, a small speculator, and Stanley Barrett and Driver altered No. 17 Balfour Mews (now No. 23 South Street) for two maiden ladies, in both cases with the help of Thackeray Turner, joint architect of the original stabling here. By 1915, on the strength of the

many applicants he had for his conversion, Matheson (as Mendelssohn now called himself) was able to report 'great demand' for what he was already speaking of as 'bijou' housing, and after the war this rapidly increased.[114] One of the first such post-war conversions, again undertaken by Matheson with Gilbert and Constanduros at No. 1 Mount Row in about 1919, was deemed worthy to be published in *Country Life* four years later.[115] Characteristically, as little as possible of the exterior was changed, but the whole of the inside was gutted and made elegantly French. As mews houses became the rage, especially among *chic* young people, many such private works of conversion were undertaken (Plate 50c, d) and many must remain unrecorded. But by 1925 the Estate was beginning to explore what might be done in three minor thoroughfares, Culross Street, Mount Row and Lees Mews (later Lees Place).

The main field of Estate endeavour was the sector of Culross Street east of Park Street, where there had always been a number of small independent houses. In 1926–9 Wimperis managed to shut up the short east-west section of Blackburne's Mews, behind the north side of Culross Street, and in its place his firm laid out a narrow little garden. Both sides of the street itself were thoroughly rebuilt, with Wimperis, Simpson and Guthrie undertaking No. 6 together with No. 64 Park Street, and Forsyth and Maule (with Mrs. Macindoe) Nos. 2 and 4, while much of the rest came under the sway of Etchells. He with his partner Gordon Pringle rebuilt or brushed up Nos. 1A and 5 and probably also Nos. 1, 3, 7 and 9 on the south side, and No. 14 on the north, all in a simple style enlivened with small fetching Regency details rather in the manner of Adshead and Ramsey's work on the Duchy of Cornwall Estate in Kennington (Plate 50a, b). Most of this took place between 1926 and 1928, and was so subtly done that it is hard to believe the transformation so complete or so modern. Further west in Culross Street there are one or two other nice mews houses (Plate 51a), for instance Ernest Cole's witty No. 25 (1929).

Having proved that an admirer of Corbusier could play a good hand in neo-Georgianism, Etchells produced another trick from his sleeve in Mount Row. Here the young T. P. Bennett in 1926–7 had designed the charming Nos. 12–14 (Wren House), with an intricate plan including a garage on the ground floor, reception rooms above, and round 'Hampton Court' windows to the bedroom storey (Plate 51c). Not to be outdone, Etchells in 1929–31 followed on with the neighbouring Nos. 6–10 (Tudor House), an irreverent group with a pair of half-hipped gables that look as though they had dropped in on Mayfair from some smart suburban estate (Plate 51d). Such slight interludes upon the staid Grosvenor scene were what Etchells loved; another, a restoration of a run of shops along Little Grosvenor (now Broadbent) Street, sadly failed to materialize, though drawings survive (Plate 51b). Further north and west in Lees Place (as Lees Mews became in 1930), his role was smaller but his spirit of paradox as present as ever. With the pleasant neo-Georgian houses built in Shepherd's Place in the 1930's he was not involved, but in Lees Place itself he probably designed No. 14 (1930) and certainly the more formal Lees House, No. 4 (1930–1) for the Hon. Evelyn FitzGerald. Etchells was determined not to let the tall symmetrical neo-Georgian façade of Lees House be taken at its face value. In a tongue-in-cheek article for *The Architectural Review*, presumably written by himself, he pleaded that Lees House was a 'modern house, built for two modern people leading a highly modern life', and that its 'faint flavour of the eighteenth century . . . is as illusive and as unimportant as when Picasso, to compare small things with great, gives the world a bold experiment in the guise of an 1870 lithograph'; and in justification he pointed to the variations he had made on the 'typical London plan'.[116] The old traditional house plan was indeed at last beginning to fade away in metropolitan London, as domestic architects learned to deal with smaller sites and cope with conversions. Though Lees House and one or two other of the mews houses mentioned do still have two staircases, in most the demise of old Mayfair patterns of living was plain to behold.

In one respect the interwar period was still a golden age, and that was for interior decoration. Fashionable families who gave up their great houses and installed themselves in flats wanted and, on the whole, could still afford some compensation for their novel anonymity in the shape of good furniture and design. In this period there was probably more originality in decorating work than ever before. One little-remembered factor in the increasing separation of architecture from interior design was the apartment block, for in a flat there was no need to employ an architect but plenty of opportunity to display good taste. Decorating firms of the 1920's and '30's are recalled usually for their contributions to country houses, but blocks of flats like those in Grosvenor Square were their staple fare. Several such schemes were chattily written up in magazines like *Vogue* and *Harper's Bazaar*.

Most of the Mayfair decorators of the day still adhered to the traditional styles, but many hankered for modernity in one form or another. Despite the occasional go-ahead client, like the one who employed Serge Chermayeff to redecorate a flat at No. 42 Upper Brook Street shortly before 1935, or Mr. Saxon Mills, who got Denham MacLaren to 'scramble' the walls of his flat at No. 52 Grosvenor Street,[117] the traditional concerns naturally got the better of the market. But gone were the days when French stucco-work was reeled out by the yard; instead, firms like White Allom or Lenygon and Morant now offered quiet, relatively scholarly interiors, with panelling of waxed oak or subdued colouring, and the emphasis all upon the furniture, pictures and carpets. Much borrowing from old houses went on at this time, which Philip Tilden speaks of as 'a period when all Mayfair panelled its walls with pine stripped from old discarded Georgian houses, and which were limed to

greyness, or waved to honey'.[118] Such was the character of Lenygon and Morant's transformation of No. 25 Upper Brook Street of 1933 (Plate 53a), of their work at No. 9 South Audley Street (1935) and of the surviving interiors at No. 45 Upper Grosvenor Street, where date and designer are unknown. Oliver Hill was, on the whole, equally reticent in his work of 1928 for Lord Forres at No. 70 Grosvenor Street (now demolished). A less individual but similar style of work could be had from the big department stores like Whiteleys, Harrods, Waring and Gillows and Maples, all of whom sported flourishing decorating sides between the wars.

For greater originality, still within a traditional framework, it was possible to go to one of a group of amateurs and ladies who did much for interior decoration in the 1920's and '30's. 'The conversion of stables and garages was an important part of Mrs. Beaver's business' in *A Handful of Dust*, and for Mrs. Beaver Evelyn Waugh could have had one or several personalities in mind. In Culross Street we have already seen a Mrs. Macindoe in operation at Nos. 2 and 4, but some more familiar names were active on and around the estate. Lady Sibyl Colefax, probably the best known of these women, began her decorating practice from rooms just out of our area in Bruton Street; her only known work on the Grosvenor estate in this period was the redecoration of No. 40A Hill Street in 1938. After the war, however, she joined forces with John Fowler in Wyatville's old house at No. 39 Brook Street, the gallery of which was separated off and redecorated as a private house for Mrs. Lancaster (doyenne of 1930's taste) in Fowler's inimitable manner, while the main house remains the headquarters of Colefax and Fowler. Another celebrated shop was that of Mrs. Guy Bethell and Mrs. Dryden, partners in an interior decorating firm called E. Elden at No. 84 Duke Street, just behind No. 10 Grosvenor Square;[119] they altered No. 9 Upper Grosvenor Street in 1928, and some surviving reliefs of this date by Gilbert Bayes in the back yard must relate to their work here.

Near Elden's shop, behind No. 9 Grosvenor Square, Somerset Maugham's wife Syrie had in the late 1920's and 1930's a 'wildly expensive corner block with "Syrie Ltd." in gold letters', where her estranged husband once uncharitably imagined her as 'on her knees to an American m-m-millionairess trying to sell her a chamber-p-p-pot'.[120] But Syrie Maugham did serious work. She is usually remembered for her obsession with white and her love of stripped furniture, though neither taste was greatly in evidence in her three known works on the Grosvenor estate—interiors at No. 48 Upper Grosvenor Street for the Whighams (1935), at Israel Sieff's flat in the new Brook House (1935), and at No. 47 Upper Brook Street (1936) for the Leveson-Gowers. Her work for the Whighams still survives, and not untypically the room with the most panache is the bathroom, that classic inner sanctum of the sybarite of the '30's, where good taste could surrender to luxury and ostentation, and modern materials come to the fore. 'Bathrooms nowadays look more expensive than any rooms in the house', commented *Vogue* in 1935.[121] There were other excellent bathrooms at nearby No. 44 Upper Grosvenor Street, as done up for Leo d'Erlanger and his very fashionable wife by Jansen of Paris, and at No. 12 North Audley Street where in 1932 the mysterious Marchesa Malacrida (with White Allom) put in for Samuel Courtauld a witty semi-circular bathroom of temple form (Plate 53d).

If wit was a prized commodity in interior decoration of the period, nobody was the readier with it than Rex Whistler, who painted a panel for Courtauld's bedroom in North Audley Street, and designed urns for the house's great gallery. More extensive were his murals of 1937 (now removed) for Lady Mountbatten's boudoir in the large double-storey penthouse at the top of the new Brook House; this had been designed specially for the Mountbattens by L. Rome Guthrie, penthouses as much as bijou mews houses being a feature of the age. At some point also Whistler sketched an interesting and in some ways prophetic suggestion for the replanting of Grosvenor Square, with formal paths converging on a central monument.

Classicism of Whistler's variety was sometimes combined with elements from the various *jazz-moderne* styles to convey freshness and humour in interiors of the 1930's. Such an instance was No. 25 South Street, a big private house built in 1932–3 by E. B. Musman for Sir Bernard Eckstein, and augmented and decorated in 1936–7 by Turner Lord and Company with flamboyant painted interiors and furniture (Plate 53c). In an appropriately lower but similar key were the various extensions to Claridge's Hotel. In 1926 Basil Ionides, a pioneer in several aspects of interior design between the wars, redecorated the restaurant and with the help of William Ranken put in some pretty engraved glass and some large modelled elephants. This scheme was not to survive for long in its entirety; in 1929 Oswald Milne constructed a new entrance foyer, remodelled the restaurant again (keeping the glass and the elephants), and followed these with large extensions east of the main hotel in 1930–1 and a penthouse on top in about 1936; in the same period many of the suites were refurnished. Milne's work (Plate 52) was carried out in a gay, up-to-the-minute manner, with copious help from subordinates like Marion Dorn for carpets and the Bath Artcraft Company, R. Burkle and Son, and Gordon Russell for the furniture. Even *Country Life* was compelled to admire 'the beauty of the freedom afforded by the revolution of the last ten years', at least in the shape that it took at Claridge's, duly denuded of too much French Cubism or German utilitarianism by the civilizing hand of 'a humanist such as Mr. Milne'.[122]

Though the façade of the Claridge's extension towards Brook Street, an essay in the stepped-back manner of the day, is less distinctive than Milne's interiors, it is more able than most of the comparable large inter-war blocks

along the main streets. At first, a majority of these had been flats, but by 1939 encroachment by office blocks was under way, especially along Grosvenor Street. The residential character of the principal streets was now under serious threat. Following their appearance on the ground floors of new blocks, shop windows were beginning to be seen upon even the major old houses; in Grosvenor Street, one (since taken out) was installed when Keeble Limited, the decorators, converted No. 34 as their Mayfair showroom in 1936, and others appeared at about this time at Nos. 18 and 58. Probably the best of these was at No. 15 North Audley Street, where Albert Richardson put in a Regency Gothick shop front for the West End branch of B. T. Batsford in 1930. There was a natural tendency for commercial concerns to move into the old houses first, because new flats often had stringent rules about occupation, whereas these had to be relaxed for the houses because only firms could fill them economically. So the influx of commerce probably saved many of these houses from destruction, though office use naturally tended to detract from their interior character, sometimes very severely.

The war of 1939–45 of course speeded up the progress of commerce and left even fewer private householders in its wake. There were not many important architectural losses by bombing, the destruction of the picture gallery and ballroom at Dudley House being the worst, but the wear and tear of war confirmed the fate of the remnants of old Grosvenor Square. Here, a number of good houses were sacrificed to the rebuilding scheme, notably Nos. 12 (1961) and 44 (1967), but outside the square few first-rate houses have disappeared since the war. Still, the onward march of commerce has led to further proliferation of office and apartment blocks. Before 1960 few of these buildings espoused an overtly modern style. Possibly the last block in the full neo-Georgian tradition was Nos. 76–78 Grosvenor Street (designed by P. Macpherson, of Hillier, Parker, May and Rowden, 1939–40), a building still in the brick manner of Wimperis, Simpson and Guthrie. A comparison with the estate's first big post-war block, the unambitious British Council headquarters on the site of St. Anselm's Church at No. 65 Davies Street, designed under austerity conditions by Howard, Souster and Partners (1948–50), shows the now pressing need for a new initiative. On the British Council *The Architectural Review* was predictably scathing, but still had to look abroad for support for the new aesthetic: 'the many foreign visitors the Council entertains will not be impressed by the heavy Georgian-style office block illustrated herewith'.[123] But the Grosvenor Estate was still a champion of neo-Georgian, as the stone-faced Drill Hall opposite the British Council at No. 56 Davies Street by Trenwith Wills (1950) testifies. Its architectural policies, if unadventurous, were at least more mannerly than in some other parts of London. As late as 1963–5 a development in Davies Street with a frontage at No. 53 Grosvenor Street was obliged to keep this façade in reasonably decorous adherence to the brick traditions of the street.

But the Modern Movement finally arrived on the Mayfair estate with a bang at the United States Embassy (1956–60), inevitably a foreign achievement. Old American associations with Grosvenor Square had been renewed when the embassy moved to the east side in 1938. Throughout the war the American presence strengthened, and was confirmed in 1947 by the replanting of the central garden as a memorial to President Franklin D. Roosevelt, which led to the felling of 'over sixty five mature trees'[124] and the setting up of a statue by Sir William Reid Dick in the centre. Then the west side, substantially complete still except for bomb damage at its north end, was after years of prevarication allotted to the new American Embassy, and a limited competition was held. Great care was taken not to outrage traditional Grosvenor sentiment, so much so that the American assessors outlined in the conditions of competition the need for an undogmatic building related in scale and materials to the rest of the square, while of the competitors it is recorded that 'some... were certainly chosen for their moderation'.[125]

The result was a win by an experienced competitor, Eero Saarinen, the runner-up being Edward D. Stone. A third participant, Minoru Yamasaki, produced a design with a strong Gothic flavour. But though Saarinen showed respect for the neo-Georgianism around him, there was nothing really Georgian about either his style or his materials. The building itself (Plate 55b) has brought a dramatic, internationalist change to the atmosphere of the very centre of the estate, still hard to assess fifteen years after completion. Many of Fello Atkinson's original criticisms in *The Architectural Review* remain as pertinent as ever. The Embassy's merits in his eyes were Saarinen's sensitivity to the square's scale and his determination to design a deeply relieved façade, which was met by slotting a complex grid of Portland stone window frames into the diagonal structural system developed after he had won the competition. On the other hand, because the huge building is set back from the street line on all three of its major sides (a condition which appears to have been part of the brief), it fails to enclose the square and therefore, paradoxically, is too small; set up on a podium as it is, it appears as an austere, free-standing temple rather than the palace or fortress that embassies traditionally have been and truly are. On a third point mentioned by Atkinson time has yet to tell: Saarinen looked forward to the day when the building would darken with dirt, and the gilded aluminium of the window frames would stand out against dark stonework.[126]

Since the American Embassy, it has never been quite so easy to be conservative on the estate again. Most big developments have taken the bull by the horns, some with reasonable success. Sir John Burnet, Tait and Partners have made a pair of lively contributions to the estate scene at Nos. 15–27 (odd) Davies Street (1963–5) and 399–405

(odd) Oxford Street (1967–70); another sizeable block is Grosvenor Hill Court between Bourdon Street and Grosvenor Hill, by Westwood, Piet and Partners (1962–6); while Fitzroy Robinson and Partners have blown the brazen trumpet of comprehensive redevelopment at Nos. 455–497 (odd) Oxford Street (1961–9). The wholesale rebuilding of this area was indeed a prominent feature of Chapman Taylor Partners' *Grosvenor Estate Strategy for Mayfair and Belgravia* (1971). Respect for 'conservation' (distinguished, however, from 'preservation') was there expressed, and also for many of the Victorian buildings. But in execution the visual transformation of the area would doubtless have been very great, not least because of the low architectural assessment in that report of the estate's numerous twentieth-century buildings of more-or-less 'period' character. In its assumptions about the successful juxtaposition of the indigenous styles of Georgian and modern times this careful and very interesting report already seems characteristic of its period. At present (1976) there has been a retreat from a number of these premises and objectives and the estate enters a period when more extensive conservation appears, for the moment, to have gained the upper hand.

APPENDICES

APPENDIX I: LEASES OF THE PRINCIPAL

This table provides information about the initial development of Brook Street, Grosvenor Square, Grosvenor Street, Upper Brook Street, Upper Grosvenor Street and the part of South Audley Street between South Street and the estate boundary: the house plots and the areas covered by building agreements are shown on Plan A in the end pocket.

The house numbers are as at present or (where sites have been merged) are those of the original sites in the present sequence. Where the present site arrangement differs substantially from the original the numbers last in use when the original sites still existed are given (as at the corners with Park Street). Where sites were merged before the present sequence of numbers was adopted, as at No. 10 Grosvenor Square or No. 75 South Audley Street, the original houses have been distinguished as, for example, 10 (*east*) and 10 (*west*) or 75 (*north*) and 75 (*south*).

The building leases were granted by the head of the Grosvenor family, or by Robert Myddelton, the guardian of Dame Mary Grosvenor (see pages 7–8, 16–17, where general information about the leases can also be found).

House No.	*Frontage in Feet*	*Date of Building Agreement*	*No. on Plan A*	*Undertaker*	*Date of Building Lease*	*Lessee*
BROOK STREET, NORTH SIDE						
36	19	3 Dec. 1720 (36–64)	9	Robert Pollard, yeoman, and Henry Avery, bricklayer	31 July 1724 (36–38)	Augustin Woollaston
38	16					
40	32				30 July 1724	Thomas Lansdell
42	16				do.	Thomas Couch
44	18				do.	do.
46	20				do.	Edward Buckingham
48	20				do.	Edward Austin
50	20				do.	John Ellis
52	20				do.	John Howorth
54	20				do.	William Head
56	19				31 July 1724 (56–62)	Ralph Harrison and Thomas Barlow
58	19					
60	19					
62	19					
64	25				30 July 1724	Thomas Hogg
Here is Davies Street						
66	36	7 Nov. 1723 (66–78)	36	Edward Shepherd, plasterer	25 Jan. 1724/5	Edward Shepherd
68	36				do.	do.
70	32				1 April 1725	Lawrence Neale
72	22½				do.	Edward Shepherd
74	26				do.	Thomas Hogg
76	20				1 April 1726 (76–78)	Colen Campbell
78	30					
Here is Gilbert Street						

STREETS ON THE ESTATE

The rent is the sum specified in the building lease except where a separate sub-lease is indicated in the table, when the rent is the sum specified in that sub-lease.

Information about the first occupants is derived mainly from the ratebooks of the parish of St. George, Hanover Square, and because of the nature of the evidence there may be inaccuracies in the dates of residence given.

Principal sources: agreements and lease books in Grosvenor Office; Middlesex Land Register in Greater London Record Office; ratebooks in Westminster City Library; *Burke's Peerage*; *The Complete Peerage*; *Dictionary of National Biography*; *History of Parliament*.

Designation	*Associated Builders and Architects*	*Rent* £	*s.*	*d.*	*First Occupant*	*Period*	*House No.*
esquire	William Barlow, bricklayer, party to lease			8	John Watts	1725–30	36
					Mr. Thickbroom	1726–8	38
joiner	do.; assigned to Daniel Marston, glazier	3	0	0	Slingsby Cressy, apothecary	1726–30	40
slater	William Barlow, bricklayer, party to lease	3	10	0	William Blackburne, shoemaker	1726–43	42
do.	do.	do.			Edward Thompson	1728–30	44
mason		4	0	0	William Winde, esq.	1728–32	46
bricklayer		do.			Mrs. Lewis	1728–30(d)	48
joiner		do.			General Joseph Sabine, M.P., Governor of Gibraltar	1728–39(d)	50
carpenter		do.			Humphrey Denby	1725–50	52
carpenter		do.			Joseph Crouchley	1725–52	54
	Sub-let 1724 to William Barlow, bricklayer, and by him to William Austin, carpenter	8	15	0	Elizabeth Allen	1728–30	56
gentleman		do.			Thomas Thickbroom	1728–30	58
carpenter	Sub-let 1724 to William Barlow, bricklayer, and by him to Thomas Lansdell, joiner	do.			Bennet Demages	1734–6	60
		do.			Ann Vincent	1728–31	62
lime merchant		5	0	0	Lady Drogheda, ?widow of 4th Earl (she d. 1735)	1731–5(?d)	64
plasterer		20	0	0	Sir Nathaniel Curzon, Bt., M.P.	1729–58(d)	66
do.	Assigned to Thomas Fayram, mason	15	0	0	Lawrence Shirley, esq.	1729–31	68
carpenter		8	0	0	Brigadier Robert Murray, M.P., s. of 1st Earl of Dunmore	1727–38(d)	70
gentleman		3	0	0	Edward Shepherd	1726–9	72
lime merchant	Assigned to Lawrence Neale, carpenter	10	8	0	William Cowper, esq.	1726–9	74
					Colen Campbell, architect	1726–9(d)	76
esquire, architect to H.R.H. the Prince of Wales	Israel Russell, painter-stainer, witness to lease	19	12	0	Hon. Henry Vane, M.P. (later 1st Earl of Darlington)	1727–34	78

House No.	Frontage in Feet	Date of Building Agreement	No. on Plan A	Undertaker	Date of Building Lease	Lessee
BROOK STREET, NORTH SIDE (continued)						
80	22				25 Aug. 1725	James Heathfield
82	25				do.	do.
84	32	27 April 1724	38	Augustin Woollaston, esquire	do.	Augustin Woollaston
Here is Binney Street						
86	32				do.	do.
88	50				26 April 1725	William Barlow jnr.
BROOK STREET, SOUTH SIDE						
39	26	12 Dec. 1720	11	Thomas Phillips, carpenter	9 March 1722/3	Thomas Phillips
41	32				22 July 1725	do.
43	35	21 Dec. 1720	20	David Audsley, plasterer	21 July 1725	David Audsley
45	38	17 Dec. 1720	13	George Pearce, plumber	10 May 1723	George Pearce
47	40	do.	14	Joseph Osborne, ironmonger (assigned to Edward Shepherd)	do.	Edward Shepherd
49	40				21 June 1725	George Pearce
51	29				22 June 1725	do.
53	30	25 May 1724	39	George Pearce, plumber	do.	George Barlow and William Head
55 (*east*)	18				do.	John Barnes
55 (*west*)	24	12 Dec. 1720	12	John Barnes, bricklayer	25 April 1724	do.
57	36				do.	do.
Here is Davies Street						
59	31				20 Aug. 1723	Edward Liney
61	18				25 Aug. 1725	William Jackling
63	30	24 Nov. 1720	7	Francis Bailley, carpenter	do.	do.
65	31				28 Feb. 1722/3	Henry Avery
67	31				do.	Francis Bailley
69	50	6 March 1724/5	50	do.	25 Aug. 1725	do.
71	31	24 Nov. 1724	44	John Simmons, carpenter	18 Feb. 1725/6	John Simmons
GROSVENOR SQUARE, EAST SIDE						
51	22				5 June 1731	John Simmons
1	30				4 June 1731	do.
2	44	24 Nov. 1724	44	John Simmons, carpenter	3 June 1731	do.
3	44				2 June 1731	do.
4	70				12 Sept. 1728	do.

Designation	*Associated Builders and Architects*	*Rent* £ s. d.	*First Occupant*	*Period*	*House No.*
carpenter	William Barlow jnr. party to lease	8 0 0	Captain (later Colonel) Mark Anthony Saurin	1727–31	80
do.	do.	do.	Eleanor Farmer	1728–41	82
esquire	Assigned to Lawrence Neale, carpenter	9 13 0	Margaret Graham	1728–36	84
do.	Assigned to Robert Umpleby, carpenter	do.	5th Earl of Northampton	1729–54(d)	86
bricklayer		22 0 0			88
carpenter		9 0 0	Thomas Phillips	1723–36(d)	39
do.		4 0 0	2nd Viscount Mountjoy	1725–8(d)	41
plasterer		9 0 0	16th Baron Abergavenny	1727–44(d)	43
plumber		do.	5th Earl of Coventry	1725–35 (moved to No. 3 Grosvenor Sq.)	45
plasterer		10 0 0	Sir John Buckworth, Bt., M.P.	1725–37 (moved to No. 13 S. Audley St.)	47
plumber		do.	Marquess of Hartington, M.P. (succ. as 3rd Duke of Devonshire in 1729)	1726–9	49
do.		4 0 0	'Sir August Humes' ? Sir Gustavus Hume, Bt.	1727–9	51
bricklayer carpenter		7 10 0	Augustus Schutz, esq., Master of the Robes and Keeper of the Privy Purse to George II	1727–57(d)	53
bricklayer		4 10 0	Mr. Parker	1726–8	55 (*east*)
do.		4 0 0	? John Shepherd, plasterer	1725	55 (*west*)
do.		6 0 0	Edward Reculest, grocer	1726–46	57
paviour		7 10 0	Hugh Williams, esq., M.P.	1726–37	59
bricklayer		6 6 0	Abigail Jones	1729–31	61
do.		10 0 0	Robert Moore, esq.	1730–48	63
do.		9 6 0	Captain (later Colonel) Martin Madan	1727–31	65
carpenter		7 14 0	Nicholas Grice, esq.	1726–9	67
do.		6 3 0	Marquis de Montandré, Field-Marshal	1734–9(d)	69
do.		9 0 0	Hon. Capel Moore, s. of 3rd Earl of Drogheda	1729–37	71
carpenter		3 14 0	Mrs. Simmons or William Mabbott, esq., Director of E. India Co.	1741 1741–8	51
do.		do.	Lady Barker	1734–9	1
do.		4 0	Lady Mary Colley, d. of 6th Earl of Abercorn and widow of Henry Colley, M.P.	1735–6	2
do.		do.	5th Earl of Coventry	1735–51(d)	3
do.		do.	9th Duke of Norfolk	1739–41	4

House No.	Frontage in Feet	Date of Building Agreement	No. on Plan A	Undertaker	Date of Building Lease	Lessee
GROSVENOR SQUARE, EAST SIDE (continued)						
5	45	24 Nov. 1724	44	John Simmons, carpenter	28 May 1728	John Simmons
6	45				2 Aug. 1727	Chrysostom Wilkins
7	51				1 Aug. 1727	John Simmons
GROSVENOR SQUARE, NORTH SIDE						
[Former No. 8 now No. 88 Brook Street]						
9	30	27 April 1724	38	Augustin Woollaston, esquire	24 May 1725	William Barlow [jnr.]
Here is Duke Street						
10 (*east*)	30	6 March 1724/5	51	do	5 May 1726	do.
10 (*west*)	36				4 May 1726	William Packer
11	34				6 May 1726	William Gray and John Brown
12	50				30 June 1727	John Kitchingman
13	32				14 Aug. 1727	Lawrence Neale
14	32				15 Aug. 1727	do.
15	44				21 Nov. 1727	Augustin Woollaston
16	32				22 Nov. 1727	Richard Davies
17	50	do.	52	do.	15 April 1729	Lawrence Neale
18	50	do.	54	Edward Shepherd, gentleman	22 July 1728	Thomas Fayram
19	60				23 July 1728	Edward Shepherd
20	50				24 July 1728	Francis Drewitt
21	20				25 July 1728	John Shepherd
Here is North Audley Street						
22	30	do.	55	Robert Andrews, gentleman, and Thomas Barlow, carpenter	28 Nov. 1728	John Kitchingman
23	21				26 Sept. 1727	Robert Andrews
GROSVENOR SQUARE, WEST SIDE						
24	33	6 Feb. 1724/5	47	Thomas Ripley, esquire (assigned to Robert Andrews, gentleman, and Robert Scott, carpenter); Isaac Ware witness of agreement	22 June 1728	Francis Bailley
25	45				21 June 1728	John Green
26	50				20 June 1728	Charles Griffith
27	42				19 June 1728	Robert Scott
28	44				18 June 1728	Benjamin Timbrell
29	44				17 June 1728	Thomas Richmond
30	36				15 June 1728	Joseph Stallwood
31	30				14 April 1729	John Sanger
32	26				15 April 1729	John Worrington

Designation	*Associated Builders and Architects*	*Rent* £ *s. d.*	*First Occupant*	*Period*	*House No.*
carpenter		22 10 0	Lady King, widow of 1st Baron King	1734–67(d)	5
plasterer		do.	Edward Chandler, Bishop of Durham	1730–50(d)	6
carpenter		25 0 0	2nd Viscount Weymouth	1731–9	7
bricklayer		18 0 0	Sir Thomas Samwell, Bt.	1727–30	9
do.	Finished according to agreement with, and assigned to, Thomas Archer, esquire [architect]	10 0 0	Thomas Bladen, esq., M.P.	1731–8	10 (*east*)
carpenter	William Barlow jnr. party to lease	14 8 0	John Campbell, esq., M.P., Lord of the Treasury	1729–67	10 (*west*)
bricklayers	William Barlow jnr. party to lease; Roger Morris supervised finishing of house	13 12 0	14th Baron (later Earl) Clinton	1729–51(d)	11
timber merchant		20 0 0	John Aislabie, esq., Chancellor of Exchequer 1718–21	1729–42(d)	12
carpenter		12 16 0	Dorothea Dashwood	1729–51	13
do.		do.	Sir William Strickland, Bt., M.P., P.C., Secretary at War	1729–35(d)	14
esquire	Assigned to Richard Davies, joiner	3 12 0	Thomas Duncombe, esq., M.P.	1729–46(d)	15
joiner		12 16 0	Lady Gowran, widow of 1st Baron Gowran	1729–44(d)	16
carpenter		20 0 0	2nd Earl of Albemarle	1730–54(d)	17
mason	John Deval, mason, did £300 worth of work in interior in 1736	25 0 0	2nd Earl of Rockingham	1737–45(d)	18
gentleman		26 0 0	7th Earl of Thanet	1730–53(d)	19
bricklayer		25 0 0	6th Earl of Mountrath, M.P.	1731–44(d)	20
plasterer		7 0 0	Sir Cecil Bishopp, 6th Bt., M.P.	1733–8	21
timber merchant		10 10 0	5th Baron (later Earl) Cornwallis	1730–9	22
gentleman	Assigned to John Worrington, paviour	6 6 0	John Evelyn, esq., M.P., Groom of the Bedchamber to Prince of Wales	1732–51	23
carpenter	Assigned to James Theobald, timber merchant	12 0 0	Lord Nassau Powlett, s. of 2nd Duke of Bolton	1735–8	24
joiner		19 2 6	Duchess of Rutland, widow of 2nd Duke	1733–51(d)	25
carpenter		21 15 0	Sir Robert Sutton, M.P., P.C., diplomat	1730–5	26
do.		17 17 0	4th Earl of Shaftesbury	1731–71(d)	27
do.		18 14 0	General Sir Charles Wills, M.P., P.C.	1730–41(d)	28
do.		do.	2nd Duke of Manchester	1732–9(d)	29
bricklayer	Thomas Richmond, carpenter, party to lease	15 6 0	Anne Jennings	1730–61	30
carpenter	do.	12 10 0	Sir Charles Gounter Nicoll, M.P.	1730–3(d)	31
paviour	do.	10 16 0	Lady Acklom or Charles Echlin, esq.	1729–30 1730–48	32

House No.	Frontage in Feet	Date of Building Agreement	No. on Plan A	Undertaker	Date of Building Lease	Lessee
GROSVENOR SQUARE, SOUTH SIDE						
33	35	18 Nov. 1725	58	Richard Andrews, gentleman	22 Aug. 1727	William Moreton
34	30				25 May 1728	Robert Scott and William Barlow snr.
Here is South Audley Street						
35	25	29 April 1725	57	Robert Grosvenor, esquire	4 Feb. 1726/7	Robert Grosvenor
36	35					
37	38					
38	39					
39	36					
40	45					
41	42					
42	38	(No building agreement found)			22 April 1725	do.
43	36					
44	36					
45	40					
46	35					
47	35	6 March 1724/5	48	Thomas Cook and Caleb Waterfield, carpenters	25 Oct. 1726	Caleb Miller
48	40				5 May 1726	Thomas Cook and Caleb Waterfield
Here is Carlos Place						
49	30	28 Jan. 1724/5	46	John Jenner, bricklayer	25 Jan. 1727/8	John Jenner
50	33				28 Jan. 1725/6	do.
GROSVENOR STREET, NORTH SIDE						
4 & 5	40	2 Sept. 1720	3	William Barlow snr., bricklayer	5 Feb. 1722/3	William Barlow and Robert Scott
6	18				do.	Robert Scott
7	18				do.	William Barlow
8	20				15 July 1721	William Mantle
9	31				8 Oct. 1722	Robert Scott
10	20				5 Feb. 1722/3	William Barlow
11	20				do.	John Cartwright

Designation	*Associated Builders and Architects*	*Rent* £ *s. d.*	*First Occupant*	*Period*	*House No.*
mason	Robert Scott, carpenter, and William Barlow snr., bricklayer, parties to lease	12 0 0	4th Earl of Inchiquin, M.P.	1731–6	33
carpenter bricklayer		5 15 0	Lady Bishopp, widow of Sir Cecil Bishopp, 5th Bt.	1729–50(?d)	34
	Sub-let 1728 to William Head, carpenter; George Barlow, bricklayer, party	8 10 0	Lady Mary Saunderson, d. of 1st Earl of Rockingham	1730–7(d)	35
	Sub-let 1727 to George Barlow, bricklayer; William Head, carpenter, party	14 0 0	Colonel (later General) Roger Handasyde, M.P.	1730–42	36
	Sub-let 1728 to Samuel Phillips, carpenter	15 0 0	2nd Earl of Scarbrough	1733–40(d)	37
esquire	Sub-let 1727 to Israel Russell, painter-stainer	14 0 0	4th Earl of Dysart	1733–9	38
	Sub-let 1728 to William East, esquire; Thomas Phillips, carpenter, party	14 8 0	William East, esq., M.P.	1727–31	39
	(Sub-let 1727 to Baron Carpenter)	13 10 0	1st Baron Carpenter, general, commander of forces in North Britain 1715	1727–32(d)	40
	Sub-let 1727 to Benjamin Timbrell, carpenter	14 14 0	Henry Bromley, esq., M.P. (later 1st Baron Montfort)	1728–34	41
	Built directly and sold in 1731 by Robert Grosvenor to Benjamin Timbrell, carpenter		Frederick Frankland, esq., M.P.	1731–7	42
	Sub-let 1727 to William Barlow [snr.], bricklayer	9 0 0	Duchess of Kendal	1728–43(d)	43
do.	Sub-let 1727 to Robert Scott, carpenter	do.	Oliver St. George, esq.	1728–31(d)	44
	Sub-let 1727 to Thomas Richmond, carpenter	1 0 0	Marquess of Blandford, M.P., g.s. of 1st Duke of Marlborough	1730–1(d)	45
	do.	13 10 0	Lord Glenorchy, M.P. (later 3rd Earl of Breadalbane)	1731–8	46
brickmaker	Assigned to Thomas Knight, joiner	17 10 0	5th Baron Baltimore, M.P.	1731–42	47
carpenters		20 0 0	Sir William Wyndham, Bt., M.P., Chancellor of Exchequer 1713–14	1738–40(d)	48
bricklayer		2 2 0	Henry Talbot, esq., b. of 1st Baron Talbot, Lord Chancellor	1728–61	49
do.		16 7 0	William Bumpsted, esq. or Hon. Anne Vane, mistress of Frederick, P. of Wales	1732 1733–6(d)	50
bricklayer carpenter		6 0 0	Richard Davies, victualler (Red Lion)	1723–32	4 & 5
do.		2 10 0	Frances Wyndham	1725–38	6
bricklayer		do.	Major James Haldane	1725–8	7
plasterer		6 0 0	Colonel Lloyd	1724–6	8
carpenter		6 10 0	Mrs. Rowe	1725–6	9
bricklayer		5 0 0	Mrs. Wallop	1724–5	10
blacksmith		6 0 0	Edward Cressett, esq.	1725–6(?d)	11

House No.	Frontage in Feet	Date of Building Agreement	No. on Plan A	Undertaker	Date of Building Lease	Lessee
GROSVENOR STREET, NORTH SIDE (continued)						
12	30				15 Nov. 1723	Israel Russell
13	20	2 Sept. 1720	6	Mathew Tomlinson, carpenter (assigned to Benjamin Timbrell, carpenter)	30 Nov. 1723	Charles Griffith
14	20				do.	John Jenner
15	30	11 Jan. 1722/3	28	John Jenner, bricklayer	3 June 1723	do.
16	55	2 Sept. 1720	5	Thomas Ripley, carpenter	25 April 1724	Thomas Ripley
17	35	do.	6a	Robert Scott, carpenter	30 Nov. 1723	Robert Scott
18	35				do.	Thomas Richmond
19	20	22 June 1723	31	John Laforey, esquire	31 Oct. 1723	John Laforey
20	20	20 July 1723	32	Benjamin Whetton, bricklayer	30 Nov. 1723	Richard Lissiman
21	19½	9 Aug. 1723	35	Samuel Phillips, carpenter	do.	John Steemson
22	19½				do.	Samuel Phillips
23	23	4 Jan. 1720/1	21	George Chamberlen, carpenter, and George Wyatt, bricklayer	28 Jan. 1724/5	George Chamberlen
24	23				do.	George Wyatt
25	25				1 Aug. 1724	John Deane
26	25	2 Sept. 1720	2	John Deane, painter	do.	do.
27	20				26 Jan. 1724/5	Richard Davies
28	31½				10 Aug. 1725	do.
Here is Davies Street						
29	18				26 Nov. 1725	Francis Commins
30	19	19 July 1723	33	Francis Commins, mason		
31	18				25 Aug. 1725	William Mantle
32	35	24 July 1724	41	Robert Scott, carpenter	20 April 1725	Robert Scott
33	35				21 July 1725	Richard Lissiman
34	43	10 July 1724	40	Richard Lissiman, mason	do.	do.
35	22				22 July 1725	do.
36	31				18 Feb. 1725/6	John Simmons
37	30				16 Feb. 1730/1	do.
38	30	24 Nov. 1724	44	John Simmons, carpenter	do.	do.
39	22				do.	do.
40	22				do.	do.
GROSVENOR STREET, SOUTH SIDE						
43	40	17 Dec. 1720	17	John Pritchard, gentleman	12 April 1726	Benjamin Hoadly
44	20				12 May 1726	John Pritchard
45	18	20 Dec. 1720	18	Stephen Whitaker, brickmaker (assigned to William and Benjamin Benson)	31 Dec. 1725	William Benson
46	18				do	Benjamin Benson
47	24	22 Jan. 1724/5	45	John Jenner, bricklayer	29 July 1726	Colonel Charles Churchill
48	36	17 Dec. 1720	16	Henry Huddle, carpenter	22 June 1726	Henry Huddle

Designation	*Associated Builders and Architects*	*Rent* £ *s. d.*	*First Occupant*	*Period*	*House No.*
painter[-stainer]		9 0 0	Earl of Burford, M.P. (succ. as 2nd Duke of St. Albans in 1726)	1725–6	12
carpenter		6 0 0	Charles Miller, esq.	1726–32	13
bricklayer		do.	William Edwards, esq.	1725–30	14
do.		7 10 0	(Rectory of St. George, Hanover Square)	1725 onwards	15
esquire		15 15 0	Baron Walpole, s. of Sir Robert Walpole (later 2nd Earl of Orford)	1725–38	16
carpenter		10 0 0	James Vernon, esq., Clerk of the Privy Council	1725–55	17
do.		do.	Elizabeth Strangeways (later Duchess of Hamilton)	1725–9(d)	18
esquire		5 0 0	? Colonel Churchill	1725	19
mason		do.	John Herring, esq.	1725–43 (?d)	20
carpenter		4 17 0	— Smith, esq.	1725–6(d)	21
do.		do.	Major (later Colonel) William Duckett, M.P.	1726–49(d)	22
do.		6 15 0	Governor Morris, ? Bacon Morris, Gov. of Landguard Fort, Suffolk	1726–7	23
bricklayer		do.	Simon Smith, esq.	1726–30	24
painter		3 0 0	Mr. Davies	1725–6	25
do.		do.	John Harrison	1725–8	26
joiner		5 0 0	Elizabeth O'Court	1726–33	27
do.		8 10 0	Mary Butler	1727–48	28
			?		29
mason		3 4	Mr. Pitts	1727–8	30
plasterer		6 10 0	William Mantle	1726–7	31
carpenter		8 10 0	Lady Edwin (and her son, Charles Edwin, esq., M.P., who d. 1756)	1726(–56(d))	32
mason		10 10 0	Baron Sparre, Swedish Envoy	1727–36	33
do.		14 10 0	Sir Paul Methuen, M.P., P.C.	1728–57(d)	34
do.		3 4	William Turner, esq.	1728–34	35
carpenter		9 0 0	Judith Ayliffe	1728–35	36
do.		5 0 0	Charles Evelyn, esq.	1733–5	37
do.		do.	Lady Gray, ? widow of Sir James Gray, Bt.	1733–44	38
do.		3 0 0	Marquess of Graham (succ. as 2nd Duke of Montrose in 1742)	1734–42	39
do.		do.	Thomas Colnit, esq.	1734–5	40
Bishop of Salisbury	John Jenner, bricklayer, party to lease; Robert Phillips, ? bricklayer, witness	15 0 0	Benjamin Hoadly, Bishop of Salisbury (later B. of Winchester)	1726–45	43
gentleman		6 0 0	John Pritchard	1726	44
esquire		5 8 0	William Benson, Surveyor-General of the King's Works 1718–19	1726–52	45
do.		do.	Benjamin Benson, brother of above	1727	46
		10 16 0	Colonel (later General) Charles Churchill, M.P.	1727–45(d)	47
carpenter		14 8 0	Lord Charles Cavendish, M.P., s. of 2nd Duke of Devonshire	1729–32	48

House No.	Frontage in Feet	Date of Building Agreement	No. on Plan A	Undertaker	Date of Building Lease	Lessee
GROSVENOR STREET, SOUTH SIDE (continued)						
49	36	9 Aug. 1723	34	Robert Herne, joiner (assigned to John Green)	21 Oct. 1725	John Green
50	36½				3 Nov. 1724	Charles Griffith
51	39½				do.	Israel Russell
		21 Dec. 1720	19	Benjamin Timbrell, carpenter		
52	50				do.	Benjamin Timbrell
53	40					
		17 Dec. 1720	15	William Waddell, plumber (assigned to Thomas Barlow, carpenter)	11 Jan. 1724/5	Thomas Barlow
54	31					
Here is Davies Street						
55	17½					
56	19					
57	25					
58	36					
59	36					
60	24					
61	18					
62	20					
63	17					
Here is Broadbent Street						
64	19					
65	21½	8 Aug. 1720	1	Thomas Barlow, carpenter	15 or 27 July 1721	Thomas Barlow
66	35					
67	28					
68	20					
69	35					
70	35					
71–72	42					
73	34					
74	34					
75	22					
76	26					

Designation	*Associated Builders and Architects*	*Rent £ s. d.*	*First Occupant*	*Period*	*House No.*
joiner		10 16 0	Earl Grandison	1727–35	49
carpenter		do.	1st Earl of Uxbridge	1726–43(d)	50
painter[-stainer]		11 14 0	Sir John Werden, Bt.: his son-in-law, 2nd Duke of St. Albans, also here 1726–7	1726–8	51
carpenter		15 0 0	Sir Thomas Hanmer, Bt., M.P., Speaker of House of Commons 1714–15	1726–46(d)	52
do.	John Prince, ? surveyor, witness to lease; sub-let 1725 to John Neale, carpenter	do.	Earl of Arran	1726–58(d)	53
	do.	12 0 0	Robert Knight, esq., M.P.	1729–36	54
	Sub-let 1724 to Samuel Phillips, carpenter	5 0 0	William Fellows, victualler (Three Tuns Tavern)	1725–39(d)	55
	do.	4 0 0	? Mrs. Robinson	1726	56
	Sub-let 1724 to Walter Lee, mason	8 0 0	Lady Stapleton, widow of Sir William Stapleton, Bt.	1725–33	57
	Sub-let 1724 to John Green, joiner	12 12 0	Baron Ranelagh	1726–54(d)	58
	Sub-let 1725 to David Audsley, plasterer	10 0 0	Sir Robert Rich, Bt., M.P.	1726–42	59
	Sub-let 1723 to John Neale, carpenter	7 0 0	Anne Oldfield, actress	1725–30(d)	60
	Sub-let 1721 to George Worrall, plasterer	4 1 0	George Worrall or Lady Allen, ? widow of Sir William Allen, Bt.	1725 1725–36	61
	Sub-let 1721 to John Neale, carpenter	5 0 0	Mr. Munday	1725–8	62
	Sub-let 1723 to Thomas Sams, joiner	3 10 0	William Robertson	1726–30	63
	Sub-let 1724 to Edward Allen, carpenter	4 0 0	Mrs. Milton	1726–56	64
carpenter	Sub-let 1725 to do.	5 0 0	Lucy Killigrew	1726–9(d)	65
	Sub-let 1723 to Joshua Fletcher, mason	10 0 0	2nd Baron Barnard	1725–9	66
	Sub-let 1723 to Caleb Waterfield and Thomas Cook, carpenters	7 16 0	Lady Strafford, widow of William, Earl of Strafford	1725–31	67
	do.	6 0 0	Mary Fox	1725–32(d)	68
	Sub-let 1723 to Benjamin Timbrell, carpenter	10 0 0	Earl of Dalkeith (later 2nd Duke of Buccleuch)	1725–9	69
	Sub-let 1722 to Robert Hearne, joiner; Benjamin Timbrell party	do.	Godfrey Clarke, esq., M.P.	1724–34(d)	70
	Sub-let 1722 to Benjamin Timbrell, carpenter	do.	Earl of Hertford (succ. as 7th Duke of Somerset in 1748)	1724–48	71–72
	Sub-let 1722 to John James, bricklayer	do.	Sir Edward Ernle, Bt., M.P.	1724–9(d)	73
	Sub-let 1722 to Stephen Whitaker, brickmaker; John James party	do.	Lord Compton (later 5th Earl of Northampton)	1725–9 (moved to No. 88 Brook St.)	74
	Built by Thomas Barlow and let at rack rent		Mrs. Herne	1725–32	75
	Sub-let 1722 to William Waddell, plumber	7 0 0	John Dobson, esq.	1727–57	76

House No.	Frontage in Feet	Date of Building Agreement	No. on Plan A	Undertaker	Date of Building Lease	Lessee
GROSVENOR STREET, SOUTH SIDE (continued)						
77, 78	37					
Here is the entrance to Grosvenor Hill						
79	19½	8 Aug. 1720	1	Thomas Barlow, carpenter	15 or 27 July 1721	Thomas Barlow
80						
81						
SOUTH AUDLEY STREET, EAST SIDE						
9	18	24 May 1736	74	John Eds, carpenter	7 Dec. 1738	John Blagrave
10	18				do.	Roger Blagrave
11	16				22 June 1737	George Thwaits
12	31	do.	73	William Singleton, plasterer	5 Aug. 1737	William Singleton
13	21				19 July 1736	do.
14	34	1 Feb. 1735/6	72	Roger Blagrave, carpenter	do.	Roger Blagrave
15	26				do.	do.
16	27				14 Feb. 1735/6	do.
SOUTH AUDLEY STREET, WEST SIDE						
71	20	24 May 1736	75	Edward Shepherd, esquire	19 July 1736	Thomas Skeat
72	19				do.	John Eds
73	20				do.	John Shepherd
74	56				do.	Edward Shepherd
75 (*north*)	26				do.	do.
75 (*south*)	19½				do.	do.
	22				do.	do.
UPPER BROOK STREET, NORTH SIDE						
1	23	6 March 1724/5	55	Thomas Barlow, carpenter, and Robert Andrews, gentleman	27 May 1728	John Evans
2	30				16 June 1730	John Neale
3	20				do.	do.
4	31				do.	David Audsley
5	31				do.	do.
6	30				19 Sept. 1732	Edward Shepherd
7	19				do.	Edward Cock
8	16				do.	do.
Here is Shepherd's Place						

Designation	*Associated Builders and Architects*	*Rent* £ s. d.	*First Occupant*	*Period*	*House No.*
	Sub-let 1722 to William Waddell, plumber	12 19 0	William Robertson	1725–6	77
			George Bickford	1723–42(?d)	78
carpenter	Sub-let 1721 to John James, bricklayer, and David Audsley, plasterer	5 0 0	Thomas Hewson	1725–8	79
	Built by Thomas Barlow and let at rack rent		Francis Minetone (Mount Coffee House)	1721–3	80
	(? originally part of No. 80)		James Martin	?1736–48	81
carpenter	Roger Blagrave, carpenter, party	4 19 0	Susannah Jennings	1739–53	9
do.	Assigned to John Blagrave, carpenter, his son	do.	Catherine Sloper, estranged wife of William Sloper of West Woodhay, Berks., M.P.	1739–99	10
gentleman		4 10 0	George Thwaits	1738–44	11
plasterer		9 0 0	Hon. James Lumley, M.P., s. of 1st Earl of Scarbrough	1740–4	12
do.		6 6 0	Sir John Buckworth, Bt., M.P.	1737–41	13
carpenter	Assigned to John Blagrave, carpenter, his son	13 12 0	Jerome de Salis, esq.	1740–5	14
do.	do.	7 16 0	Barbara Cavendish, estranged wife of William Cavendish, g.s. of 1st Duke of Devonshire	1738–50	15
do.		4 1 0	John Tubb, chandler	1738–61	16
bricklayer		6 0 0	Samuel Greathead, esq., M.P.	1739–56	71
carpenter		8 0 0	Hon. Colonel Charles Ingram, M.P., s. of 3rd Viscount Irwin	1738–43	72
plasterer		10 8 0	George Ogle, esq., classicist and Chaucerian scholar	1738–46(d)	73
esquire		20 0 0	(Portuguese Embassy)	1747 onwards	74
do.		7 12 0	2nd Earl of Halifax	1739–46	75 (*north*)
do.		5 0 0	Hon. John St. John (later 2nd Viscount St. John of Battersea)	1738–48(d)	75 (*south*)
do.		6 0 0			
joiner		6 4 0	Mary Fox	1732–4	1
carpenter		8 10 0	Archibald Hutcheson, esq., lawyer and economist	1732–40(d)	2
do.		6 6 0	Colonel Francis Byng, b. of Admiral Sir George Byng, 1st Viscount Torrington	1732–3	3
plasterer		10 10 0	Mrs. Trenchard	1733–8	4
do.		do.	Richard Powys, esq., M.P.	1734–7	5
esquire	John Shepherd, plasterer, party to lease	10 7 0	Edward Shepherd	1734–5	6
carpenter	do.	5 5 0	Lady Betty Lowther (and/or Sir Thomas Lowther, Bt., M.P.)	1735–7(d)	7
do.	do.	4 7 6	Thomas Burke	1733–6	8

House No.	Frontage in Feet	Date of Building Agreement	No. on Plan A	Undertaker	Date of Building Lease	Lessee
UPPER BROOK STREET, NORTH SIDE (continued)						
9	20				14 Oct. 1729	John Shepherd
9A	20				13 Oct. 1729	do.
10	34				25 May 1732	Edward Cock
11	15				26 May 1732	do.
12	38				1 March 1728/9	Elizabeth Alleyne
13	22	6 March 1724/5	55	Thomas Barlow, carpenter, and Robert Andrews, gentleman	28 Nov. 1728	William Davis
80 Park St.	20				22 Nov. 1728	Thomas and Samuel Gough and Richard Peacy
Here is Park Street						
14	22				23 July 1728	William Barlow jnr.
15A	18				1 April 1729	William Davis
15	20				2 April 1729	John Barlow
16	20				10 Oct. 1729	William Bennett
17	23				do.	John Panton
18	30					
19	30					
20	30					
21	30	6 March 1724/5	53	Augustin Woollaston, esquire (assigned to Robert Andrews, gentleman)		
22	31					
23	27				19 Sept. 1732	Robert Andrews
24	32					
25	30					
26	28					
27	18					
28	23					
29	46				16 May 1729	Francis Bailley

Designation	*Associated Builders and Architects*	*Rent* £ *s.* *d.*	*First Occupant*	*Period*	*House No.*
plasterer		5 5 0	John Dickins, coffee house keeper	1730–48	9
do.	Assigned to John Barnes, bricklayer	do.	Elizabeth Jenkins	1733–56	9A
carpenter		14 0 0	Sir Francis Head, Bt.	1732–41	10
do.		6 0 0	Catherine Hewsham	1734–8	11
widow		13 6 0	Elizabeth Alleyne	1730–7	12
carpenter	Daniel Marston, glazier, Thomas and Samuel Gough, bricklayers, and Richard Peacy, carpenter, parties to lease; assigned to Francis Jackman, timber merchant	4 0 0	Dr. Lovell	1736–7	13
bricklayers carpenter	Daniel Marston, glazier, party to lease; assigned to Francis Drewitt, bricklayer	3 0 0	Lady Vane, ? widow of 1st Viscount Vane	1739–41	80 Park St.
bricklayer	George Barlow, bricklayer, party to lease; William Allison, carpenter, witness	6 0 0	James Liverpoole, victualler (Barley Mow)	1736–46(?d)	14
carpenter	George Barlow and William Barlow jnr., bricklayers, parties to lease; assigned to William Jayne, carpenter	4 10 0	Thomas Marsh	1734–5	15A
bricklayer	George Barlow and William Barlow jnr., bricklayers, parties to lease; assigned to latter	5 0 0	Captain John Aldred, R.N.	1733–40(d)	15
carpenter	George Barlow, bricklayer, party to lease	8 0 0	'Lord Peters', ? 8th Baron Petre	1741–2	16
do.	do.	9 4 0	Major Weldon and/or Lady Charlotte Weldon	1734–8	17
	Sub-let 1737 to John Simmons, carpenter	12 0 0	1st Earl of Pomfret	1740–7	18
	do.	do.	3rd Viscount Doneraile, M.P.	1742–4	19
	Sub-let 1737 to William Atlee, painter; John Simmons, carpenter, mortgagee	do.	Mr. Fortnam, ? Richard Fortnam, bricklayer, son-in-law of John Simmons	1744–5	20
	Sub-let 1737 to John Simmons, carpenter	do.	Sir Edmund Thomas, Bt., M.P., Groom of the Bedchamber to Prince of Wales	1742–51	21
	Sub-let 1742 to Joshua Fletcher, mason	12 8 0	3rd Earl of Marchmont	1744–63	22
gentleman	Sub-let 1742 to Thomas Barratt, brickmaker, and John Barlow, bricklayer	10 16 0	Trafford Barnston, esq.	1747	23
	Sub-let 1742 to Lawrence Neale, carpenter	12 16 0	2nd Duke of Chandos	1746–54	24
	do.	12 0 0	Lady Frances Bland, widow of Sir John Bland, Bt.	1744–58(?d)	25
	Sub-let 1746 to Elizabeth Simmons, widow of John Simmons	11 4 0	Sir Francis Eyles(-Stiles), Bt.	1747–50	26
	Sub-let 1742 to do.	7 4 0	Samuel Spencer, esq.	1744–50	27
	Sub-let 1742 to Joshua Ransom, John Smith and Griffin Ransom, [timber] merchants; Richard Fortnam, bricklayer, a witness	9 4 0	Lady Sidney Beauclerk, widow of Lord Sidney Beauclerk and mother of Topham Beauclerk	1745–53	28
carpenter	Assigned to Thomas Phillips, carpenter, and eventually vested in his nephew, John Phillips, carpenter	4 0	14th Earl of Morton	1747–9	29

House No.	*Frontage in Feet*	*Date of Building Agreement*	*No. on Plan A*	*Undertaker*	*Date of Building Lease*	*Lessee*
UPPER BROOK STREET, SOUTH SIDE						
30	51					
31	23					
32	29					
33	31				25 Sept. 1736	William Barlow and Robert Scott (as execs. of Stephen Whitaker)
34	20					
35	28					
36	28					
37	28				do.	do.
		11 May 1721	26	Stephen Whitaker, brickmaker		
38	25				do.	Isaac Mansfield
39	20				do.	John Simmons
40	30				do.	do.
41	35				do.	William Barlow and Robert Scott (as execs. of Stephen Whitaker)
42	27				11 Dec. 1735	John Brown
43	23					William Barlow and Robert Scott (as execs. of Stephen Whitaker)
44	21				do.	
45	19					
46	17				14 Dec. 1734	William Arnott
Here is Park Street						
47	36					
48	19					
49	31½					
50	32½					
		6 Feb. 1724/5	47	Thomas Ripley, esquire (assigned to Robert Andrews, gentleman, and Robert Scott, carpenter); Isaac Ware witness to agreement	1 June 1728	Robert Andrews
51	31½					
52	20					
53	21					
Here is Blackburne's Mews						

Designation	*Associated Builders and Architects*	*Rent* £ s. d.	*First Occupant*	*Period*	*House No.*
	Sub-let 1756 to William Timbrell, esq., and John Spencer, carpenter, co-partners; Alexander Rouchead, mason, party	8 10 0	Mrs. Stanley	1757–64	30
	do.	do.	Thomas Ramsden, esq.	1759–91(d)	31
	Sub-let 1756 to John Barlow, bricklayer; Timbrell, Spencer and Rouchead (as above) parties	10 3 0	Sir Charles Hanbury Williams, M.P.	1758–9	32
bricklayer carpenter	Sub-let 1756 to Edmund Rush, mason; Timbrell, Spencer and Rouchead (as above) parties	12 8 0	Lady Anne Jekyll	1757–66(d)	33
	do.	5 9 0	Thomas Sanders, esq.	1757–75	34
	Sub-let 1737 to Anthony Cross, mason; Alexander Rouchead, mason, party	8 14 0	Duchess of Atholl	1746–8	35
	do.	7 5 0	6th Baron Ward (later 1st Viscount Dudley and Ward)	1742–57	36
do.	Sub-let 1736 to Stephen John Whitaker, brickmaker, and assigned by him to Lawrence Neale, carpenter	2 0	Lord Mark Kerr, general, s. of 1st Marquis of Lothian	1742–52(d)	37
plasterer	William Barlow, bricklayer, and Robert Scott, carpenter, parties to lease	8 15 0	Lady Delorain, widow of 3rd Earl of Delorain	1741–53 and 1773–94(d)	38
carpenter	do; Isaac Mansfield, plasterer, witness	7 0 0	2nd Viscount Vane	1742–3	39
do.	do.	10 10 0	Hon. Nicholas Herbert, M.P., s. of 8th Earl of Pembroke	1742–75(d)	40
bricklayer carpenter	Sub-let 1736 to John Brown, bricklayer, and Anthony Cross, mason	12 5 0	Lady Georgiana Spencer, widow of Hon. John Spencer (later Countess Cowper)	1747–61	41
bricklayer	William Barlow, bricklayer, and Robert Scott, carpenter, parties to lease	8 2 0	Anthony Chute, esq., M.P.	1739–47	42
do. carpenter	Sub-let 1736 to William Arnott, carpenter	1 0	Lady Anne Cavendish	1739–80	43
	do.	6 16 0	Robert Bragg, esq.	1739–43	44
	Sub-let 1735 to do.	4 10 0	Robert Bogg	1738–47	45
do.		4 0 0	William Davis, cheesemonger	1737–69	46
	Sub-let 1730 to John Barnes, bricklayer	do	Thomas Mitchell	1732–4	47
	do.	do.	John Gill	1732–3	48
	do.	9 9 0	Duchess of Bolton	1731–49	49
gentleman	Sub-let 1730 to Israel Russell, painter[-stainer]; John Barnes, bricklayer, party	9 15 0	Countess of Shaftesbury, widow of 3rd Earl	1733–51(d)	50
	Sub-let 1730 to Edward Cock, carpenter; John Barnes, bricklayer, party	9 9 0	Arthur Stafford, esq., and/or Lady Stafford	1732–5	51
	do.	4 0 0	Robert Sheppard, tailor	1732–54	52
	Sub-let 1730 to John Barnes, bricklayer	3 0 0	Daniel Fitzpatrick, victualler (Cock and Bottle)	1730–40(?d)	53

House No.	Frontage in Feet	Date of Building Agreement	No. on Plan A	Undertaker	Date of Building Lease	Lessee
UPPER BROOK STREET, SOUTH SIDE (continued)						
54	38½	6 Feb. 1724/5	47	Thomas Ripley, esquire (assigned to Robert Andrews, gentleman, and Robert Scott, carpenter); Isaac Ware witness to agreement	19 Sept. 1729	John Green
55	20					
56	41½				8 Sept. 1729	do.
UPPER GROSVENOR STREET, NORTH SIDE						
1	28	6 Feb. 1724/5	47	Thomas Ripley, esquire (assigned to Robert Andrews, gentleman, and Robert Scott, carpenter); Isaac Ware witness to agreement	16 April 1729	Thomas Richmond
2	20					
3	18					
4	17					
5	17					
Here is Blackburne's Mews						
6	24				1 June 1728	Robert Scott
7	20					
8	20					
9	30					
10	33					
11	31					
12	36					
Here is Park Street						
37 Park St.	17	25 April 1724	37	Robert Andrews, gentleman	14 Feb. 1726/7	Robert Andrews
13	20					
14	33					
15	32					
16	25					
17	34					
18	34					
19	30					
20	30					

Designation	Associated Builders and Architects	Rent £ s. d.	First Occupant	Period	House No.
joiner		1 2 6	Jonathan Scull	1730–8	54
			? Joseph Reeve	1739	55
do.		17 6	(Originally added to curtilage of 25 Grosvenor Sq.; separate house not built here until 1810–13)		56
	Sub-let 1729 to Thomas Fry, carpenter	9 2 0	Lady Frances Erskine, widow of 22nd Earl of Mar	1736–42	1
	do.	6 10 0	George Ogle, esq., classicist and Chaucerian scholar	1737–8 (moved to No. 73 S. Audley St.)	2
carpenter					
	Sub-let 1729 to John Worrington, paviour; Thomas Fry, carpenter, party	5 17 0	John Gillard	1733–41	3
	do.	5 10 6	William Gillett	1731–55	4
	Sub-let 1729 to Thomas Fry, carpenter	5 0 0	Evan Brotherton	1731–4	5
	Sub-let 1728 to John Worrington, paviour	4 0 0	John Stokes, victualler (Oval)	1729–53	6
	Sub-let 1729 to William Waddell, plumber	6 0 0	John Lamp, esq.	1734–6	7
		do.	Captain Robert Hale	1732–50	8
do.	Mortgaged by Scott to Charles Serena, Italian plasterer	7 0 0	William Edwards, esq., Treasurer of New River Co.	1731–7(d)	9
	Sub-let 1728 to Benjamin Timbrell, carpenter	8 10 0	(Sir) Robert Grosvenor, M.P.	1730–3	10
	do.	8 0 0	Captain (later Major) Humphry Watson	1731–41(d)	11
	do.; Henry Flitcroft [architect], mortgagee	do.	Benjamin Timbrell	1729–51	12
	Sub-let 1732 to Richard Davies, joiner; John Mackreth, lime merchant, and Stephen Whitaker, brickmaker, parties	4 0 0	John Hughes	1737–46	37 Park St.
	do.	6 0 0	Thomas Miller	1734–6	13
	do.; assigned to Lawrence Neale, carpenter	13 0 0	6th Viscount Irwin	1736(d)	14
	do.	do.	Hon. Bussy Mansell, M.P. (later 4th Baron Mansell)	1736–50(d)	15
gentleman	Sub-let 1730 to Joshua Fletcher, mason; Mackreth, Whitaker (as above) and Thomas Hipsley, bricklayer, parties	10 12 6	Thomas Whichcot, esq., M.P.	1741–8	16
	Sub-let 1732 to Lawrence Neale, carpenter; Mackreth and Whitaker (as above) parties	13 12 0	Hon. Lawrence Shirley, s. of 1st Earl Ferrers	1734–8	17
	do.	do.	Thomas Boothby Skrymsher, esq.	1735–51(d)	18
	do.	12 0 0	Viscount Blundell	1734–56(d)	19
	do.	do.	John Nightingale, esq.	1735–6	20

House No.	Frontage in Feet	Date of Building Agreement	No. on Plan A	Undertaker	Date of Building Lease	Lessee
UPPER GROSVENOR STREET, NORTH SIDE (continued)						
21	29	25 April 1724	37	Robert Andrews, gentleman	14 Feb. 1726/7	Robert Andrews
22	21					
23	20					
24	19					
UPPER GROSVENOR STREET, SOUTH SIDE						
(Former 28 Park Lane)	28	12 April 1728	65	Richard Lissiman, mason	8 April 1729	William Hale and Richard Lissiman
25	18				9 April 1729	do.
26	28				16 Aug. 1729	Richard Lissiman
27	19				15 Aug. 1729	do.
28	20				14 Aug. 1729	do.
29	21				19 Sept. 1732	do.
30	34				do.	do.
31	19	(no building agreement found)			5 June 1731	1st Viscount Chetwynd
32	57					
33						
34	40					
35	26	5 June 1727	61	Thomas Goff, blacksmith (assigned to Robert Grosvenor)	11 Dec. 1735	Thomas Skeat
36	24				do.	John Eds
Here is Park Street						
56 Park St.	16	18 Nov. 1725	58	Richard Andrews, gentleman	4 Oct. 1731	Richard Andrews
37	21					
38	33					
39	34					
40	36					
41	36					
42	33				2 Oct. 1731	John Green
43	33				1 Oct. 1731	do.
44	25				3 Nov. 1727	William Draycott

Designation	*Associated Builders and Architects*	*Rent* £ s. d.	*First Occupant*	*Period*	*House No.*
	Sub-let 1732 to Lawrence Neale, carpenter; Mackreth and Whitaker (as above) parties; assigned to Benjamin Denne, mason	11 12 0	Leonard Smelt, esq., M.P.	1734–40(d)	21
gentleman	Sub-let 1732 to John Clarkson, carpenter; Lawrence Neale, carpenter, party	5 5 0	John Emmett	1737–51 (intermittently)	22
	Sub-let 1730 to John How, carver; Lawrence Neale, carpenter, party	4 15 0	? Mrs. Atheton or Lady Hubbard	1735 1736–44	23
	Sub-let 1730 to Lawrence Neale, carpenter; Richard Davies, joiner, a witness	3 10 0	Lawrence Neale	1730–45	24
masons		5 0 0	Richard Burket, victualler (Wheatsheaf)	1730–7	(Former 28 Park Lane)
do.		4 10 0	Rev. Thomas Clark(e)	1730–45	25
mason		7 0 0	William Hale, mason, son-in-law of Lissiman	1730–6	26
do.		4 0 0	Captain Lawrence	1733–40	27
do.		5 0 0	Mrs. Burroughs	1734–8	28
do.		5 5 0	Charles Carter, esq.	1732–8	29
do.		9 7 0	Hon. Frances Bruce	1739–51	30
			Mary Hutchenson	1736–42	31
			George Wright, esq.	1736–42	32
	(Large mansion set back from road; later called Grosvenor House)	76 13 0	1st Viscount Chetwynd, M.P.	1732–6(d)	33
	Sub-let 1731 to Benjamin Timbrell, carpenter	8 0 0	Colonel Richard Pyott and/or Mrs. Pitts	1732–7	34
bricklayer	John Eds, carpenter, party to lease	9 10 0	2nd Viscount Chetwynd, M.P.	1738–41	35
carpenter		4 10 0	? John Powis	1737–9	36
	Sub-let 1731 to James Jenner, bricklayer; assigned to William Allison, carpenter	do.	John or Thomas Baswick	1731–4	56 Park St.
	Sub-let 1731 to Colonel Francis Williamson; James Jenner, bricklayer, party	5 10 0	Colonel Francis Williamson	1731–8	37
esquire	Sub-let 1731 to James Jenner, bricklayer	13 10 0	Richard Edgcumbe, esq., M.P. (later 1st Baron Edgcumbe)	1733–58(d)	38
	Sub-let 1731 to John Neale, carpenter; Charles Griffith, carpenter, party	13 12 0	3rd Earl of Jersey	1733–43	39
	Sub-let 1731 to Israel Russell, painter[-stainer]; John Eds, carpenter, party	13 4 0	Lord Lynne (later 3rd Viscount Townshend)	1735–41	40
	Sub-let 1731 to John Eds, carpenter	14 8 0	Hon. Henry Vane, M.P. (later 1st Earl of Darlington)	1734–9	41
joiner		13 4 0	7th Viscount Falkland	1734–6	42
do.		do.	Marquess of Carnarvon, M.P. (later 2nd Duke of Chandos)	1735–9	43
esquire	Charles Griffith, carpenter, party to lease	8 15 0	— Jolliffe, esq.	1731–2	44

House No.	Frontage in Feet	Date of Building Agreement	No. on Plan A	Undertaker	Date of Building Lease	Lessee
UPPER GROSVENOR STREET, SOUTH SIDE (continued)						
45	25	18 Nov. 1725	58	Richard Andrews, gentleman	2 Nov. 1727	William Draycott
46	40				12 Sept. 1728	Edward Cock
47	20				do.	Robert Phillips
48	20				28 Aug. 1727	William Hanmer

Designation	Associated Builders and Architects	Rent £ s. d.	First Occupant	Period	House No.
esquire	Charles Griffith, carpenter, party to lease	8 15 0	Sir George Oxenden, Bt., M.P., Lord of the Treasury	1732–7	45
carpenter		15 0 0	Lady Isabella Scott, d. of Anne, Duchess of Buccleuch	1733–48(d)	46
bricklayer		3 0 0	Francis Blake Delaval, esq., of Seaton Delaval	1732–8	47
esquire	Robert Phillips, bricklayer, party to lease and builder of house	10 0 0	Colonel William Hanmer	1729–41(d)	48

APPENDIX II

Schedule of Fixtures at No. 45 Grosvenor Square, 1733

This schedule is contained in a lease in the Grosvenor Office dated 3 December 1733 from Thomas Richmond, carpenter, to Philip Dormer, Earl of Chesterfield.

IN the Six Garretts—Eight Sash Windows compleatly glazed with inside Shutters thereto Three Portland Chimney pieces and Slabs and Hearths, Five Closetts with Doors to the same also Six Doors to the Garretts, A Skylight at the head of the great Stairs.

IN the two front Rooms on the two pair of Stairs Floor—Five Sash Windows compleatly glazed with inside Shutters and Iron fastnings thereto, The Rooms compleatly wainscotted, Two Marble Chimney pieces and Slabs with firestone Hearths and Covings, Three Closetts with Shelves and Doors to the same and two Doors to the Rooms.

IN the back Room next the Garden—Two Sash Windows compleatly glazed with inside Shutters and Iron fastnings thereto, The Room compleatly wainscotted, a Marble Chimney piece and Slab with firestone Hearth and Covings, Two Doors to the Room and two Closetts with Shelves and Doors to the same.

IN the two Rooms and dressing Room adjoining Six Sash Windows compleatly glazed with inside Shutters and Iron fastnings thereto, Two Marble Chimney pieces and Slabs compleat A Portland one compleat, seven Cupboards with Doors and Shelves, The Rooms compleatly wainscotted, four Doors to the Rooms, Brass Knobs to all the Sashes and Shutters in this Floor.

IN the Room one pair of Stairs forward—Three Sash windows compleatly glazed with inside Shutters and Iron fastnings thereto, The Room compleatly wainscotted with Modillion Cornish & Dentill Bedmold around the same, Two Ionic Pillasters next the Chimney with the Entablature over them, A Marble Chimney piece with Slab Slips and Nosings with a Cornish over the Mantle, Firestone Hearth and Covings, Two Doors with Pediments over them.

IN the Room adjoining next the Garden—Two Sash windows compleatly glazed with inside Shutters and Iron fastnings thereto, The Room compleatly wainscotted, A Marble Chimney piece with Slab Slips and Nosings Firestone Hearth & Covings, A Door to the Room

IN the Middle Room—One Sash Window compleatly glazed with inside Shutters and Iron fastnings thereto The Room compleatly wainscotted, A Marble Chimney piece Slab Slips, firestone Hearth and Covings, a Door to the Room.

IN the Wing—Five Sash Windows compleatly glazed with inside Shutters and Iron fastnings thereto, the Rooms compleatly wainscotted with A Modillion Cornish around the same, Two Ionic Pillasters with the Entablature over them A Marble Chimney piece and Slab Slips and Nosings with a Cornish over the Mantle, Firestone Hearth and Covings Four Doors to the Rooms, A Water Closett adjoining to the Garden with a Marble Bason Bosses and Seat Compleat a Leaden Cistern on the Top of the same, Brass Knobs to all the Sashes and Shutters in this Floor.

IN the fore Parlour—Three Sash Windows compleatly glazed with inside Shutters and Iron fastnings thereto, The Room compleatly wainscotted, Two Doric Pillasters with the Entablature over them, A Marble Chimney piece and Slab Slips and Nosings, firestone Hearth and Covings, The Jaumbs continued above the Mantle with a Cornice over them.

IN the back Parlour—Two Sash Windows compleatly glazed with inside Shutters and Iron fastnings thereto the Room compleatly wainscotted, A marble Chimney piece with Slab Slips and Nosings, Firestone Hearth and Covings, two Doors to the Room.

IN the Middle Room—One Sash Window compleatly glazed with inside Shutters and Iron fastnings thereto the Room compleatly wainscotted A Marble Chimney piece with Slab and Slips, Firestone Hearth and Covings A Book press with Shelves and folding Doors to the same, A Door to the Room.

IN the Wing or great Room next the Garden—Five Sash Windows compleatly glazed with inside Shutters and Iron fastnings thereto, The Room compleatly wainscotted, Two Doric Pillasters with the Entablature over them A Marble Chimney piece with a Cornice over the Mantle Slab Slips and Nosings, Firestone Hearth and Covings one Door to the Room, and a Pair of Pedestall folding Doors.

IN the Hall and Staircase—Three Sash Windows compleatly glazed with inside Shutters and Iron fastnings thereto The Hall wainscotted compleat, Two Ionic Pillasters with the Entablature carved around the Hall (The Staircase Painted) A Wainscot Staircase with Twist Rails & Ballisters carved Bracketts, also the Caps of Columns and Pillasters a Portland Chimney piece Brass Knobs to all the Shutters and Sashes in this Floor.

IN the Housekeeper's Room below Stairs next the front Arey—Three Sash windows compleatly glazed with outside Shutters and plate Bolts, The Room compleatly wainscotted, a Closet with Door to the same, a Portland Chimney piece with Slab and Hearth, Three firestone Stoves with Grates and Boxes fixt to them, a Leaden Cistern with Pipes and Brass Cock to the same, a Door to the Room.

IN the Pantry next the fore Arey—One Sash Window compleat with outside Shutters and Plate Bolts thereto The Rooms wainscotted, A Portland Chimney piece and Slab, Two Closetts with Shelves, two Doors to the same, a Door to the Room, a Leaden Cistern with Pipes and a brass Cock to the same.

IN the Steward's Room—Two Sash windows compleatly glazed with inside Shutters thereto, The Room wainscotted about six foot high, a Portland Chimney piece and Slab, with firestone hearth, a Door to the Room.

Two Wine Vaults next the Passage with Binns, a Pantry with Shelves

IN the Servants Hall—Four Windows with inside Shutters Kirb and Iron Bars over Ditto in the Garden, The Hall wainscotted about six foot high, a Portland Chimney piece, Two Appartments divided off with Partions Story high, Leaden Pipes laid from the force Pump to the Marble Bason in the Middle Room Ground Floor, with a Brass Cock to one of them.

IN the Front Arey—Four Vaults with Doors.

IN the back Arey—A Vault with a Door, a Flatt covered with Lead leading to the Kitchen Passage in which is a Wine Vault with Binns, and a Door to the same.

IN the Kitchen Arey—a Cool Larder with a Bressimer Front wired, a Door to the same and two Dressers, a Deal Dresser in the Washhouse, a Pump compleat, and Elm Dresser and Sash Window in the Scullery, The flat over the Washhouse and Arey leaded, a Door to the same and Scullery, a Large Leaden Cistern with water pipes, Brass Cocks and Bosses with a Ball Cock to the same, a Pipe laid from the Cistern to the force pump in the Garden to convey the water into the Cistern at the Top of the water Closet

IN the Garden—A Boghouse wainscotted with a Door to the same, a leaden Bason with Bosses and wast pipes and Seat compleat.

IN the Kitchen—Three Sash Windows compleat, Two large Dressers and Shelves with Drawers under Ditto A Cool Larder adjoining with Dressers and Shelves, a Sash Window to the same, An Oven with an Iron Door, a Portland Chimney piece, four Stoves with Grates and Boxes set in Brick work with an Iron Rim around the same a Door to the Coal Vault and two Kitchen Doors, a Leaden Sink with a Pipe and brass Cock.

The Water laid from the Tree to serve the Cisterns in the front Arey, housekeeper's Room and Butler's Pantry, also the back Arey, the Kitchen Arey, washhouse and Sink in Kitchen.

IN the Rooms over the Scullery—A Sash Window with inside Shutters thereto, a Portland Chimney piece & Slab and Hearth, a Door to the Room.

IN the Room over the last mentioned Room—Two Sash Windows with inside Shutters thereto a Portland Chimney piece Slab and firestone hearth, a Door to the Room.

IN the Landry—Three Sash windows with inside Shutters and Iron fastnings thereto, a Portland Chimney piece and Slab, a Door to the Room

IN the Stables—Standings for twelve horses with turn'd Columns, Bailes, Rings, Chains, Staples, Racks and Mangers compleat, Two Corn Binns, outside Shutters to the Window, three Coach houses divided, a Hay loft over the Stables with a Window and Shutters to the same, three Windows with Shutters to the same belonging to Coachmen and Grooms Rooms over the Coachhouses, a Crane to the Hay loft Door, a Lead water trough to convey the wast water into the Stable Yard, The water laid into the Cistern in the Stables.

ABOUT the Outside of the House—Stone Steps and Iron Rails in the Front Arey, Iron Pallasades to Ditto and back Arey, Rain Lead Waterpipe, with proper Fastnings to all the outside Doors and Shutters.

APPENDIX III

Problems of short-term leasing: an episode

Short-term speculation and improvement played a vital part in the leasehold system, especially in the complex period at the end of one lease and the beginning of another one. But though they were essential for the needs of fashionable society in the eighteenth and nineteenth centuries, short-term occupiers could also by their nature, habits and interests dissuade other potential lessees from taking on the longer tenancies that were the life-blood of the system. Nowhere is this better highlighted than by the history of No. 51 Brook Street in 1802–6, as recorded chiefly in letters (now in the North Yorkshire County Record Office) from the architect P. F. Robinson to Mrs. Osbaldeston of Hutton Buscel, Yorkshire, a prospective lessee.

The head lease of No. 51 Brook Street, due to run out at Lady Day (25 March) 1804, was held by General Thomas Davies, who for some years had been sub-letting to tenants, the last of them a Frenchman, Mr. Grillion, who may have been running the house as a private hotel. Since the renewal terms offered by the Estate were high, both Davies and Grillion successively declined them. But Robinson, hearing of the house through an agent and having after inspecting it received 'very satisfactory answers' about the 'disagreeables to which Houses are liable', clinched the terms verbally on behalf of his client Mrs. Osbaldeston early in January 1803. Mrs. Osbaldeston was to have a sixty-two-year term from Lady Day 1804. Though the fine was higher than he had at first been led to believe, Robinson still thought the house a bargain, telling Mrs. Osbaldeston 'if I had money to lay out I do not know a speculation I would more willingly engage in than that of purchasing Houses in the neighbourhood of Grosvenor Square, improving and selling them. I think I could make a fortune. Houses in this quarter are so much sought after that the value encreases rather than otherwise.'

Nevertheless the fine was never paid and the deal was to fall through for two connected reasons. Firstly, Mrs. Osbaldeston was primarily interested in a town house which she could occupy for short periods, at most for the duration of the London Season, and not as the long-term investment which her architect was urging upon her. So much is clear from Robinson's letters of subsequent years about other London houses he looked into for her. Secondly, the subtenants were left in a confusing situation during the last year of General Davies's term.

Grillion's sub-lease expired in March 1803 and he was anxious to be relieved of his tenancy before that date if possible. But though Mrs. Osbaldeston herself took on a sub-lease of the following six months from April to September under General Davies, so as to be able to have a house for the Season of 1803 while postponing her final decision about a new lease, she declined to take over Grillion's last two months as well. This put Grillion 'in so great a rage', Robinson reported, 'that he swears neither I nor any person on your account shall enter the House while he has any power to prevent it. I calculate however upon his getting cool and seeing his interest a little better.' This duly occurred; Grillion performed some minor repairs and made over these two months to Mr. Polton, an upholsterer, who in his turn prepared to refurbish the house and looked for a short-term tenant. Polton naturally wanted the house for a longer period than two months; thinking of letting it for the Season, he applied to Robinson for the ensuing six months (April–September 1803). But Robinson advised against this unless Mrs. Osbaldeston were herself to live in the house as furnished by Polton during the period, 'as we otherwise shall get possession of the House at a Season when it will be impossible to put workmen in it [i.e. too late in the year] and you would have it on your hands during a winter in its present state.'

Mrs. Osbaldeston therefore kept these six months in reserve with a possible view to living in the house for the Season of 1803, while Polton found a two-month tenant in the shape of the Danish Ambassador. But in February 1803, Robinson was reporting gloomily that the house was 'dirty enough indeed, I believe it is in vain to look for cleanliness from a Frenchman and if Grillion or his agents are so unwise as to neglect their interest in not rendering it tolerable, we must search for another house pro tempora [*sic*]'. Whether Mrs. Osbaldeston actually did take the house for the Season is unclear, but the likelihood is that in the light of these reports she did not. Her enthusiasm for a long lease was also beginning to wane. In June 1803 Robinson sent sketches to her for proposed permanent alterations in stages and attempted to reconcile her to taking on the lease with the thought that the house could be easily sold at any time. 'The present time has the effect of encreasing the value of Houses' he argued; 'I have had some conversation with intelligent Builders, who agree in believing that Rents will universally be raised.' But by August Mrs. Osbaldeston had taken fright, and by Autumn 1803 she had definitely decided against taking the long lease. Though this led to difficulties with the Grosvenor Board and some talk in December 1803 of litigation, the subsequent immediate history of No. 51 Brook Street suggests that she was right and her architect wrong. After General Davies had surrendered the house empty in April 1804, it hung heavy on the Estate's hands for several years. Despite various proposals, one to convert it into a bookshop, no permanent tenant could be found until December 1806, when Sir Joseph Copley agreed to take a new long lease from Lady Day 1807. Even then the house remained private for only a few years, for in 1813 it was to become the first of a series of houses to be taken over as Mivart's Hotel, chief ancestor of the modern Claridge's.

References

ABBREVIATIONS

B.A.	Building Act case, Greater London Council.
B.L.	British Library, Reference Division.
Colvin	H. M. Colvin, *A Biographical Dictionary of English Architects, 1660–1840*, 1954.
D.N.B.	*Dictionary of National Biography*.
E.H.P.	Eaton Hall Papers, archives of the Grosvenor family at Eaton Hall, Cheshire.
GBA	Grosvenor Building Agreements in Grosvenor Office (numbered sequence, 1–92).
GBM	Grosvenor Board Minutes, 46 volumes, 1789–*c.* 1920, in Grosvenor Office.
G.E.C.	*The Complete Peerage*, ed. G.E.C., 1910–59.
GLB	Grosvenor Lease Books, 45 volumes, 1721–1834, in Grosvenor Office.
G.L.R.O.(L)	Greater London Record Office (London Records), County Hall.
G.L.R.O.(M)	Greater London Record Office (Middlesex Records), Dartmouth Street.
G.O.	Grosvenor Office, 53 Davies Street, W.1.
M.L.R.	Middlesex Land Register in Greater London Record Office.
P.O.D.	*Post Office Directories.*
P.P.	*Parliamentary Papers.*
P.P.R.	Principal Probate Registry, Somerset House.
P.R.O.	Public Record Office.
R.B.	Ratebooks of the parish of St. George, Hanover Square, in Westminster City Library, Buckingham Palace Road.
R.I.B.A.	Royal Institute of British Architects.
W.C.L.	Westminster City Library, Buckingham Palace Road.

CHAPTER I (pp. 1–5)

The Acquisition of the Estate

1. P.R.O., C66/880, m. 32.
2. William Loftie Rutton, 'The Manor of Eia, or Eye next Westminster', in *Archaeologia*, vol. LXII, 1910, pp. 31–58, from which most of the information about the early history of the manor is derived.
3. 28 Henry VIII, c. 49 in *Statutes of the Realm*, vol. III, 1817, pp. 709–12.
4. Rutton, *op. cit.*, p. 33.
5. E.g. G.O., early deeds and papers, no. 242.
6. Rutton, *op. cit.*, p. 34.
7. G.O., early deeds..., no. 11.
8. B. H. Johnson, *Berkeley Square to Bond Street*, 1952, pp. 10–21.
9. 27 Car. II, c. 2, private.
10. M.L.R. 1738/4/11.
11. *Calendar of Letters and Papers of Henry VIII*, vol. XVII, p. 392.
12. GBA 75.
13. G.O., early deeds, no. 15.
14. For Ossulston see Charles T. Gatty, *Mary Davies and the Manor of Ebury*, 1921, vol. I, pp. 51–60 and G.O., London Scrapbooks, vol. I, pp. 47–89.
15. G.O., early deeds, nos. 5–12, 15: B.L., Add. MS. 38104 (reproduced by London Topographical Society as *A Plan of the Manor of Ebury*, c. *1663–1670*, 1915).
16. G.O., early deeds, nos. 26–7: Menna Prestwich, *Cranfield, Politics and Profits under the Early Stuarts*, 1966, pp. 258–9.
17. Prestwich, *op. cit.*, pp. 591, 601: B.L., Add. MS. 38104 (see ref. 15).
18. P.R.O., C66/3032, no. 8, m. 6.
19. G.O., early deeds, nos. 33–4.
20. *Ibid.*, no. 38: Gatty, *op. cit.*, vol. I, pp. 76–155 *passim.*
21. Prestwich, *op. cit.*, pp. 478–9.
22. B.L., Add. MS. 38104 (see ref. 15): Gatty, *op. cit.*, vol. I, pp. 97–8.
23. G.O., early deeds, nos. 101–2.
24. *Ibid.*, no. 107.
25. Gatty, *op. cit.*, vol. I, p. 119.
26. 27 Car. II, c. 2, private: Gatty, *op. cit.*, vol. I, p. 169.
27. G.O., early deeds, nos. 111–12.
28. *Ibid.*, no. 135.
29. G.O., chest B, bundle 9, 22 and 23 April 1763.
30. *Ibid.*, unnumbered early deeds, agreement of 12 Dec. 1672.
31. *Ibid.*, misc. box 3, 'An Acount at the Marage of my Daughter Grosvenor', quoted in Gatty, *op. cit.*, vol. II, pp. 186–92.
32. Johnson, *op. cit.*, pp. 51–9.
33. Gatty, *op. cit.*, vol. I, p. 222.
34. G.O., early deeds, nos. 170–1.
35. *Ibid.*, MS. vol. called 'Title Deeds', deed of 31 Oct. 1677.
36. *Ibid.*, early deeds, no. 242.
37. *Ibid.*, nos. 166, 181.
38. G.O., unnumbered early deeds, bundle of deeds of 1681; early deeds, nos. 242, 328.
39. *Ibid.*, early deeds, no. 242: *Survey of London*, vol. XI, 1927, p. 5.
40. Gatty, *op. cit.*, vol. II, pp. 54–182.
41. E.H.P., personal papers, 4th Bt., petition to Chancery, *c.* 1720; 3rd Bt., copy of will.
42. G.O., chest B, bundle 6, 12 June 1708.
43. 9 Anne, c. 22, private.
44. G.O., misc. box 21, abstract of title, [*c.* 1730].
45. *Ibid.*, London Scrapbooks, vol. II, p. 35.

CHAPTER II (pp. 6–33)

The Development of the Estate 1720–1785

1. Daniel Defoe, *A Tour Thro' London about the year 1725*, ed. Sir Mayson M. Beeton and E. Beresford Chancellor, 1929, pp. 97–8.
2. *Ibid.*, p. 21.
3. *Mist's Weekly Journal*, 17 July 1725.
4. M. Dorothy George, *London Life in the Eighteenth Century*, 1925, pp. 23–5: George Rudé, *Hanoverian London 1714–1808*, 1971, p. 4.
5. Defoe, *op. cit.*, p. 98.
6. Corporation of London Record Office, 'The City's Estate in Conduit Mead', [*c.* 1742–3].
7. Romney Sedgwick, *The House of Commons 1715–1754*, 1970, vol. I, pp. 64–5, 113, 203–4, vol. II, pp. 87–8.
8. P.R.O., E112/1181/954.
9. E.H.P., box 42/2, 23 Nov. 1732 and 9 Jan. 1732/3.
10. R.B.: M.L.R. 1731/2/382–3.
11. GLB II/66, IV/114.
12. G.E.C.: *D.N.B.*
13. E.H.P., personal papers, 1st Earl, letters from W. Pitt, 1759–60.
14. Sir Lewis Namier and John Brooke, *The House of Commons 1754–1790*, 1964, p. 557.
15. E.H.P., box 42/4, 14 Nov. 1772, 20 Feb. 1781, 17 May [? 1784].
16. GBA 1.
17. *Ibid.*, 2–7, 9–20.
18. GLB I/1, II/55.
19. G.O., chest B, bundle 6, 2 June 1721.
20. GLB I/2.
21. E.H.P., box 77/2, 'A Particular of Ground-Rents, and other Leasehold Premises, Late the Estate of Mr. Richard Barlow, deceased.'
22. G.O., chest B, bundle 6, 10 July 1723: E.H.P., item 1193, lease and plan book, p. 5.
23. G.O., misc. box 3, draft petition with accompanying letter of 27 Nov. 1725.
24. 12 Geo. I, c. 23, private.
25. G.O., chest B, bundle 7, 9–10 April and 11 May 1730.
26. P.R.O., PROB 11/655/284.
27. G.O., chest B, bundle 9, 14 Nov. 1755.
28. E.H.P., personal papers, 4th Bt., undated petition to Ld. Chancellor and letter from J. Sharp of 17 April 1722.
29. GBA *passim*.
30. G.L.R.O.(L), W.C.S. 51, pp. 229, 275, 378.
31. G.O., cash book no. 1.
32. GBA 87.
33. E.g. *Ibid.*, 13.
34. W.C.L., deed 143/1 (copy: original in possession of Williams and Glyn's Bank Ltd.).
35. G.O., agreement of 11 Nov. 1725, J. Alston and Sir Rd. Grosvenor; rent book, 'Old Estate', 1725–9.
36. *Ibid.*, 'The State of the Accot. for making up Grosvenor Sq.'.
37. *Ibid.*, chest B, bundle 6.
38. *Ibid.*, misc. box 3, draft petition with accompanying letter of 27 Nov. 1725: E.H.P., personal papers, 4th Bt., letter from Rbt. Grosvenor of 27 May 1725.
39. G.O., chest B, bundle 7.
40. E.H.P., personal papers, 3rd Bt., 'An Account of Lady Grosvenor's Personal Estate made up to 12 Jan. 1729'.
41. *Ibid.*, box 77/2, rough note of receipts and expenditure up to 1737: G.O., chest B, bundle 7, 19 May 1730: M.L.R. 1731/3/65.
42. G.O., Sir Rbt. Grosvenor's Trust Estate boxes, bundles of deeds relating to purchase of ground rents in Grosvenor Square.
43. *Ibid.*, bundle of deeds concerning leaseholds purchased from E. Bennett.
44. E.H.P., box 77/2, 'An account of the late Sir Robert Grosvenor's several Securities and Moneys due to him in Middlesex'.
45. G.O., rent books, Mayfair estate, 1724–9, 1730–2.
46. *Ibid.*, 1733–47.
47. *Ibid.*, 1755–63.
48. Lambeth Palace Library, MS. 2714, f. 12.
49. G.O., misc. box 3, deposition of Rd. Andrews [*c.* 1714].
50. E.H.P., personal papers, 4th Bt., letters of 10 June, 6 Nov. 1706 and 15 May 1716.
51. G.O., cash book no. 2.
52. Inner Temple Admissions Register, vol. II, p. 251, f. 1378: P.R.O., C24/1588/54, deposition of Rbt. Andrews.
53. G.O., misc. box 6, solicitor's bills.
54. R.B.: M.L.R. 1730/4/301.
55. W.C.L., C767, p. 34; C768, pp. 1, 106.
56. P.R.O., E112/1181/954: Inner Temple Admissions Register, vol. II, p. 252, f. 1379.
57. E.g. GBA 37, 58: GLB IV/115, IX/247–51: M.L.R. 1725–63 *sub* Andrews, Rd. and Rbt.
58. GLB IV/115, XI/278: M.L.R. 1726–47 *sub* Andrews, Rbt. (sub-leases).
59. GLB IX/236: W.C.L., C766a (at rear): M.L.R. 1751/1/567–8.
60. E.g. M.L.R. 1729/6/95; 1736/5/337.
61. E.H.P., item 1194, account book 1756–63.
62. P.R.O., PROB 11/891/415; C12/1086/1: *The Gentleman's Magazine*, vol. XXXIII, Sept. 1763, p. 465.
63. P.R.O., C12/1086/1; C12/1092/3.
64. R. E. Megarry and H. W. R. Wade, *The Law of Real Property*, 3rd ed., 1966, pp. 237, 508–9.
65. *Parish Register of the Holy and Undivided Trinity in the City of Chester 1532–1837*, ed. L. M. Farrell, 1914, p. 175.
66. G.O., misc. box 5, solicitor's bills.
67. Inner Temple Admissions Register, vol. II, p. 316, f. 1476.
68. M.L.R. 1750/3/117.
69. GLB XVI/412.
70. *Harleian Society Publications, Registers XI, St. George's, Hanover Square, Marriages*, vol. I, *1725–1787*, 1886, p. 53.
71. R.B.
72. P.R.O., PROB 11/1203/146.
73. G.O., chest C, bundle 10, 'State of Lord Grosvenor's Affairs', 1779.
74. GLB XVII/434.
75. R.B.: *P.O.D.*
76. P.R.O., C54/4883, no. 8.
77. B. H. Johnson, *Berkeley Square to Bond Street*, 1952, pp. 131, 147.
78. W.C.L., ratebooks of St. Paul's, Covent Garden.
79. *Survey of London*, vol. XXXVI, 1970, pp. 39n., 107, 107n., 312–13.
80. Lambeth Palace Library, MS. 2690, p. 206; MS. 2714, f. 7.

81. B. H. Johnson, 'Note on the early development of the sites of the buildings in Hanover Square and St. George Street, Westminster', typescript in possession of G.L.C. *Survey of London* section: Lambeth Palace Library, MS. 2714, f. 3.
82. Johnson, 'Note...', *ut supra*, pp. 13-14, 17.
83. *Ibid.*, p. 14: Lambeth Palace Library, MS. 2691, pp. 95, 97, 100-1, 118.
84. P.R.O., PROB 11/635/26.
85. Corporation of London Record Office, 'The City's Estate in Conduit Mead', [*c.* 1742-3], p. 2.
86. E.H.P., personal papers, 4th Bt., copy of undated petition to Ld. Chancellor with Order dated 11 Feb. 1720/1 entered on it.
87. *Ibid.*: G.O., cash books nos. 1 and 2.
88. *The Daily Post*, 22 Jan. 1730.
89. GBA 46.
90. E.H.P., item 1193, lease and plan book, pp. 2, 6-7.
91. M.L.R. 1721/6/196-7; 1722/3/337; 1723/5/294: GLB II/53.
92. GBA I: GLB I/2.
93. G.O., misc. box 13, abstract of title to estate of Bird's trustees: E.H.P., box 77/2, 'A Particular of Ground-Rents...', *ut supra* (see ref. 21).
94. E.H.P., item 1193, lease and plan book, p. 32.
95. W.C.L., WBA 343/1.
96. *Ibid.*, C766, pp. 325-30.
97. P.R.O., C12/2201/2.
98. *Ibid.*, *loc. cit.*; PROB 11/635/26.
99. Norman G. Brett-James, *The Growth of Stuart London*, 1935, pp. 274-5, 281.
100. P.R.O., MPH 258; C11/2430/38: G.L.R.O.(M), L.V.(W) 68/33: G.O., plan of Oliver's Mount public house, *c.* 1816.
101. G.O., building agreements, bundle 5, 8 June 1722; chest B, bundle 6, 10 July, 26 Oct. 1723.
102. Johnson, 'Note...', *ut supra*, pp. 13, 15: M.L.R. 1719/5/267-8.
103. E.g. GBA 30: GLB I/9.
104. E.H.P., item 1193, lease and plan book.
105. G.O., John Mackay's map of the Grosvenor estate, 1723.
106. GBA 26: G.O., chest B, bundle 6, 10 July 1723.
107. GLB XVII/450-3, XVIII/454-60.
108. GBA 36: M.L.R. 1755/3/503; 1757/1/362.
109. John Gwynn, *London and Westminster Improved*, 1766, p. x, note.
110. GBA 26, 27, 37.
111. R. Horwood, *Plan of the Cities of London and Westminster* ..., 1792-9: G.O., estate surveyor's plans, vol. I, p. 79.
112. M.L.R. 1726/2/407; 1727/5/394; 1730/4/340; 1732/3/322-4: R.B.
113. GBM 1/156.
114. E.H.P., item 1193, lease and plan book, p. 20.
115. Jacob Larwood, *The Story of the London Parks*, 1881 ed., p. 59.
116. G.O., misc. box 6, papers relating to Grosvenor Gate, 1724-5.
117. The information in this section is largely based on GBA *passim*.
118. GLB II/66, IV/120: M.L.R. 1719/6/36; 1727/1/62.
119. G.O., Sir Rbt. Grosvenor's Trust Estate boxes, agreement of 5 June 1727 with T. Goff and endorsement.
120. E.g. GLB V/132-3.
121. *Ibid.*, XVII/444-53, XVIII/454-60.
122. E.g. GBA 10 and GLB X/275, XI/276-7: GBA 16 and GLB VII/191: GBA 38 and GLB III/90.
123. GLB II/67, III/70, IV/109.
124. GBA 51: GLB V/142.
125. G.O., early deeds and papers, no. 149.
126. GBA 1, 23.
127. *Ibid.*, 75.
128. B.L., Add. MS. 18,238, ff. 30-2: *Survey of London*, vol. XXXVI, 1970, p. 38.
129. GBA 29, 30.
130. *Ibid.*, 36, 38.
131. *Ibid.*, 85, 87.
132. *Ibid.*, 30.
133. *Ibid.*, 36.
134. *Ibid.*, 72, 74, 81.
135. *Ibid.*, 9.
136. *Ibid.*, 53.
137. *Ibid.*, 57.
138. *Ibid.*, 48, 52.
139. The information in this section is largely based on GLB I-XVIII/1-460.
140. GLB XIII/348.
141. *Ibid.*, IV/115.
142. *Ibid.*, II/37, III/70.
143. *Ibid.*, XI/295, 297, 300, XII/301.
144. GBA 2, 5-7, 12-13, 16-21.
145. *Ibid.*, 25, 36.
146. *Ibid.*, 38.
147. *Ibid.*, 10, 22, 24, 30, 42-3, 49, 56, 59, 62-4, 66.
148. *Ibid.*, 16-18, 23, 29.
149. W.C.L., C766, pp. 1-120 *passim*.
150. GBA 44.
151. *Ibid.*, 47.
152. *Ibid.*, 51-2, 54.
153. GLB II/66, IV/114: G.O., Sir Rbt. Grosvenor's Trust Estate boxes, building agreements of 3 Aug. 1725 and 6 April 1726.
154. GBA 72-5.
155. *Ibid.*, 92.
156. Information kindly provided by Mr. G. C. Berry, archivist to the Thames Water Authority.
157. GBA 27.
158. E.H.P., box 42/2, 31 June 1726.
159. *Ibid.*, box 77/2, letter of 19 Sept. 1734 from Rbt. Andrews.
160. G.O., chest B, bundle 6, 10 July 1723.
161. GBA 68-71.
162. Johnson, *Berkeley Square*, *ut supra*, pp. 103-7.
163. *Survey of London*, vol. XXXII, 1963, p. 452.
164. Corporation of London Record Office, 'The City's Estate in Conduit Mead', [*c.* 1742-3], inset report of sub-committee of 2 Nov. 1742, p. 16.
165. G.O., misc. box 13, abstract of title to estate of Bird's trustees; Bird v. Lefevre, sale particulars of 1792: Williams and Glyn's Bank Ltd., same sale particulars: E.H.P., box 77/2, 'A Particular of Ground-Rents...', *ut supra* (see ref. 21).
166. E.g. GLB III/90.
167. *Ibid.*, VI/156, VII/178.
168. *Ibid.*, IV/98.
169. *Ibid.*, XVII/450-3, XVIII/454-8.
170. *Ibid.*, IV/98: R.B.: *The St. James's Evening Post*, 9-11 Sept. 1729.

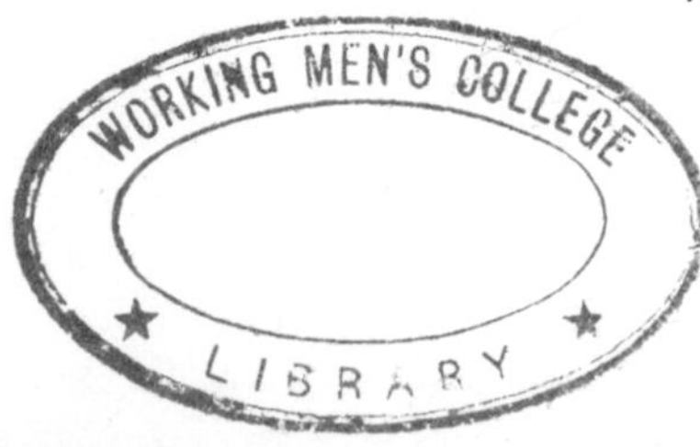

171. GBA 63-6.
172. John Summerson, *Architecture in Britain 1530 to 1830*, 1969 ed., p. 230.
173. *Catalogue of the Drawings Collection of the Royal Institute of British Architects. Colen Campbell*, 1973, [13], 1-2.
174. GLB II/66: G.O., Sir Rbt. Grosvenor's Trust Estate boxes, building agreements of 3 Aug. 1725.
175. GBA 54.
176. *R.I.B.A. Drawings Catalogue: Colen Campbell*, [13], 3-4.
177. GLB V/121: M.L.R. 1729/4/40; 1742/2/318: R.B.
178. Colvin.
179. GLB IV/94-5.
180. G.O., chest B, bundle 8, 26 March 1732.
181. GLB I/13: Colvin.
182. GLB II/50.
183. M.L.R. 1729/6/248: Hoare's Bank, Ledger K/98.
184. P.R.O., C105/32/1, agreement of 6 April 1728, E. Shepherd and F. Drewitt.
185. Robert Morris, *Lectures on Architecture*, [Part I], 1734, preface.
186. *Ibid.*, p. 85.
187. GBA 51-2.
188. GLB IV/102-3.
189. P.R.O., C105/32/1, manuscript plan of E. Shepherd's estate in N. Audley St.: M.L.R. 1735/1/285: R.B.
190. *Architectural Drawings in the Library of Elton Hall by Sir John Vanbrugh and Sir Edward Lovett Pearce*, ed. Howard Colvin and Maurice Craig, for Roxburghe Club, 1964, p. xliii and Catalogue, no. 6.
191. GBA 5: GLB I/28.
192. GLB VI/162.
193. M.L.R. 1730/4/178-9; 1731/5/13: R.B.
194. GBA 76: GLB XIII/342, XIV/360: M.L.R. 1738/5/29-30.
195. M.L.R. 1738/4/52: R.B.: P.R.O., PROB 11/812/334.
196. M.L.R. 1728/1/245; 1728/6/174: R.B.
197. M.L.R. 1735/5/10.
198. *Survey of London*, vol. XXXII, 1963, p. 477.
199. Guildhall Library, MS. 3045/2, entry of 1 Feb. 1704/5.
200. *Ibid.*, entry of 24 May 1715.
201. GLB II/67, III/70.
202. W.C.L., C766, pp. 5-6, 22.
203. GBA 67.
204. Rev. William Betham, *The Baronetage of England*..., vol. V, 1805, pp. 536-9.
205. W.C.L., C766, pp. 1, 16, 237, 325-30; C768, p. 172.
206. M.L.R. 1756/1/393-4, 505-8.
207. P.R.O., C12/356/33.
208. W.C.L., C766, pp. 1, 16, 120, 325-30.
209. GLB I/11: R.B.: Colvin.
210. P.R.O., PROB 6/151, Farrant, Nov. 1775; PROB 11/1016/87: M.L.R. 1776/3/353: Colvin.
211. GBA 92: GLB XVII/446: Northamptonshire Record Office, BH(K) 1185-6.
212. Information kindly provided by the Clerk of the Merchant Taylors' Company: P.R.O., PROB 11/689/103.
213. Colvin *sub* Gibbs.
214. G.O., rent book, 'Old Estate', 1730-2: W.C.L., ratebooks of St. Margaret's parish.
215. P.R.O., PROB 11/817/203; PROB 11/994/28: M.L.R. 1778/1/334: Badminton MSS., III·1·1, abstract of title to D. of Beaufort's stables.
216. Guildhall Library, MS. 5305/3, 12 Jan. 1691/2: P.R.O., PROB 6/109, f. 193v.: M.L.R. 1733/3/111.
217. GLB IX/245: *The Weekly Miscellany*, 15 July 1737.
218. M.L.R. 1762/3/10; 1772/3/237; 1773/2/453: R.B.: P.R.O., B4/21, S.22.
219. John Summerson, *Georgian London*, 1962 ed., p. 77.
220. P.R.O., C105/32/1, agreement of 11 March 1724/5, E. Shepherd and T. Fayram.
221. GLB VII/176.
222. M.L.R. 1728/4/47.
223. GLB VI/172.
224. G.O., building agreements, bundle 5, 20 Oct. 1755.
225. M.L.R. 1756/3/207, 230, 296, 482-3; 1756/4/133.
226. G.O., building agreements, bundle 5, 22 March 1741/2.
227. P.R.O., C105/21.
228. Corsham Court Archives, deed of 2 March 1727/8.
229. M.L.R. 1723/2/366; 1727/2/189.
230. *Ibid.*, 1733/2/162.
231. *Ibid.*, 1729/6/157.
232. *Ibid.*, 1727/4/212; 1728/2/67; 1728/4/132; 1728/5/449: G.O., chest B, bundle 7, 17 Oct. 1728.
233. M.L.R. 1721/4/94; 1725/3/233, 415; 1727/2/202; 1728/4/395; 1729/4/32; 1730/1/67; 1731/1/308; 1732/2/298; 1733/2/206; 1734/4/347; 1736/4/583; 1736/5/583; 1737/1/397; 1740/4/20.
234. *Ibid.*, 1724/4/227-8; 1728/2/336.
235. *Ibid.*, 1725/4/99; 1729/6/157; 1736/5/358; 1737/5/139; 1740/3/334.
236. *Ibid.*, 1723/3/129; 1723/6/414; 1725/1/442; 1725/2/74; 1726/4/111.
237. *Ibid.*, 1729/1/3; 1729/5/79.
238. *Ibid.*, 1723/2/366; 1727/2/189; 1728/1/257; 1728/2/67; 1737/5/324; 1738/5/30.
239. *Ibid.*, 1741/3/445.
240. *Ibid.*, 1736/4/47; 1738/4/258; 1738/5/206; 1751/2/676: Hoare's Bank, M/L 1743-73/13.
241. *The Gentleman's Magazine*, vol. X, Sept. 1740, p. 469.
242. M.L.R. 1731/3/278-81; 1732/5/414; 1734/2/24.
243. GLB VII/199 (variations vol.): R.B.
244. P.R.O., PROB 11/704/240.
245. M.L.R. 1728/5/299; 1728/6/398; 1729/3/174; 1729/4/325; 1730/6/4.
246. *Ibid.*, 1725/4/511; 1726/6/412; 1728/2/338; 1730/1/381.
247. *Ibid.*, 1728/1/420; 1728/2/336; 1737/1/279.
248. P.R.O., PROB 11/635/26; PROB 11/700/3.
249. M.L.R. 1725/2/181; 1726/3/70, 82; 1727/4/339; 1729/3/173.
250. P.R.O., B4/10, p. 280, no. 1791; C12/2200/59.
251. M.L.R. 1728/6/152.
252. *Ibid.*, 1728/1/181.
253. P.R.O., B1/17, p. 299.
254. M.L.R. 1728/6/159.
255. *Ibid.*, 1724/1/263-4, 266-9; 1725/1/48.
256. *Ibid.*, 1725/4/320.
257. *Ibid.*, 1726/6/168.
258. *Ibid.*, 1728/1/246.
259. P.R.O., C105/21, copy of deed of 12 Dec. 1728, J. Montigny to H. Huddle.
260. *Ibid.*, undated paper listing value of J. Jenner's property, and deed of 12 June 1729, J. Montigny to F. Commins.
261. M.L.R. 1739/2/252.
262. GLB XVII/444.
263. Northamptonshire Record Office, BH(K)1185.
264. GLB V/133.
265. *The Builder*, 23 Nov. 1867, p. 861.

266. GLB II/44.
267. Wiltshire Record Office, Radnor MSS., 490/630.
268. Suffolk Record Office, Bury St. Edmunds, Bunbury Papers, E 18/660.2.
269. GLB III/76: Corsham Court Archives, deed of 2 March 1727/8.
270. Corsham Court Archives, memo. of 2 March 1727/8.
271. *Ibid.*, bills, 1728.
272. M.L.R. 1726/3/301.
273. P.R.O., C11/1690/29.
274. M.L.R. 1727/1/410.
275. *The London Daily Post, and General Advertiser*, 19 June 1738; 7, 8, 9, 11 June 1739: *The Daily Post*, 16 Feb. 1739: *The Daily Gazetteer*, 11 June 1739: *The Gentleman's Magazine*, vol. IX, 1739, pp. 325, 437: Northamptonshire Record Office, Fitzwilliam (Milton) MSS., tin box 10, Mx, parcel 3.
276. Kent Archives Office, U455/T136: *The St. James's Evening Post*, 30 April–2 May 1730.
277. M.L.R. 1731/5/187.
278. Kent Archives Office, U791/T236: G.L.R.O.(L), O/179/4: M.L.R. 1729/4/40; 1730/4/37: *The London Daily Post*, 29 April 1738.
279. M.L.R. 1730/2/15.
280. Essex Record Office, D/DCc T55.
281. *The London Daily Post*, 23 Jan. 1737/8: Hoare's Bank, Ledger K/98.
282. M.L.R. 1726/1/134: Sedgwick, *op. cit.* (ref. 7 above), vol. II, p. 6.
283. Warwickshire Record Office, CR 114/Rag. iii/4: R.B.: Colvin.
284. Lambeth Palace Library, MS.2691, pp. 245, 254.
285. M.L.R. 1728/2/131.
286. W.C.L., deed 21/7.
287. M.L.R. 1725/3/443; 1725/5/400.
288. *Ibid.*, 1737/3/503.
289. *Ibid.*, 1726/5/198–9; 1730/1/91.
290. *Ibid.*, 1740/4/55.
291. G.O., chest B, bundle 8, 3 Dec. 1733.
292. M.L.R. 1731/5/187: lease of 15 Aug. 1733, E. Shepherd to R. Barlow, formerly in possession of Williams and Glyn's Bank Ltd.
293. P.R.O., C11/2430/38.
294. *Ibid.*, C11/2501/16.
295. *Ibid.*, C13/2851, Bevan v. Pearce.
296. *Ibid.*, C12/356/33.
297. *The Weekly Miscellany*, 15 July 1737.
298. *The Daily Post*, 10 Feb. 1739.
299. P.R.O., B4/3–21 *passim.*
300. G.O., misc. box 6, letter of 1 March 1744, E. Biscoe to Rbt. Andrews.
301. P.R.O., C54/5236, no. 7.
302. Lambeth Palace Library, MS. 2691, p. 254; MS. 2714, f. 59.
303. GLB VI/161.
304. W.C.L., C766, pp. 207, 210, 212–13, 229, 245; C766a, copies of deeds at back.
305. G.O., Park Street Chapel box, agreements of 13 July 1762.
306. GLB XXI/551–69: GBM 1/42–3, 211, 230, 262, 266, 290, 297: G.O., box Q, bundle 35; box S, bundle 157.
307. GLB IV/99.
308. G.O., box S, bundle 157, undated petition.
309. G.L.R.O.(M), TC/St.G/1–2.
310. M.L.R. 1721/6/196–7.
311. GLB VIII/219.
312. *The London Daily Post*, 13 June 1739.
313. Information kindly provided by Mr. G. C. Berry: Jacob Larwood, *The Story of the London Parks*, 1881 ed., p. 95.
314. G.L.R.O.(L), W.C.S. 53, p. 322.
315. A. Morley Davies, 'London's First Conduit System: A Topographical Study', in *Transactions of the London and Middlesex Archaeological Society*, n.s., vol. II, 1913, pp. 9–59: G.O., early deeds and papers, no. 44; misc. box 17, papers re conduit house, 1865–6: GBA 91–3: GLB IV/120; XVI/428–53; XVIII/454–60: GBM 14/8, 389–90, 400; 15/78–9, 182, 264: W.C.L., watercolour, C138 Oxford St. (6).
316. G.L.R.O.(L), W.C.S. 53, p. 308.
317. W.C.L., C 769, p. 82.
318. M.L.R. 1737/4/249; 1756/1/394.
319. John Summerson, *Architecture in Britain 1530 to 1830*, 1969 ed., pp. 229–30.
320. John Strype, *A Survey of the Cities of London and Westminster*, 1754–5 ed., vol. II, p. 688.
321. Lease of 15 Aug. 1733, E. Shepherd to R. Barlow, formerly in possession of Williams and Glyn's Bank Ltd.
322. P.R.O., C105/21; C11/2430/38.
323. GLB VII/183.
324. M.L.R. 1730/6/156.
325. GBM 9/420: G.O., lease particulars book A, No. 8 Green Street.
326. G.O., box P, bundle 133, 28 Dec. 1816.
327. GLB XIV/360.
328. *Ibid.*, XVI/413–14.
329. G.O., expired leases, 29 Oct. 1700 and 4 Dec. 1716.
330. *Ibid.*, box B, bundle 8, 28 Sept. 1743.
331. *Ibid.*, rent book, Mayfair estate, 1764–88.
332. *Ibid.*, rent books of Sir Rbt. Grosvenor's Trust Estate.
333. E.H.P., box 42/4, 20 Feb. 1781, 17 May [? 1784].
334. G.O., chest C, bundle 11, 5 April 1785.

CHAPTER III (pp. 34–66)

The Administration of the Estate 1785–1899

1. Gervas Huxley, *Victorian Duke. The Life of Hugh Lupus Grosvenor, First Duke of Westminster*, 1967, p. 101.
2. G.E.C.
3. Romney Sedgwick, *The House of Commons 1715–1754*, 1970, vol. I, p. 203; vol. II, pp. 87–8: Sir Lewis Namier and John Brooke, *The House of Commons 1754–1790*, 1964, vol. II, pp. 557–9: J. Vincent and M. Stenton, *McCalmont's Parliamentary Poll Book. British Election Results 1832–1918*, 1971, *passim*: G.E.C.
4. Richard Rush, *The Court of London from 1819 to 1825*, 3rd ed., 1873, pp. 8–10: see also Prince Pückler-Muskau, *Tour in England, Ireland and France in the Years 1826, 1827, 1828 and 1829*, 1940, pp. 40–1.
5. John Langton Sanford and Meredith Townsend, *The Great Governing Families of England*, 1865, vol. I, p. 112.

6. Hermione Hobhouse, *Thomas Cubitt, Master Builder*, 1971, p. 561.
7. G.O., box Q, bundle 143.
8. R.B.: *Boyle's Court Guide*.
9. P.P.R., will of John Boodle, 1859.
10. *Harleian Society Publications, Registers XXIV, St. George's, Hanover Square, Marriages*, vol. IV, *1824–1837*, 1897, p. 257: *Boyle's Court Guide*.
11. *P.O.D.*
12. P.P.R., will of H. M. Boodle, 1878.
13. *Ibid.*, will of Edward Partington, 1883.
14. *Ibid.*, will of W. C. Boodle, 1887.
15. *Ibid.*, will of H. T. Boodle, 1901.
16. *Ibid.*, index to wills: *P.O.D.*: *Boyle's Court Guide*.
17. G.O., memo. of 5 Jan. 1807.
18. *Ibid.*, Hailstone corresp., Grosvenor to H., 6 March 1809; Moore letter books, vol. 7, 2 March 1809.
19. *Ibid.*, Hailstone corresp., H. to Grosvenor, 27 Nov. 1808.
20. *P.P.*, 1887, XIII, *Report from the Select Committee on Town Holdings*, p. 319.
21. G.L.R.O.(M), TC/St.G/2.
22. G.O., box A, *passim*.
23. *Ibid.*, Hailstone corresp., Grosvenor to H., 27 Dec. 1795; Moore letter books, vol. 7, Aug. 1806.
24. *Ibid.*, Moore letter books, vol. 3, 5 April 1799.
25. *Ibid.*, Moore's accounts, 1809 17.
26. *Ibid.*, Moore letter books, *passim*, and especially vol. 8, Dec. 1811.
27. *Ibid.*, Hailstone corresp., Grosvenor to H., 2 Aug. 1821.
28. *Ibid.*, misc. box 21, abstract of title 1878, p. 39.
29. *Ibid.*, misc. box 15, 14 Aug. 1828.
30. E.H.P., box 76.
31. G.O., Hailstone corresp., H. to Grosvenor, 28 Jan. 1808.
32. Royal Bank of Scotland, Drummonds Branch, ledgers, Grosvenor accounts, 1815–45 *passim*.
33. G.O., misc. box 15, Grosvenor to Empy, 1822–8.
34. R.B.
35. P.R.O., PROB 11/2042/652.
36. *P.O.D.*: *Robson's Directory*, 1843.
37. P.P.R., index to wills, 1864.
38. G.O., misc. box 17, memo. re Mr. Burge, 16 Sept. 1864.
39. Royal Bank of Scotland, Drummonds Branch, ledgers, Grosvenor accounts, 1875.
40. *Ibid.*, Grosvenor accounts, 1855, 1865.
41. *Ibid.*, Grosvenor accounts, 1885, 1895.
42. P.P.R., index to wills, 1902.
43. Royal Bank of Scotland, Drummonds Branch, ledgers, Grosvenor accounts, 1875, 1895.
44. P.P.R., index to wills, 1922: *P.O.D.*
45. E.H.P., box 42/4, 17 May [? 1784]; 42/6, 2 Feb. 1814.
46. Information kindly supplied by Mr. H. M. Colvin.
47. W.C.L., C774, pp. 117–18.
48. G.O., misc. box 13, Porden valuations: E.H.P., box 42/6, 2 Feb. 1814.
49. G.O., box Q, bundle 35.
50. E.H.P., box 42/6, 24 Sept. 1809, 10 Nov. 1810; box 76, receipts *passim*.
51. G.O., account books of first Marquess, vol. 10, 1839–44 *passim*: Royal Bank of Scotland, Drummonds Branch, ledgers, Grosvenor accounts, 1875, 1885.
52. G.O., Cundy papers, 1864–6: GBM 15/3–4.
53. P.P.R., wills of H. M. Boodle, 1878, F. Boodle, 1891, and T. Cundy, 1895.
54. *Survey of London*, vol. XXXVI, 1970, pp. 41–2, 47, 49.
55. G.O., misc. box 12, Taylor and Shakespear's receipt, 1782.
56. GLB XXI/545–8.
57. E.H.P., box 42/4, 14 Nov. 1772.
58. G.O., chest C, bundle 10, 'State of Lord Grosvenor's Affairs', 1779, and mortgage, 1 April 1779.
59. *Ibid.*, Hailstone corresp., Grosvenor to H., 2 Sept. 1796.
60. E.H.P., box 42/4, 20 Feb. 1781.
61. *Ibid.*, box 42/4, 17 May [? 1784].
62. G.O., chest C, bundle 11, 5 April 1785.
63. *Survey of London*, vol. XXIX, 1960, p. 11.
64. *Ibid.*, vol. XXXVI, 1970, p. 36.
65. *Ibid.*, vol. XXXI, 1963, p. 13.
66. GLB XXI/549.
67. GLB *passim*.
68. G.O., chest D, 6 Feb. 1808.
69. *Ibid.*, box S, bundle 156, 15 Feb. 1817.
70. E.H.P., box 42/6, 10 Nov. 1810.
71. G.O., box R, bundle 147, 1 Feb. 1812.
72. GBM 1/45.
73. *Ibid.*, 1/156.
74. *Ibid.*, 1/141, 145; 2/218.
75. G.O., box Q, bundle 142, Jan. 1796.
76. GBM 2/95; 7/325.
77. Francis Baily, *Tables for the purchasing and renewing of Leases...*, 3rd ed., 1812, preface (B.L. pressmark 8506 f 13): Colvin *sub* William Inwood.
78. Baily, *op. cit.*, p. 4.
79. *Ibid.*, pp. 90–3.
80. *Ibid.*, p. 49.
81. GBM 1/116.
82. G.O., box Q, bundle 143, 14 Feb. 1814.
83. GBM 7/325.
84. *Ibid.*, 15/415, 492.
85. *Ibid.*, 17/470, 505; 18/90.
86. *Ibid.*, 18/275; 19/38.
87. *Ibid.*, 1/234.
88. *Ibid.*, 2/95.
89. *Ibid.*, 1/160: G.L.R.O.(M), TC/St.G/1.
90. GBM 2/204.
91. *Ibid.*, 1/161; 2/143; 3/172, 178.
92. *Ibid.*, 2/289.
93. G.O., chest C, bundle 12, 20 Aug., 3 Dec. 1791.
94. *Ibid.*, Moore letter books, vol. 3, 13 Feb. 1799.
95. *Ibid.*, vol. 2, 5, 12 Jan., 31 Aug., 5 Nov. 1798 and *passim*.
96. *Ibid.*, vol. 3, 1 May 1799.
97. *Ibid.*, vol. 2, 22 Nov. 1798.
98. *Ibid.*, vol. 7, Aug. 1806.
99. *Ibid.*, vol. 3, 3 Jan. 1800.
100. *Ibid.*, vol. 4, 18 July 1801.
101. *Ibid.*, box P, bundle 133, 11 Dec. 1804.
102. *Ibid.*, chest D, deed of 6 Feb. 1808 and endorsement of 12 April 1809.
103. *Ibid.*, Moore letter books, vol. 7, Aug. 1806: GLB *passim*.
104. GLB XXIV/678.
105. *Survey of London*, vol. XXXVI, 1970, p. 40.
106. G.O., chest D, bundle 14, 10 Oct. 1804: GLB *passim*.
107. GLB XXVIII/780.
108. *Ibid.*, XXI/575.
109. G.L.R.O.(M), TC/St.G/1.
110. GLB XXIV/678: GBM 1/188, 212.
111. GBM 2/204.
112. *Ibid.*, 2/309; 3/21: GLB XXV/701.

113. GBM 7/144.
114. *Ibid.*, 2/160–1; 3/160, 178: R.B.
115. GBM 4/83, 158: R.B.
116. GBM 3/288; 4/82; 5/273: G.O., box R, bundles 147–8, 27 Aug. 1812 and 11 May 1813.
117. P.R.O., HO 107/733/5, 6, 12.
118. GLB xxv/696–7.
119. GBM 4/85.
120. *Ibid.*, 6/215.
121. *Ibid.*, 1/13, 57; 2/76, 256; 3/34; 4/259.
122. GLB xxiv/683.
123. GBM 2/222; 5/275, 289, 308; 6/326: G.O., box P, bundle 133, 29 Aug. 1812.
124. GBM 3/22, 177.
125. *Ibid.*, 1/51.
126. *Ibid.*, 6/130.
127. *Ibid.*, 9/126.
128. *Ibid.*, 1/132.
129. G.L.R.O.(M), WR/LV, register 1793–1813.
130. GBM 2/309; 3/21, 65; GLB xxv/701.
131. GBM 5/25.
132. *Ibid.*, 6/87; 7/50, 319; 8/276; 9/35.
133. *Ibid.*, 8/464; 9/123.
134. *Ibid.*, 6/113, 139, 143–4.
135. *Ibid.*, 6/141–2, 163, 170.
136. *Ibid.*, 6/163–4; 8/263, 468.
137. *Ibid.*, 7/443; 8/210, 212, 249.
138. G.L.R.O.(M), WR/LV, St. Geo. Han. Sq. 1828.
139. GBM 4/315: G.O., box Q, bundle 143, 3 Sept. 1814.
140. GBM 5/322: G.O., misc. box 14, 8 April 1808.
141. GBM 4/148; 5/36, 303, 338.
142. *Ibid.*, 3/9.
143. *Ibid.*, 2/110; 5/101; 6/246; 7/25, 84, 453; 8/54.
144. *Ibid.*, 1/156.
145. *Ibid.*, 1/198, 212; 2/176; 4/232.
146. *Ibid.*, 3/74; 4/210.
147. *Ibid.*, 1/28, 235.
148. *Ibid.*, 2/37, 46, 163.
149. *Ibid.*, 3/204, 241; 7/178.
150. M.L.R. 1824/8/392.
151. GBM 1/288.
152. *Ibid.*, 1/187.
153. *Ibid.*, 5/281.
154. Sanford and Townsend, *op. cit.* (ref. 5 above), vol. 1, pp. 122–3: G.E.C.
155. G.O., chest D, bundle 14, 10 Oct. 1804; box S, bundle 153, 11 Oct. 1804.
156. Colvin.
157. G.O., chest D, bundle 14, 2 Aug. 1806.
158. Gervas Huxley, *Lady Elizabeth and the Grosvenors, Life in a Whig Family, 1822–1839*, 1965, p. 58: GBM 4/299–300.
159. G.O., Hailstone corresp., Grosvenor to H., 11 Oct. 1802, and *passim* 1808–10.
160. Huxley, *Lady Elizabeth*, *ut supra*, pp. 6, 8, 59: G.O., misc. box 15, Jones to Grosvenor, 17 Aug. 1825.
161. W.C.L. and G.O., Grosvenor rent books.
162. G.O., lease particulars book A.
163. *Ibid.*, chest D, deeds 1829–36.
164. *Ibid.*, Hailstone corresp., H. to Grosvenor, 23, 27 Feb. 1807, 3 Feb. 1808.
165. *Ibid.*, 17 Feb. 1808, 10 March 1813.
166. E.H.P., box 42/6, 12 Nov. 1803.
167. G.O., Hailstone corresp., H. to Grosvenor, 23 Feb. 1807.
168. *Ibid.*, *ut supra*, Grosvenor to H., 29 Aug. 1808, 15, 19 Nov. 1810.
169. GBM 8/491.
170. E.H.P., box 42/6 *passim*.
171. P.R.O., PROB 11/1665/35.
172. *Ibid.*, PROB 11/1708/72.
173. Huxley, *Lady Elizabeth*, *ut supra*, p. 17.
174. G.O., lease particulars book A: GBM 4/315: Hertfordshire Record Office, Grimston MSS., D/EV, F331.
175. G.O., box Q, bundle 143, 3 Sept. 1814.
176. *Ibid.*, misc. box 17, 'Remarks upon granting Leases...', 1845.
177. GBM 8/326.
178. *Ibid.*, 1/288.
179. G.O., box R, bundle 149, Sept. 1815.
180. GBM 9/295.
181. *Ibid.*, 8/3.
182. *Ibid.*, 12/33: 8 and 9 Vict., c. 33, private.
183. G.O., box Q, bundle 143, 14 Feb. 1814.
184. GBM 6/186.
185. *Ibid.*, 8/326.
186. *Ibid.*, 9/2.
187. *Ibid.*, 12/373, 375: G.O., misc. box 17, 'Remarks upon granting Leases...', 1845.
188. GBM 12/178; 13/541: G.O., misc. box 17, 'Remarks upon granting Leases...', 1845.
189. G.O., lease particulars book 1.
190. GBM 15/162.
191. *Ibid.*, 15/436; 18/88–9, 285, 352.
192. *Ibid.*, 2/122.
193. *Ibid.*, 5/245; 6/22, 124; 7/69, 247.
194. *Ibid.*, 7/479; 8/215.
195. *Ibid.*, 8/396.
196. *Ibid.*, 9/57, 215.
197. *Ibid.*, 9/75, 528: G.O., lease particulars book A.
198. GBM 12/73.
199. G.O., misc. box 17, 'Remarks upon granting Leases...', 1845.
200. GBM 12/117.
201. Huxley, *Lady Elizabeth*, *ut supra*, pp. 13, 14, 22, 52, 54, 56.
202. *The Times*, 2 Nov. 1869, p. 7.
203. Huxley, *Lady Elizabeth*, *ut supra*, p. 14: Huxley, *Victorian Duke* (see ref. 1 above), pp. 11, 13, 71–4.
204. Huxley, *Lady Elizabeth*, *ut supra*, p. 162.
205. Recited in 8 and 9 Vict., c. 33, private.
206. Huxley, *Victorian Duke*, *ut supra*, pp. 16, 73.
207. Huxley, *Lady Elizabeth*, *ut supra*, p. 167.
208. GBM 14/498.
209. Huxley, *Victorian Duke*, *ut supra*, pp. xi, xii, 67, 93, 95, 105, 114–18, 176–94: G.E.C.
210. Huxley, *Victorian Duke*, *ut supra*, pp. 76–80, 100, 150–1, 154, 160–5, 168–9.
211. *The Times*, 23 Dec. 1899, p. 6.
212. Huxley, *Victorian Duke*, *ut supra*, pp. 91–2.
213. *Ibid.*, pp. 34, 74, 92, 96, 130.
214. *Ibid.*, pp. 67, 120, 126: G.O., Trustees' accounts, 1893.
215. GBM 18/248.
216. G.O., misc. box 21, abstract of title, 1918: M.L.R. 1874/10/646.
217. G.O., misc. box 21, deed of resettlement, 1901.
218. *Ibid.*, lease particulars books 1 and 2.

219. *Ibid.*, Trustees' accounts; misc. box 21, deed of resettlement, 1901.
220. 8 and 9 Vict., c. 33, private.
221. GBM 15/438–9.
222. *The Building News*, 13 Oct. 1865, p. 712.
223. Papers of John Liddell, architect, in stock of B. Weinreb, Architectural Books Ltd., Lord Westminster to Lord Carnarvon, 22 May 1845.
224. GBM 12/178.
225. G.O., misc. box 17, bonds.
226. GBM 12/426–7.
227. *Ibid.*, 13/324.
228. *Ibid.*, 13/326, 348.
229. *Ibid.*, 12/353.
230. *Ibid.*, 13/312–13, 368: G.O., lease particulars books A and I.
231. *Survey of London*, vol. XXXVII, 1973, pp. 304–5.
232. GBM 14/305–6: G.O., lease particulars book I.
233. G.L.R.O.(L), M.B.W. Minutes, 10 May 1867, p. 565.
234. GBM 12/240, 480; 13/14–15, 62–3: G.O., misc. box 17, papers attached to elevation of No. 41 Upper Brook Street.
235. GBM 13/541; 14/9, 239, 261.
236. *Ibid.*, 15/282, 308, 352; 16/182.
237. *Ibid.*, 20/295.
238. *Ibid.*, 18/437.
239. *Ibid.*, 12/178.
240. W.C.L., WBA 429, see for instance bundle 98, lease of 65 Grosvenor Street, 20 Sept. 1854, and bundle 99, lease of 46 Grosvenor Street, 5 Aug. 1873.
241. GBM 13/76.
242. *Ibid.*, 13/291.
243. *Ibid.*, 13/516–20; 24/34–5: W.C.L., WBA 429, bundle 93, lease of 41 Grosvenor Square, 29 Sept. 1865.
244. GBM 15/178.
245. W.C.L., WBA 429, bundle 99, lease of 46 Grosvenor Street, 5 Aug. 1873.
246. *Ibid.*, bundle 93, lease of 13 Grosvenor Square, 1837.
247. *Ibid.*, bundle 93, lease of 15A Grosvenor Square, 7 Aug. 1848.
248. *Ibid.*, bundle 93, lease of 41 Grosvenor Square, 29 Sept. 1865; bundle 99, lease of 46 Grosvenor Street, 5 Aug. 1873.
249. *Ibid.*, bundle 189, lease of premises in Brook's Mews, 20 May 1887.
250. *Ibid.*, lease of No. 19 North Audley Street, 25 Feb. 1846.
251. *Ibid.*, bundle 189, lease of premises in Brook's Mews, 22 May 1862.
252. *Ibid.*, bundle 189, Brook's Mews leases, 1887, 1891, 1905.
253. *Ibid.*, bundle 189, Brook's Mews lease, 20 May 1887; bundle 93, lease of 45 Grosvenor Square, 1 July 1895.
254. GBM 12/373, 375.
255. *Ibid.*, 15/178.
256. *Ibid.*, 13/383–4, 389; 14/120, 122, 149.
257. *Ibid.*, 14/495.
258. *Ibid.*, 13/181.
259. *Ibid.*, 16/239–40, 253, 286.
260. *Ibid.*, 15/150.
261. *Ibid.*, 12/426; 15/402.
262. *Ibid.*, 15/200, 269, 441, 458–9, 513; 16/4: G.O., improvement account book, 1864–82.
263. GBM 14/195–7.
264. *Ibid.*, 14/290–1.
265. *Ibid.*, 17/220.
266. *Ibid.*, 18/423.
267. *Ibid.*, 27/498.
268. *Ibid.*, 13/446, 459–60; 19/280–1.
269. *Ibid.*, 27/487.
270. *The Builder*, 7 Dec. 1895, p. 426.
271. GBM 20/171–2; 21/383–4.
272. *Survey of London*, vol. XXXVIII, 1975, Plate 89b.
273. *The Builder*, 17 Feb. 1911, p. 222.
274. GBM 24/40.
275. *Who Was Who 1897–1915*.
276. GBM 35/470; 37/489–90: *The Builder*, 17 Feb. 1911, p. 222.
277. GBM 23/306; 24/20, 169.
278. G.O., Duke's instruction book, 1905–8, pp. 7–12.
279. GBM 18/248.
280. *P.P.*, 1884–5, XXX, *R.C. on the Housing of the Working Classes*, p. 52.
281. G.O., Trustees' accounts, 1874–1901.
282. GBM 24/322, 376; 25/312, 347, 455, 495–6.
283. *Ibid.*, 19/245; 20/379.
284. *Ibid.*, 21/518.
285. *Ibid.*, 20/371, 379; 21/19, 219; 25/2–3.
286. *Ibid.*, 22/467–8.
287. *P.P.*, 1887, XIII, *S.C. on Town Holdings*, p. 351.
288. GBM 22/402, 437–8, 539.
289. *Ibid.*, 23/385–6, 429; 24/40, 45: *P.P.*, 1887, XIII, *S.C. on Town Holdings*, p. 321.
290. GBM 25/82.
291. *P.P.*, 1887, XIII, *S.C. on Town Holdings*, pp. 325, 350.
292. *Ibid.*, p. 352.
293. GBM 24/127–8.
294. *Ibid.*, 22/397: *P.O.D.*
295. GBM 22/129.
296. *Ibid.*, 22/320.
297. *P.P.*, 1887, XIII, *S.C. on Town Holdings*, pp. 326, 354.
298. *Ibid.*, pp. 245–6, 326–8, 354, 361–2, 370–1.
299. *Ibid.*, p. 370: GBM 24/279–80.
300. GBM 26/407–8.
301. *Ibid.*, 26/451, 453.
302. *Ibid.*, 27/195–6.
303. *Ibid.*, 27/210.
304. *Ibid.*, 23/364.
305. *Ibid.*, 27/289.
306. *Ibid.*, 26/17.
307. *Ibid.*, 26/415–16.
308. *Ibid.*, 27/101–2.
309. *Ibid.*, 22/474, 486; 23/123.
310. *Ibid.*, 27/112.
311. *Ibid.*, 26/387–8.
312. *Ibid.*, 26/441.
313. *Ibid.*, 21/133–6; 22/320; 24/358.
314. *Ibid.*, 26/95, 376.
315. *Ibid.*, 24/480.
316. *Ibid.*, 27/112, 171.
317. *Ibid.*, 22/320.
318. *Ibid.*, 23/183–4; 24/463; 25/77; 27/209–10.
319. *Ibid.*, 24/171; 25/233.
320. *Ibid.*, 24/437, 477–8; 25/356; 26/263.
321. *Ibid.*, 25/509–10; 26/59–60.
322. *Ibid.*, 22/339–40.
323. Frank Banfield, *The Great Landlords of London*, [1888], p. 59.

324. *Annual Report of the Vestry of the Parish of Saint George Hanover Square*, 1883–4, p. 44; 1884–5, p. 34: GBM 21/463.
325. GBM 22/152–4.
326. *Annual Report*, *ut supra*, 1887, p. 38.
327. GBM 23/463–4; 25/199–200, 315–16.
328. *Ibid.*, 25/115–18, 225.
329. *Ibid.*, 25/127–8, 369–70.
330. *Ibid.*, 21/120, 122.
331. *Ibid.*, 22/402.
332. *R.I.B.A. Journal*, 3rd ser., vol. VII, 1900, p. 450.
333. GBM 22/398.
334. *Ibid.*, 23/99–100, 303–4.
335. *Ibid.*, 25/432, 511–12; 26/119–20.
336. *Ibid.*, 26/407–8.
337. *Ibid.*, 26/329–30; 27/67–8.
338. *P.P.*, 1887, XIII, *S.C. on Town Holdings*, p. 332.
339. GBM 20/212.
340. *P.P.*, 1887, XIII, *S.C. on Town Holdings*, pp. 333, 461–2.
341. GBM 23/107–8, 469: G.O., lease particulars book 2.
342. GBM 25/4.
343. *Ibid.*, 18/224.
344. *Ibid.*, 19/491.
345. *Ibid.*, 25/4.
346. *P.P.*, 1887, XIII, *S.C. on Town Holdings*, p. 335.
347. GBM 22/15.
348. *Ibid.*, 23/106, 428.
349. *Ibid.*, 24/17.
350. *The Architect*, 29 Aug. 1902, illustr. facing p. 136.
351. GBM 20/143; 23/213–14.
352. *Ibid.*, 17/61.
353. *Ibid.*, 20/38.
354. *Ibid.*, 26/301, 529: W.C.L., WBA 429, bundle 237, agreement of 16 Dec. 1895.
355. W.C.L., WBA 429, bundle 279, lease of 1 July 1881.
356. *P.P.*, 1887, XIII, *S.C. on Town Holdings*, pp. 329, 371.
357. GBM 18/11; 26/40.
358. *Ibid.*, 20/378.
359. *Ibid.*, 23/306.
360. *Ibid.*, 25/2–3.
361. *Ibid.*, 23/28.
362. *Ibid.*, 21/4; 26/15–16, 19–20.
363. *Ibid.*, 18/345; 19/331; 20/378; 21/222.
364. *Ibid.*, 18/246; 25/45, 333.
365. *Ibid.*, 16/458; 18/415–16, 477; 21/18; 24/12; 26/43–4.
366. *Ibid.*, 18/122, 124; 21/4, 6, 7.
367. *Ibid.*, 21/205–6, 249–50, 353, 358.
368. *Ibid.*, 16/365; 21/20, 217; 24/49, 401.
369. *Ibid.*, 26/1, 26.
370. G.L.R.O.(L), M.B.W. 1727/5, no. 152.
371. GBM 33/473.
372. *Ibid.*, 22/6; 26/18.
373. *P.P.*, 1899, XXXVI, *R.C. on Local Taxation*, pp. 277–82.
374. *Ibid.*, 1839, XIII, *First Report from S.C. on Metropolis Improvements*, plan 6.
375. *The Architect*, Supplement 2, 6 Jan. 1899, pp. 24–5.
376. *P.P.*, 1884–5, XXX, *R.C. on the Housing of the Working Classes*, pp. 468–9.
377. GBM 18/320: *Annual Report of the Vestry of Saint George's Hanover Square*, 1889, p. 41; 1890, p. 44.
378. *P.P.*, 1887, XIII, *S.C. on Town Holdings*, p. 332.
379. *Ibid.*, pp. 324–5.
380. *Ibid.*, p. 323.
381. GBM 27/270.
382. *P.P.*, 1899, XXXVI, *R.C. on Local Taxation*, p. 280.
383. *P.P.*, 1887, XIII, *S.C. on Town Holdings*, p. 336: GBM 22/77; 26/480.
384. *P.P.*, 1887, XIII, *S.C. on Town Holdings*, pp. 325, 347.
385. *Ibid.*, pp. 322, 352: GBM 23/332.
386. *P.P.*, 1899, XXXVI, *R.C. on Local Taxation*, p. 279.
387. GBM 26/149; 27/305.
388. *Ibid.*, 27/9.
389. *Ibid.*, 25/133; 26/337.
390. *P.P.*, 1887, XIII, *S.C. on Town Holdings*, p. 322.
391. GBM 19/170–1, 175, 262.
392. *Ibid.*, 23/487–8.
393. *Ibid.*, 20/388–9; 23/306; 24/169.
394. *Ibid.*, 24/20, 22; 25/34–5: *The Times*, 6, 9, 10, 12, 13, 15, 17 Feb. 1892: Frank Banfield's articles in *The Sunday Times*, published *c.* 1888 in book form as *The Great Landlords of London.*
395. GBM 26/23.
396. *Ibid.*, 25/382.
397. Banfield, *op. cit.*, pp. 60–1, 68, 71.
398. GBM 22/393.
399. *P.P.*, 1887, XIII, *S.C. on Town Holdings*, pp. 325, 326, 332, 362.
400. *Ibid.*, pp. 245–6.
401. GBM 17/143–4.
402. *P.P.*, 1887, XIII, *S.C. on Town Holdings*, p. 325.
403. *Ibid.*, p. 352.

CHAPTER IV (pp. 67–82)

The Estate in the Twentieth Century

1. John Macdonnell, *The Land Question*, 1873, p. 84.
2. G.E.C.
3. *The Times*, 21 July 1953, pp. 7, 8.
4. *Chips. The Diaries of Sir Henry Channon*, ed. Robert Rhodes James, 1967, p. 477.
5. *The Times*, 22 July 1953, p. 8.
6. G.O., misc. box 21, resettlement of 15 Feb. 1901.
7. *Ibid.*, Trustees' accounts, 1901–21.
8. GBM 28/33; 29/537.
9. *Ibid.*, 32/237–40.
10. *Ibid.*, 29/216.
11. *Ibid.*, 31/374.
12. G.O., Duke's instruction book, 1905–8, pp. 7–12.
13. GBM 34/333.
14. *Ibid.*, 34/384; 35/130, 139.
15. *Ibid.*, 31/398; 35/471.
16. *Ibid.*, 35/495; 36/355–6.
17. *Ibid.*, 35/470.
18. G.O., Duke's instruction book, 1900–4, p. 25.
19. GBM 33/345–6.
20. *Ibid.*, 32/172, 310; 34/345.
21. G.O., Duke's instruction book, 1905–8, pp. 7–12, 19.
22. GBM 32/161, 241.
23. *Ibid.*, 33/414.
24. *Ibid.*, 38/219.
25. *Ibid.*, 32/356.
26. *Ibid.*, 38/391.
27. *Ibid.*, 29/225–6.

28. *Ibid.*, 32/162.
29. *Ibid.*, 33/217-18.
30. *Survey of London*, vol. XXIX, 1960, pp. 12-13, 13n.
31. GBM 34/125, 264, 342.
32. *Ibid.*, 38/517.
33. *Ibid.*, 20/380.
34. *Ibid.*, 38/239-40.
35. *Ibid.*, 41/119-23, 223-4, 247-8.
36. *Ibid.*, 42/302-9.
37. *Ibid.*, 31/269-70.
38. *Ibid.*, 34/122, 124.
39. G.O., Duke's instruction book, 1900-4, p. 17.
40. GBM 35/418-19.
41. *Ibid.*, 35/227-8.
42. *Ibid.*, 35/429.
43. Loelia, Duchess of Westminster, *Grace and Favour*, 1961, p. 183.
44. G.O., Duke's instruction book, 1905-8, pp. 7-12.
45. GBM 38/240.
46. *Ibid.*, 34/124.
47. *Ibid.*, 35/429.
48. 'The Work of Mr. Detmar Blow and Mr. Fernand Billerey', in *Architectural Supplement to Country Life*, 26 Oct. 1912, pp. v-ix.
49. Loelia, Duchess of Westminster, *op. cit.*, p. 186.
50. GBM 31/411.
51. *Ibid.*, 35/419.
52. *Ibid.*, 36/193-5.
53. *Ibid.*, 35/539.
54. *Ibid.*, 37/221-2.
55. *Ibid.*, 31/264.
56. *Ibid.*, 39/344.
57. *Ibid.*, 37/536; 39/342-4.
58. *Ibid.*, 39/389-90.
59. *Ibid.*, 39/414.
60. *Ibid.*, 39/421-2.
61. *Ibid.*, 39/429.
62. *Ibid.*, 34/125, 263-4: G.O., Duke's instruction book, 1905-8, pp. 114-15, 133.
63. Reginald Colby, '44 Grosvenor Square, The Residence of Lady Illingworth', in *Country Life*, 27 July 1961, pp. 193-4.
64. GBM 35/152; 36/335-40, 372, 382, 384, 393.
65. Desmond Fitz-Gerald, 'The Mural from 44 Grosvenor Square', in *Victoria and Albert Museum Yearbook*, no. 1, 1969, p. 145.
66. R.B.
67. GBM 37/411-14.
68. *Ibid.*, 19/440.
69. *Ibid.*, 39/286, 328, 370: G.O., Duke's instruction book, 1912-14, p. 189.
70. GBM 42/209; 44/413.
71. G.O., Duke's instruction books, 1900-4, p. 146; 1905-8, p. 6; 1909-11, pp. 14-15; 1912-14, p. 85.
72. GBM 31/175.
73. G.O., Duke's instruction book, 1912-14, pp. 23-4.
74. *The Times*, 26 Jan. 1911, p. 6.
75. G.O., misc. box 21, printed abstract of title, 1918.
76. *The Times*, 24 Jan. 1911, p. 15; 15 Dec. 1911, p. 10; 20 June 1912, p. 20.
77. GBM 39/304-9; 42/218.
78. F. M. L. Thompson, *English Landed Society in the Nineteenth Century*, 1963, p. 332.
79. G.O., Trustees' accounts, 1901-21, 1921-7.
80. Loelia, Duchess of Westminster, *op. cit.*, p. 86.
81. G.O., Duke's instruction book, 1919-22, pp. 94-6, 142-4.
82. *Ibid.*, Duke's instruction book, 1923-5, p. 218.
83. Christopher Hussey, *The Life of Sir Edwin Lutyens*, 1950, p. 14: *Country Life*, 23 Sept. 1911, pp. 7*-10*: *R.I.B.A. Journal*, 3rd ser., vol. XLVI, 1939, p. 571.
84. *The Architectural Review*, vol. V, 1898-9, p. 173.
85. Hussey, *op. et loc. cit.*
86. Information kindly supplied by Madame V. H. Billerey and Mr. L. V. A. Billerey.
87. R.I.B.A. Drawings Collection, Blow drawings, No. 28 South St., sheet signed by Billerey Sept. 1902.
88. London County Council Minutes, 18 July 1905, p. 520: *P.O.D.*
89. *The Times*, 8 Feb. 1939, p. 16.
90. *The Architectural Review*, vol. 138, 1965, p. 263.
91. *Ibid.*, vol. LIII, 1923, p. 31.
92. Information kindly supplied by Mr. Jonathan Blow: Company House, file 249,996.
93. Sir George Arthur, *Life of Lord Kitchener*, 1920, vol. 1, p. 11.
94. 'The Work of Mr. Detmar Blow and Mr. Fernand Billerey', in *Architectural Supplement to Country Life*, 26 Oct. 1912, pp. xx-xxvii.
95. GBM 40/375-6, 381-4.
96. *Ibid.*, 43/213.
97. *Ibid.*, 42/225.
98. *Ibid.*, 44/496.
99. *Ibid.*, 45/483-4.
100. G.O., Wimperis correspondence, Jan. 1920.
101. *Ibid.*, Duke's instruction books, 1923-5, pp. 180-6; 1926-8, part II, pp. 563-5.
102. *Ibid.*, Duke's instruction book, 1926-8, part I, pp. 156-8.
103. *Ibid.*, Duke's instruction book, 1926-8, part II, pp. 419, 563-5.
104. P.P.R., index to wills, 1946.
105. Loelia, Duchess of Westminster, *op. cit.*, pp. 160, 163, 183, 198.
106. G.O., Blow letterbooks, 1918-19, Nov. 1919.
107. *Ibid.*, Duke's instruction books, 1923-5 to 1931-2, *passim*.
108. B.A. 41564.
109. London County Council Minutes, 4 June 1935, pp. 795-6.
110. GBM 39/23, 550: *P.O.D.*
111. *Ibid.*, 39/170, 455-7.
112. *Ibid.*, 40/165-6.
113. Loelia, Duchess of Westminster, *op. cit.*, p. 187.
114. GBM 44/406, 460, 463.
115. *Ibid.*, 44/463.
116. Sir Edwin Lutyens, 'What I think of Modern Architecture', in *Country Life*, 20 June 1931, p. 775.
117. Christopher Hussey, 'The Great Estates of London and their Development: The Grosvenor Estate', in *Country Life*, 21 April 1928, pp. 558-65.
118. B.A. 80871, in G.L.R.O.(L).
119. G.O., typescript of evidence given by A. C. H. Borrer to a public inquiry conducted for the Minister of Health, *c.* 1934, pp. 32-4.
120. GBM 45/67: *The Times*, 31 March 1926, p. 16.
121. *The Times*, 20 May 1924, p. 11; 31 March 1926, p. 16; 16 Feb. 1927, p. 7; 24 July 1929, p. 12.
122. *Ibid.*, 20 March 1928, p. 18; 31 Jan. 1929, p. 9.
123. G.O., Trustees' accounts, *passim*.

124. *Ibid.*, drafts of evidence given by A. C. H. Borrer to a public inquiry conducted for the Minister of Health, *c.* 1934, pp. 2–3, 29.
125. *Ibid.*, Trustees' accounts, 1922–33.
126. *Ibid.*, Duke's instruction books, 1923–5, pp. 108–9; 1926–8, part i, pp. 96–7.
127. *Ibid.*, Trustees' accounts, 1921–7.
128. Christopher Hussey, *The Life of Sir Edwin Lutyens*, 1950, p. 482.
129. G.O., Duke's instruction book, 1926–8, part ii, p. 527.
130. *Ibid.*, Duke's instruction book, 1929–30, p. 184: B.A. 55136.
131. G.O., Trustees' accounts, 1928–33; Duke's instruction book, 1929–30, p. 409.
132. *Ibid.*, Estate Surveyor's unnumbered letterbooks, 21 July 1933: Hussey, *op. cit.*, 1950, p. 482.
133. G.O., Trustees' accounts, 1927–36.
134. *Ibid.*, solicitor's fee books, G37/455.
135. *Ibid.*, misc. letterbook, Codd to Billerey, 29 May 1929.
136. *Ibid.*, Estate Surveyor's letterbooks, 20/109, 143.
137. *Ibid.*, solicitor's fee books, G39/470.
138. *Ibid.*, solicitor's fee books, G41/433.
139. *Ibid.*, solicitor's fee books, G41/231, 277; Estate Surveyor's unnumbered letterbooks, 25 March 1936, p. 211.
140. Greater London Council, Building Regulation case 109691.
141. G.O., improvement accounts, Sept. 1923.
142. *Ibid.*, Duke's instruction book, 1933–4, p. 197.
143. *Ibid.*, Estate Surveyor's unnumbered letterbooks, Codd to Etchells, 25 March 1936.
144. *Ibid.*, Duke's instruction books, 1931–2, pp. 462–4; 1933–4, p. 358.
145. *Ibid.*, Trustees' accounts, Jan. 1929.
146. *Ibid.*, Duke's instruction book, 1926–8, part ii, p. 373.
147. *The Times*, 26 Oct. 1932, p. 4.
148. G.O., Duke's instruction book, 1931–2, pp. 392–7.
149. *Ibid.*, Duke's instruction books, 1926–8, part ii, pp. 506–7; 1931–2, p. 128.
150. Information kindly supplied by Mr. Geoffrey Singer.
151. *Ex. inf.* Mr. Singer: *The Times*, 21 July 1953, pp. 7, 8.
152. *The Times*, 21 July 1953, p. 7; 23 Oct. 1953, p. 5: P.P.R., will of Duke of Westminster, 1953.
153. *The Daily Telegraph*, 4 Nov. 1971.
154. P.P.R., will of Duke of Westminster, 1953: *The Times*, 23 Oct. 1953, p. 5.
155. *The Times*, 27 Feb. 1967, p. 3.
156. G.O., Duke's instruction book, 1933–4, p. 358.
157. *The Times*, 9 June 1966, p. 15: *The Director*, Aug. 1974.
158. *The Daily Telegraph*, 19 June 1967.
159. G.L.R.O.(L), L.C.C. file AR/TP/2/48.
160. *The Times*, 6 Oct. 1960, p. 9.
161. Michael Hanson, 'Private Houses Return to Mayfair', in *Country Life*, 15 Nov. 1973, p. 1601.
162. *The Grosvenor Estate Strategy for Mayfair and Belgravia*, 1971, Foreword.
163. *The London Gazette*, 8 May 1969, p. 4863.
164. *The Grosvenor Estate Strategy for Mayfair and Belgravia. Second Revision*, 1974, para. 4.
165. *Strategy*, 1971, p. 76.
166. *Ibid.*, pp. 88, 96.
167. *Ibid.*, pp. 148, 161.
168. *Ibid.*, pp. 78, 162.
169. *Ibid.*, pp. 99, 100, 103.
170. *Ibid.*, pp. 106, 108.
171. *Ibid.*, p. 78.
172. *The Guardian*, 4 Nov. 1971: *The Observer*, 31 Oct. 1971.
173. *Official Architecture and Planning*, Dec. 1971.
174. *Strategy*, 1971, p. 174.
175. Westminster City Council Minutes, 30 April 1973, adopting T.P. Committee Report of 15 March 1973: *Strategy... Second Revision*, 1974, para. 1.
176. *Strategy... Second Revision*, 1974, para. 12.
177. *The Grosvenor Estate Strategy Progress Oxford Street West One*, 1976.
178. *Strategy... Second Revision*, 1974, para. 11.
179. Leasehold Reform Act, 1967, c. 88, sec. 19.
180. *Strategy... Second Revision*, 1974, letter of 6 Sept. 1974.

CHAPTER V (pp. 83–102)

The Social Character of the Estate

1. Suffolk Record Office, Bury St. Edmunds, Bunbury Papers, E18/660.2: *Survey of London*, vol. xxxii, 1963, p. 557.
2. R.B.
3. *The Court Kalendar*, 1733, 1741: *The Court and City Register for 1751*.
4. Warwickshire Record Office, CR114A/253.
5. *The World*, 14 Jan. 1790.
6. *The Autobiography and Correspondence of Mary Granville, Mrs. Delany*, ed. Lady Llanover, part i, vol. i, 1861, p. 492.
7. R.B.: Ambrose Heal, *The London Furniture Makers from the Restoration to the Victorian Era 1660–1840*, 1953, p. 33.
8. G.L.R.O.(M), WR/PP, Reg. 5, 1749.
9. Romney Sedgwick, *The House of Commons 1715–1754*, 1970, vol. i, p. 287.
10. G.L.R.O.(M), L.V.(W) 68/449–56.
11. M. Dorothy George, *London Life in the Eighteenth Century*, 1925, p. 155.
12. G.L.R.O.(M), TC/St.G./1,2.
13. *Edward Jerningham and His Friends*, ed. Lewis Bettany, 1919, pp. 187–8.
14. E.H.P., box 42/6, Porden to Lord Grosvenor, 6 Nov. 1805.
15. F. G. Hilton Price, *A Handbook of London Bankers*, 1890–1, p. 53.
16. E.g. GLB xvii/435.
17. GBM 3/167.
18. *The World*, 15 May 1787, 23 Sept. 1789.
19. *Memoirs of Sir Nathaniel William Wroxall*, ed. H. B. Wheatley, vol. i, 1884, pp. 374–5.
20. GBM 3/160: R.B.
21. *The Morning Post*, 5 April 1841.
22. *Ibid.*, 3 April 1841.
23. *Ibid.*, 26 July 1841.
24. John Bateman, *The Great Landowners of Great Britain and Ireland*, 1971 ed., p. 457.
25. P.R.O., HO 107/733/12, f.38r, v.
26. *Ibid.*, HO 107/438/11, ff. 15–17.
27. G.E.C.
28. P.R.O., HO 107/733/12, f.26v.
29. *Ibid.*, HO 107/545/9, ff. 2–3.

30. *Ibid.*, HO 107/588/2, f. 43.
31. *Ibid.*, HO 107/470/17, f. 24.
32. The enumerators' books for 1841 are in P.R.O., HO 107/733/4-6, 8-16, and HO 107/734/5-6, 8-9. Those for 1871 are in P.R.O., RG 10/92 95, 97 99, 101-102.
33. R. Price-Williams, 'The Population of London 1801-81', in *Journal of the Statistical Society*, vol. 48, 1885, p. 389.
34. *P.P.*, 1843, XXII, *Abstract of the Answers and Returns: Enumeration Abstract*, p. 3n.
35. W. H. Mallock, *Memoirs of Life and Literature*, 1920, p. 71.
36. *Survey of London*, vol. XXXVI, 1970, p. 82.
37. *Ibid.*, vol. XXXI, 1963, p. 143; vol. XXXIII, 1966, p. 45; vol. XXXIV, 1966, pp. 424, 428-30.
38. *Ibid.*, vol. XXXII, 1963, pp. 442, 453, 454.
39. GBM 21/518; 20/371, 379; 21/19, 219; 25/2-3; 22/467-8.
40. *P.O.D.*
41. GBM 39/23, 550; 39/170, 455-7; *P.O.D.*
42. GBM 27/9; 25/133; 26/337.
43. *Ibid.*, 26/256.
44. *Ibid.*, 20/380.
45. *Ibid.*, 32/480.
46. *Ibid.*, 37/249, 254.
47. *Ibid.*, 42/116.
48. *P.P.*, 1887, XIII, *Report from the Select Committee on Town Holdings*, pp. 325-6.
49. P.R.O., RG 10/101, f.81v.
50. *P.P.*, 1887, XIII, *S.C. on Town Holdings*, p. 352.
51. GBM 42/223.
52. *Ibid.*, 27/195-6.
53. *Ibid.*, 33/473.
54. *Ibid.*, 38/219.
55. *Ibid.*, 35/50-1, 57, 70, 94; 36/45: G.L.R.O.(L), LCC/AR/BA/4/185/40/233.
56. *The Grosvenor Estate Strategy for Mayfair and Belgravia*, 1971, para. 83.
57. *Harper's Bazaar*, Jan. 1933, pp. 44-5; Feb. 1933, pp. 16-17; May 1933, p. 26.
58. *Strategy*, p. 37.
59. *The Times*, 6 Oct. 1960, p. 9.
60. *The Evening News*, 13 Sept. 1929.
61. *Strategy*, p. 201.
62. *Strategy*, pp. 201-2.

CHAPTER VI (pp. 103-70)

The Architecture of the Estate

1. John Summerson, *Georgian London*, 1962 ed., pp. 98-100, 105-111.
2. P. Lavedan, *Histoire de l'Urbanisme*, vol. II, 1959, fig. 193, p. 383.
3. GLB V/140-1: M.L.R. 1728/4/135.
4. P.R.O., C105/32/1, manuscript plan of E. Shepherd's estate in N. Audley St.
5. J. Ralph, *A Critical Review of the Publick Buildings...In, and about London and Westminster*, 1734, pp. 108-9.
6. Robert Morris, *Lectures on Architecture*, [Part I], 1734, preface.
7. *Survey of London*, vol. XXXII, 1963, fig. 92, p. 499.
8. Isaac Ware, *A Complete Body of Architecture*, 1777 ed., p. 320.
9. E.H.P., box 42/6, Porden to Lord Grosvenor, 6 Nov. 1805.
10. O. E. Deutsch, *Handel, A Documentary Biography*, 1955, p. 830.
11. Guildhall Library, MS. 8766: Wiltshire Record Office, Longleat MSS. 845/Schedule III/bundle 16.
12. Ware, *op. cit.*, p. 346.
13. Lincolnshire Archives Office, ANC 2B/19/2/6.
14. Bodleian Library, MS. North b. 24, f. 268.
15. Helen Sard Hughes, *The Gentle Hertford*, 1940, p. 63.
16. Warwickshire Record Office, CR114A/254.
17. *Horace Walpole's Correspondence with Sir Horace Mann*, vol. VI, 1960, ed. W. S. Lewis, Warren Hunting Smith and George L. Lam, pp. 138-41.
18. Suffolk Record Office, Bury St. Edmunds, Bunbury Papers, E18/660.2.
19. G.O., chest B, bundle 8, 3 Dec. 1733.
20. Ware, *op. cit.*, p. 469.
21. Northamptonshire Record Office, BH(K)1185.
22. *Letters of a Grandmother, 1732-1735*, ed. Gladys Scott Thomson, 1943, p. 78.
23. Bodleian Library, MS. North e.40.
24. P.R.O., C105/32/1, agreement of 6 April 1728, E. Shepherd and F. Drewitt.
25. Corsham Court Archives, memo. of 2 March 1727/8.
26. Desmond Fitz-Gerald, 'The Mural from 44 Grosvenor Square', in *Victoria and Albert Museum Yearbook*, no. 1, 1969, pp. 148-50: Staffordshire Record Office, D1161/1/2/2: Lincolnshire Archives Office, ANC 2B/19/2/6.
27. Nottinghamshire Record Office, DD4P 52/108.
28. Badminton MSS., 110.1.43.
29. *The Autobiography and Correspondence of Mary Granville, Mrs. Delany*, ed. Lady Llanover, vol. I, 1861, p. 476.
30. Cecil Aspinall-Oglander, *Admiral's Wife. Being the Life and Letters of The Hon. Mrs. Edward Boscawen from 1719 to 1761*, 1940, p. 80; and *Admiral's Widow. Being the Life and Letters of The Hon. Mrs. Edward Boscawen from 1761 to 1805*, 1942, p. 164.
31. John Harris, *Sir William Chambers*, 1970, p. 222.
32. E.H.P., box 42/6, Porden to Lord Grosvenor, [Nov. 1805].
33. Mount Stuart, Bute MSS., letter of Sir Thomas Robinson to Lord Bute, 15 Aug. 1762.
34. R.I.B.A. Drawings Collection, MS. G5/6.
35. A. E. Richardson, *Robert Mylne*, 1955, pp. 57-220 *passim.*
36. North Yorkshire Record Office, Dawnay Collection, ZDS.
37. J. M. Robinson, 'Samuel Wyatt', D.Phil. thesis, University of Oxford, 1973, pp. 426-7.
38. Leeds Archives Department, Ramsden Archives (Rockingham Letters), vol. 3b, nos. 128 and 142.
39. *The Works in Architecture of Robert and James Adam*, vol. II, 1779, Explanation of Plate I.
40. Sir John Soane's Museum, Soane Lectures, vol. X, no. 21.
41. Sheffield Central Library, Wentworth Woodhouse Muniments, R 185/3.
42. Cecil Aspinall-Oglander, *Admiral's Wife...*, 1940, pp. 68, 72.
43. G.L.R.O.(L), B/TRL/9, pp. 28, 31, 93, 206, 273, 307, 313, 381, 383.
44. Patricia Anne Kirkham, 'The Careers of William and John Linnell', in *Furniture History*, vol. 3, 1967, pp. 29-44: C. Proudfoot and D. Watkin, 'A Pioneer of English Neo-Classicism—C. H. Tatham', and 'The Furniture

of C. H. Tatham', in *Country Life*, 13/20 April 1972, pp. 918–21, and 8 June 1972, pp. 1481–6: R.B.
45. W.C.L., C775, pp. 20–1.
46. GBM 8/2.
47. *Ibid.*, 8/75, 135, 254; 9/125.
48. University of Nottingham, Newcastle MSS., Ne c 7009a.
49. GBM 2/279, 309; 3/20, 131, 234; 5/78.
50. Ann Saunders, *Regent's Park*, 1969, pp. 95–101, 178.
51. *The Works of David Ricardo*, ed. P. Sraffa, vol. 6, 1962, p. 52; vol. 7, 1962, pp. 16–17.
52. E.H.P., box 42/6, Porden to Lord Grosvenor, 9 Dec. 1807.
53. *The Times*, 2 June 1808, p. 3.
54. E.g. GBM 7/185, 205, 207, 208, 209.
55. R.B.: *Survey of London*, vol. XXXI, 1963, p. 279.
56. GBM 5/180 et seq.: Hermione Hobhouse, *Thomas Cubitt, Master Builder*, 1971, pp. 88–9.
57. Hobhouse, *op. cit.*, chapters V–VII: GBM 9/90; 10/1.
58. GBM 10/1.
59. G.O., Moor Park box, bills.
60. *Survey of London*, vol. XXVI, 1956, p. 12.
61. P.P.R., will of John Elger, 1888: M.L.R. 1826/1/571; 1844/8/969: R.B.: *P.O.D.*
62. *The Times*, 11 April 1832, p. 3: *Autobiography of James Gallier, Architect*, 1864: William R. Cullison and Roulhac Toledano, 'Our Architectural Heritage from the Brothers Gallier', in *New Orleans*, July 1970, pp. 30–5.
63. P.P.R., will of Wright Ingle, 1865.
64. GBM 12/426–7.
65. Papers of John Liddell, architect, in stock of B. Weinreb, Architectural Books Ltd., Lord Westminster to Lord Carnarvon, 22 May 1845.
66. GBM 12/426–7.
67. *The Builder*, 5 May 1855, p. 216: University College, London, Library, William Brougham MSS., letters from T. Cundy, 1854–9.
68. The John Rylands University Library of Manchester, Crawford MSS.
69. *Timber Trades Journal, Annual Special Issue*, Jan. 1965, p. 170: P.P.R., will of John Newson, 1873.
70. *Survey of London*, vol. XXXVIII, 1975, p. 17.
71. P.P.R., will of John Newson, 1873.
72. Henry Roberts, *The Progress and Present Aspect of the Movement for Improving the Dwellings of the Labouring Classes*, 1861, pp. 10–11.
73. Edward Hubbard, 'The Work of John Douglas (1830–1911)', M.A. thesis, University of Manchester, 1974.
74. Victoria and Albert Museum, Library, Diary of Henry Cole, 7 July 1863. Consulted by courtesy of Mrs. Cynthia Dutnall.
75. *The Builder*, 11 June 1864, p. 440. Drawings by Garling, Kerr and Street survive at the Grosvenor Office. For Barry's design see Sotheby's Belgravia Sale Catalogue, 11 March 1975, item 27.
76. GBM 14/523; 15/198; 16/39: *The Building News*, 6, 13 Oct. 1865, pp. 695, 712: *The Builder*, 23 Feb. 1867, pp. 121–3.
77. GBM 15/388–9.
78. *Ibid.*, 17/308.
79. *The Builder*, 25 Dec. 1875, p. 1153.
80. *P.P.*, 1874, vol. X, *Report and Minutes of Evidence of Select Committee of the House of Commons on the Metropolitan Buildings and Management Bill*, pp. 130–1, 180–1.
81. GBM 23/213–14.
82. *Ibid.*, 26/95, 376.
83. *Ibid.*, 23/364.
84. *Ibid.*, 25/27.
85. *Ibid.*, 24/411.
86. *Ibid.*, 26/17.
87. *Ibid.*, 26/297; 27/18–19, 285, 288–9.
88. Lady Frances Balfour, *Ne Obliviscaris*, 1930, vol. 2, p. 104. For Cecil Parker see Edward Hubbard, *op. cit.*
89. R.I.B.A. Library, Biographical File 774, H. S. Goodhart-Rendel to W. W. Begley, 8 Feb. 1938.
90. GBM 21/383–4.
91. Lord and Lady Aberdeen, '*We Twa*', vol. 1, 1925, pp. 280–2.
92. GBM 26/545.
93. Information supplied to Sir Nikolaus Pevsner by Mr. Clifford C. Makins, in April 1954.
94. Papers in the possession of Mr. H. D. Steiner of Steiner and Co.
95. GBM 32/328.
96. For No. 42 Upper Brook Street see *The Architect*, 4 April 1919, pp. 242 et seq.
97. GBM 38/203.
98. *The Building News*, 9 June 1905, p. 815.
99. GBM 38/239–40.
100. *The Builder*, 20 Dec. 1851, pp. 805–6.
101. GBM 34/291–2.
102. *The Builder*, 26 Feb. 1910, p. 240.
103. *The Times*, 10 Aug. 1974, p. 14.
104. Cuthbert Headlam, *George Abraham Crawley, A Short Memoir*, 1929.
105. *R.I.B.A. Journal*, 3rd ser., vol. XLIV, 1936–7, p. 1071.
106. GBM 39/200.
107. G.O., Duke's instruction book, 1919–22, pp. 133–5.
108. Information kindly supplied by Mrs. Loeb and Mrs. Carvalho, daughters of L. Rome Guthrie, and by J. R. Wilcox, Esq., assistant to Messrs. Wimperis, Simpson and Guthrie.
109. K. Jones and T. Hewitt, *A. H. Jones of Grosvenor House*, 1971, p. 24.
110. Christopher Hussey, *The Life of Sir Edwin Lutyens*, 1950, p. 460.
111. A. S. G. Butler, *The Architecture of Sir Edwin Lutyens*, vol. III, 1950, p. 35.
112. *The Times*, 6 Aug. 1930, p. 11.
113. B.A. 3440, note from Etchells on behalf of Blow and Billerey, 21 Sept. 1911.
114. GBM 42/225.
115. 'No. 1, Mount Row, W. and its conversion by Messrs. Gilbert and Constanduros', by R.R.P., in *Country Life*, 28 July 1923, pp. 131–2.
116. *The Architectural Review*, vol. LXXII, Sept. 1932, pp. 96–8.
117. Madge Garland, *The Indecisive Decade*, 1968, pp. 23–4.
118. Philip Tilden, *True Remembrances*, 1954, p. 162.
119. John Fowler and John Cornforth, *English Decoration in the 18th Century*, 1974, p. 17.
120. Beverley Nicholls, *A Case of Human Bondage*, 1966, pp. 51–2.
121. *Vogue*, 13 Nov. 1935, p. 69.
122. 'New Rooms at Claridge's Hotel', by C. H., in *Country Life*, 11 June 1932, pp. 663–5.
123. *The Architectural Review*, vol. CVIII, Oct. 1950, p. 274.
124. *Ibid.*, vol. 141, Feb. 1967, p. 133.
125. *Ibid.*, vol. 129, April 1961, p. 254.
126. *Ibid.*, pp. 252–65.

Index

NOTE

The symbols in the left-hand margin distinguish those persons who have worked, or are thought to have worked, on the fabric of the area, and the authors of unexecuted designs:

[a] Architects, designers, engineers, and surveyors
[b] Builders and allied tradesmen
[c] Artists, craftsmen, and decorators

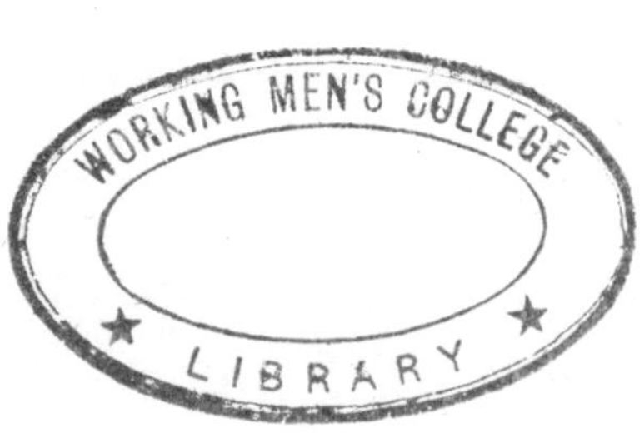

PLATES

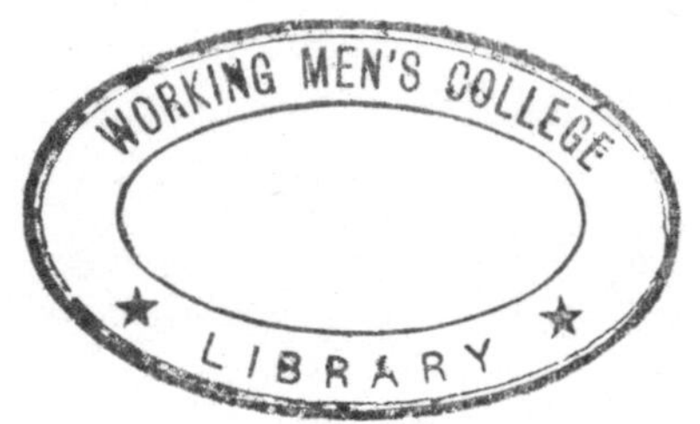

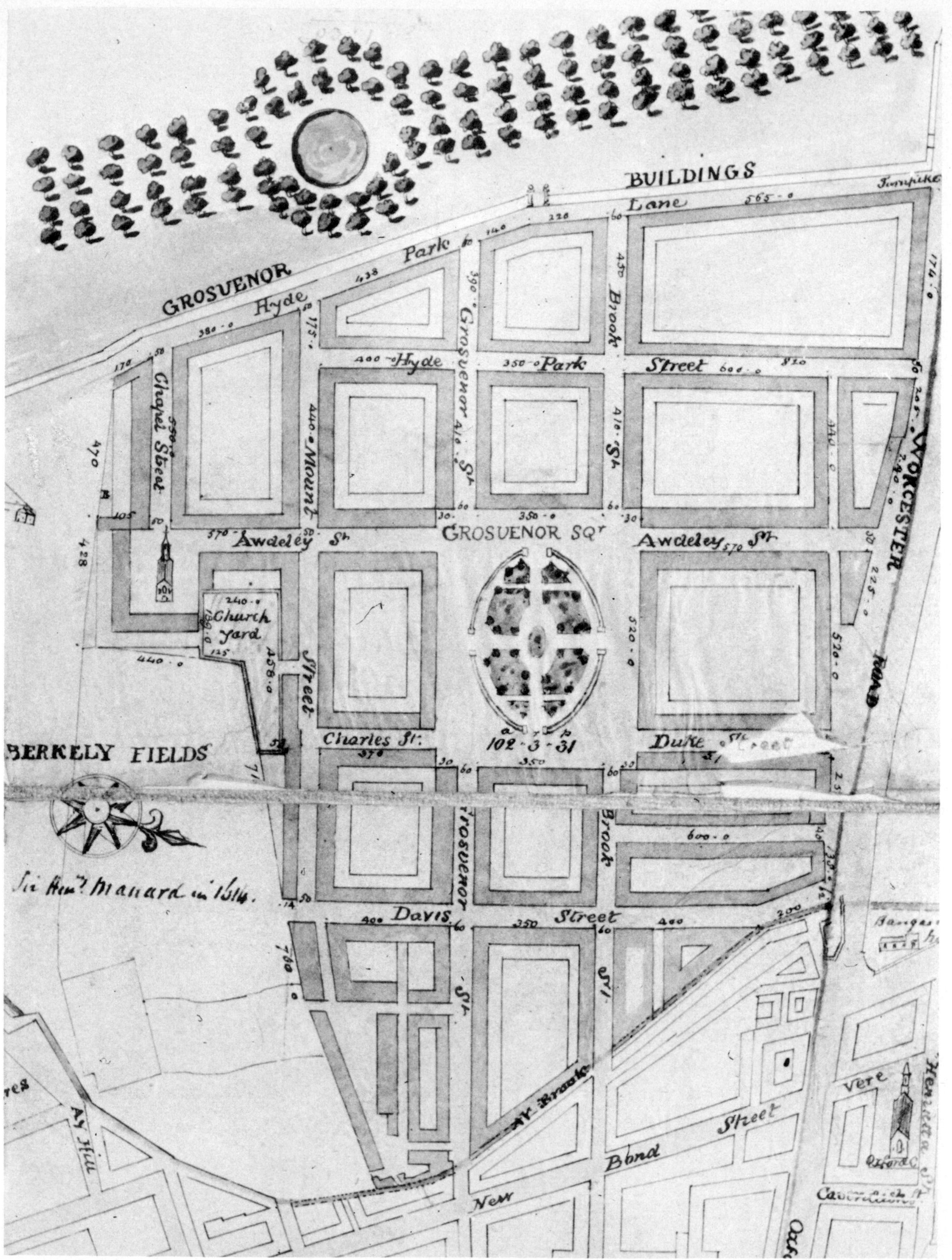

The intended layout of the estate as shown on John Mackay's map of 1723

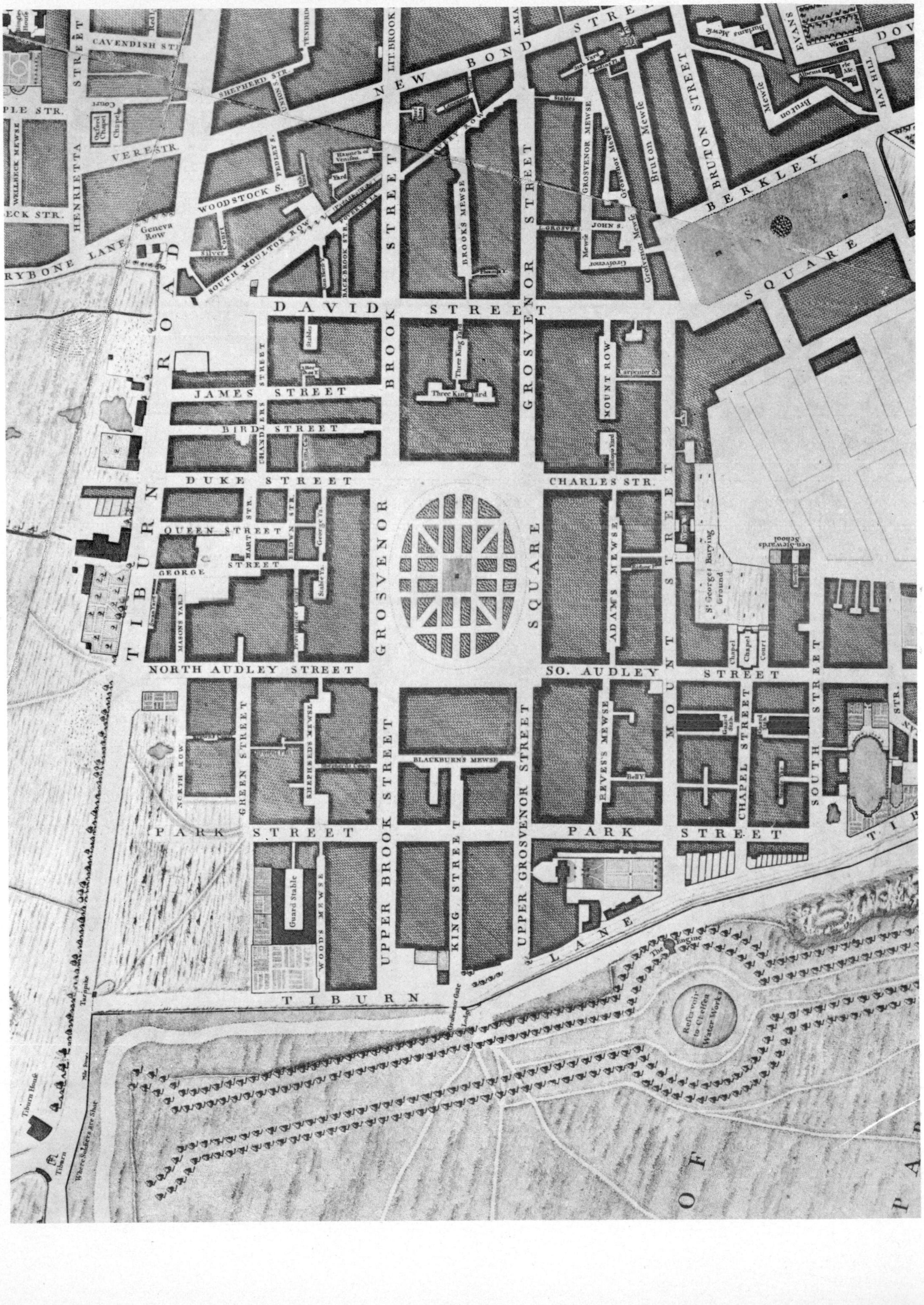

Extract from John Rocque's map of 1746

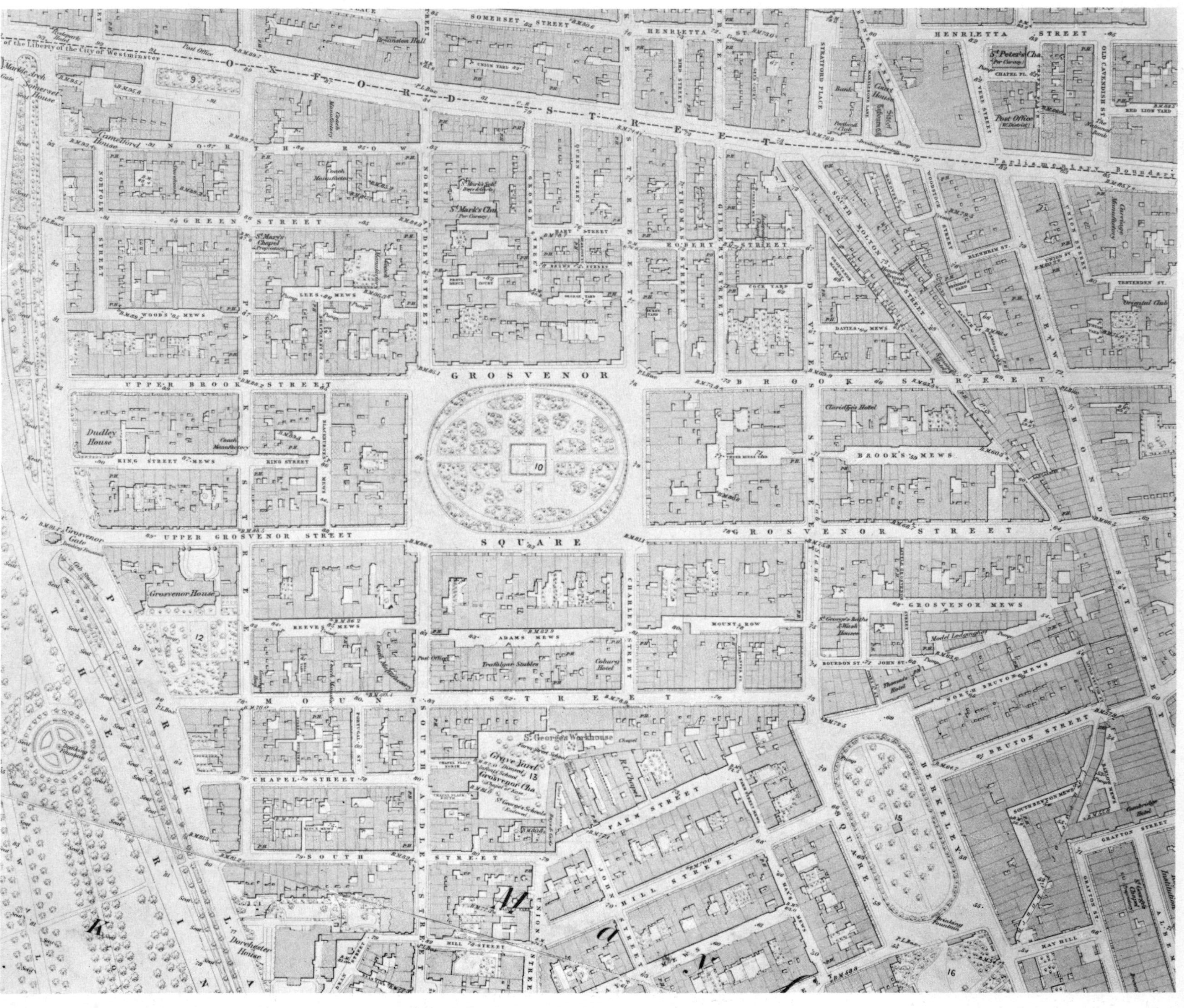

Extract from the Ordnance Survey map surveyed in 1869–70

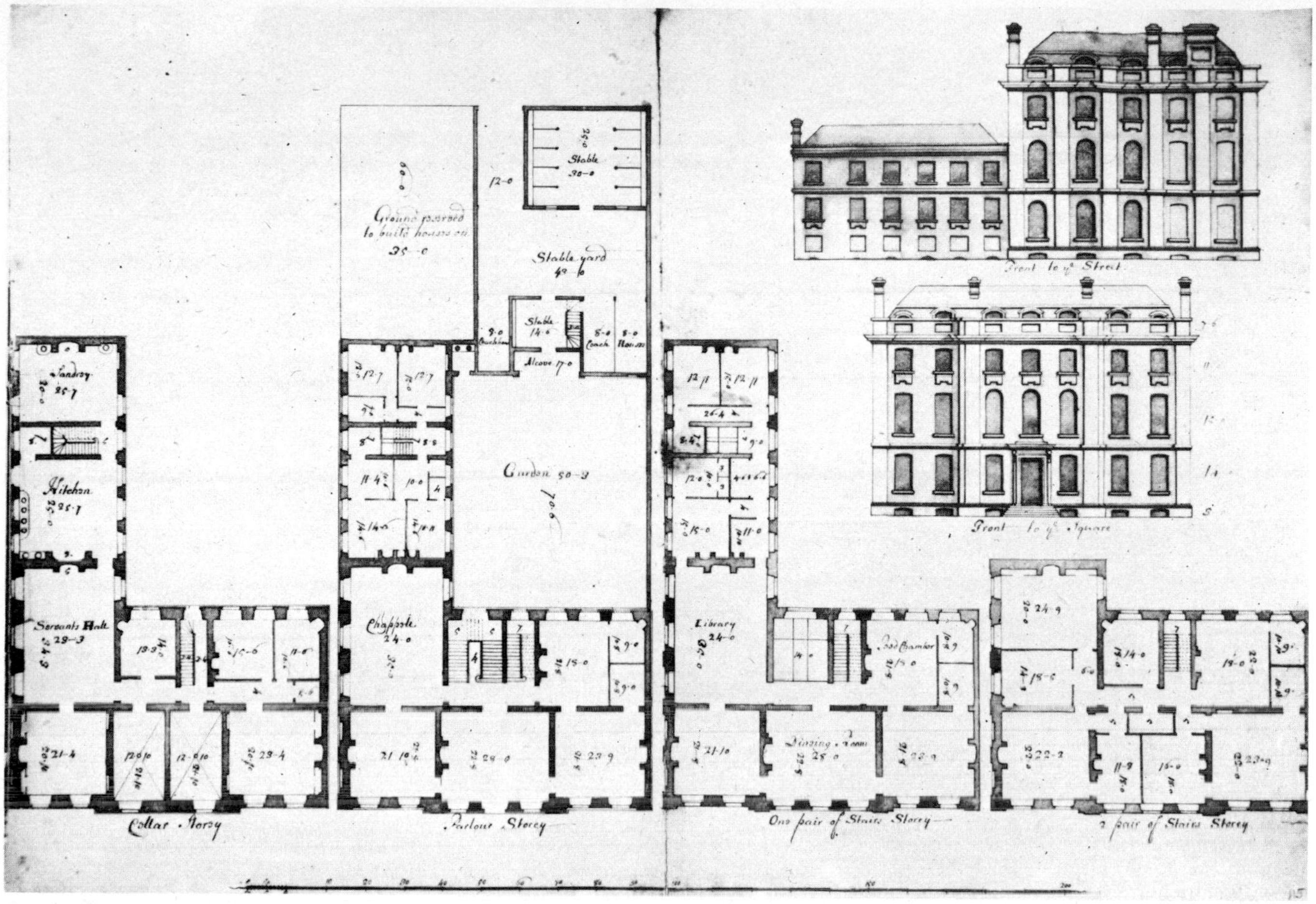

a. Undated plans and elevations of a proposed house, presumably for the square (pp. 103–4). *Not executed*

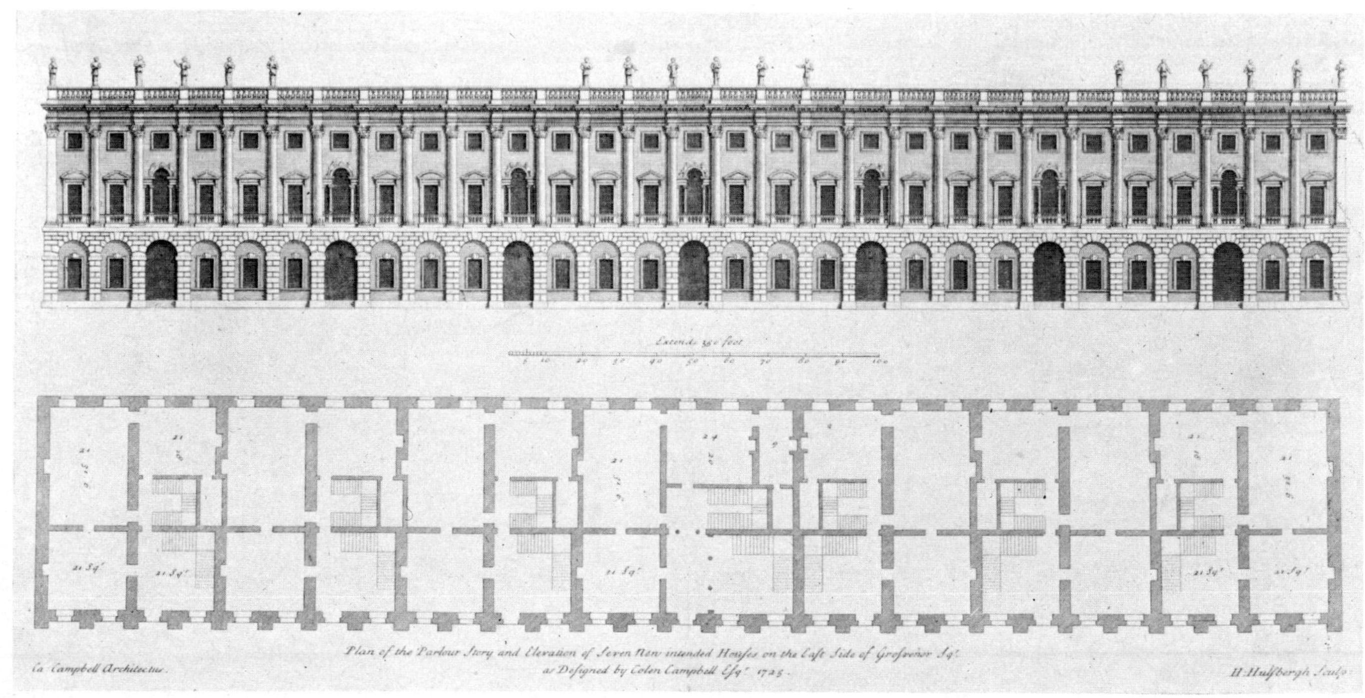

b. Ground-plan and front elevation for the east side of the square as proposed by Colen Campbell in 1725 (pp. 20, 104–5). *Not executed*

EARLY DESIGNS FOR GROSVENOR SQUARE

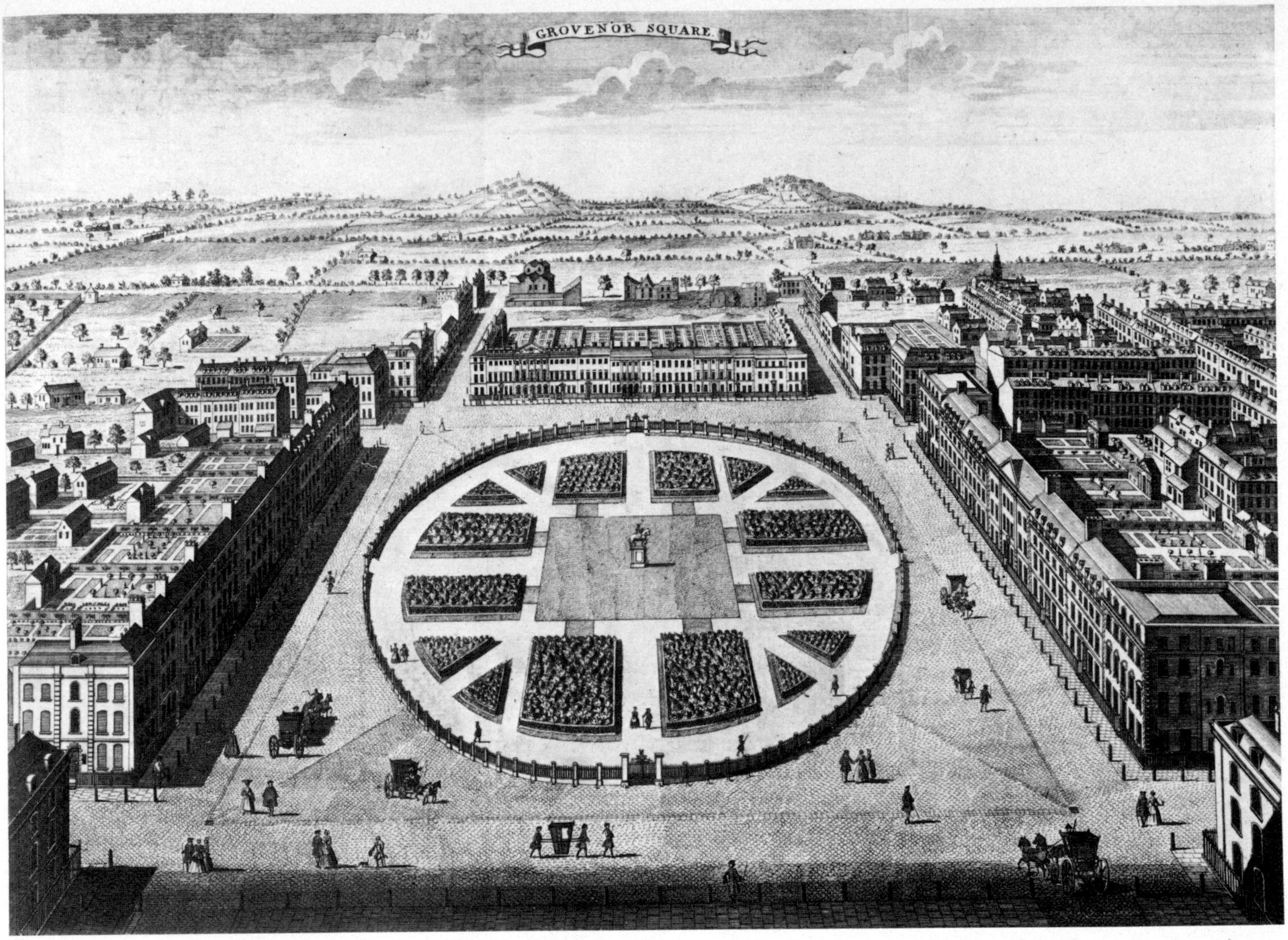

a. View looking north, *c*. 1730–5. The background appears to date from *c*. 1730 or earlier, the house fronts in the square from *c*. 1735

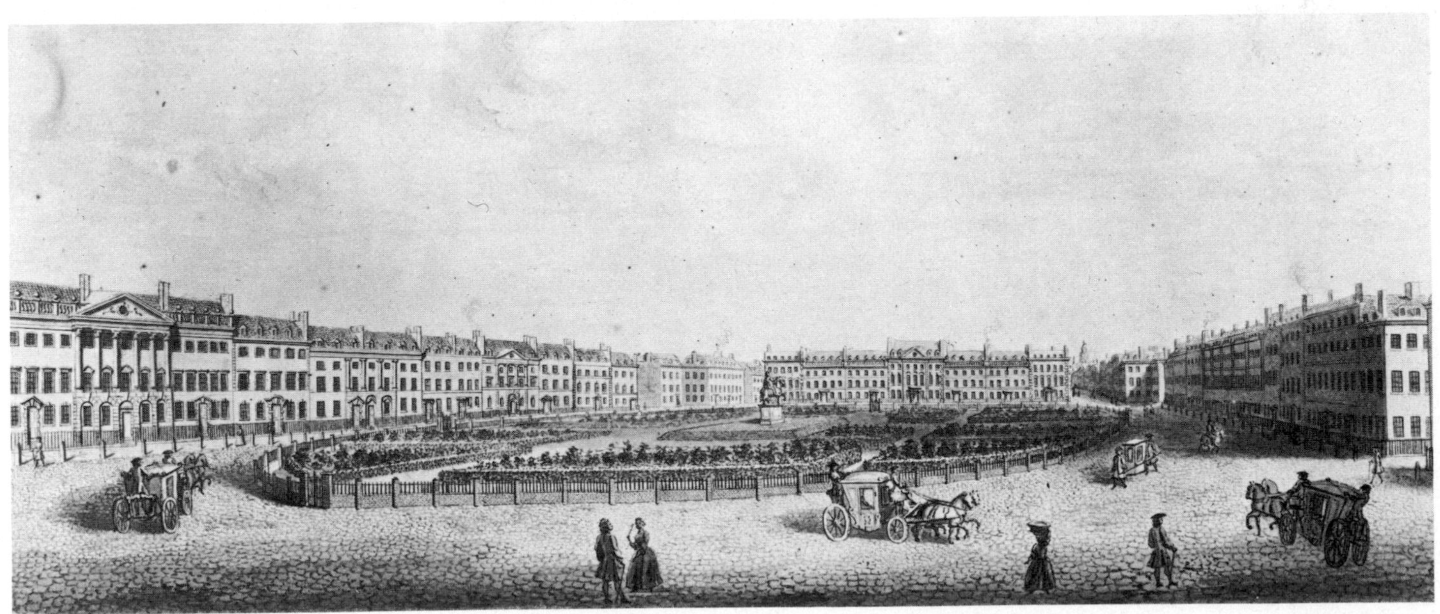

b. View looking east, *c*. 1741

EARLY VIEWS OF GROSVENOR SQUARE

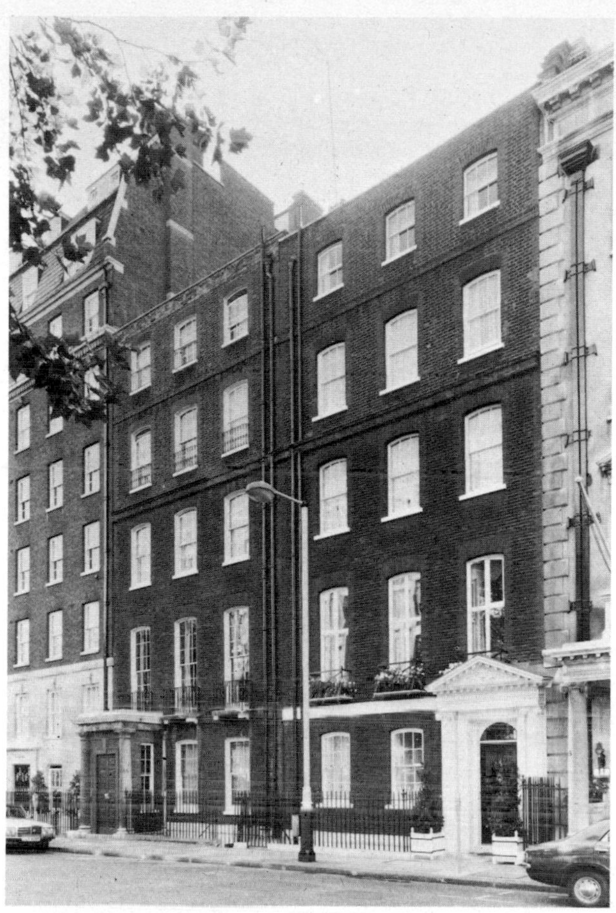

a. Nos. 44–45 Upper Grosvenor Street in 1976. William Draycott (esquire) lessee, 1727. ?Charles Griffith (carpenter) builder

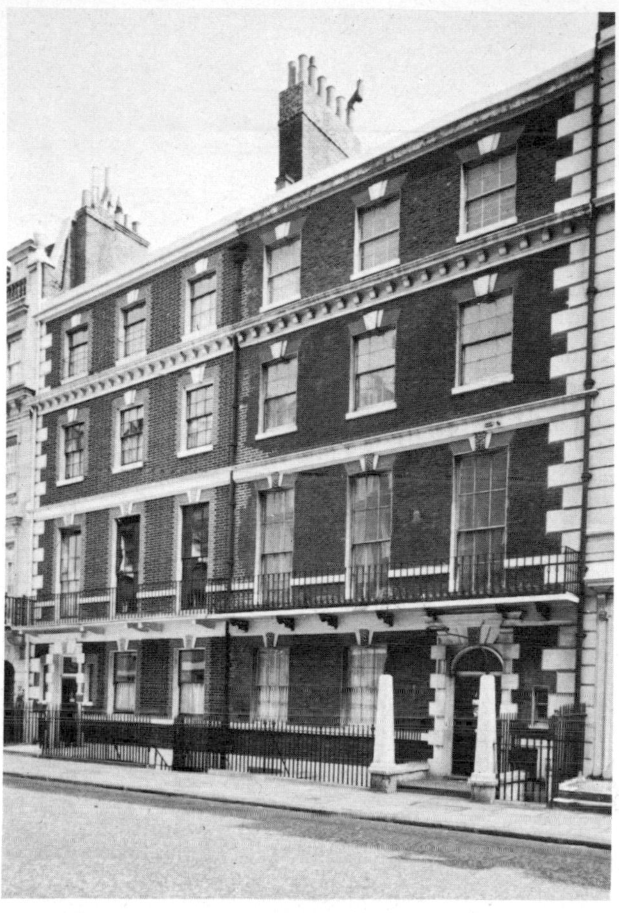

b. Nos. 35–36 Upper Brook Street in 1958. Anthony Cross (mason) sub-lessee, 1737

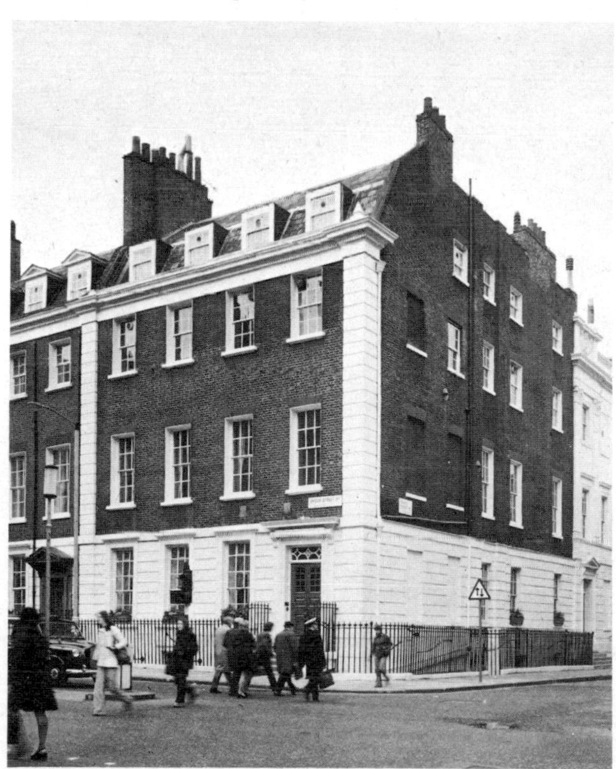

c. No. 66 Brook Street in 1973. Part of No. 68 on left. Edward Shepherd lessee of both houses, 1725. *Now the Grosvenor Office*

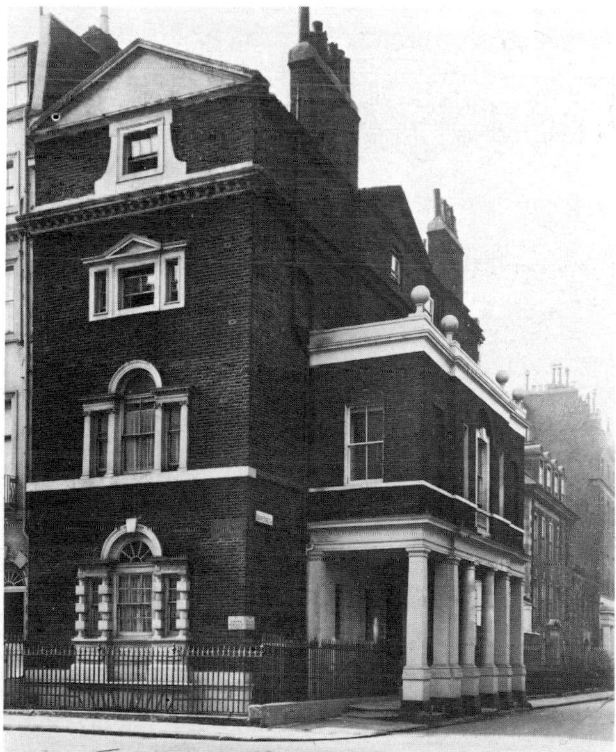

d. No. 71 South Audley Street in 1933. Thomas Skeat (bricklayer) lessee, 1736

EARLY-GEORGIAN EXTERIORS

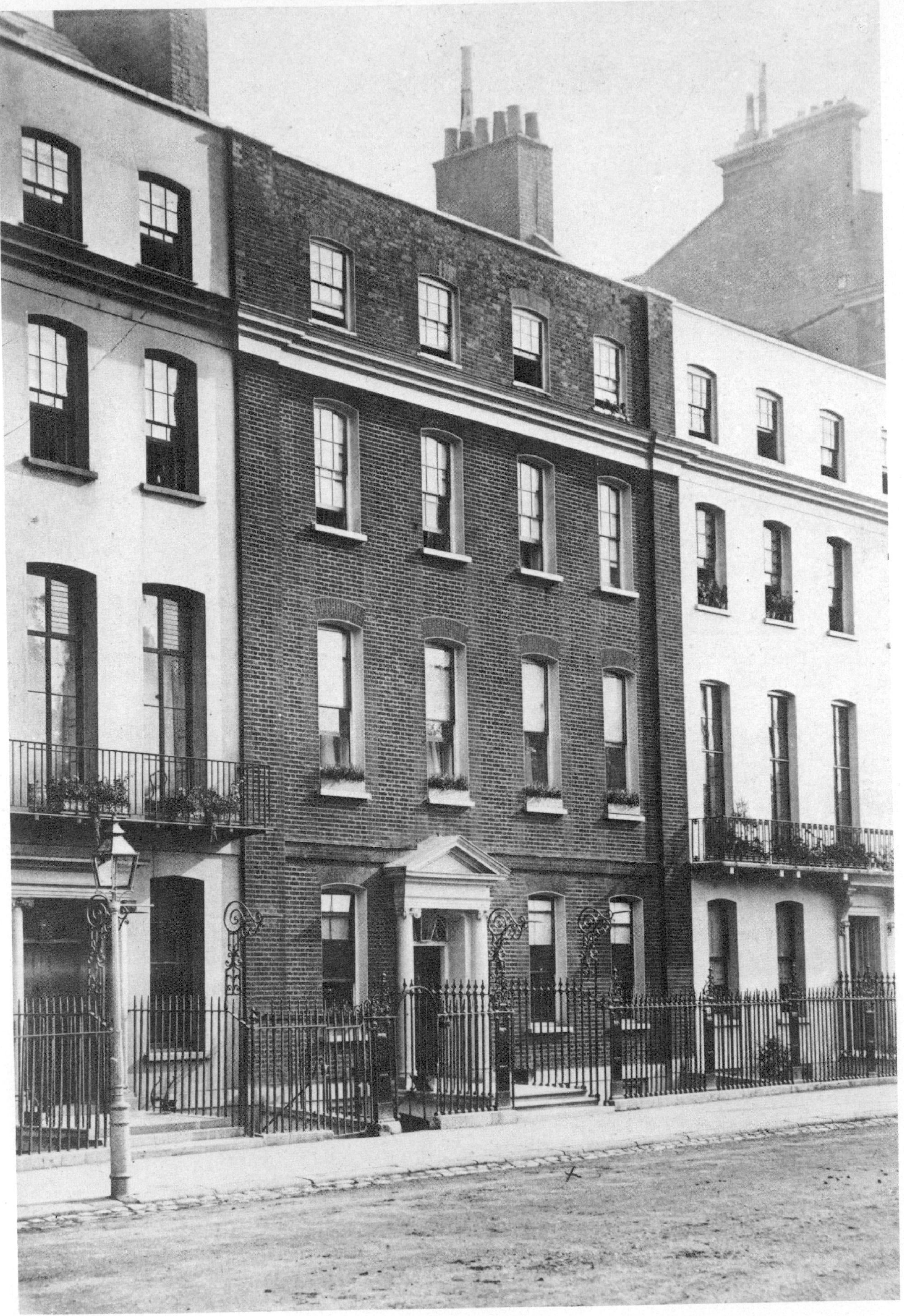

No. 44 Grosvenor Square in *c.* 1874, with No. 43 (right) and No. 45 (left). Robert Scott (carpenter) sub-lessee of No. 44, 1727. *Demolished*

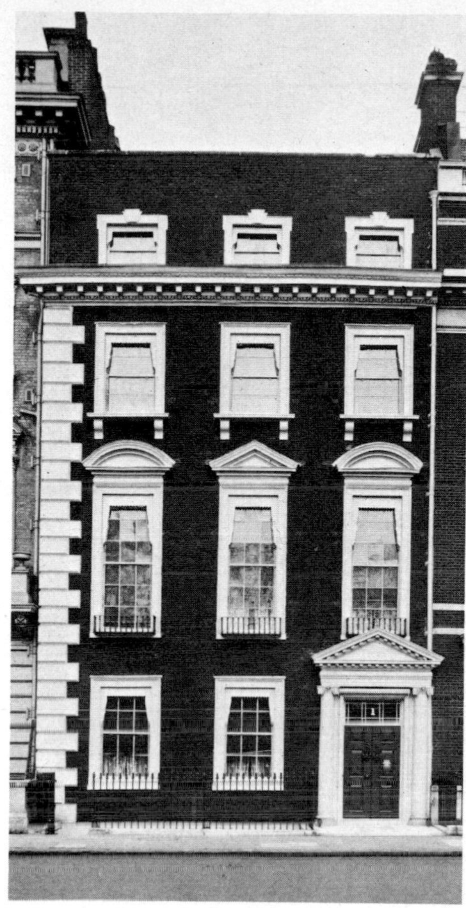

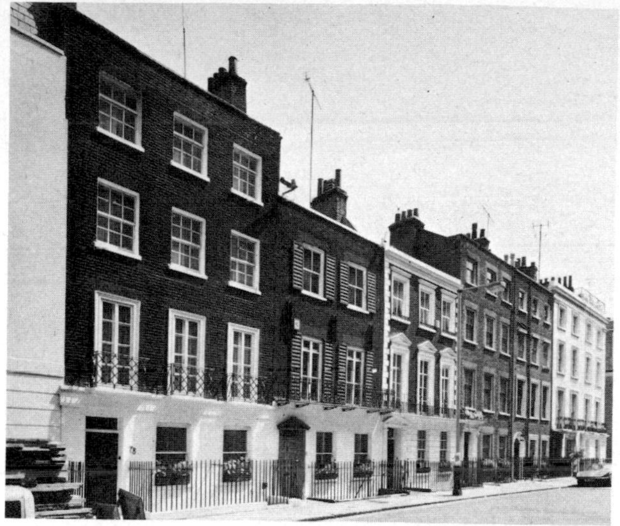

b. Nos. 70–78 (even) Park Street, *c.* 1730, in 1974 (No. 78 on left). Nos. 66 and 68 (on right) rebuilt in 1845–6

a (*above*). No. 1 Grosvenor Square in 1932. John Simmons (carpenter) lessee, 1731. *Demolished*

c (*right*). No. 53 Grosvenor Street with No. 52 (right) in *c.* 1809. Benjamin Timbrell (carpenter) lessee of No. 52, 1724: John Neale (carpenter) sub-lessee of No. 53, 1725. *No. 53 demolished*

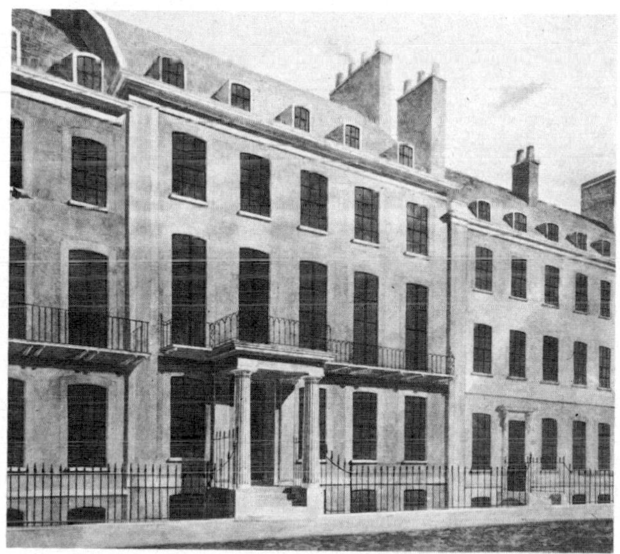

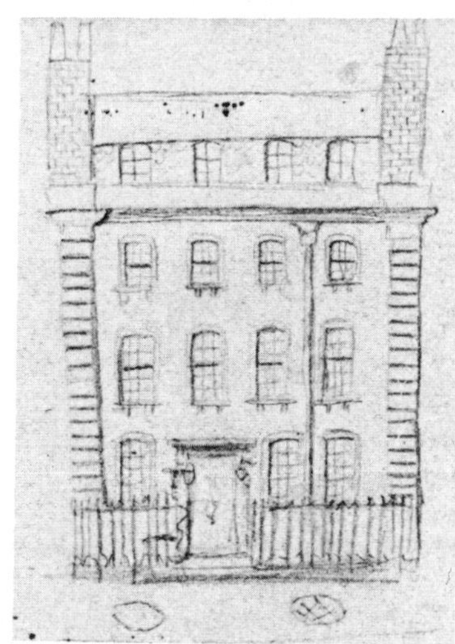

d. No. 50 Grosvenor Street in *c.* 1770–4. Charles Griffith (carpenter) lessee, 1724

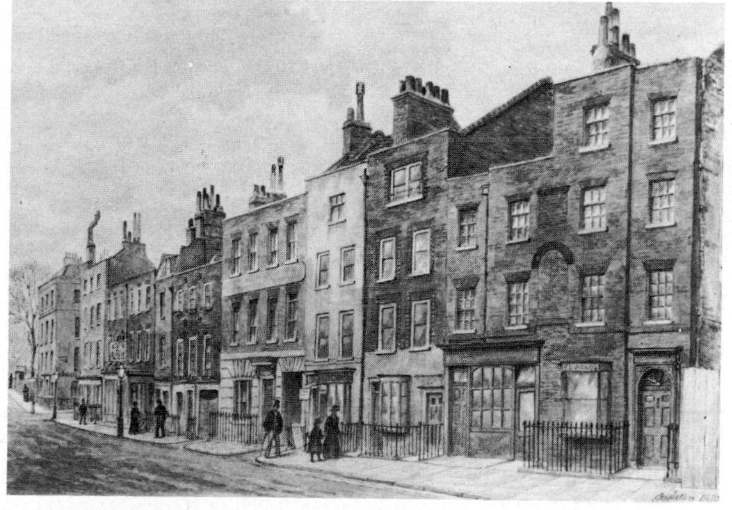

e. Mount Street, west end of north side, in 1889. *Demolished*

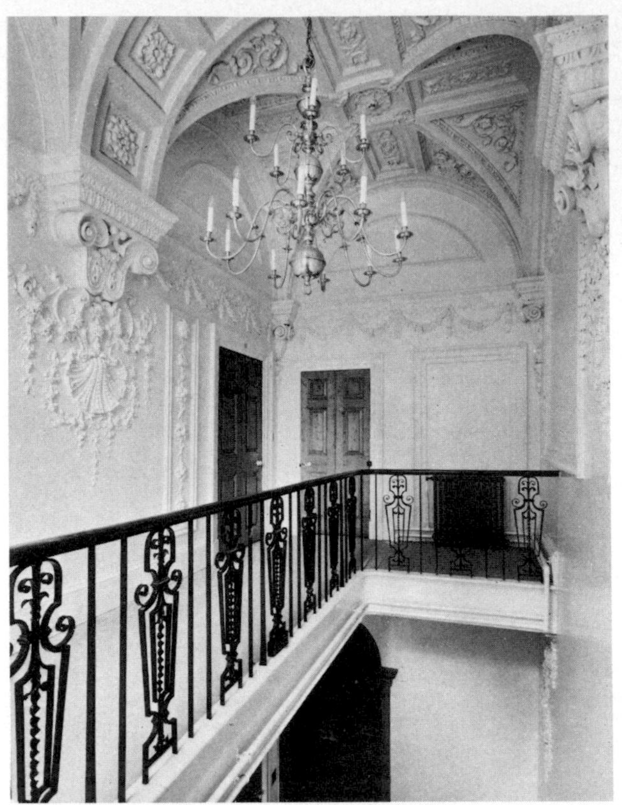

a. No. 66 Brook Street, first-floor landing to main staircase in 1974. Edward Shepherd lessee, 1725. *Now the Grosvenor Office*

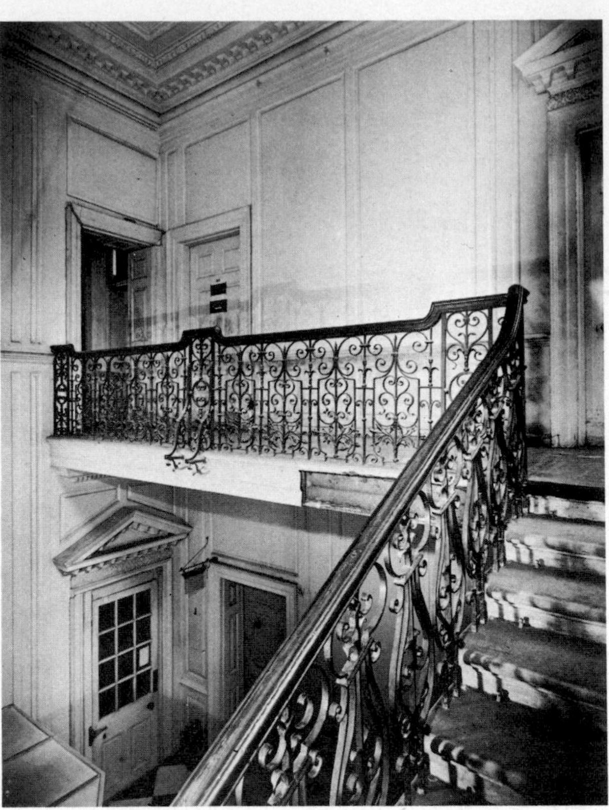

b. No. 34 Grosvenor Street, main staircase and landing in 1950. Richard Lissiman (mason) lessee, 1725

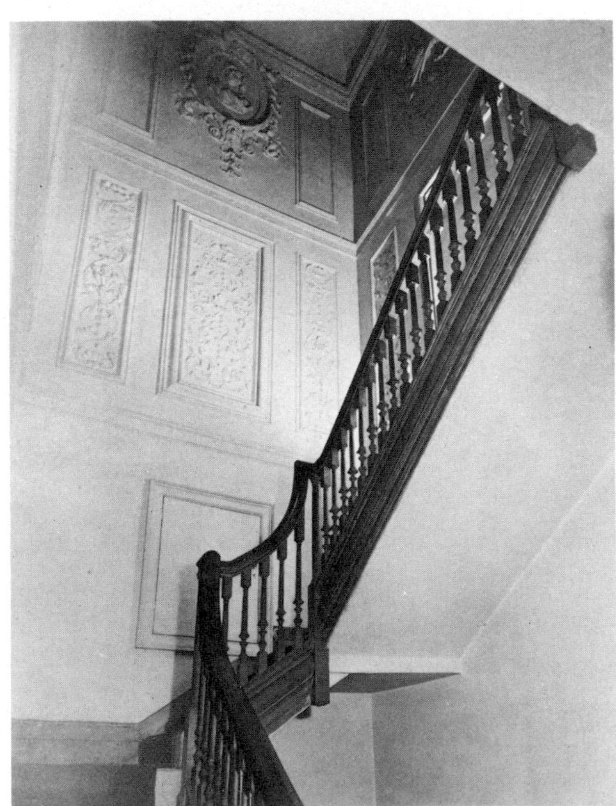

c. No. 13 South Audley Street, upper part of staircase in 1948. William Singleton (plasterer) lessee, 1736. *Plasterwork destroyed*

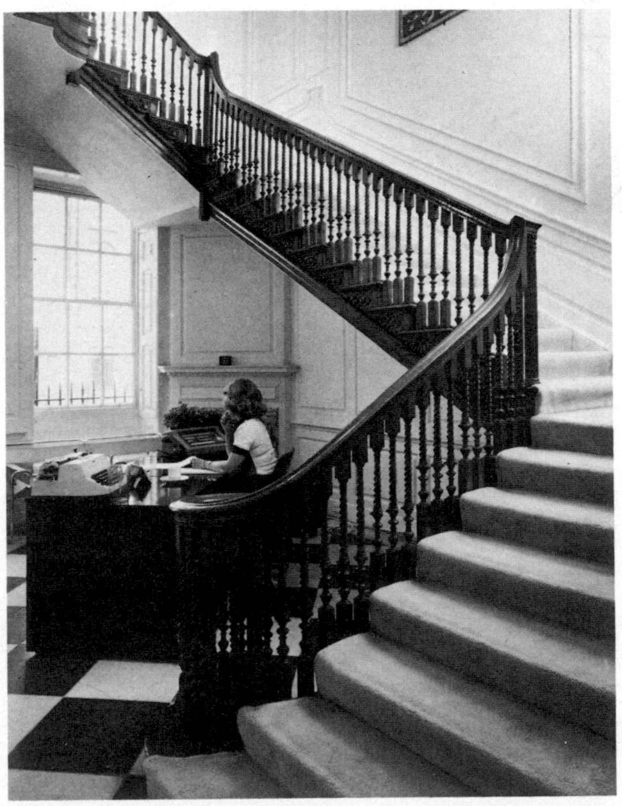

d. No. 59 Grosvenor Street, entrance hall and staircase in 1975. David Audsley (plasterer) sub-lessee, 1725. Woodwork of the staircase much restored

EARLY-GEORGIAN STAIRCASES

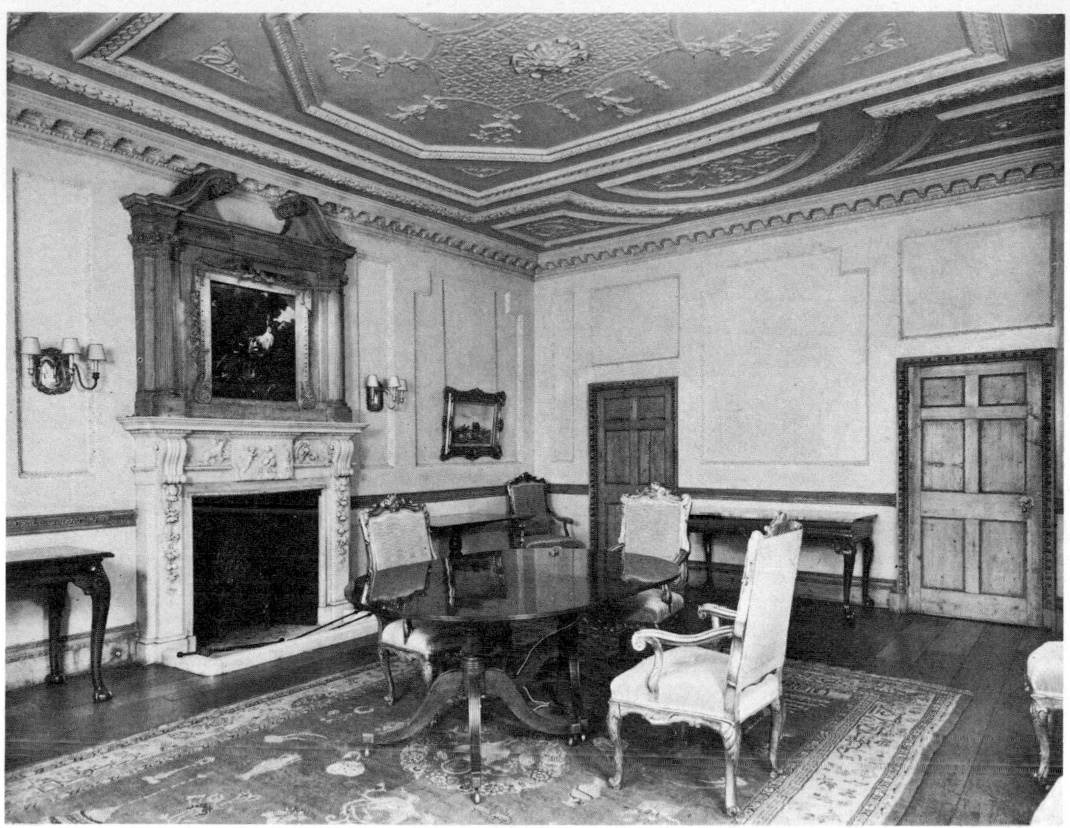

a. No. 71 South Audley Street, dining-room (ground-floor back room) in 1933. Thomas Skeat (bricklayer) lessee, 1736. Plasterwork of ceiling and walls probably by Edward Shepherd

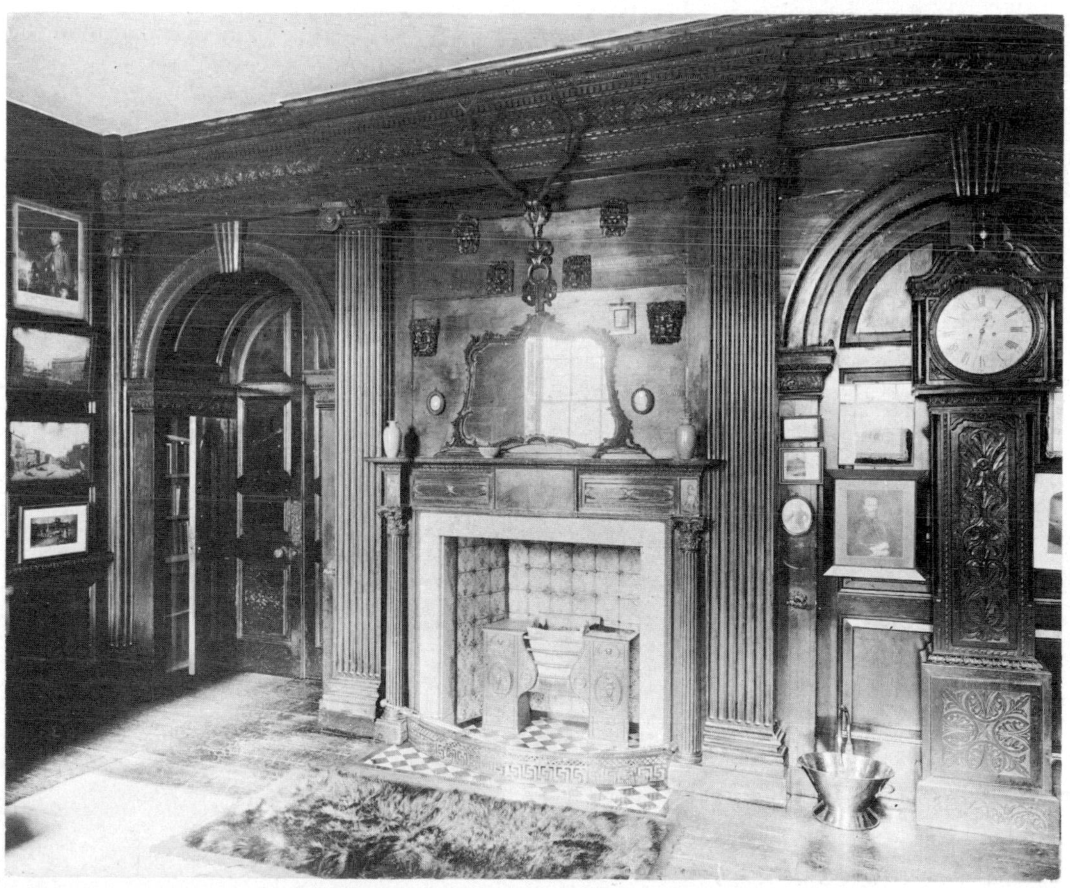

b. Bourdon House, Davies Street, 'ante-dining-room' in 1909. William Bourdon (esquire) sub-lessee, 1723. Panelled throughout in wood. Fireplace of later date

Early-Georgian Interiors: Plastering and Panelling

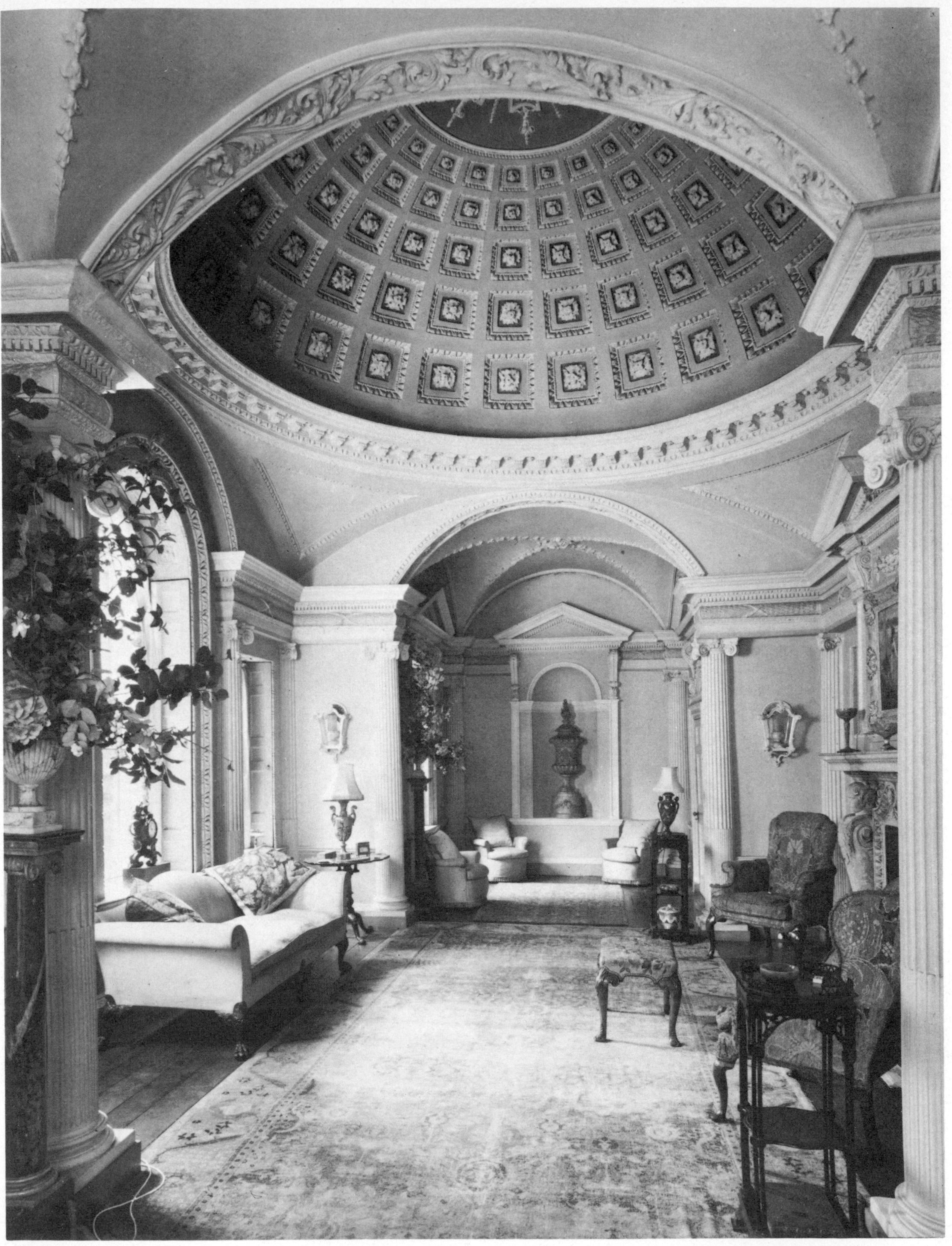

No. 12 North Audley Street, gallery in 1962, looking south. Columns and other ornamental details of plaster

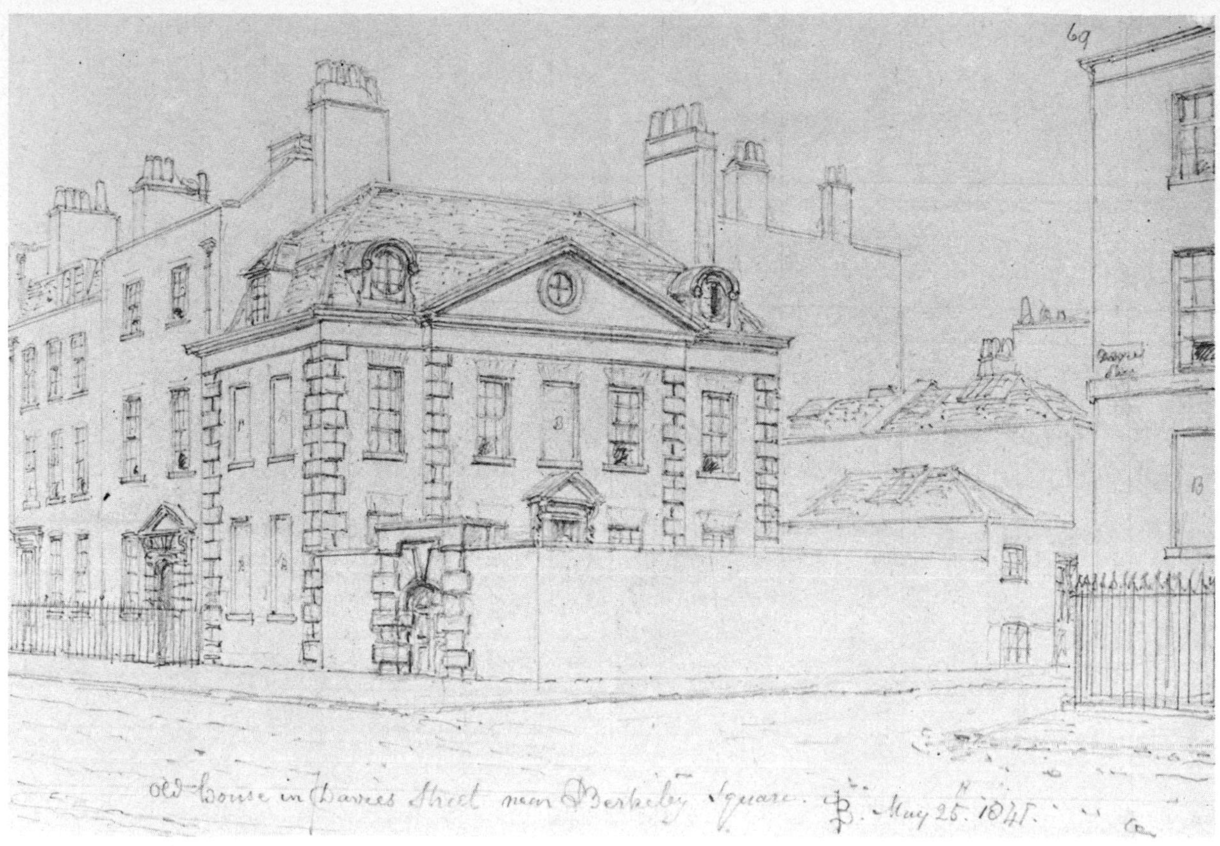
Old House in Davies Street near Berkeley Square. B. May 25th 1841.

a. Bourdon House, Davies Street, in 1841, from south-west. William Bourdon (esquire) sub-lessee, 1723

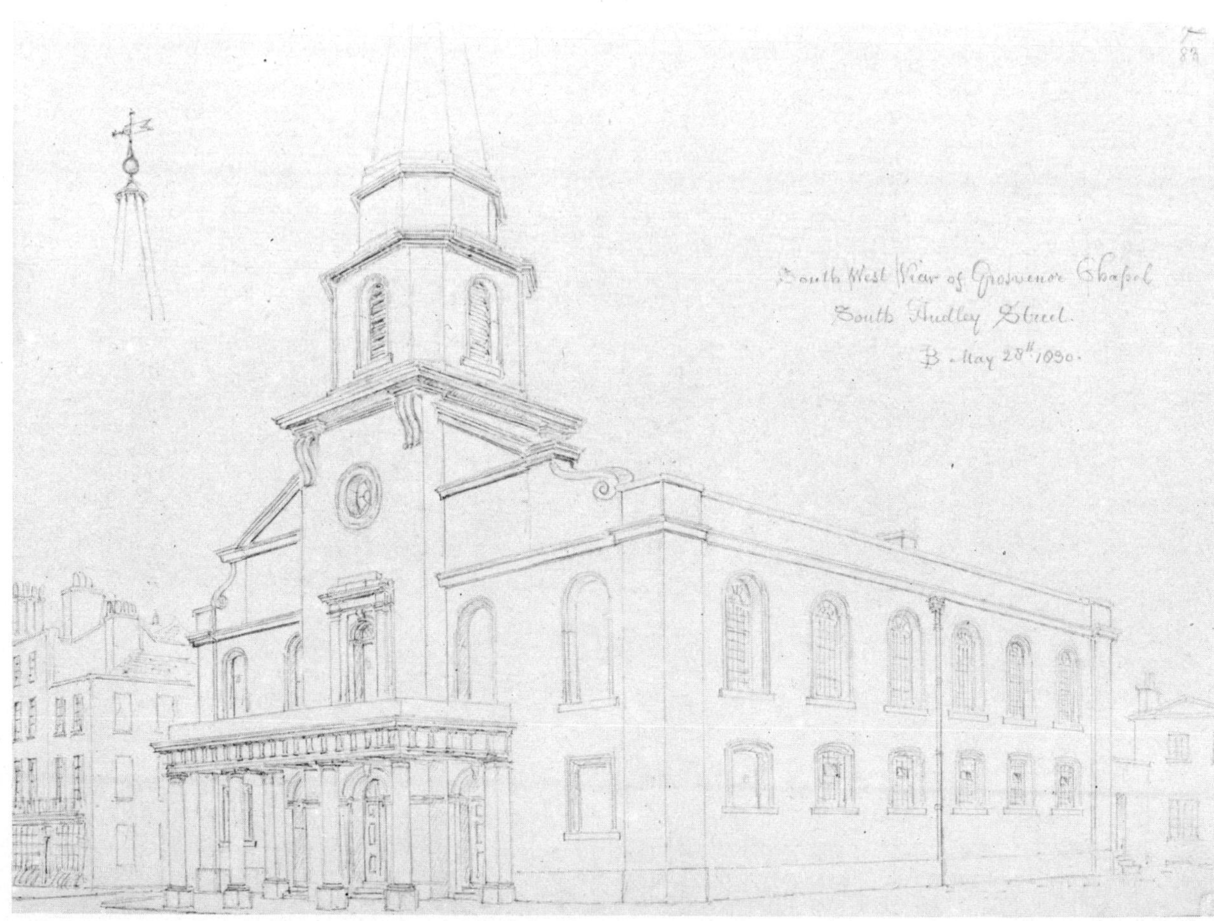
South West View of Grosvenor Chapel
South Audley Street.
B. May 28th 1830.

b. Grosvenor Chapel, South Audley Street, in 1830, from south-west. *For the presumed original state of the chapel see fig. 7 on p. 119*

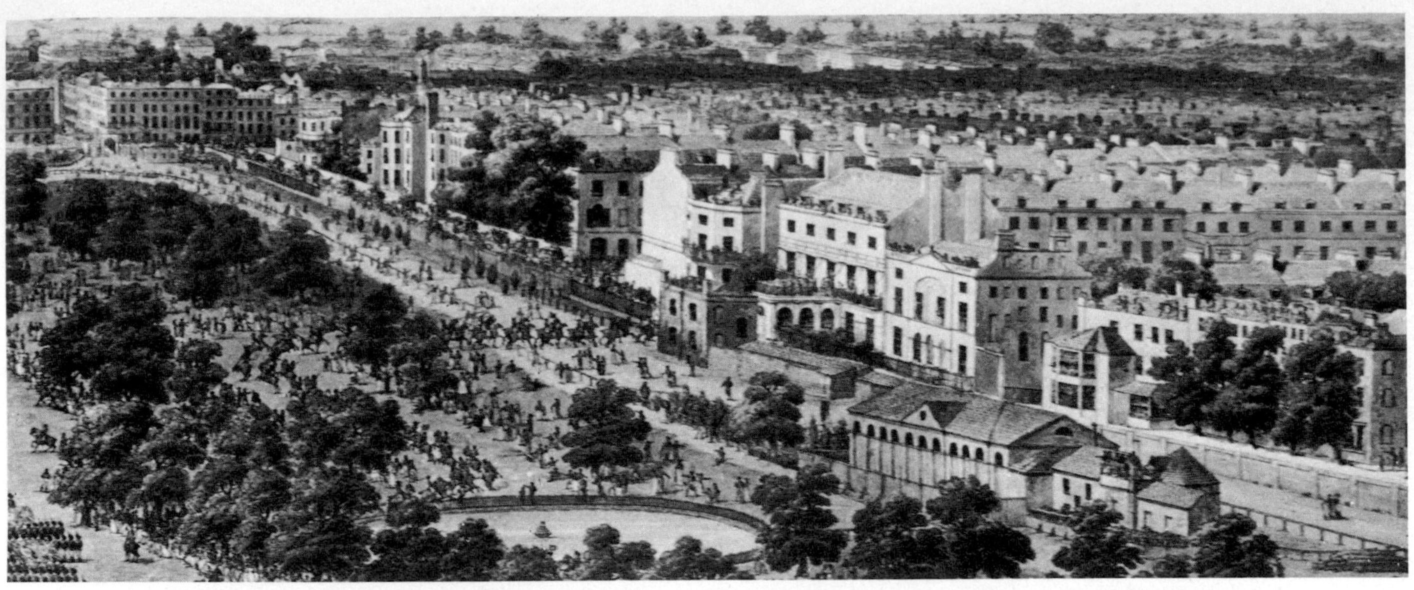

a. Park Lane, northern end from Hyde Park in 1799, showing King's Row (extreme right), the old Dudley House (right of centre with projecting porch), the end of Upper Brook Street (centre) and in the middle distance to left, the junction with Oxford Street. *Mostly demolished*

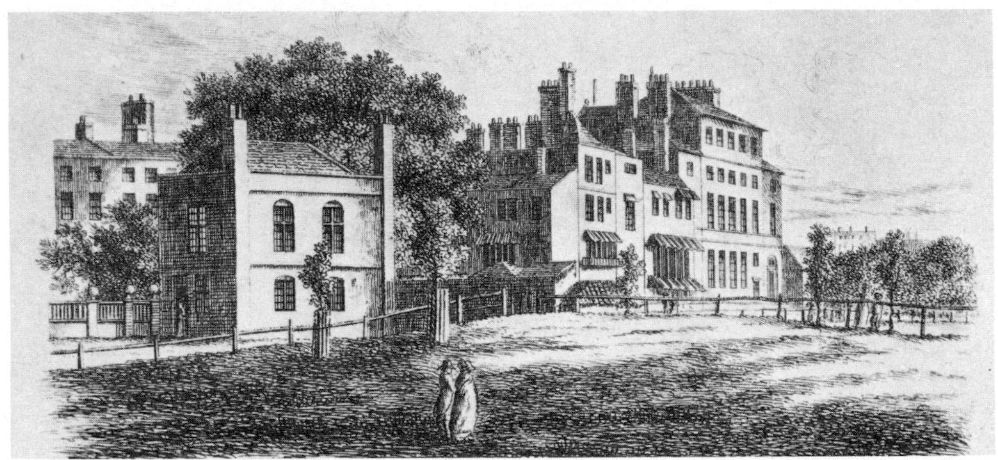

b. Park Lane, view looking south-east in *c*. 1807, showing houses in King's Row (left, behind trees), the south corner with Upper Grosvenor Street, and Breadalbane House (right). Grosvenor Gate lodge in foreground. *All demolished*

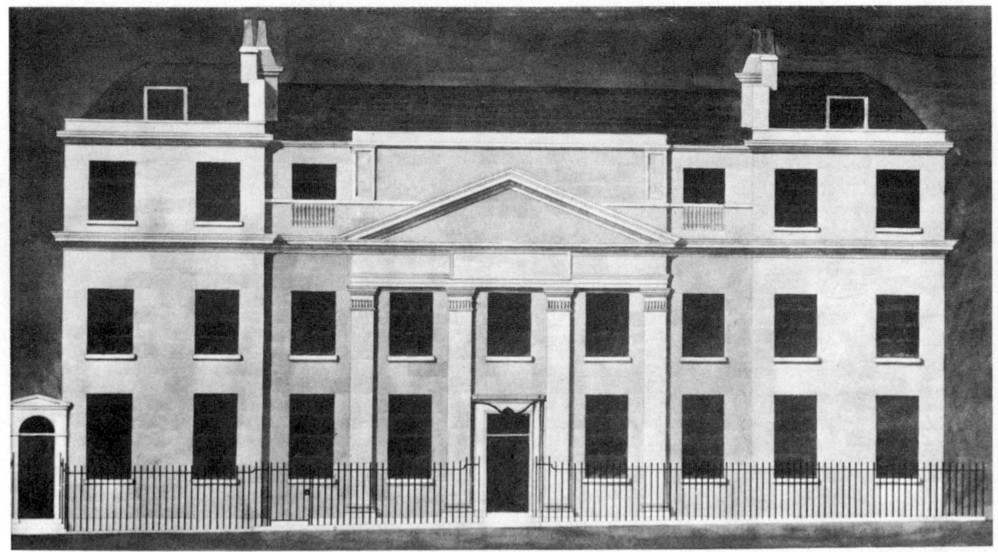

c. Park Street, elevational drawing of 1820 showing houses on west side between Hereford Street and North Row. John Crunden, architect, 1778. *Demolished*

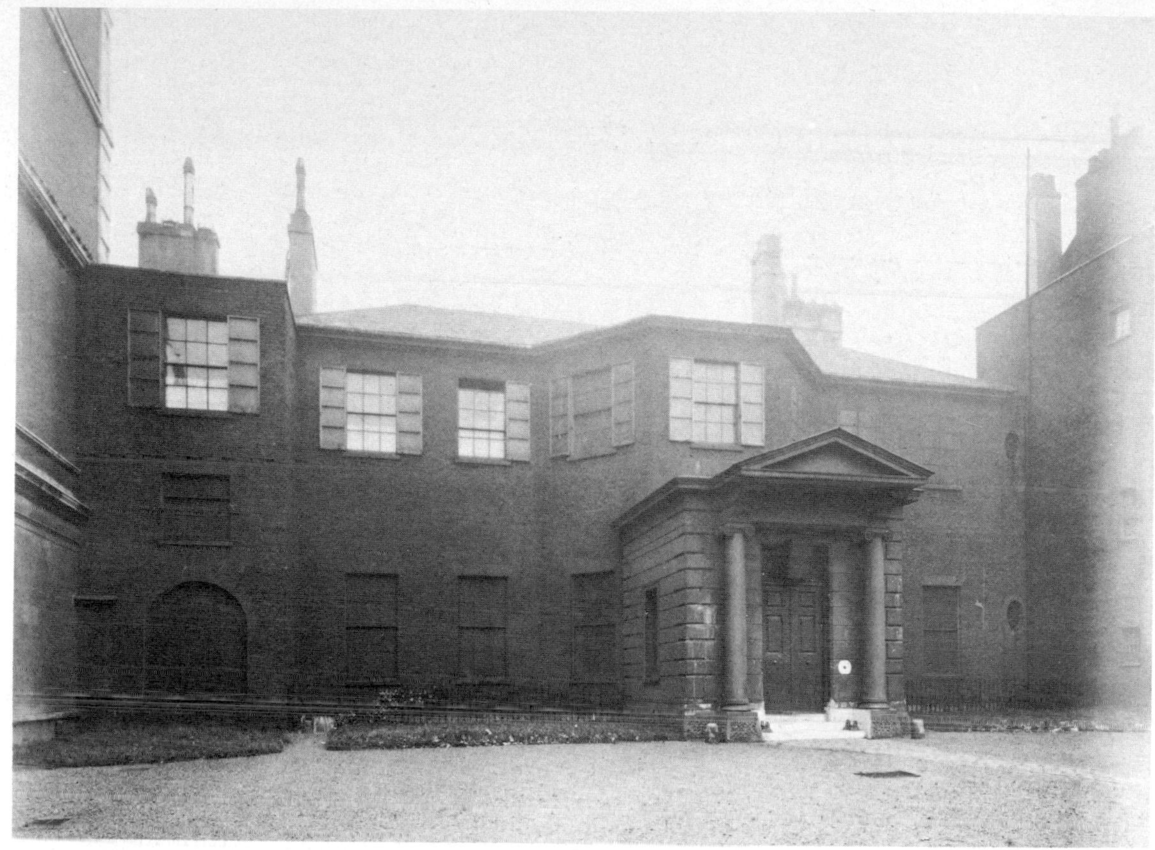

a. Camelford House, Park Lane: north front in 1912. Hereford Gardens abuts to the left, Somerset House to the right. *Demolished*

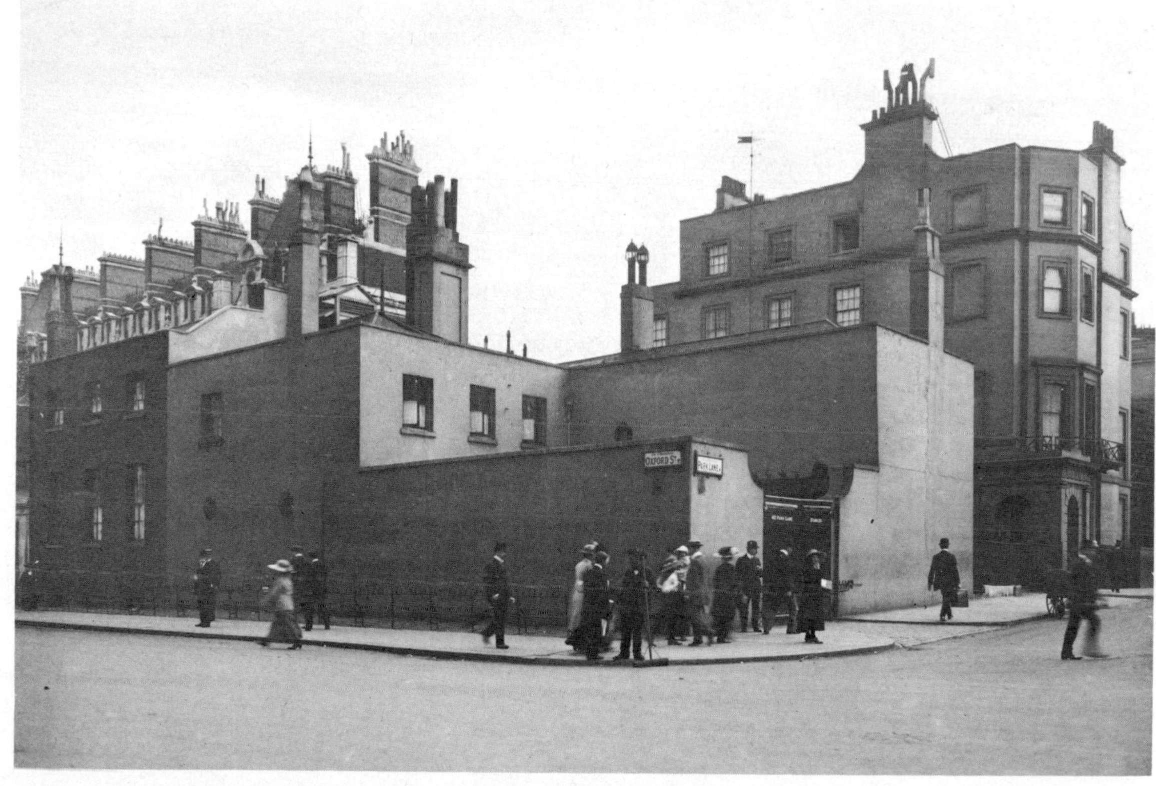

b. Somerset House, Park Lane: house (right) and stables (centre) in 1912, from junction of Park Lane and Oxford Street. Outbuildings of Camelford House in left foreground with roofs of Hereford Gardens behind. *All demolished*

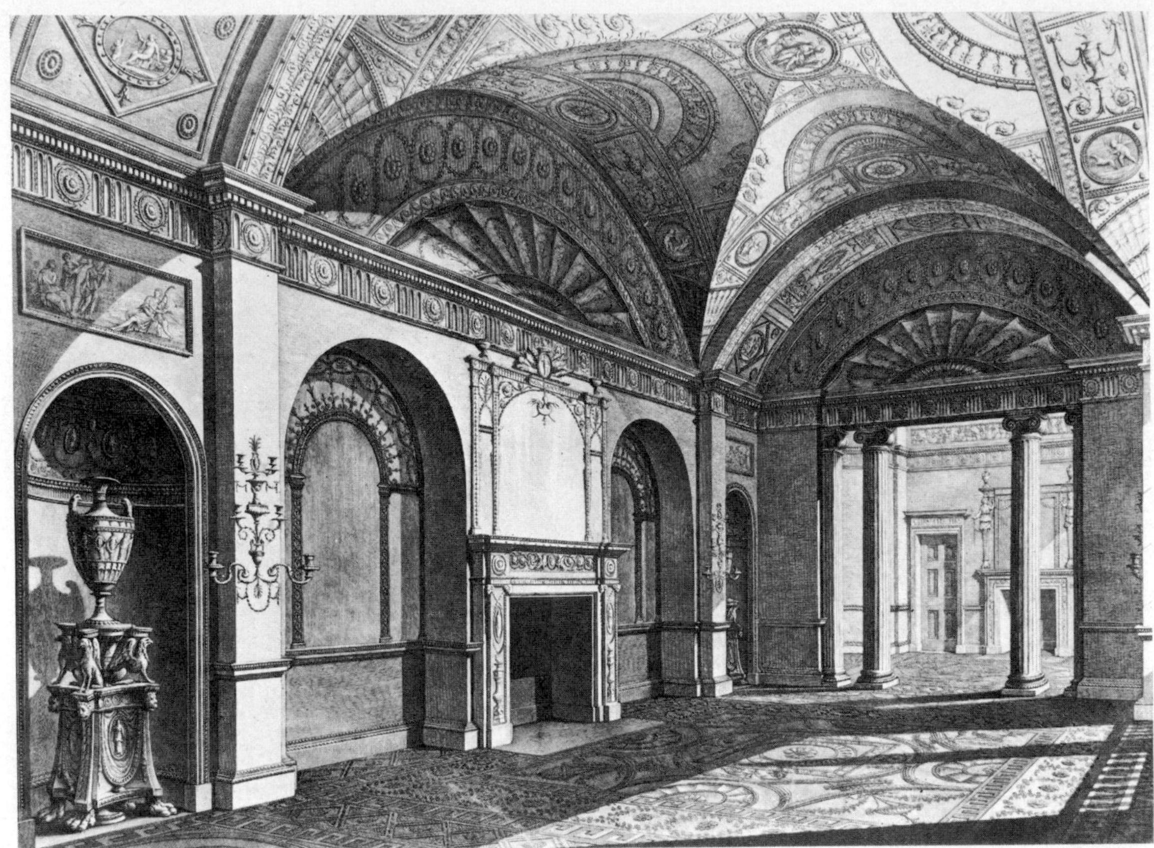

a. No. 26 Grosvenor Square (Derby House), perspective view of 'third drawing-room' in 1777. Robert Adam, architect, 1773–4. *Demolished*

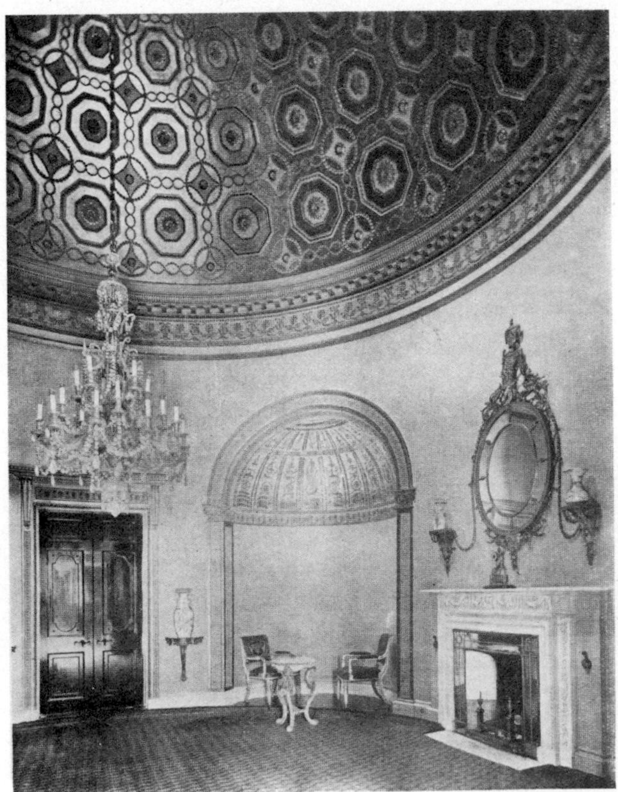

b. No. 19 Grosvenor Square, the dome room in 1919. Robert and James Adam, architects, *c.* 1764–5. *Demolished*

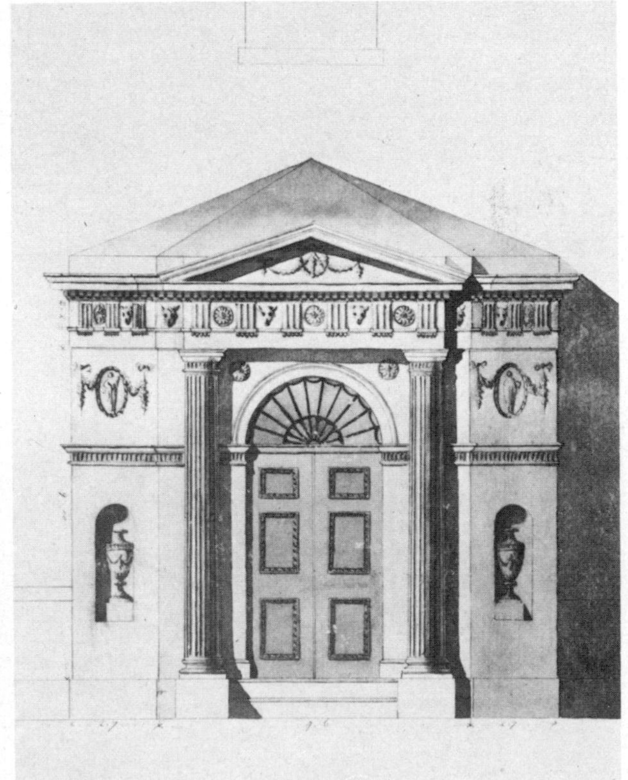

c. Design for porch at Claudius Amyand's house, corner of Mount Street and Berkeley Square. Robert or James Adam, architect, probably *c.* 1761. *Either demolished or not executed*

a. Lord Petre's house, Park Lane (later Breadalbane House), engraving of drawing-room ceiling, 1783. James Paine, architect, 1766–70. *Demolished*

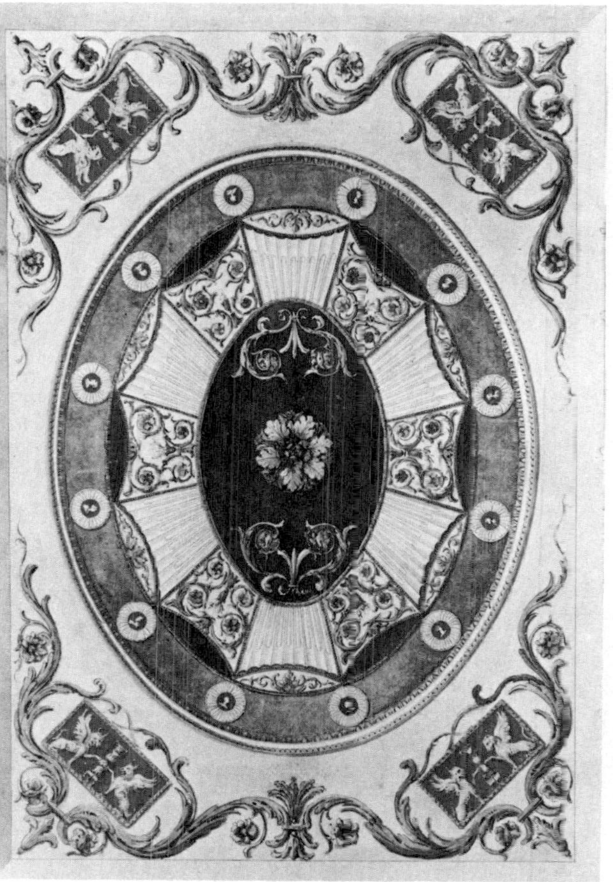

b. No. 16 Grosvenor Street, design by Robert Adam for drawing-room ceiling, 1761. *Possibly not executed*

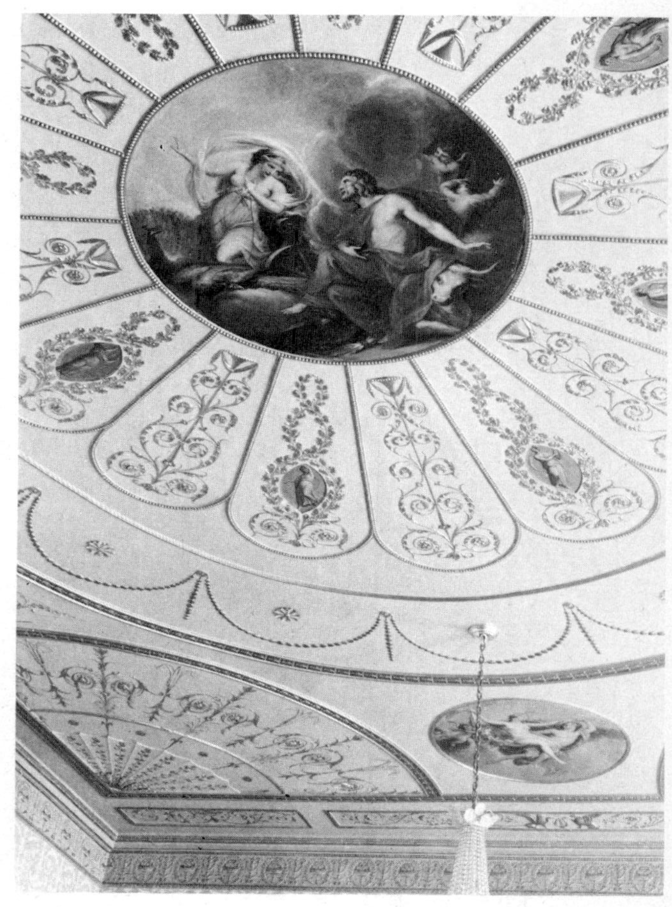

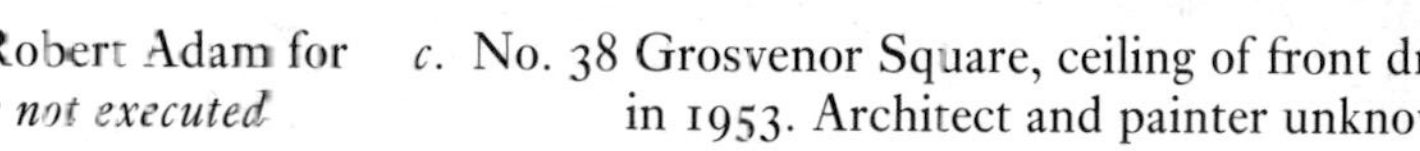

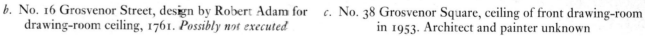

c. No. 38 Grosvenor Square, ceiling of front drawing-room in 1953. Architect and painter unknown

MID-GEORGIAN CEILINGS

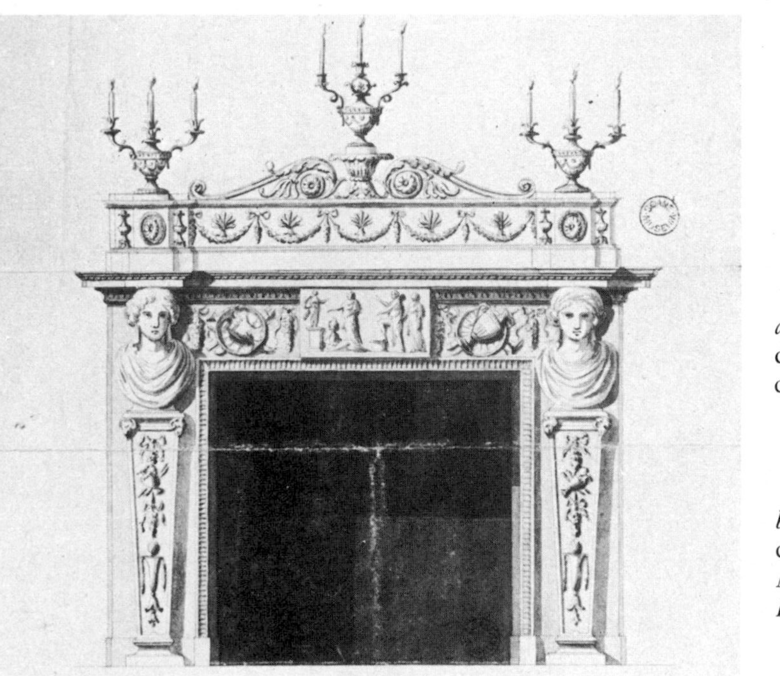

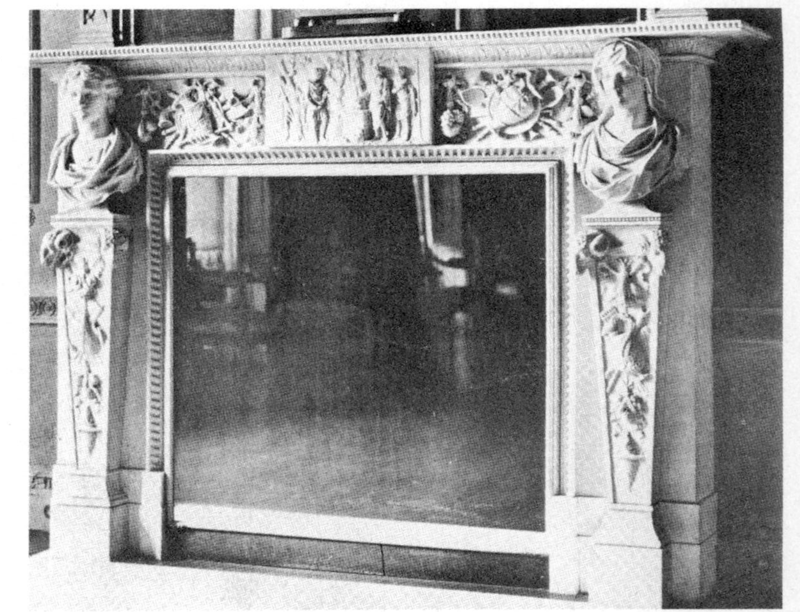

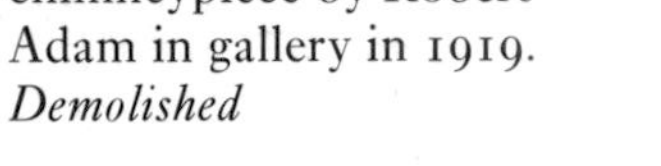

a. No. 19 Grosvenor Square, design by Robert Adam for chimneypiece in gallery, 1764

b. No. 19 Grosvenor Square, chimneypiece by Robert Adam in gallery in 1919. *Demolished*

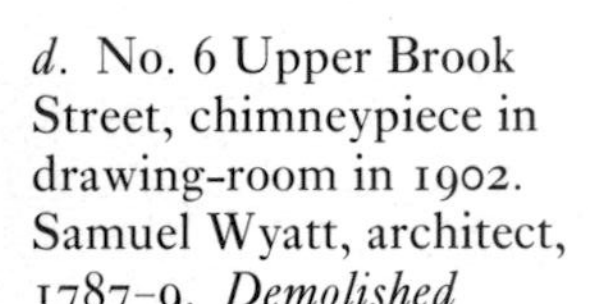

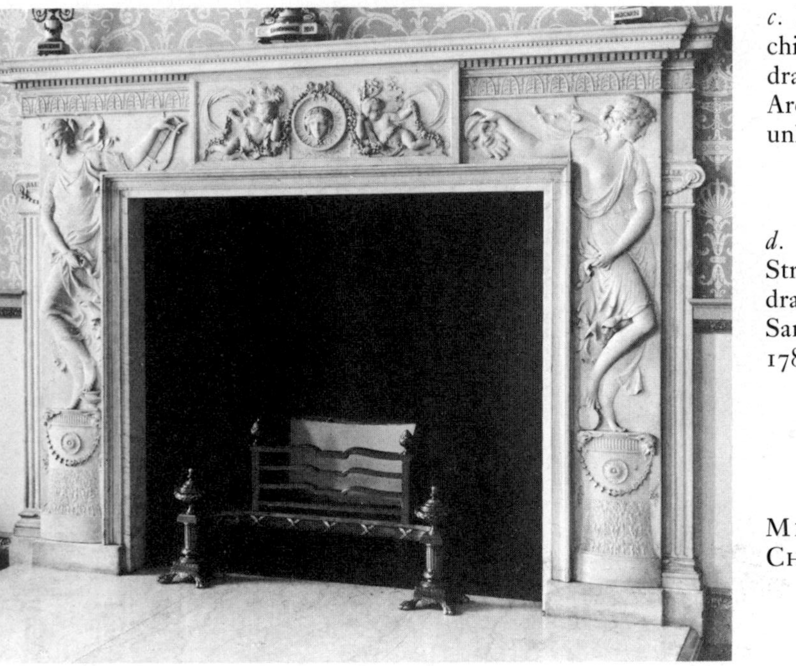

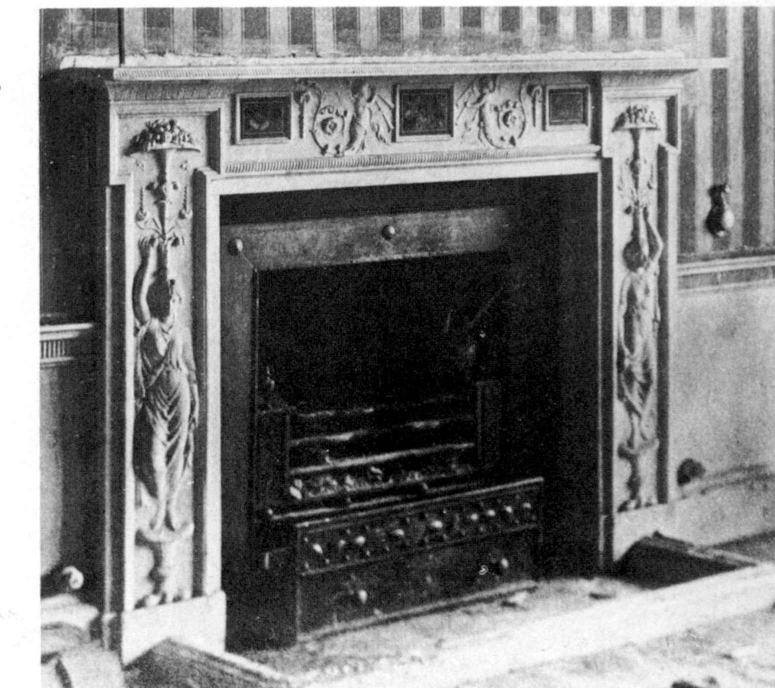

c. No. 38 Grosvenor Square, chimneypiece in front drawing-room in 1953. Architect and carver unknown

d. No. 6 Upper Brook Street, chimneypiece in drawing-room in 1902. Samuel Wyatt, architect, 1787–9. *Demolished*

MID-GEORGIAN CHIMNEYPIECES

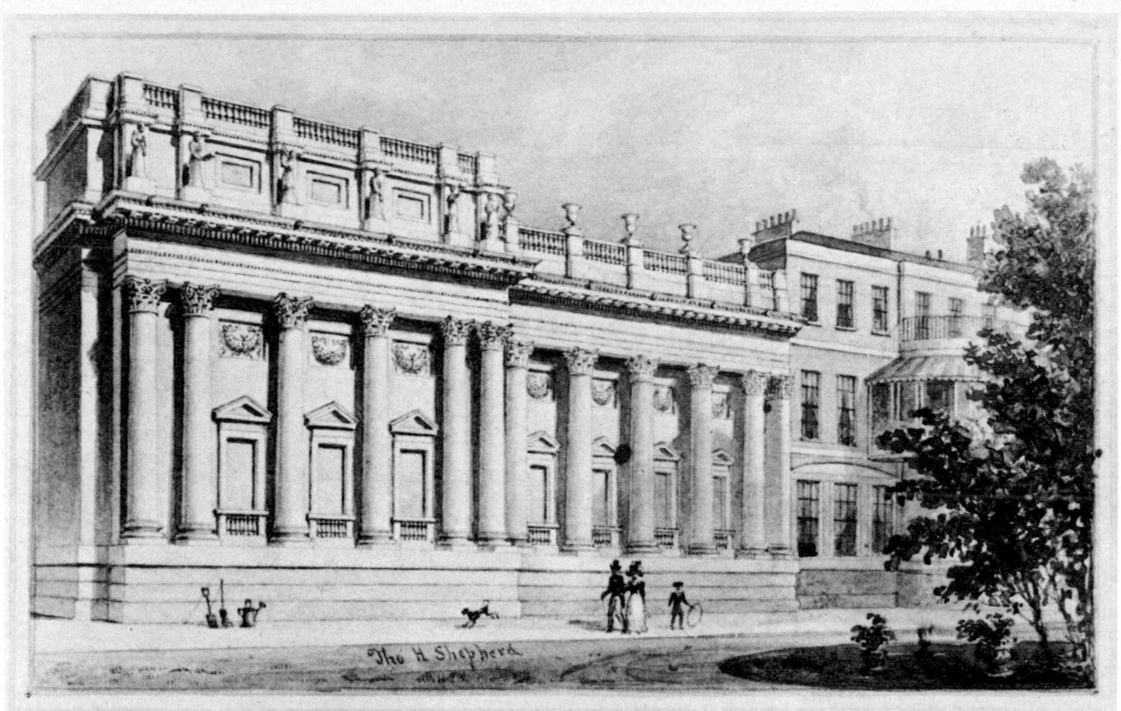

a. South front in *c*. 1827–8, showing new gallery by Thomas Cundy I and II (1826–7), and (right) old house as altered by William Porden (1806–8). *Demolished*

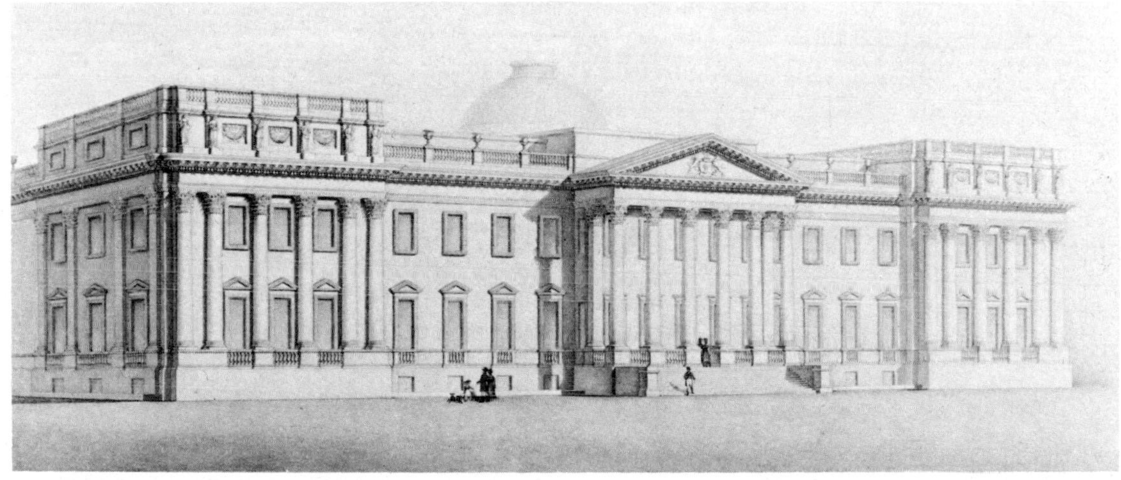

b. Design of 1827 by Thomas Cundy II for enlargement, showing proposed new entrance front on south side masking gallery shown above. *Not executed*

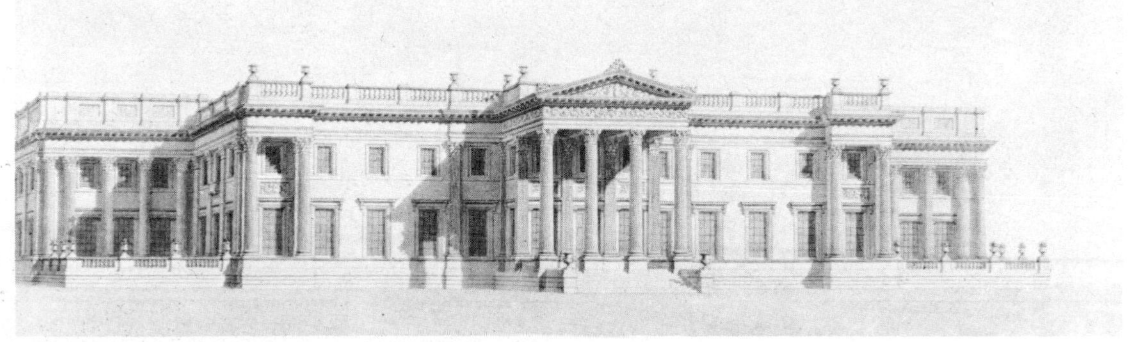

c. Design of 1827 by Robert Smirke for enlargement, showing south front. *Not executed*

GROSVENOR HOUSE

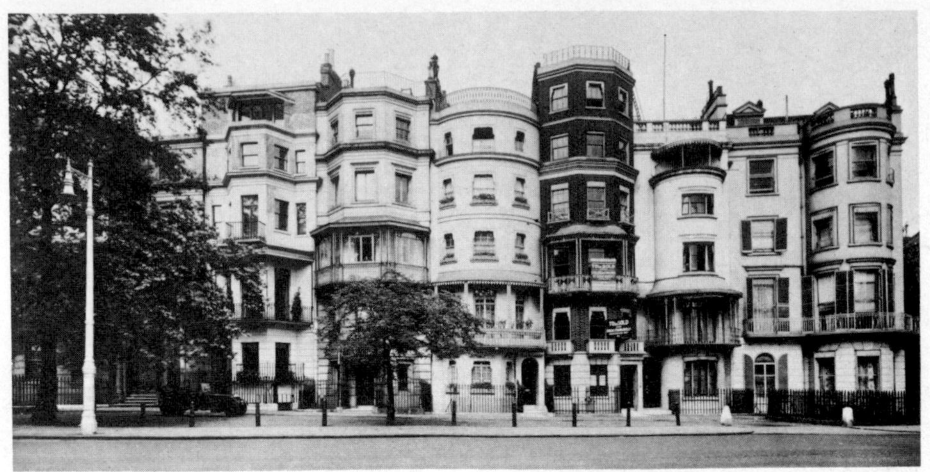

a. Nos. 93–99 (consec.). The houses are numbered from right to left, and mostly date from the 1820's, with later additions

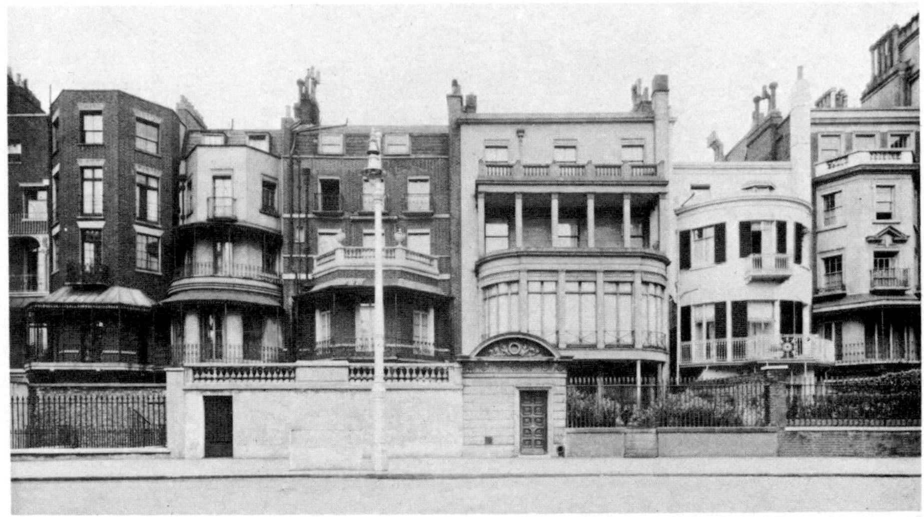

b. Nos. 26–31 (consec.) Dunraven Street, backs facing the park. Mid-Georgian houses with later additions, numbering from left to right. *All demolished*

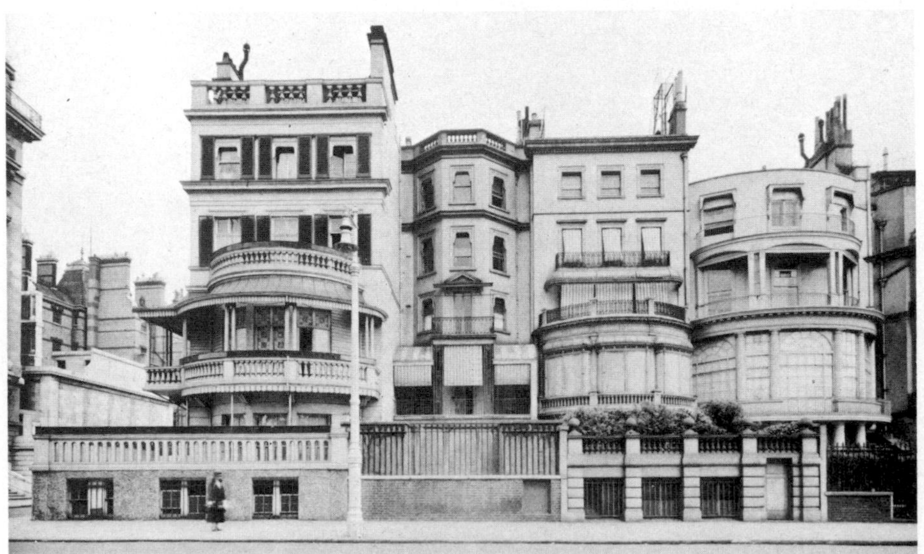

c. No. 138 Park Lane (left) and Nos. 20–22 (consec.) Dunraven Street, backs facing the park. Mostly mid-Georgian houses with later additions. No. 138 Park Lane rebuilt by John Elger in 1831–2; No. 22 Dunraven Street (right) altered by (Sir) John Soane, 1801

PARK LANE, HOUSES FACING HYDE PARK IN 1927

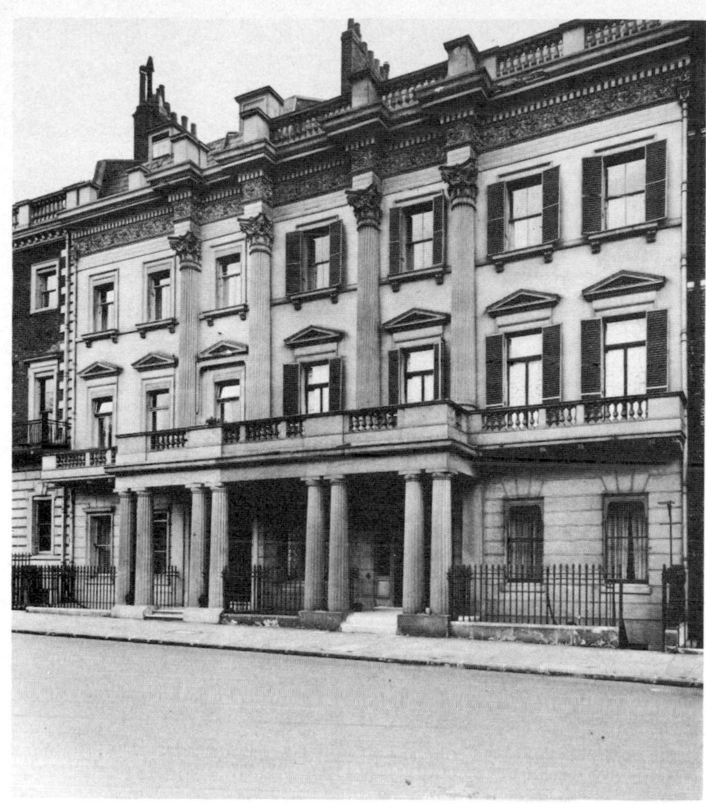

a. Nos. 15 and 16 Grosvenor Square (Belgrave House), in *c*. 1932. Fronts by Thomas Cundy II, 1822–4. *Demolished*

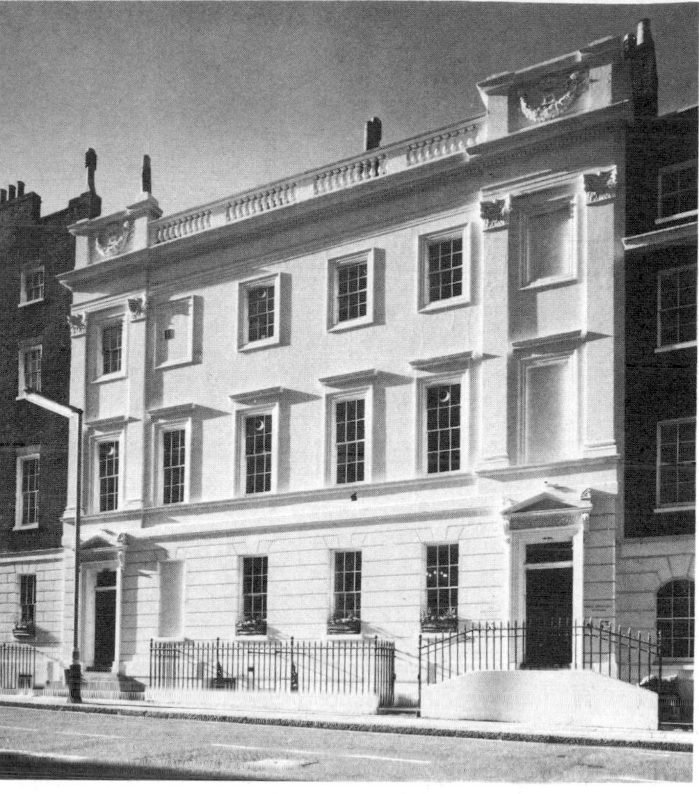

b. No. 53 Davies Street (the Grosvenor Office), in 1973. Façade probably by Thomas Cundy II, *c*. 1836

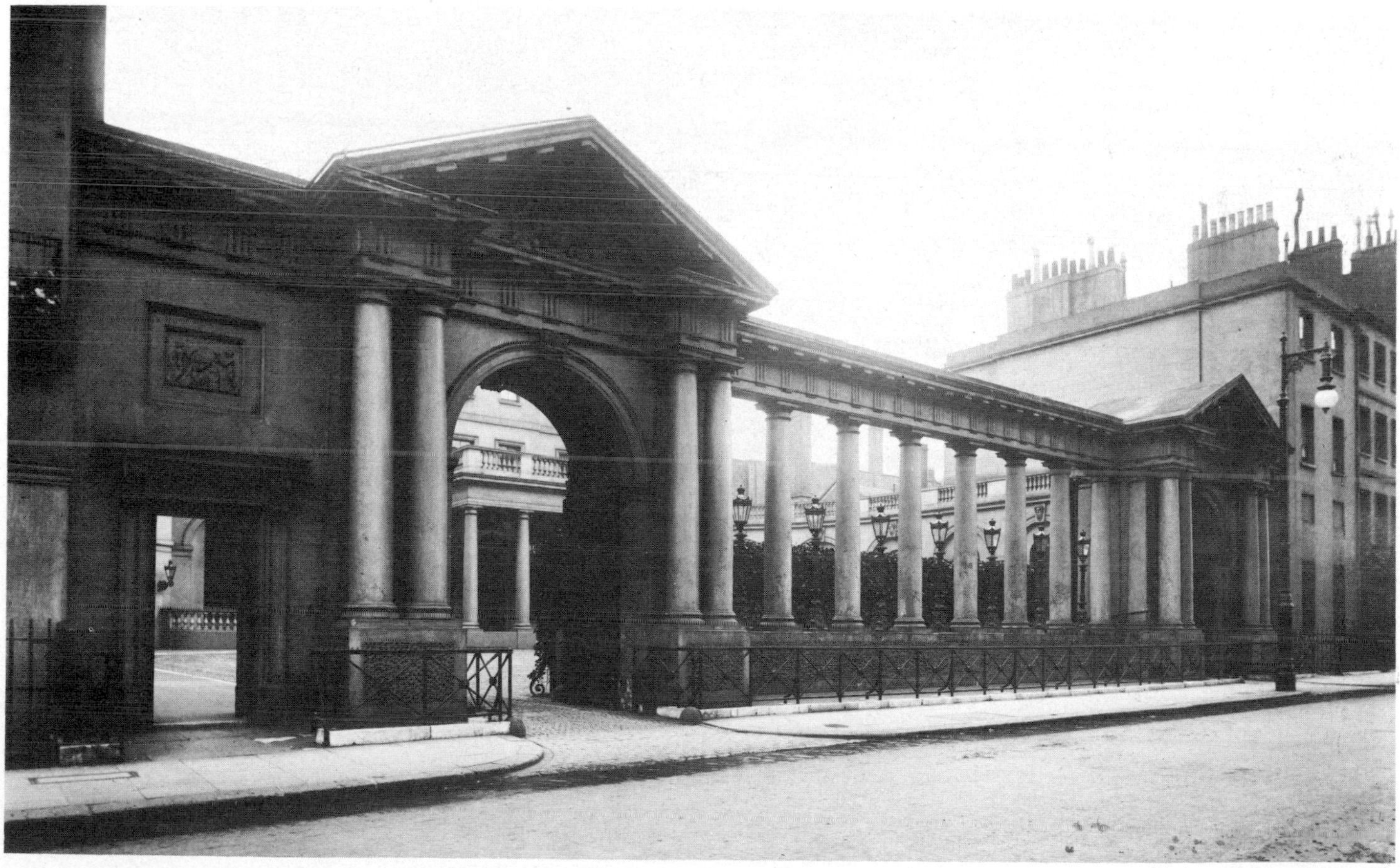

c. Grosvenor House, screen to Upper Grosvenor Street in early 20th century. Thomas Cundy II, architect, and John Elger, builder, 1842–3. *Demolished*

EARLY WORKS BY THOMAS CUNDY II

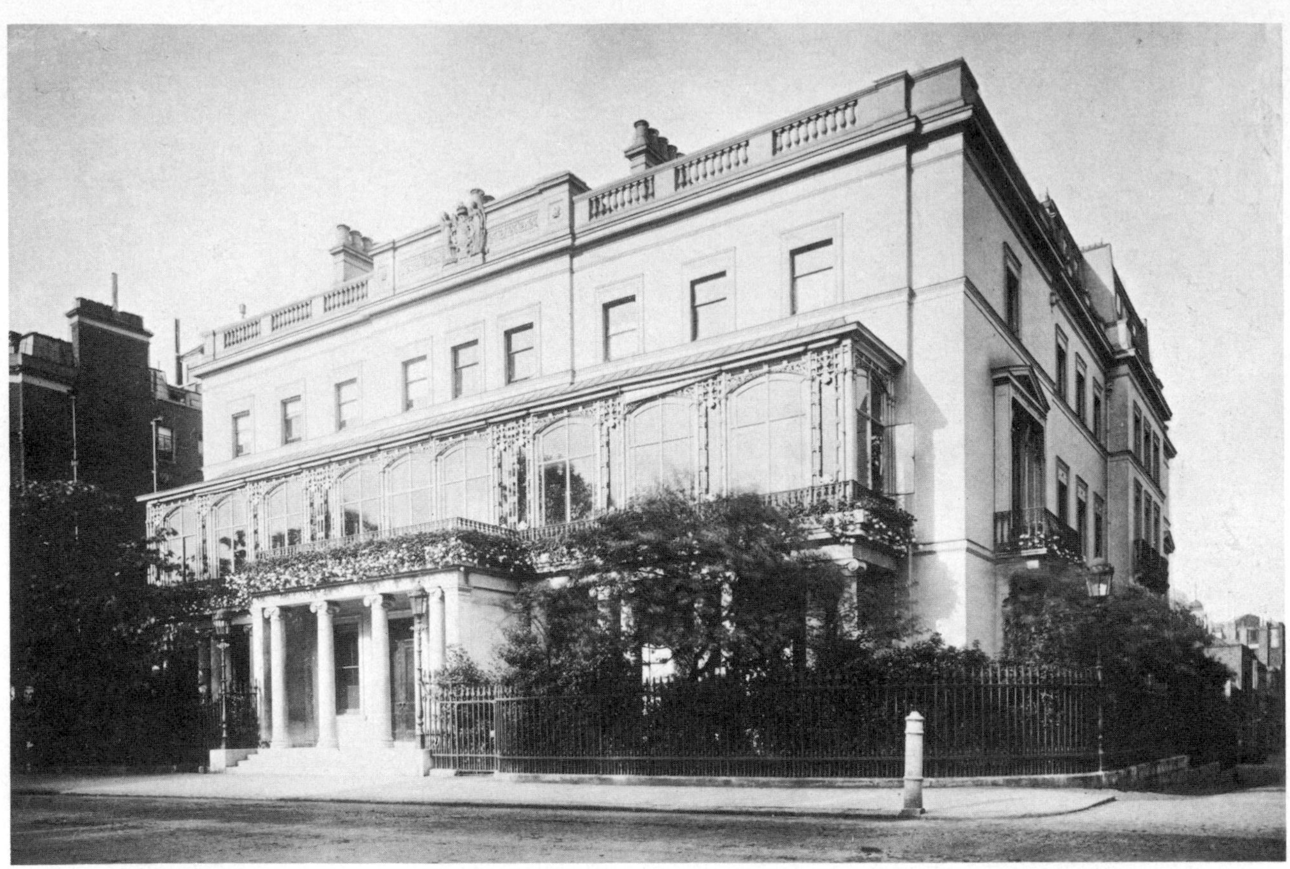

a. Park Lane front in 1890. The veranda is Victorian

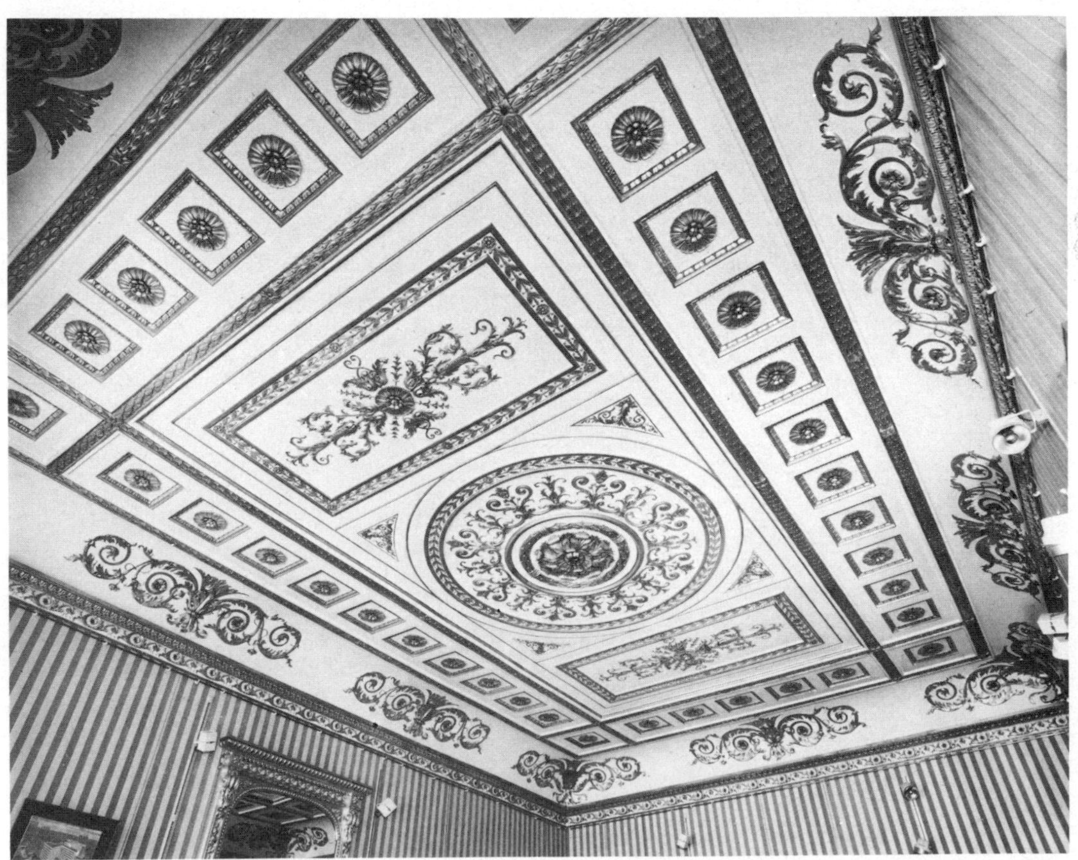

b. Ceiling in old dining-room, ground floor, in 1975

DUDLEY HOUSE, PARK LANE. William Atkinson, architect, 1827–8

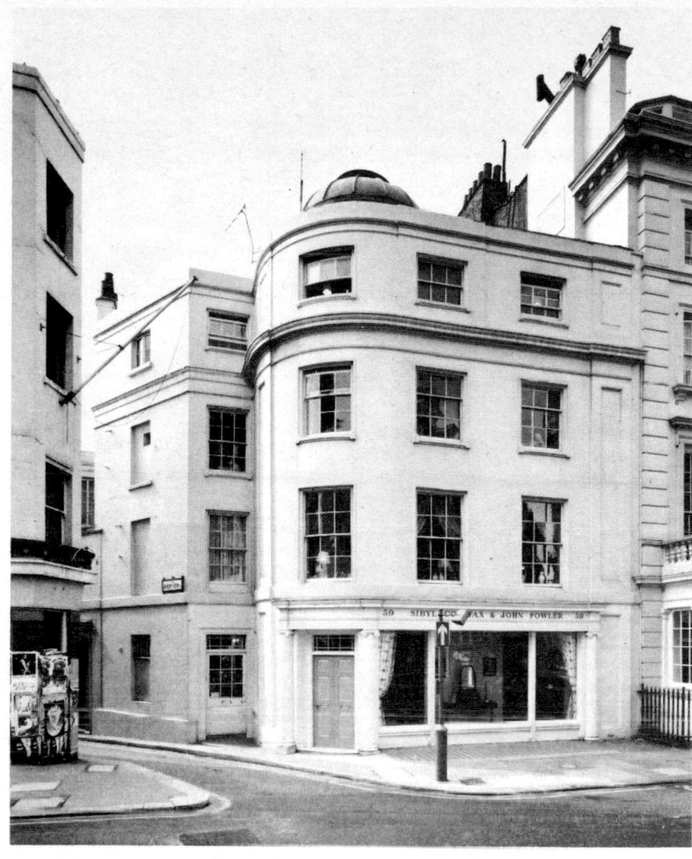

a. No. 39 Brook Street in 1971, showing front as altered by Jeffry Wyatt, *c*. 1821. The shop front is of *c*. 1927

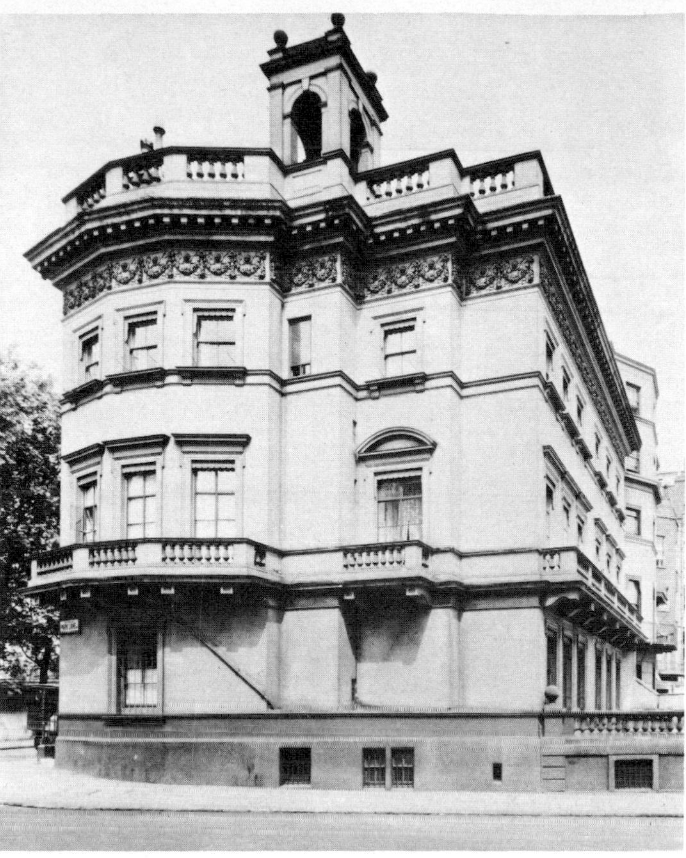

b. No. 2 South Street in 1927, from Park Lane. Façades designed by Sir Charles Barry, 1852. *Demolished*

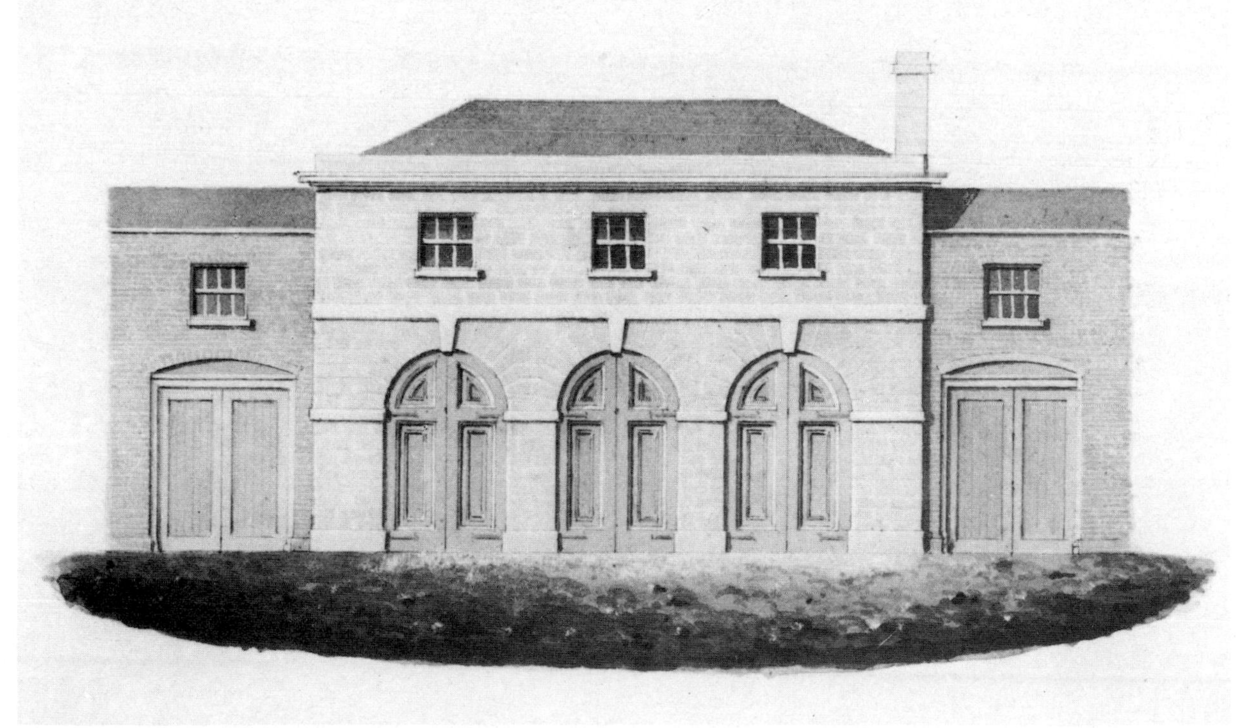

c. Wood's Mews, design for stables for S. J. Loyd by George Stanley Repton, *c*. 1823

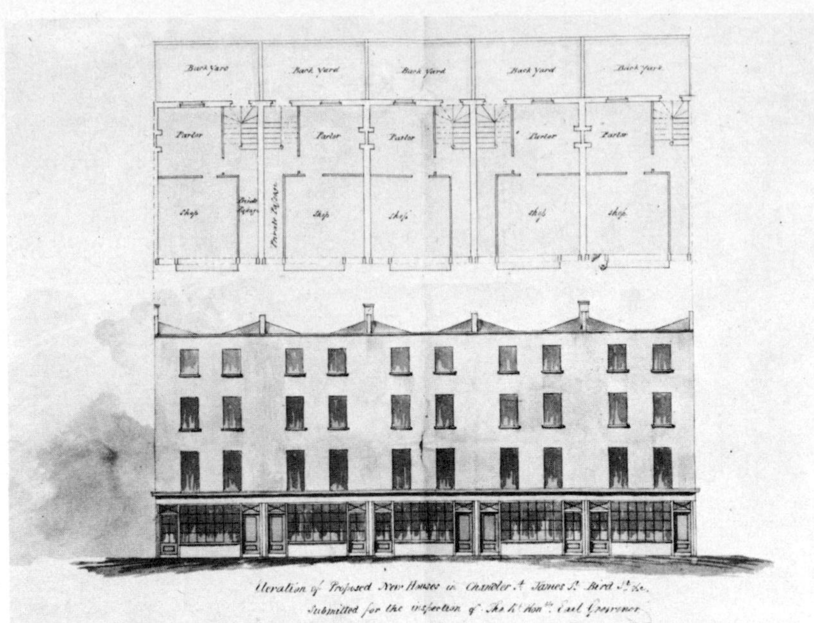

a. Ground-plan and elevation for houses and shops to be built by Seth Smith in the Gilbert Street and Weighhouse Street area. Drawing signed by [Seth] Smith and [?William] Maberley, 1821. *Demolished*

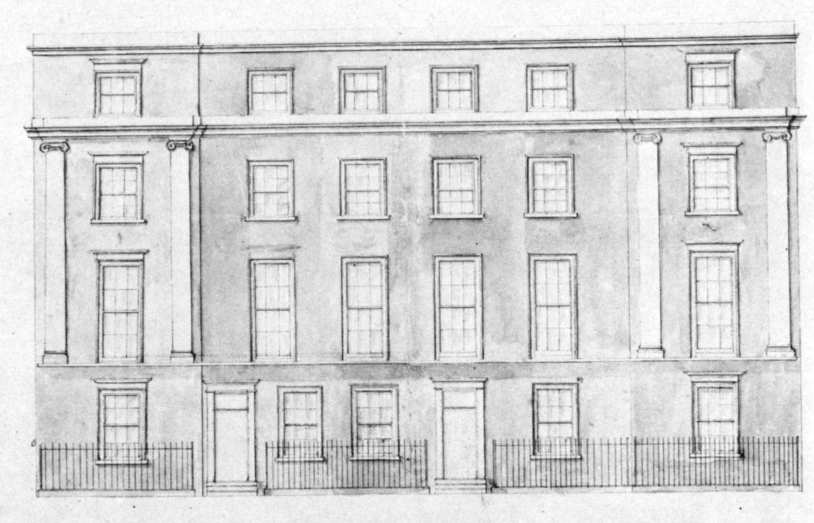

b. Elevation of houses to be built by William Skeat at the west end of Mount Street, *c.* 1830. *Demolished*

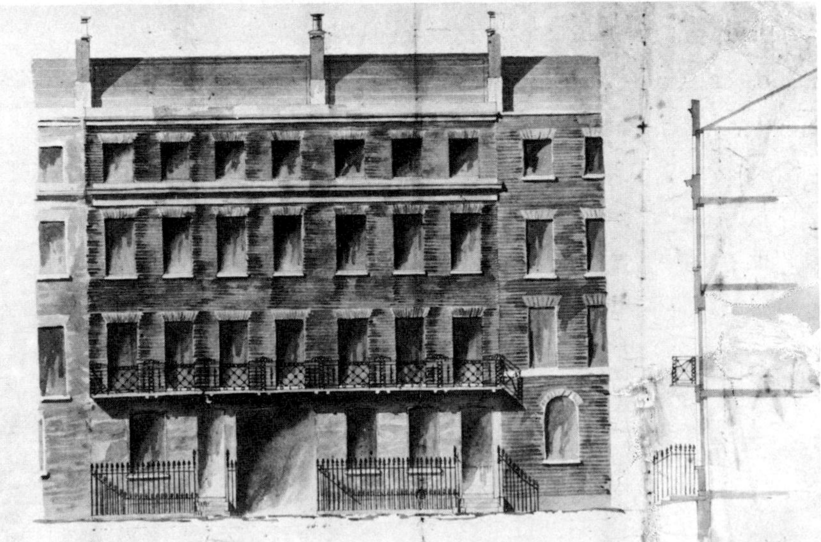

c. Elevation with section of houses to be built by John Elger in Green Street, *c.* 1825. *Demolished*

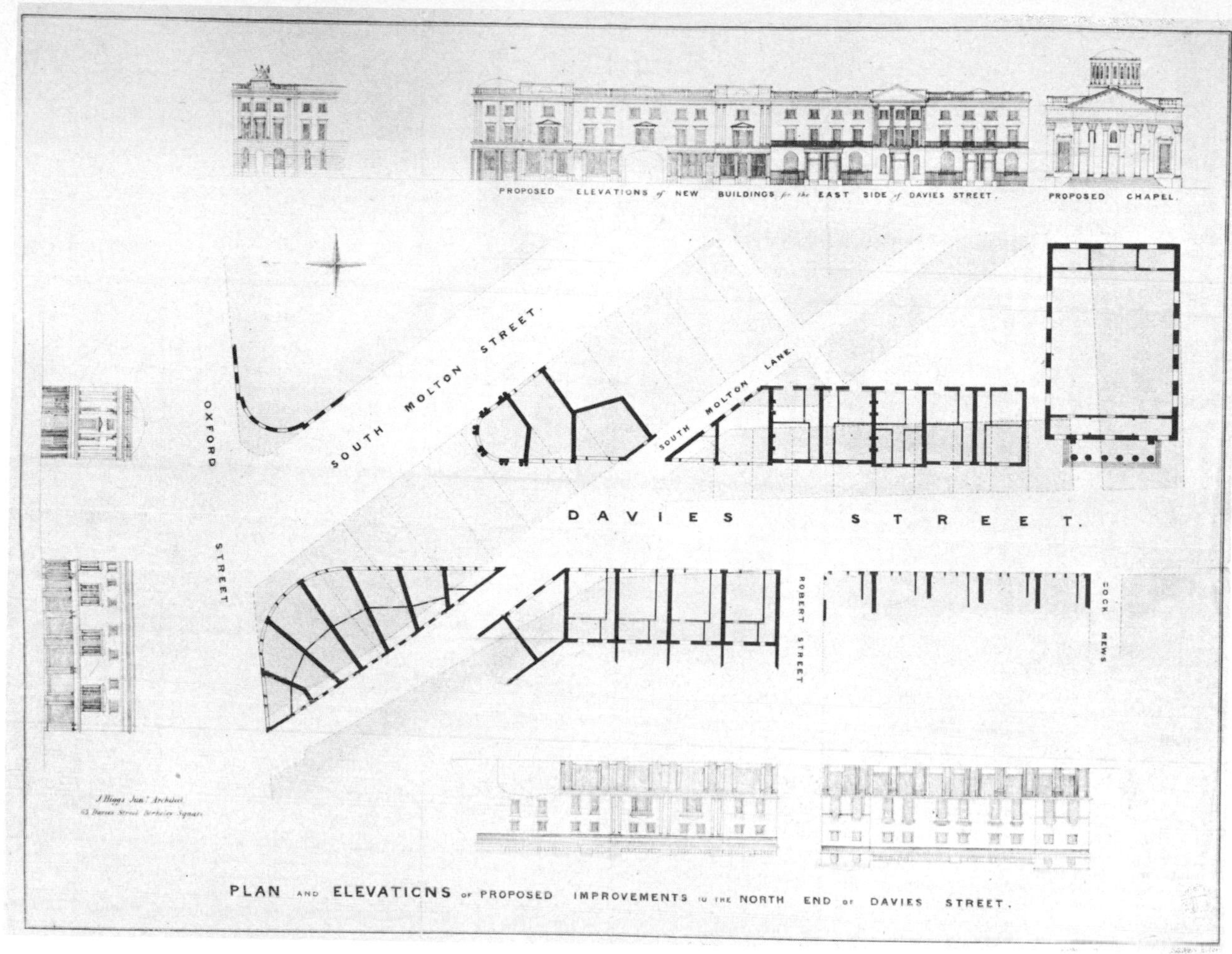

a. Davies Street, plan and elevations to show improvements at north end suggested by Joshua Higgs junior, 1839. *Not executed*

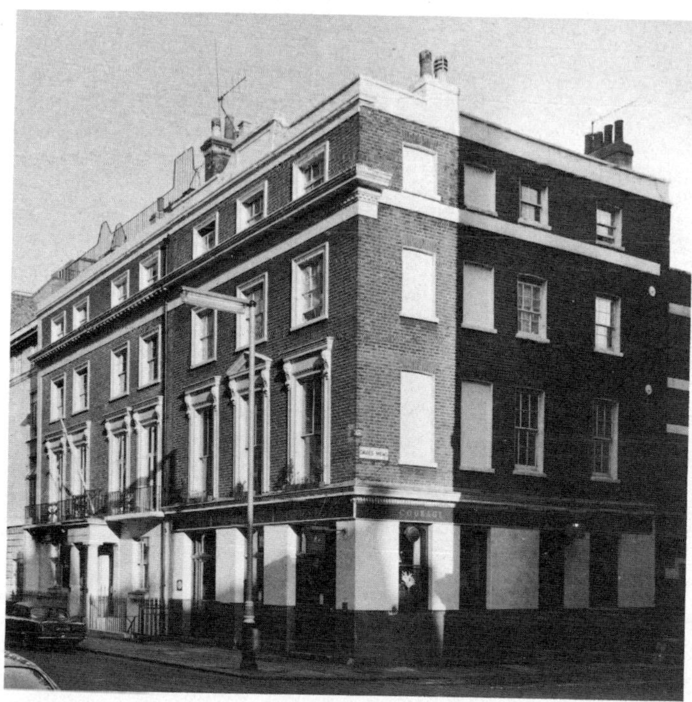

b. Nos. 50 (Running Horse), 52 and 54 Davies Street in 1968. Joshua Higgs, builder, 1839–40

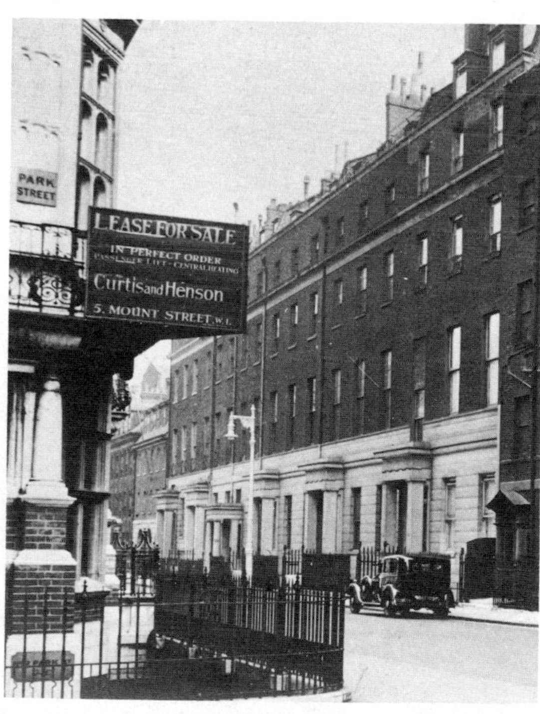

c. Nos. 14–24 (even) South Street (right to left) in *c.* 1931. J. P. Gandy-Deering, architect, *c.* 1825–35. *Mostly demolished*

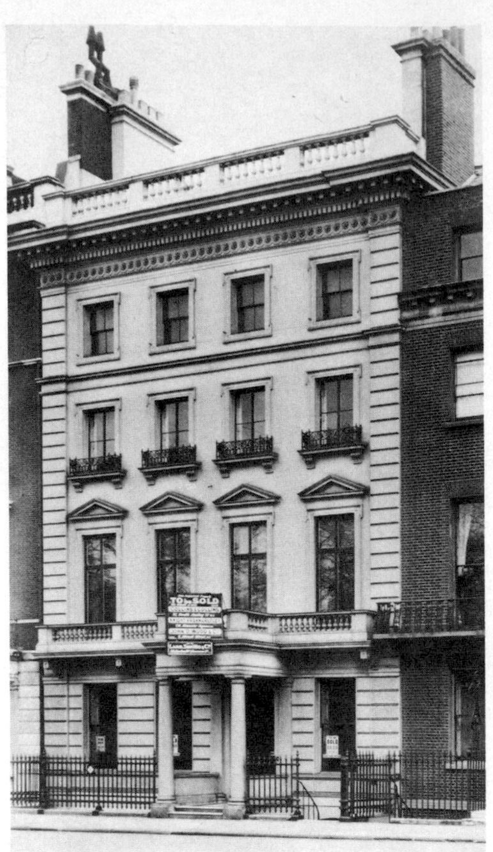

a. No. 38 Grosvenor Square in *c*. 1931. Front altered in 1854–5

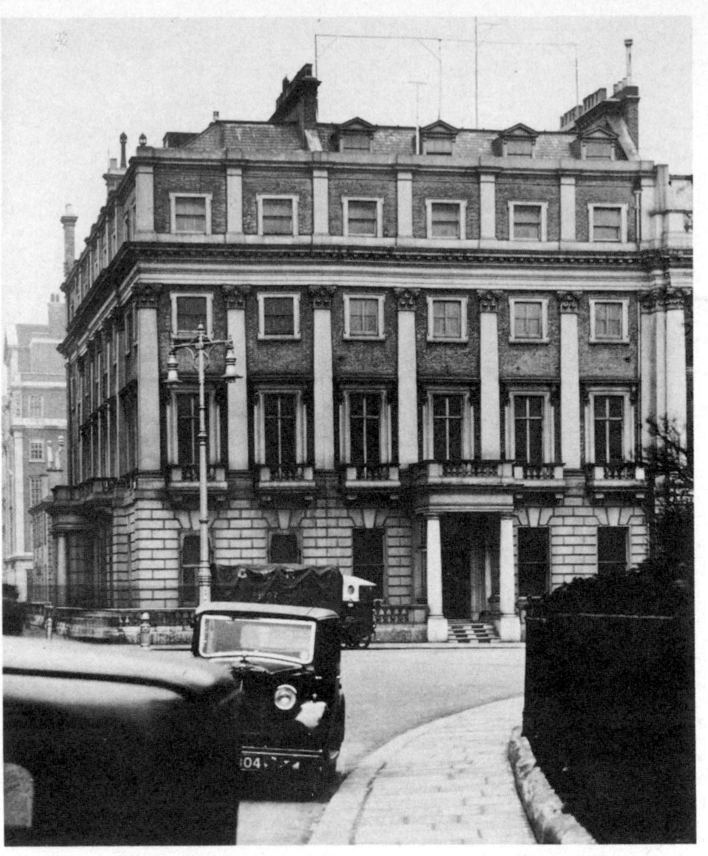

b. Nos. 20 and 21 Grosvenor Square in *c*. 1932–3. Complete rebuilding by John Kelk, 1855–8. *Demolished*

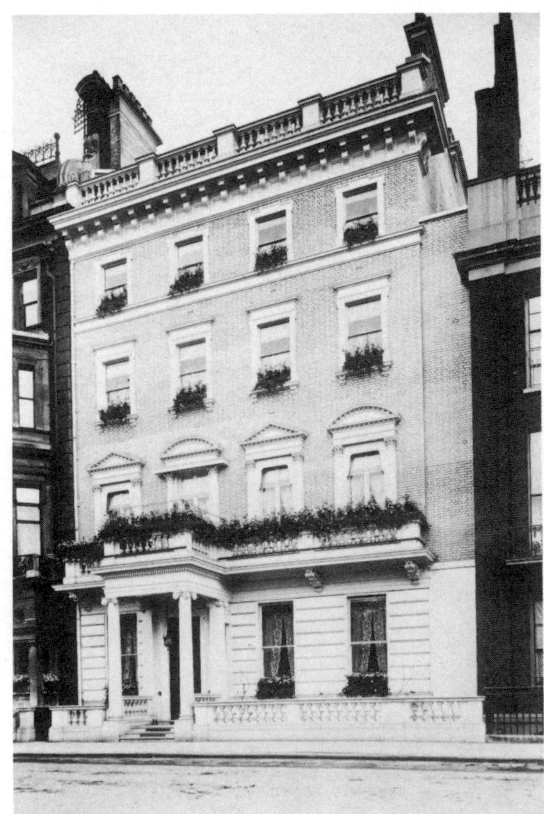

c. No. 26 Grosvenor Square in 1902. Complete rebuilding by C. J. Freake, 1861–2. *Demolished*

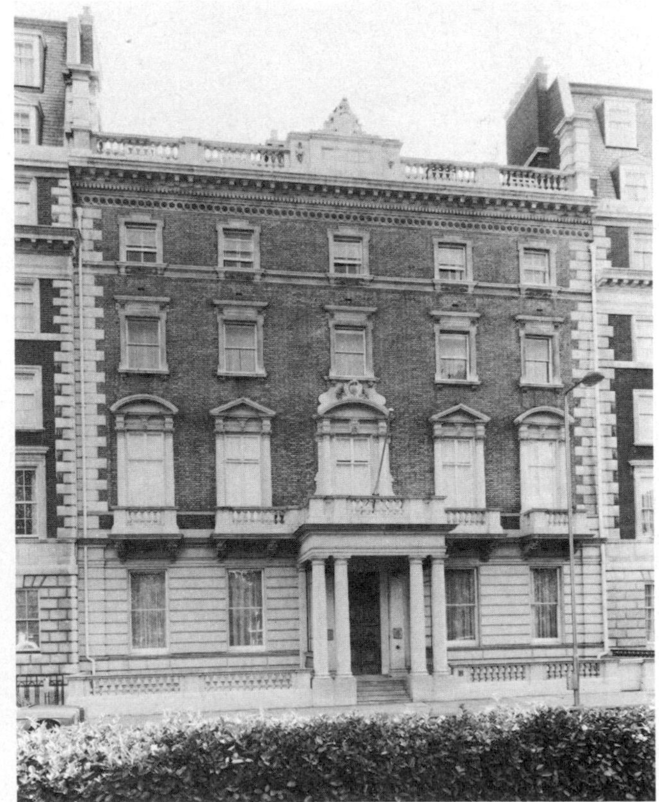

d. No. 4 Grosvenor Square in 1976. Complete rebuilding by C. J. Freake, 1865–8

FRONTS DESIGNED BY THOMAS CUNDY II AND III

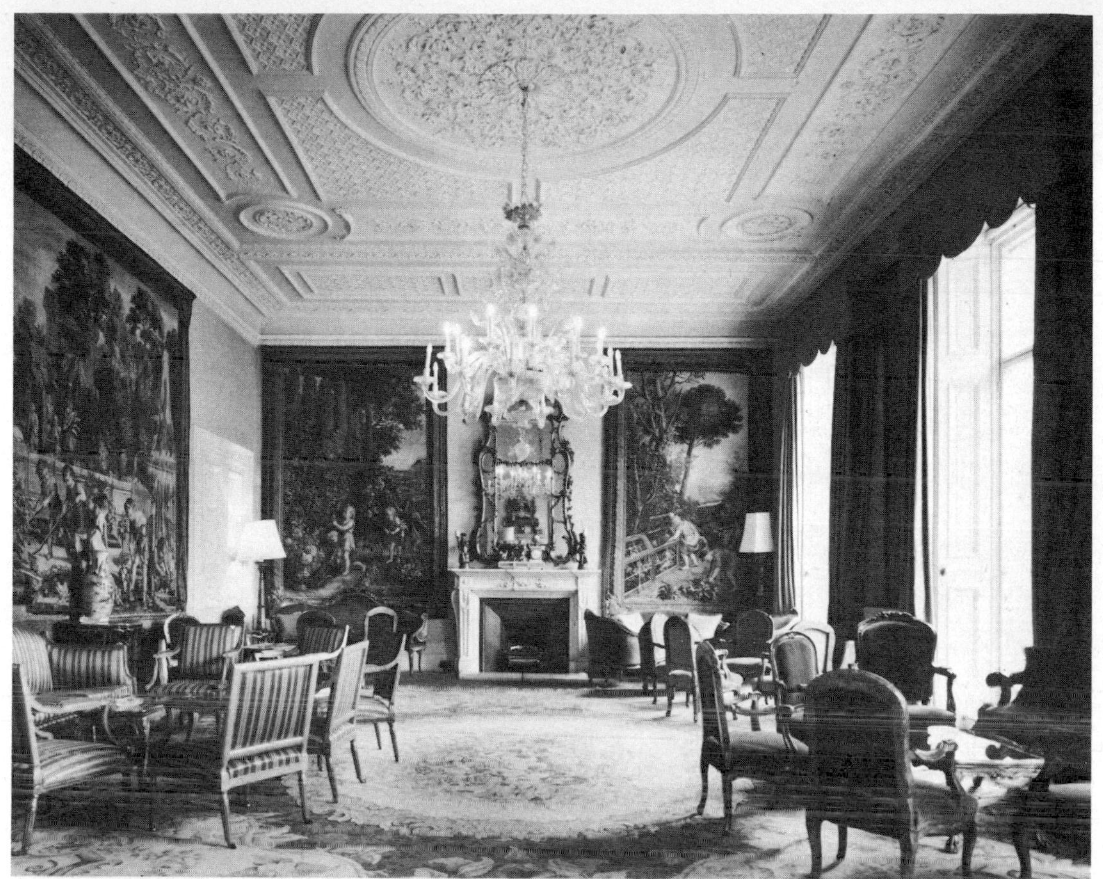

a. Front drawing-room in 1975

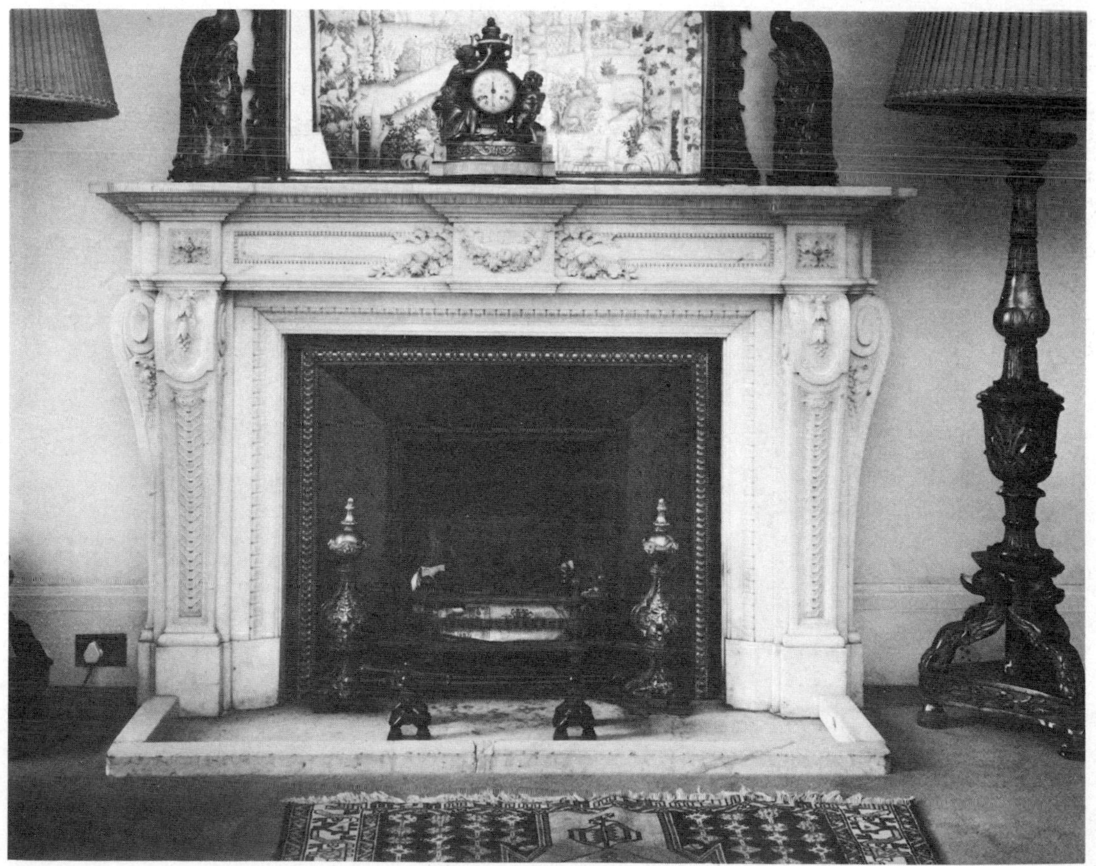

b. Chimneypiece in 1975

No. 4 Grosvenor Square, Interiors. C. J. Freake, builder, 1865–8

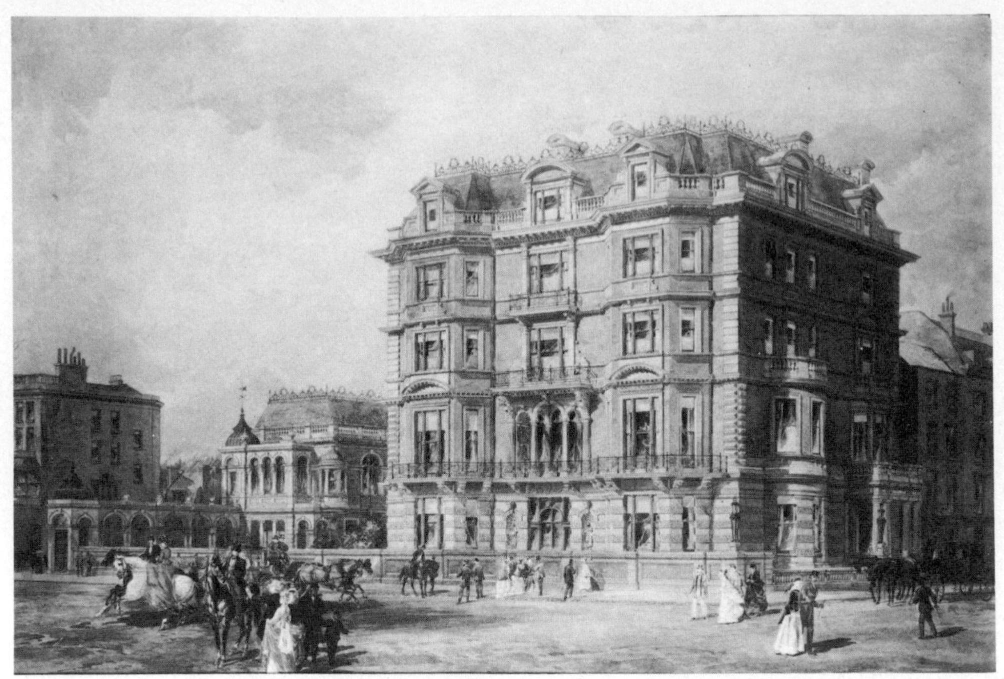

a. Brook House, Park Lane, 1866–9. Perspective view by T. H. Wyatt, architect, showing fronts to Park Lane and Upper Brook Street (right). *Demolished*

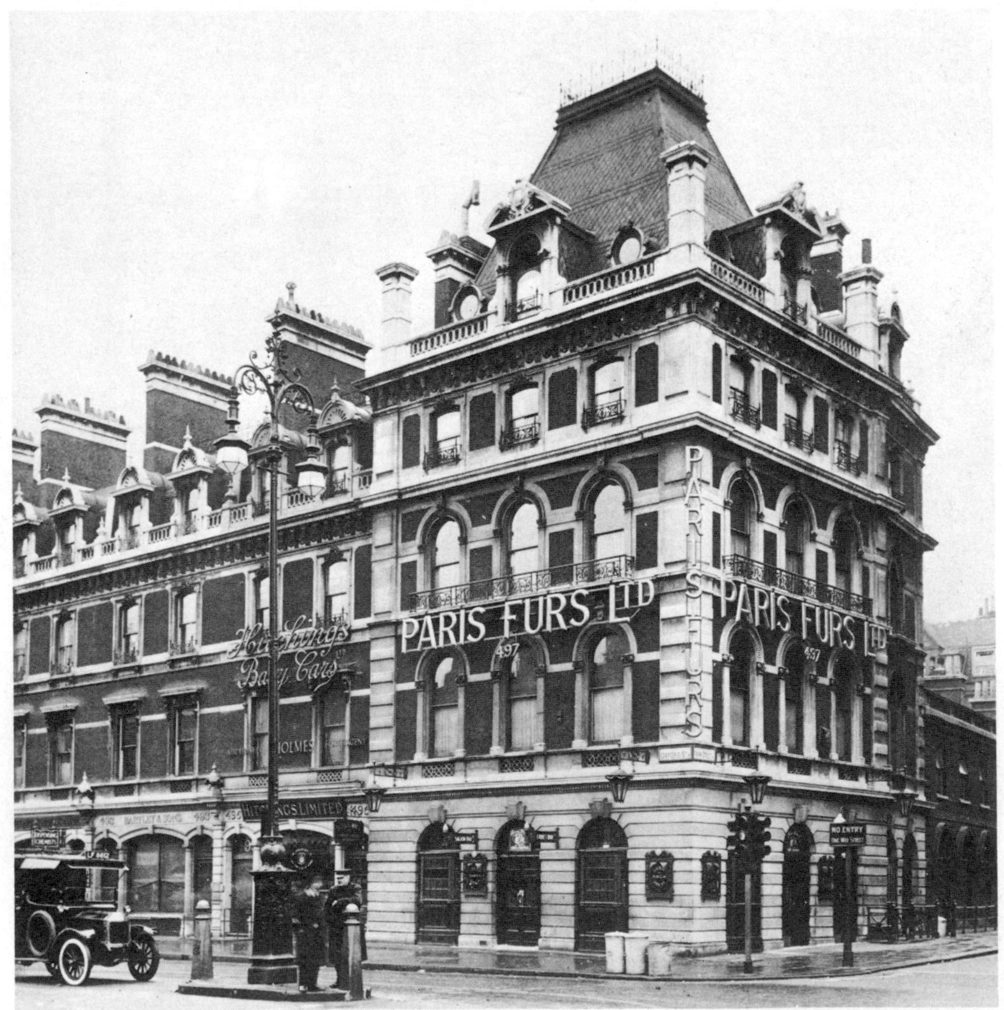

b. Nos. 491–497 (odd) Oxford Street in *c*. 1931. Thomas Cundy III, architect, 1865–6. *Demolished*

THE FRENCH STYLE IN THE 1860'S

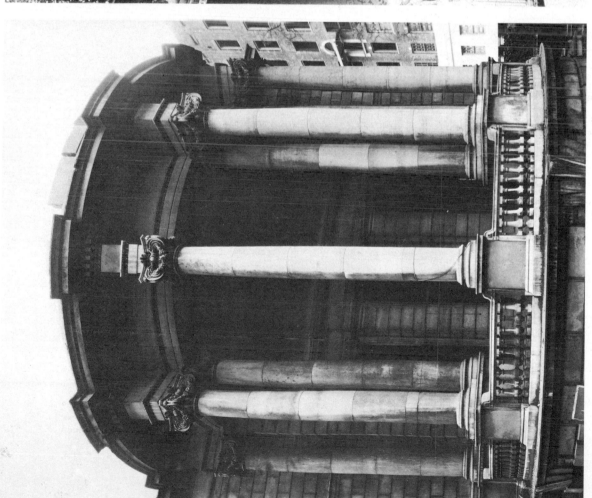

a. The loggia at the west end, added in 1880–1, from Park Lane, shortly before demolition in 1927

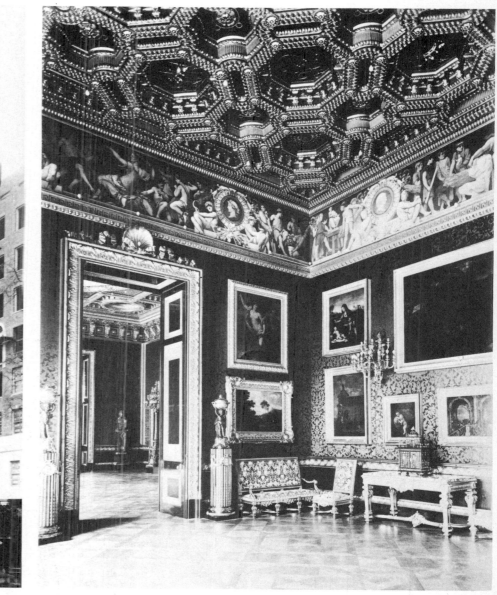

b. The gallery, with the Rubens room beyond, in 1889. Frieze painted by F. J. Barrias, 1872. *Demolished*

GROSVENOR HOUSE, REMODELLING BY HENRY CLUTTON, 1870–2 AND 1880–1

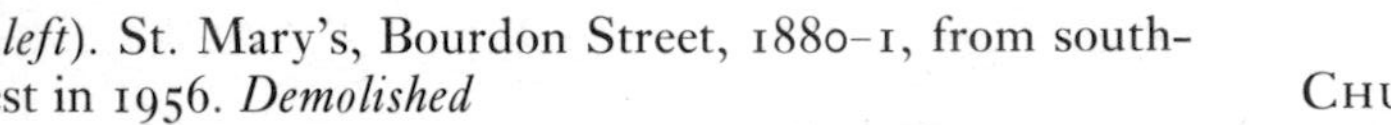

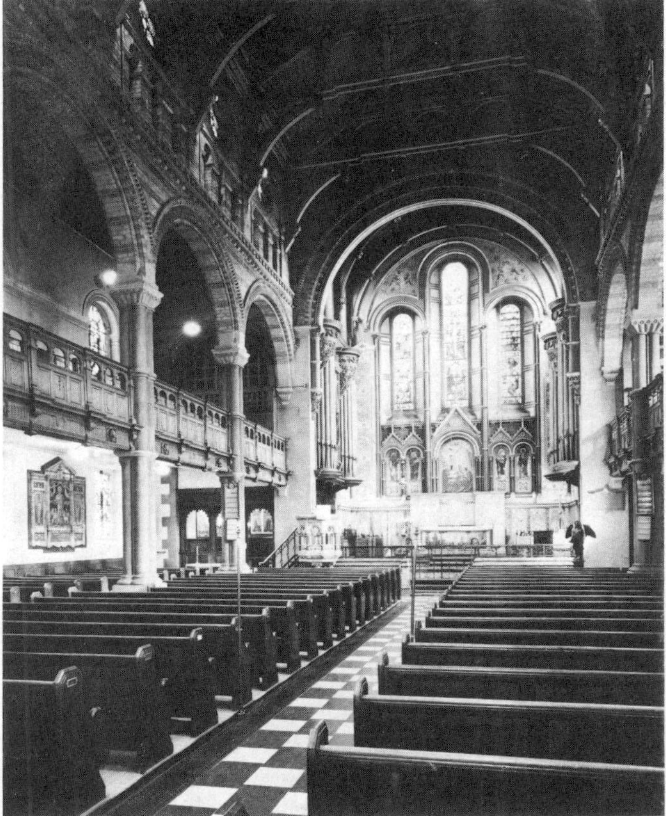

b. St. Mark's, North Audley Street, interior as remodelled by Blomfield in 1878: view looking east in 1971

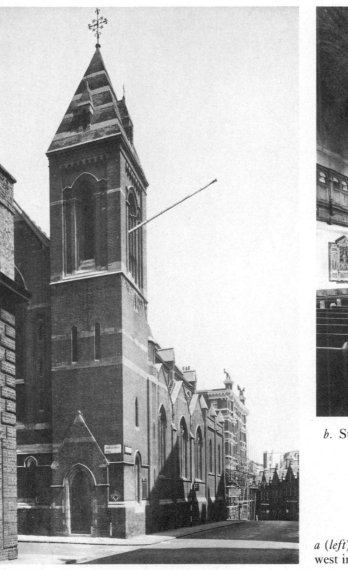

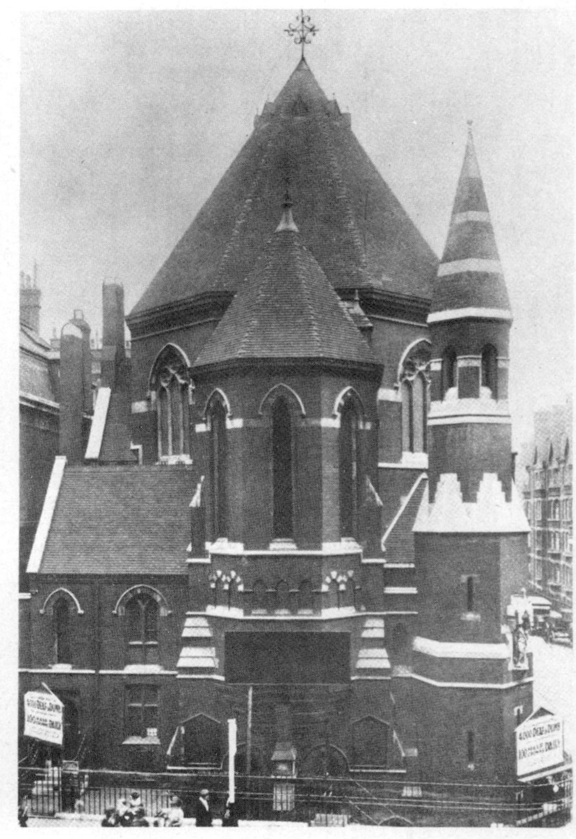

c. St. Saviour's, Oxford Street, 1870–3, from north in *c.* 1922. *Demolished*

a (*left*). St. Mary's, Bourdon Street, 1880–1, from south-west in 1956. *Demolished*

CHURCHES DESIGNED BY ARTHUR BLOMFIELD

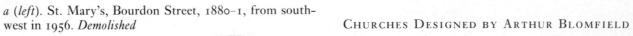

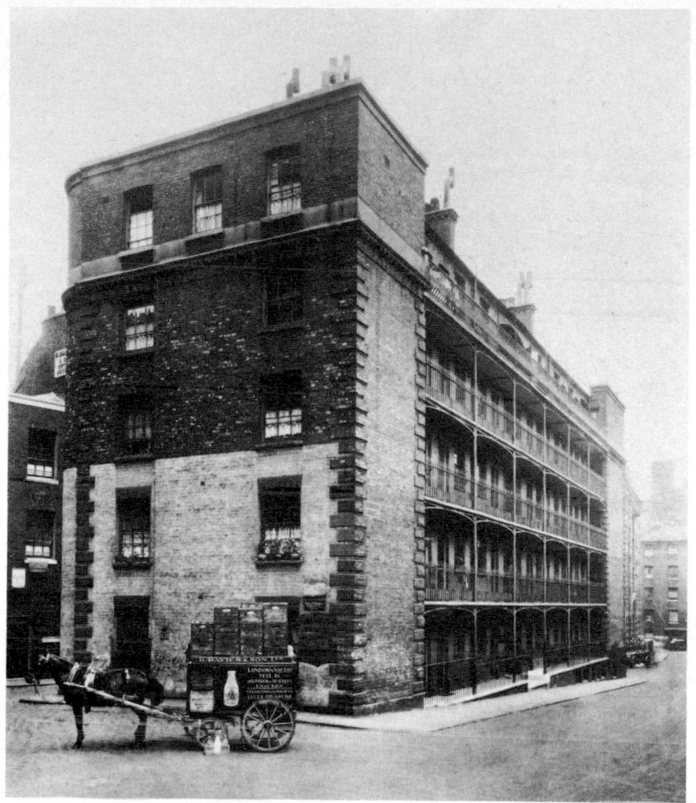

a. St. George's Buildings, Bourdon Street, from west. Henry Roberts, architect for plan, and John Newson, builder, 1852–3

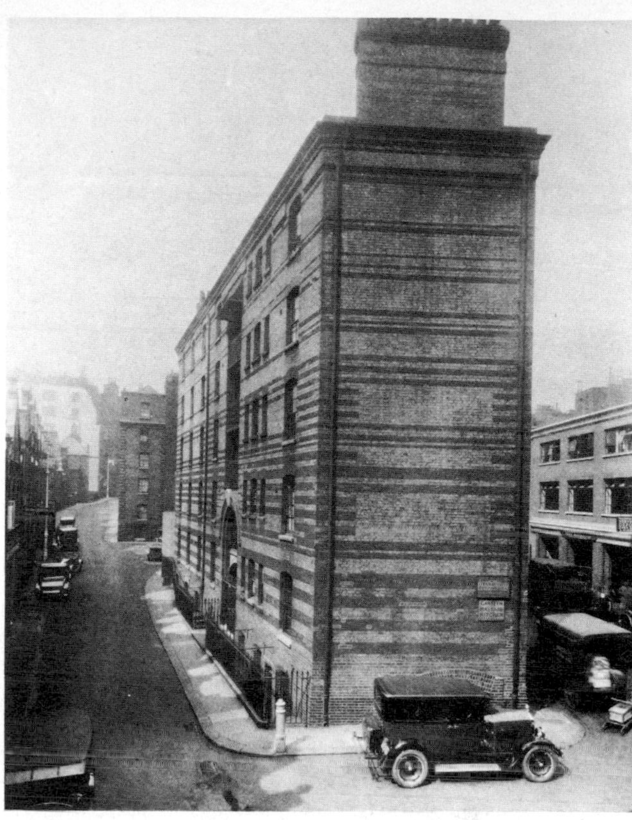

b. Grosvenor Buildings, Bourdon Street, from east, with Grosvenor Hill to right. R. H. Burden, architect, 1868–9

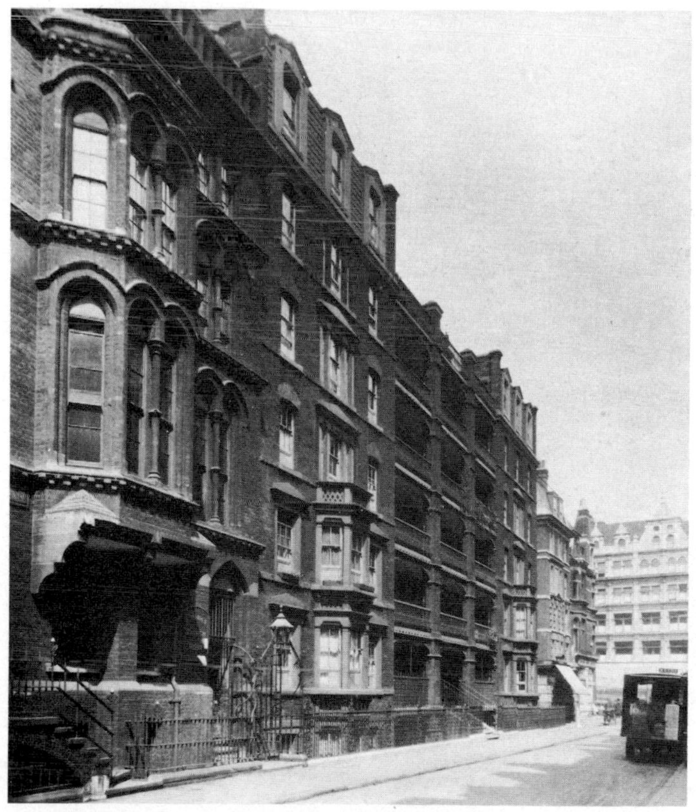

c. Clarendon Flats, Balderton Street (Improved Industrial Dwellings Company, 1871–2), from south, with St. Mark's Mansions (R. J. Withers, architect, 1872–3) on left

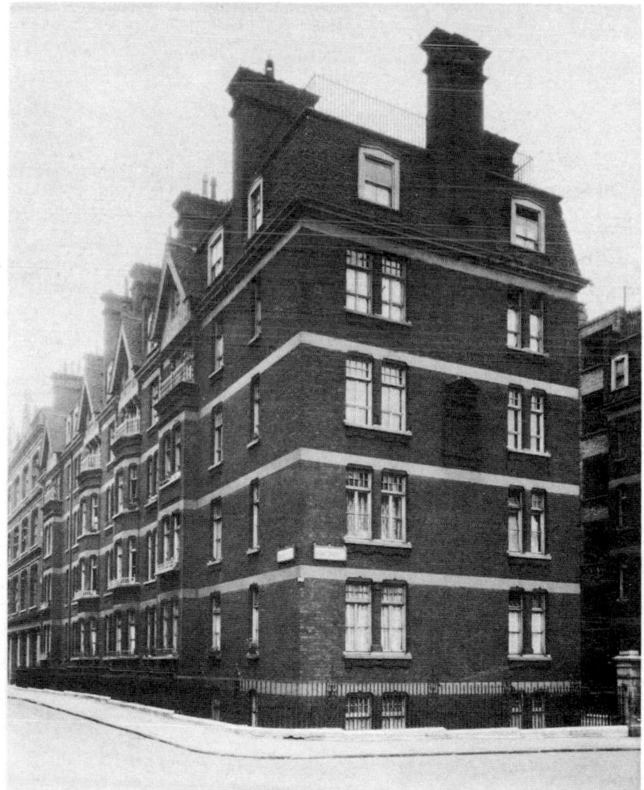

d. Balderton Flats, Balderton Street and Brown Hart Gardens (Improved Industrial Dwellings Company, 1887), from south-west

WORKING-CLASS HOUSING. Photographs of the early 1930's

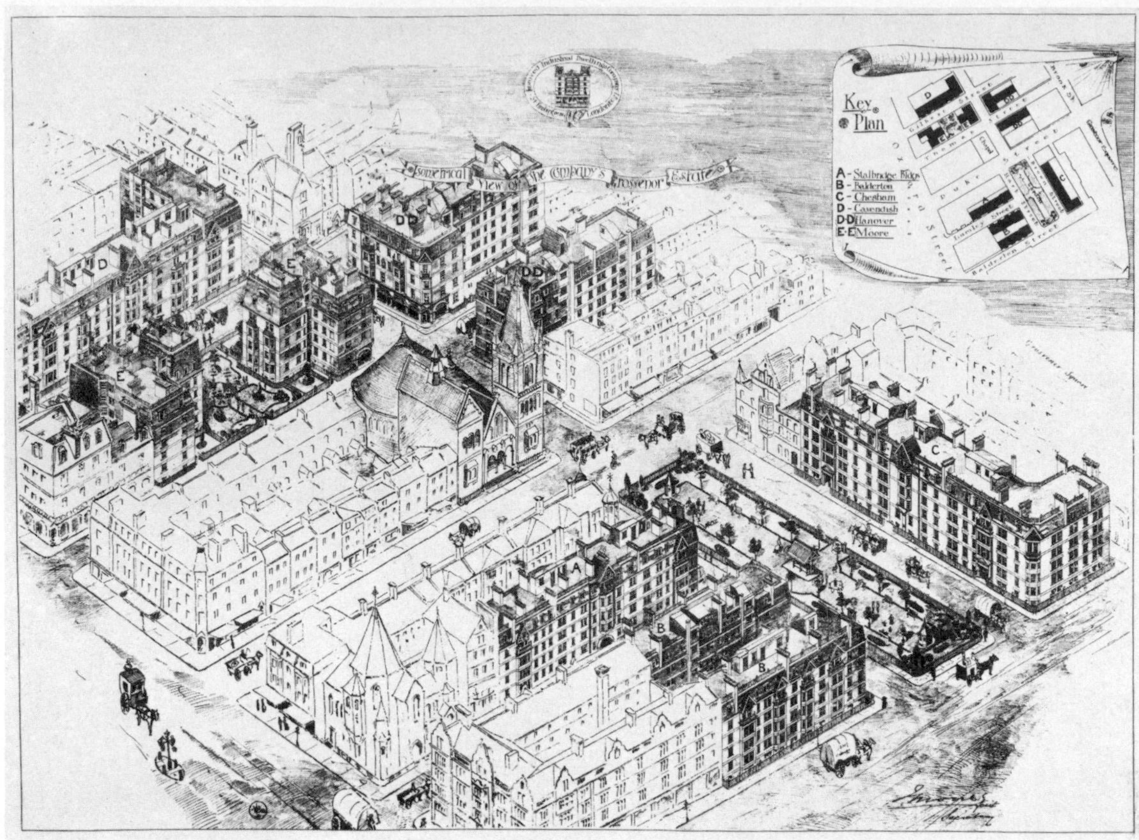

a. Plan and bird's-eye view of the Improved Industrial Dwellings Company's estate east and west of Duke Street, 1886–92

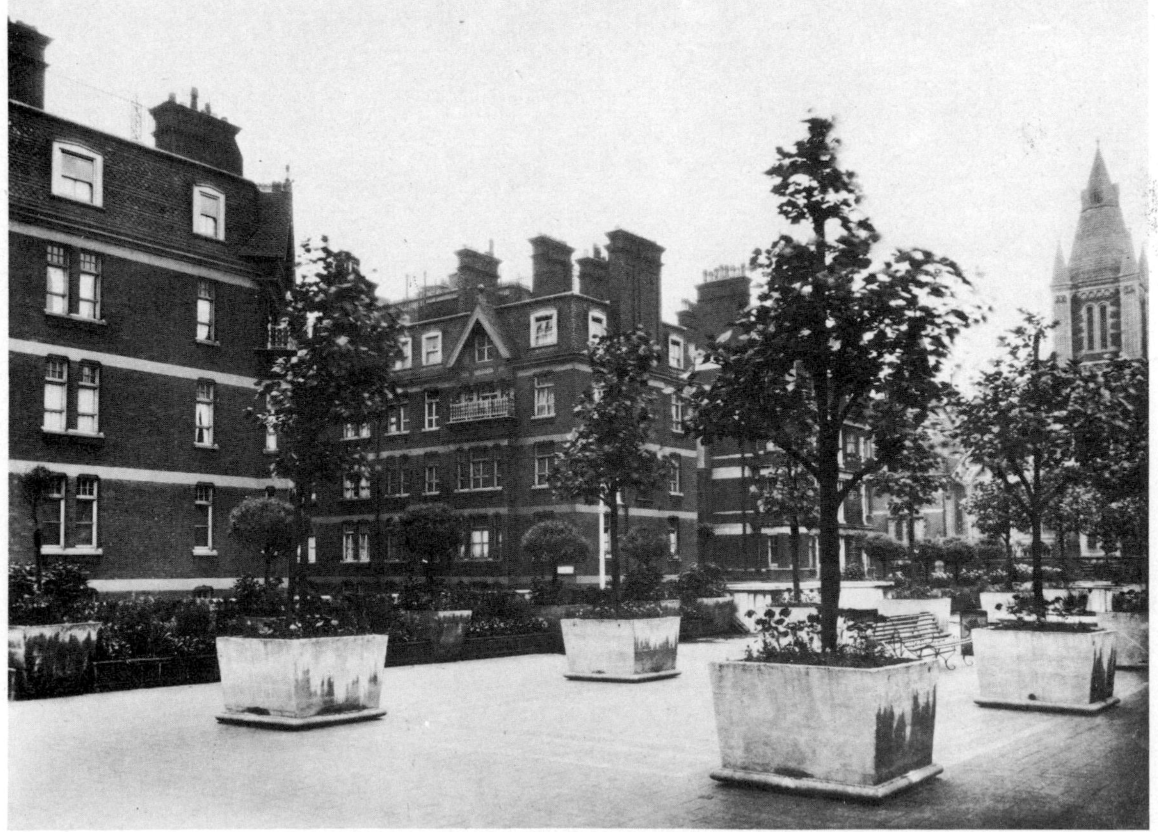

b. Improved Industrial Dwellings Company's estate, in *c.* 1930, showing blocks on north side of Brown Hart Gardens and (right) King's Weigh House Chapel, from garden of Duke Street Electricity Sub-station

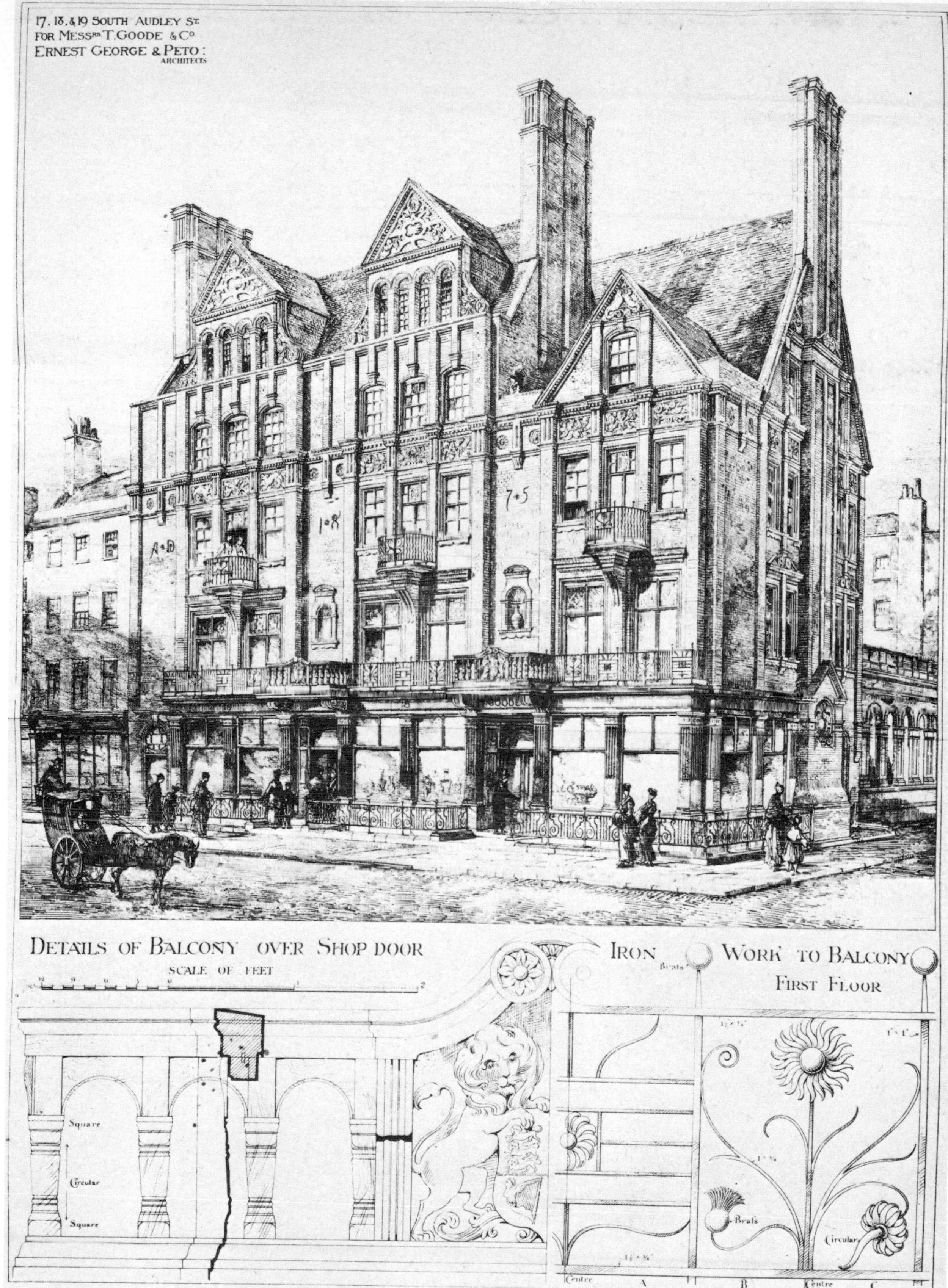

Nos. 17–19 (consec.) South Audley Street. Perspective and details, showing extent of rebuilding by Ernest George and Peto, architects, in 1875–6

GOODE'S, SOUTH AUDLEY STREET

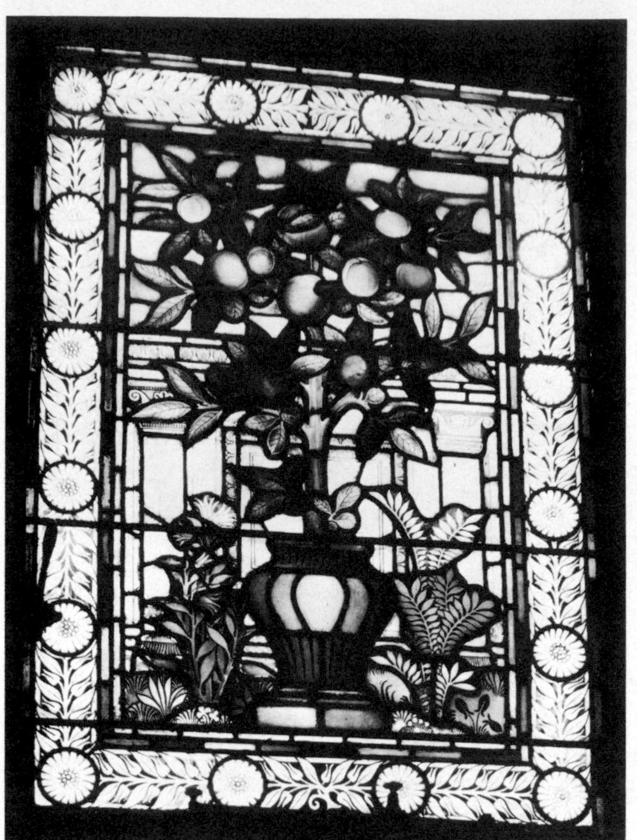

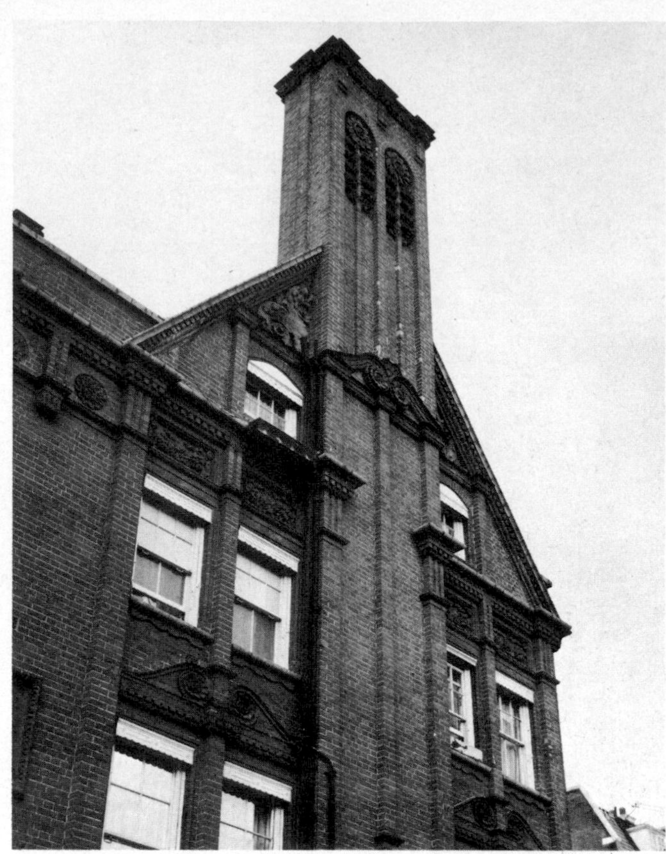

a, *b*. Goode's, South Audley Street, details in 1975: *a* (*left*), detail of stained glass window, *b* (*right*), chimney facing South Street. Ernest George and Peto, architects, 1875–6

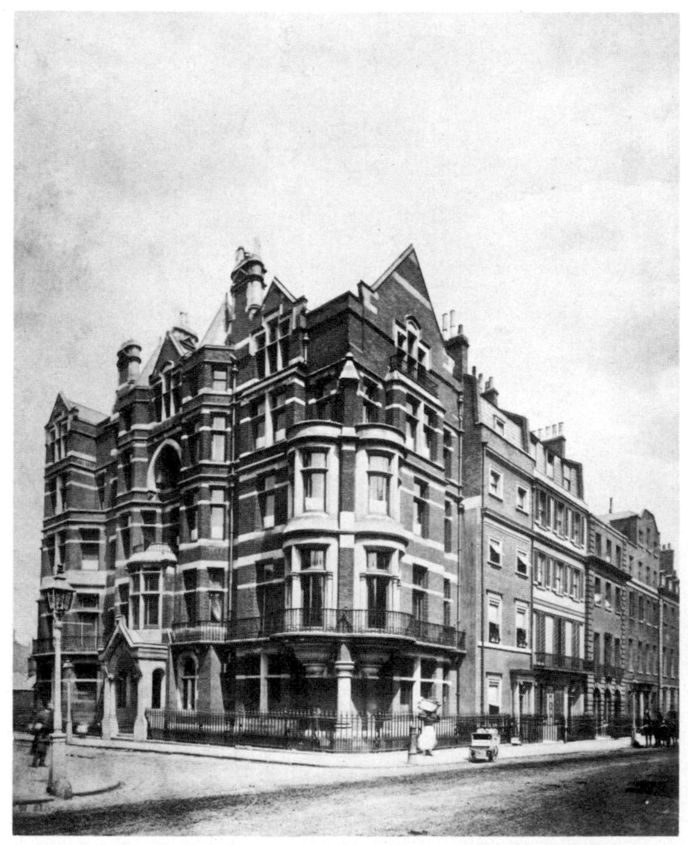

c. No. 78 Brook Street, with Nos. 76–68 (even) to right, in 1875. C. F. Hayward, architect of No. 78, 1873–5

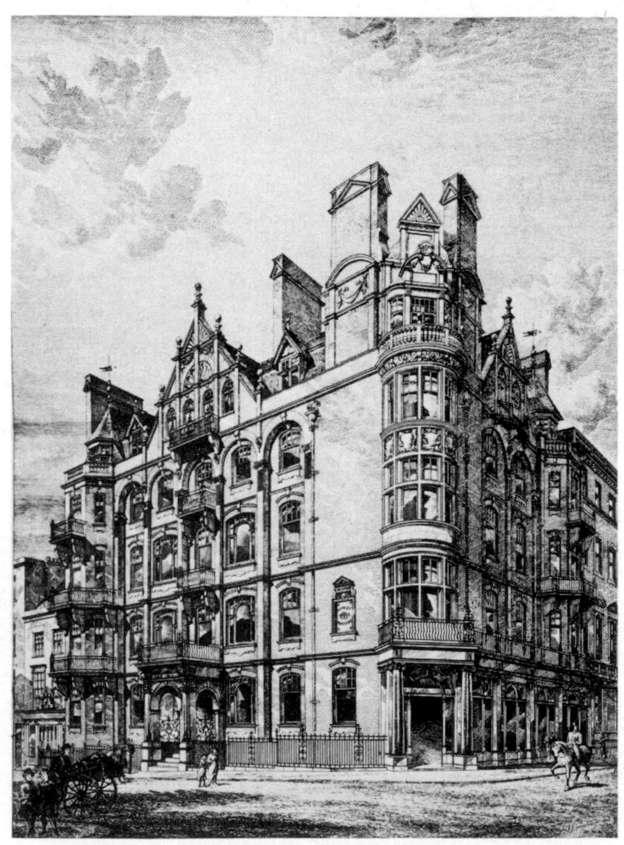

d. Audley Mansions, Nos. 56 South Audley Street and 44 Mount Street, perspective view of 1885. J. T. Wimperis, architect, 1884–6

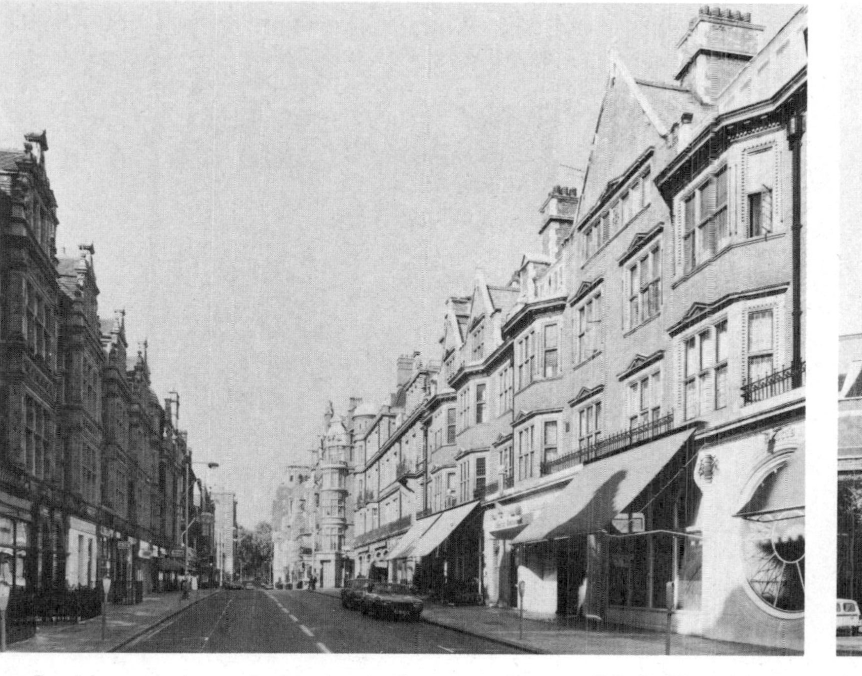

a. Looking west in 1976, showing in foreground parts of (left) Nos. 87–102 (A. J. Bolton, architect, 1889–95) and (right) Nos. 14–26 (Read and Macdonald, architects, 1896–8)

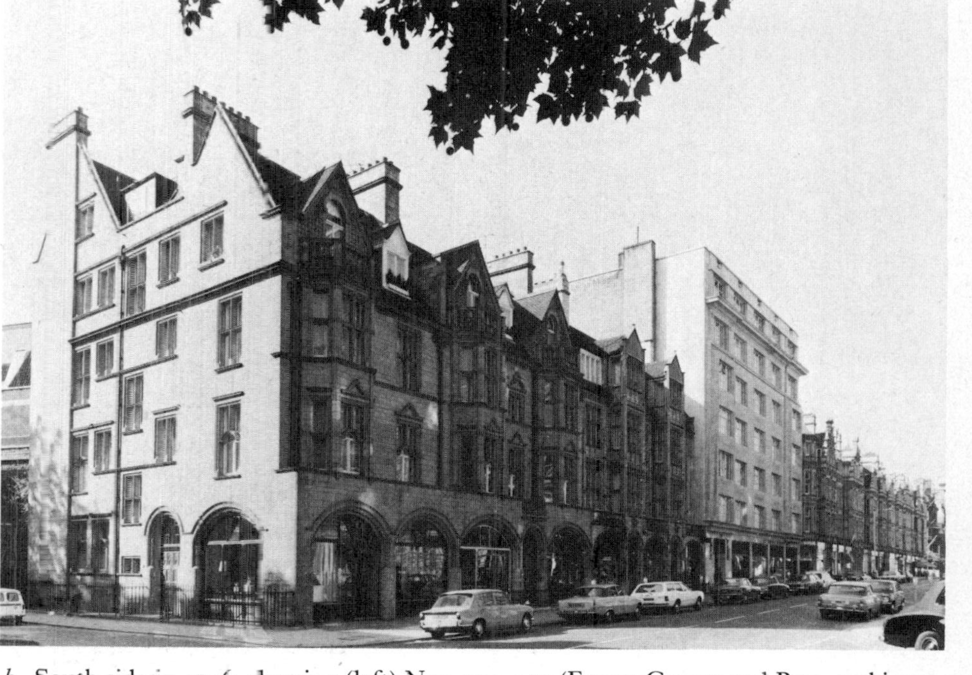

b. South side in 1976, showing (left) Nos. 104–113 (Ernest George and Peto, architects, 1885–92); (centre right) No. 103 (Wimperis, Simpson and Guthrie, architects, 1936–8); and (far right), Nos. 87–102 (A. J. Bolton, architect, 1889–95)

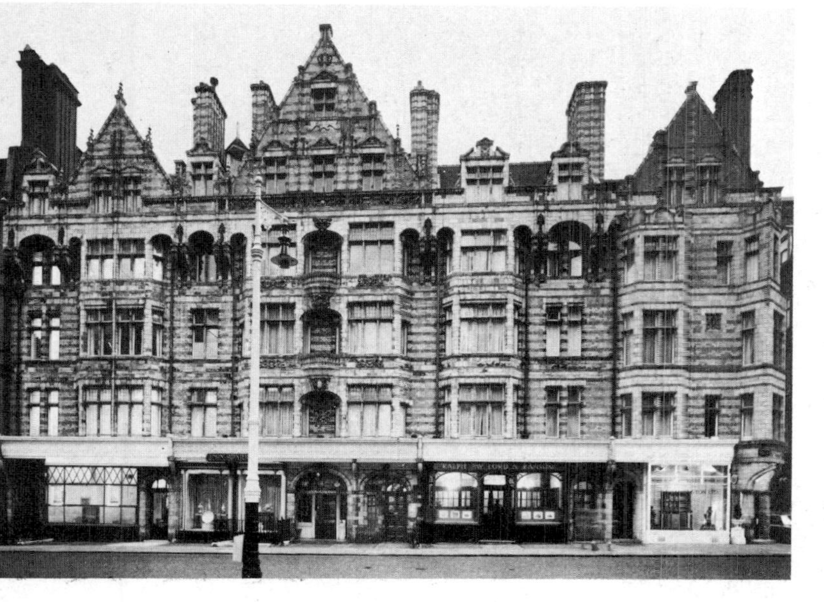

c (left). Nos. 125–129 in 1968, from Carpenter Street. W. H. Powell, architect, 1886–7

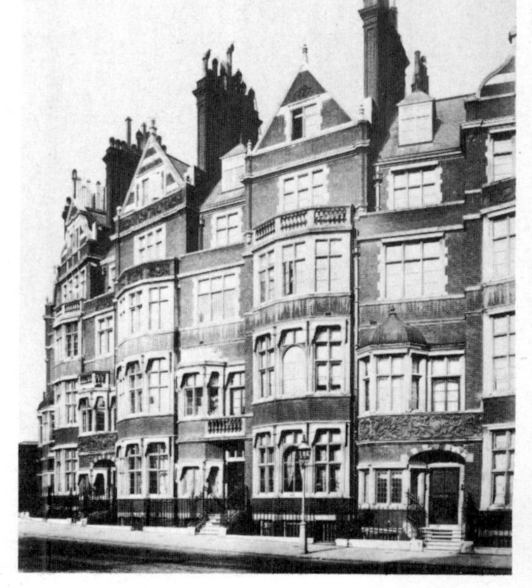

d (right). Nos. 4–7 Carlos Place, from south-west in *c.* 1897. Giles, Gough and Trollope, architects, George Trollope and Sons, builders, 1891–3

Mount Street Reconstruction

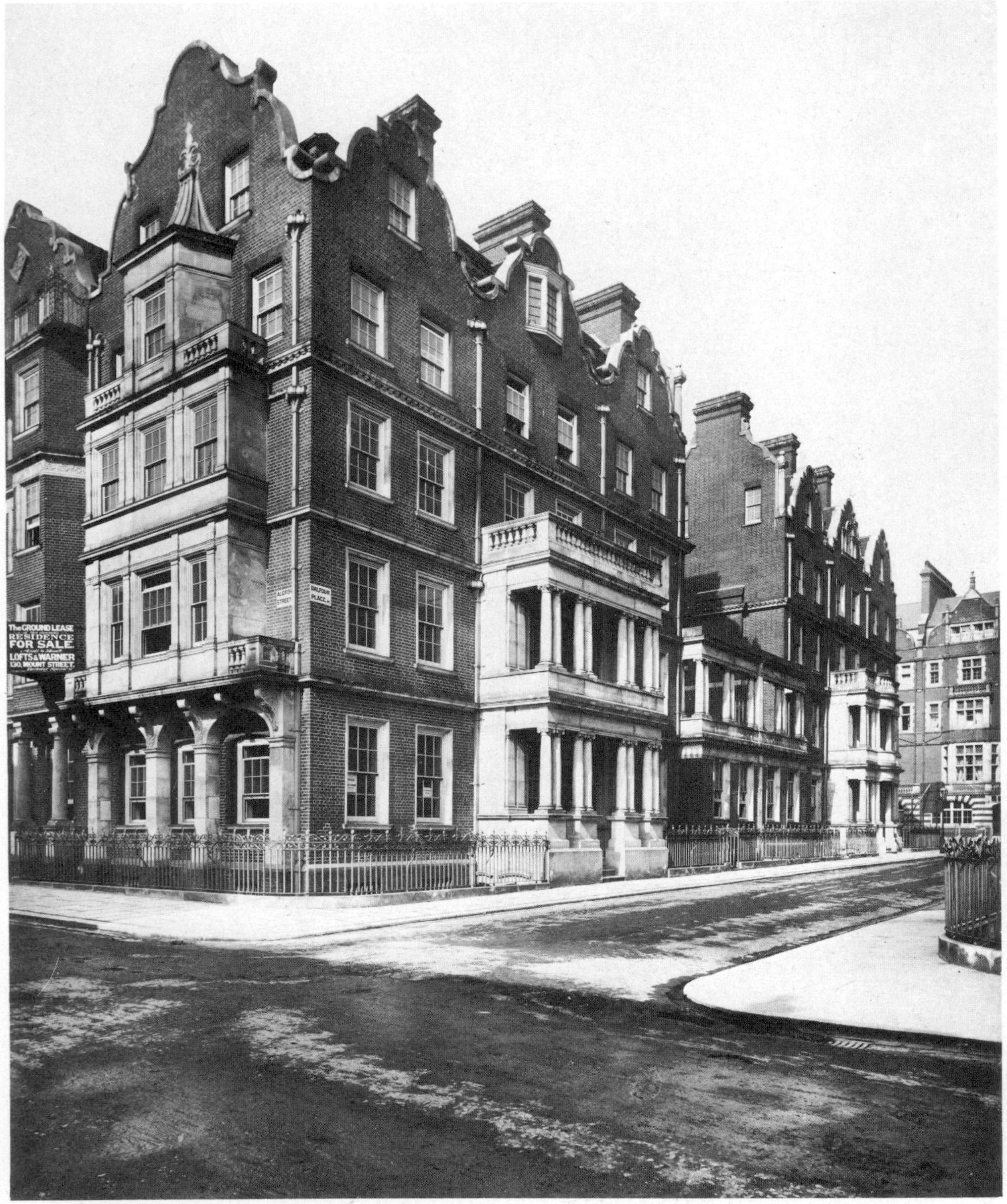

a. Nos. 7 and 8 Balfour Place, from south-east in 1894, with part of return to Aldford Street. Balfour and Turner, architects, 1891–4

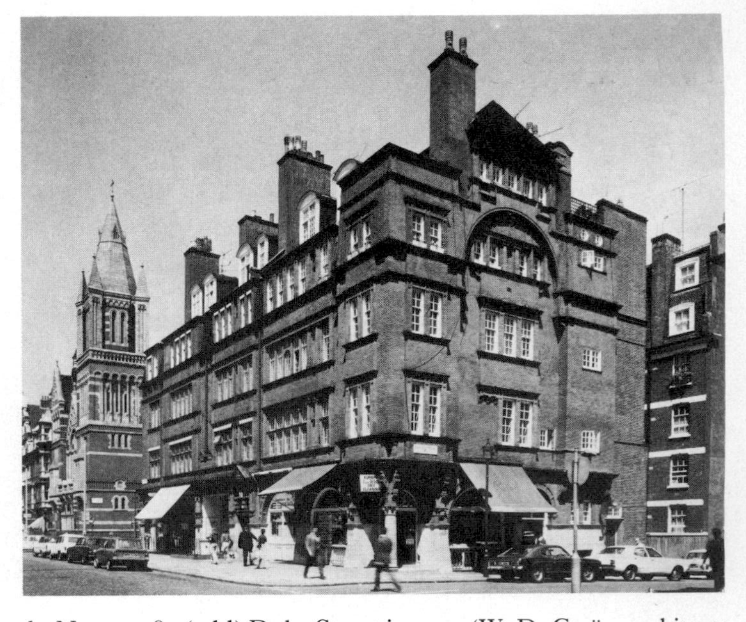

b. Nos. 75–83 (odd) Duke Street in 1975 (W. D. Caröe, architect, 1893–5), with King's Weigh House Chapel to left

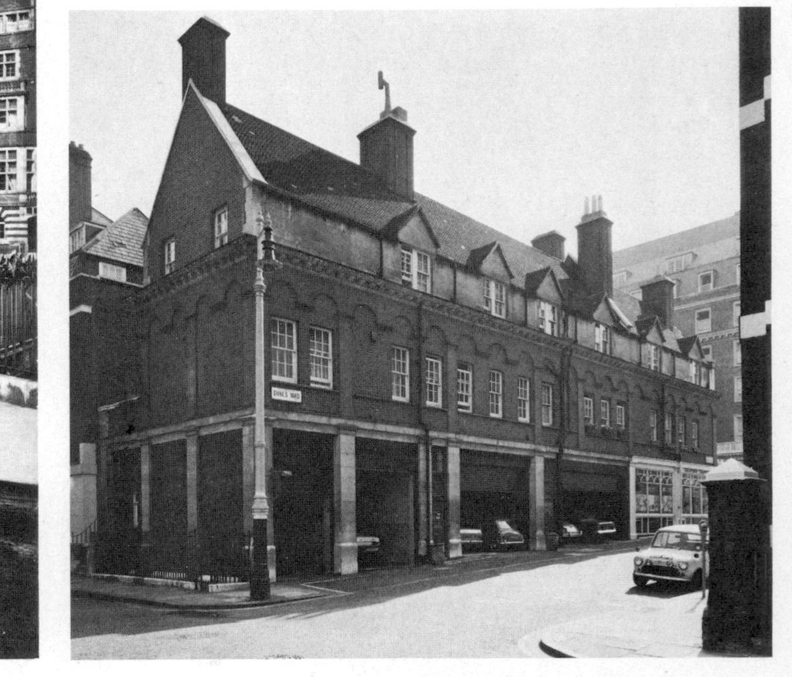

c. Duke's Yard: stable block on south side from Binney Street in 1968. Balfour and Turner, architects, 1900–2

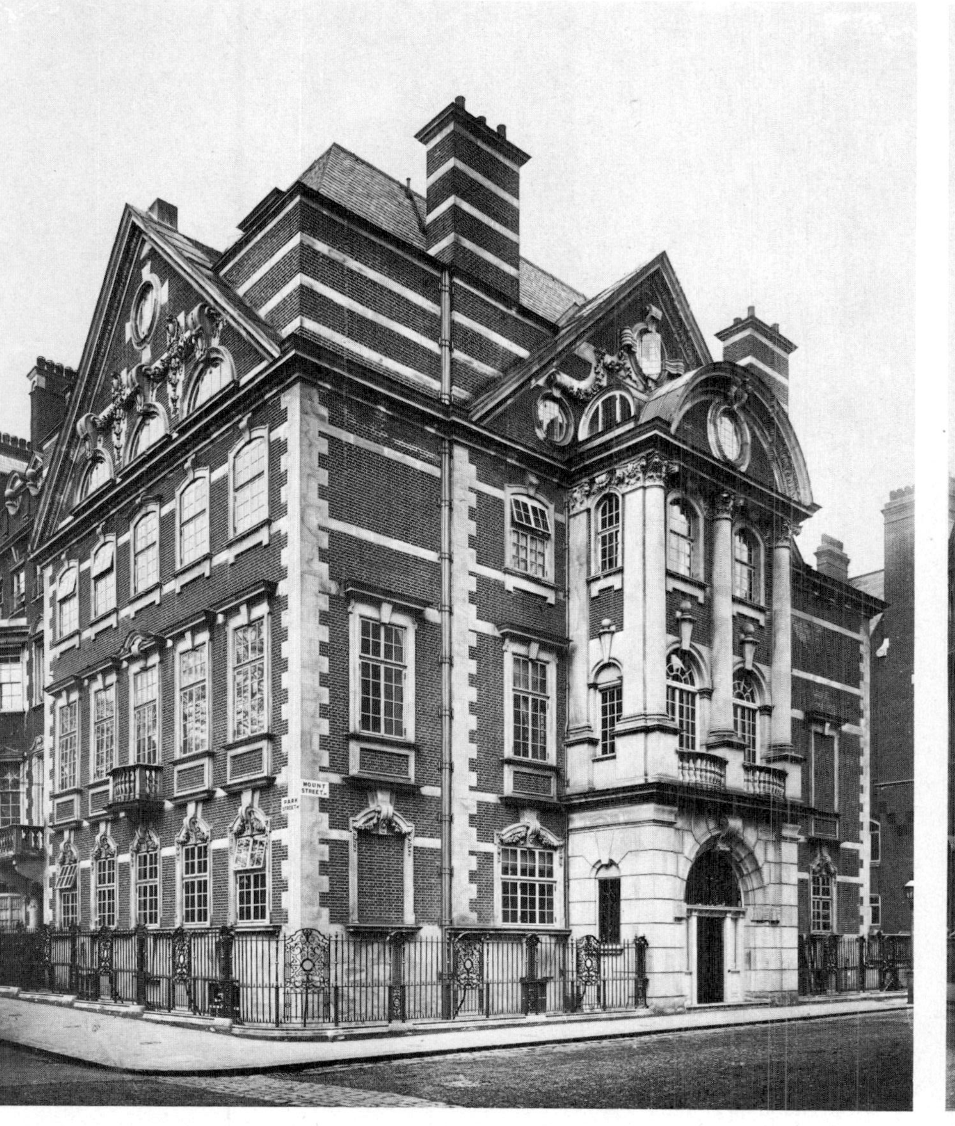

a. No. 54 Mount Street, from south-west in 1897, before completion of interior. Fairfax B. Wade, architect, 1896–9

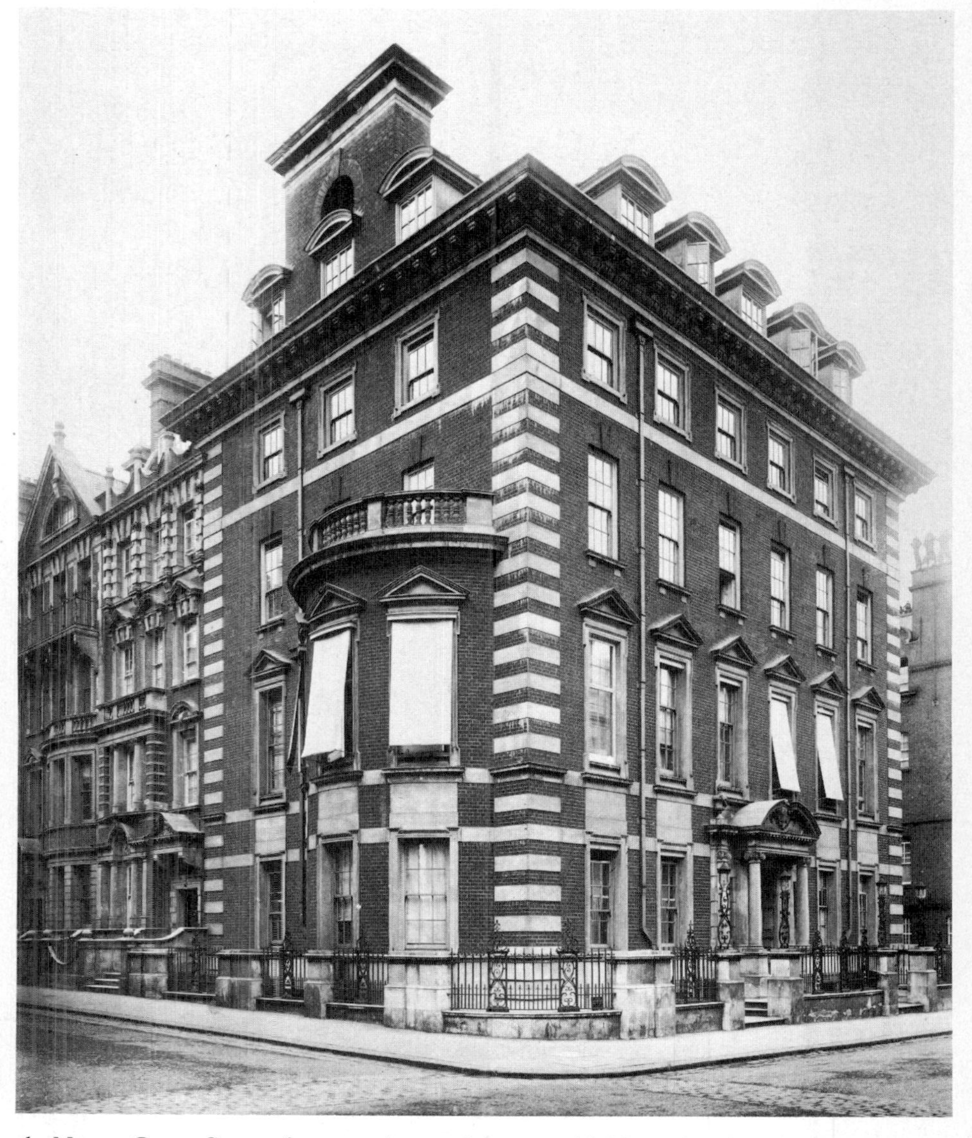

b. No. 32 Green Street, from south-west in 1901, with Nos. 16 and 17 Dunraven Street to left. Sidney R. J. Smith, architect, 1897–9

Town Houses of the 1890's

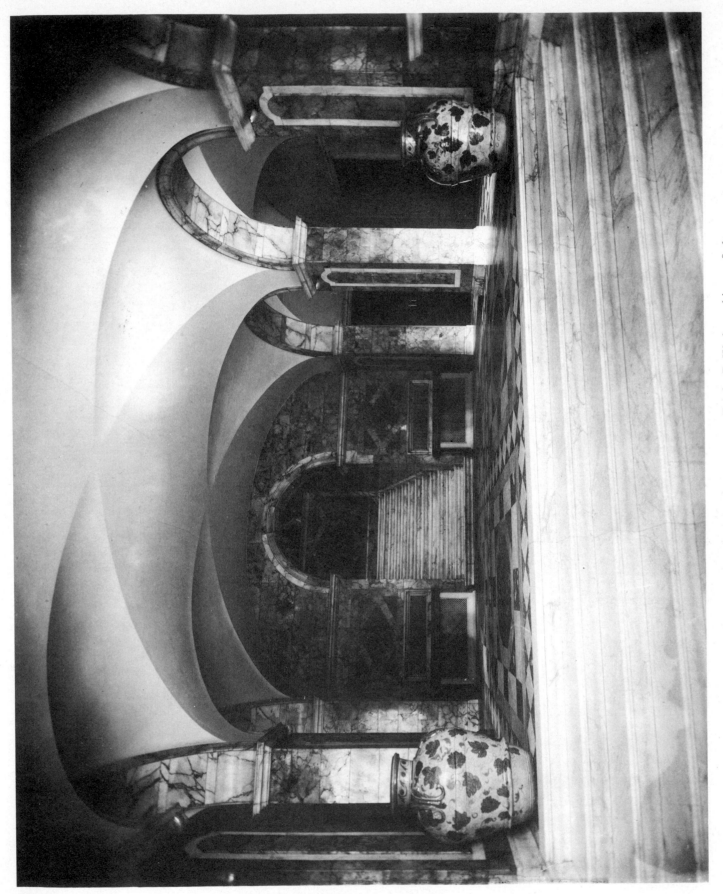

No. 54 Mount Street, entrance hall in *c.* 1911. Fairfax B. Wade, architect, 1896–9

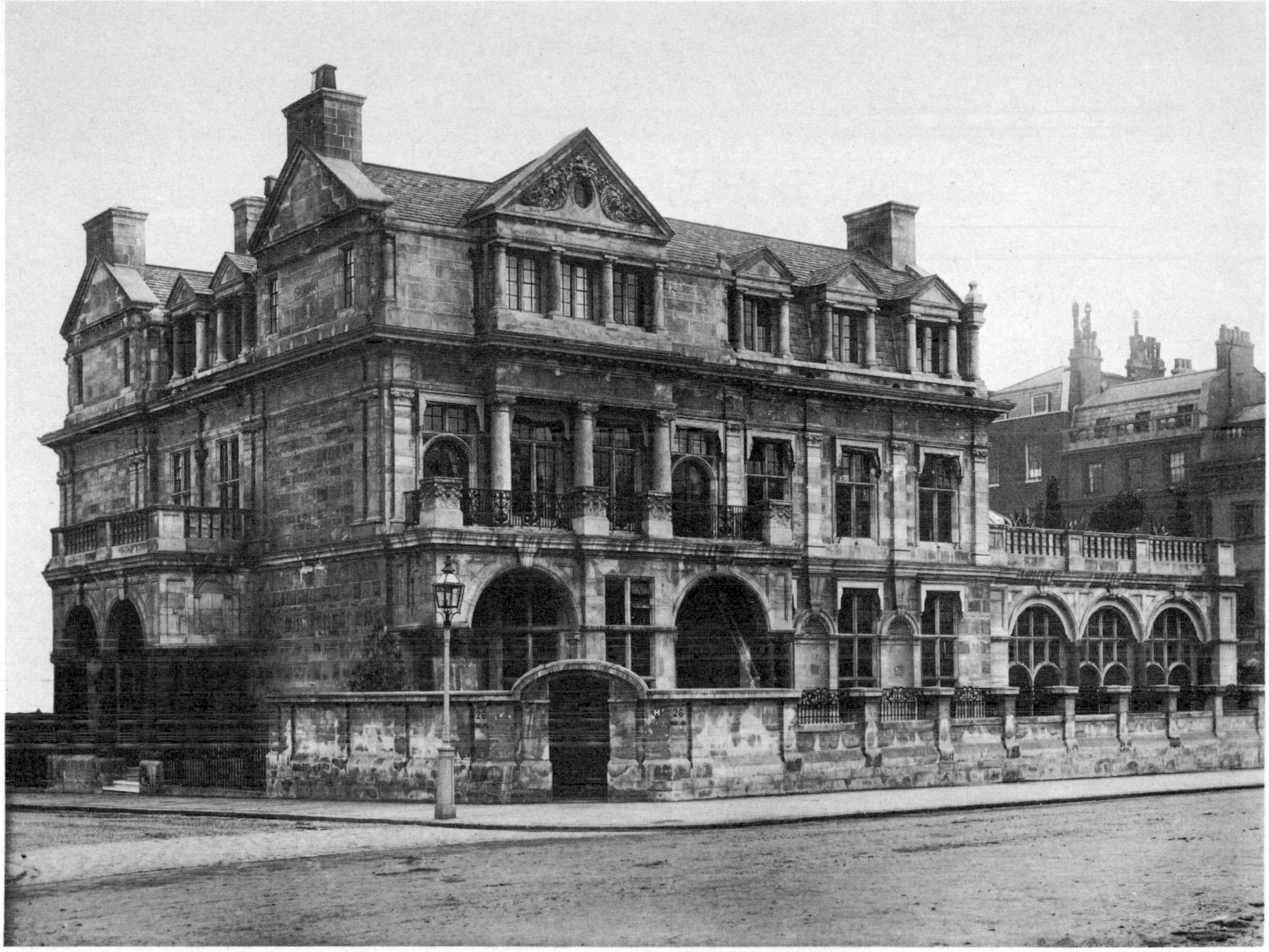

a (*above*). Aldford House, Park Lane (1894–7), fronts to Aldford Street (left) and Park Lane (centre) in 1897. *Demolished*

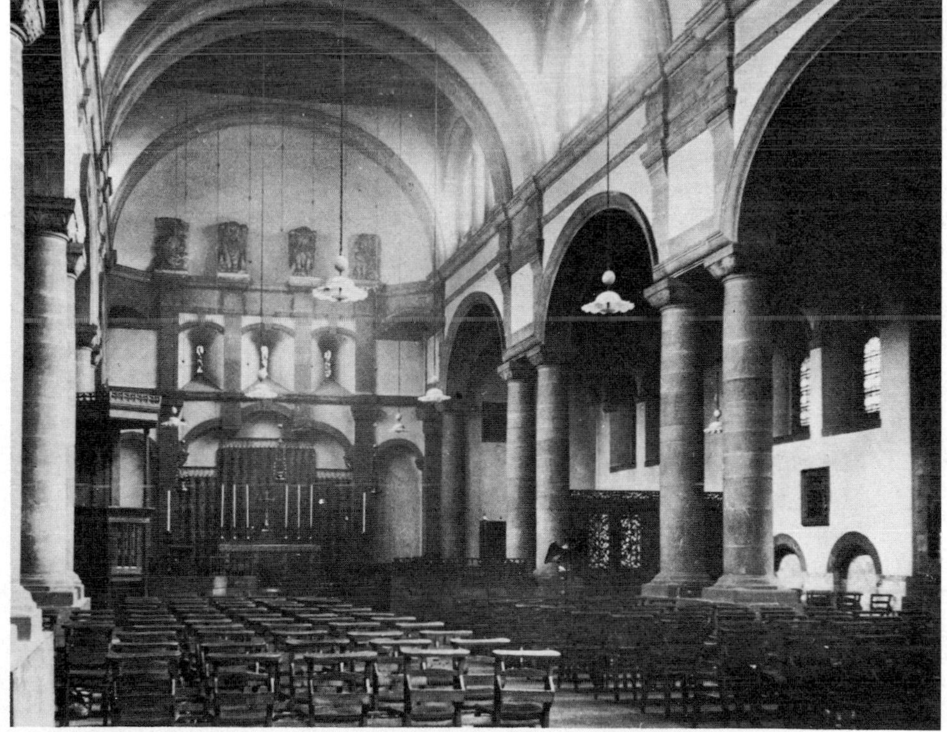

b (*left*). St. Anselm's Church, Davies Street (1894–6), interior looking east in *c.* 1938. *Demolished*

Buildings Designed by Balfour and Turner

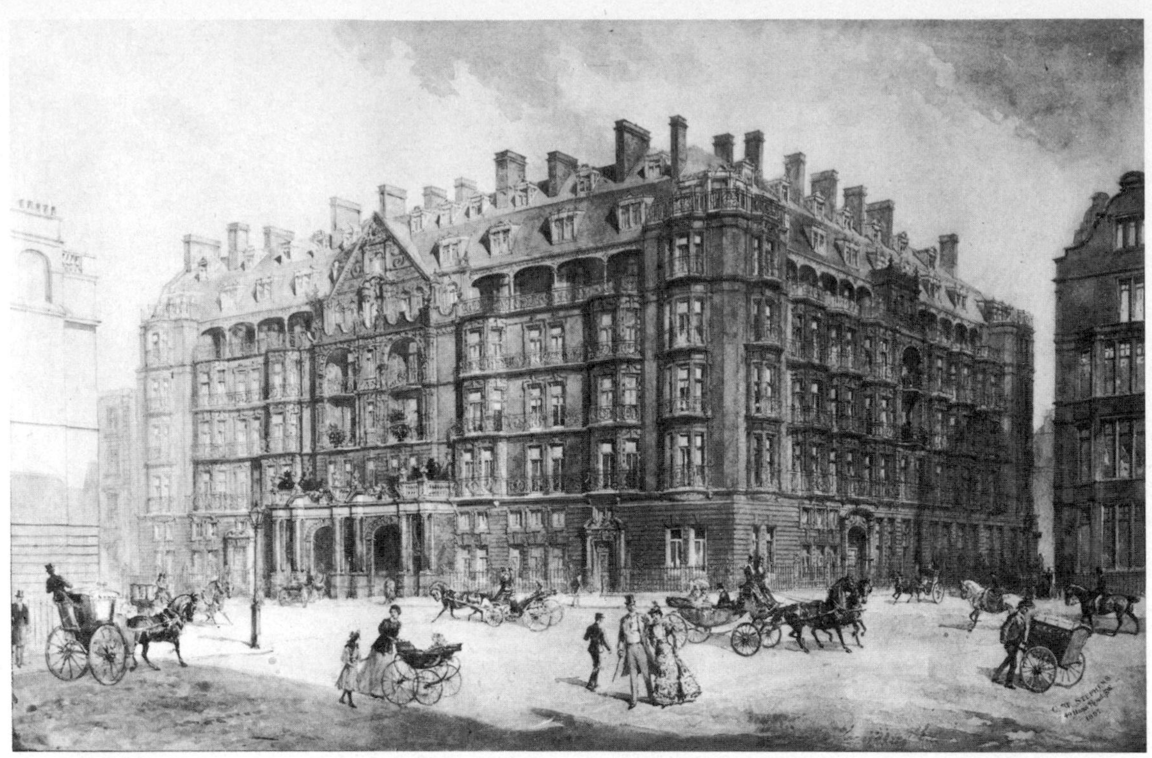

a. Perspective view showing entrance front in Brook Street and return front in Davies Street, by C. W. Stephens, architect, 1897

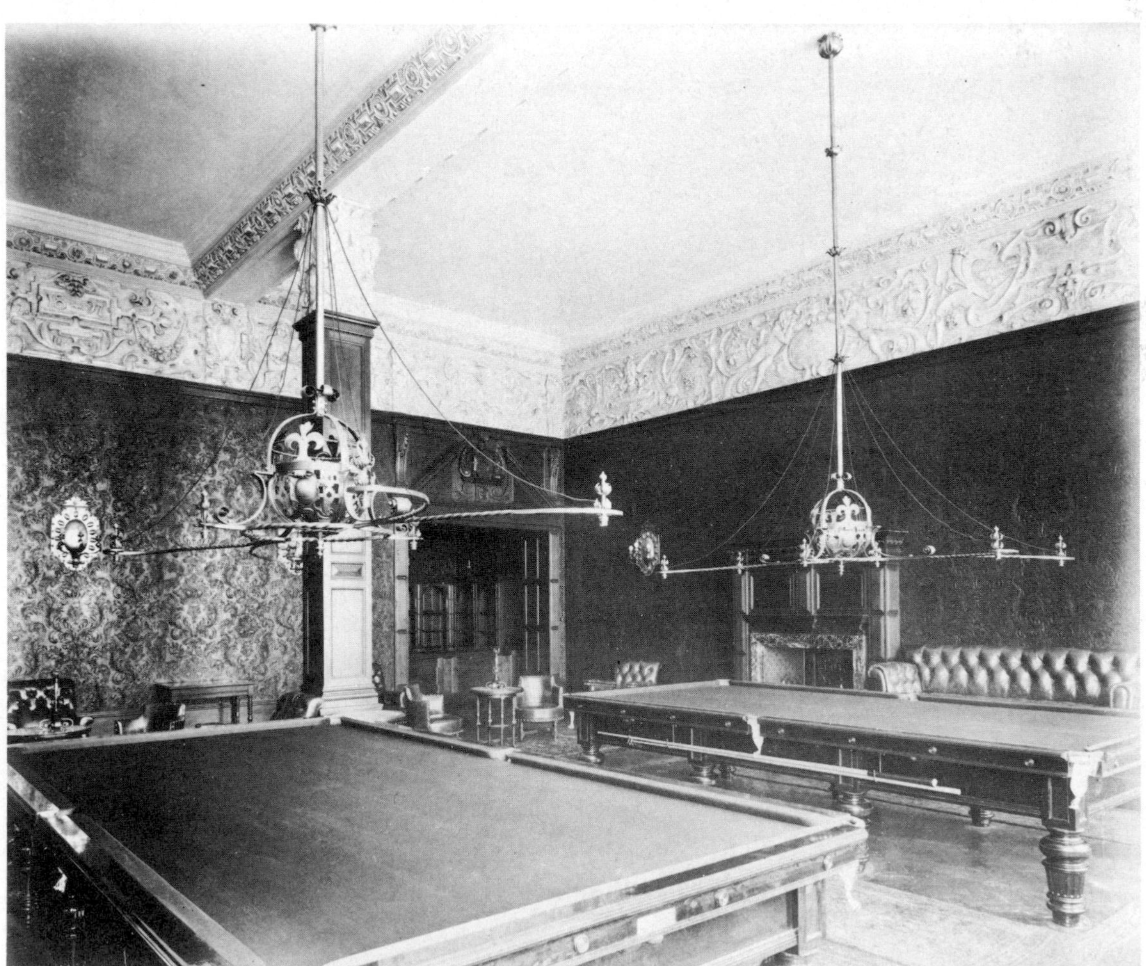

b. The billiard-room in 1898. Interior decorations by Ernest George and Yeates, architects, 1896–8. *Destroyed*

CLARIDGE'S HOTEL, NEW BUILDING

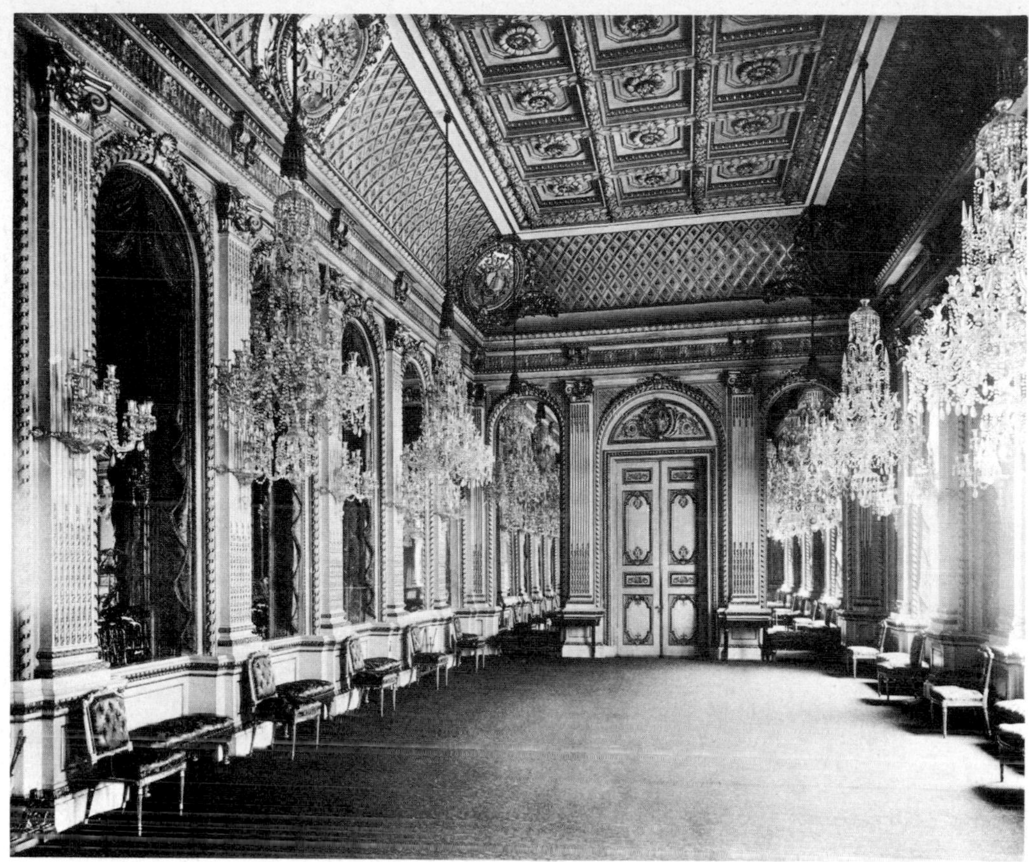

a. Dudley House, Park Lane, ballroom in 1890. Samuel Daukes, architect, and Laurent and Haber, decorators, *c*. 1858. *Destroyed*

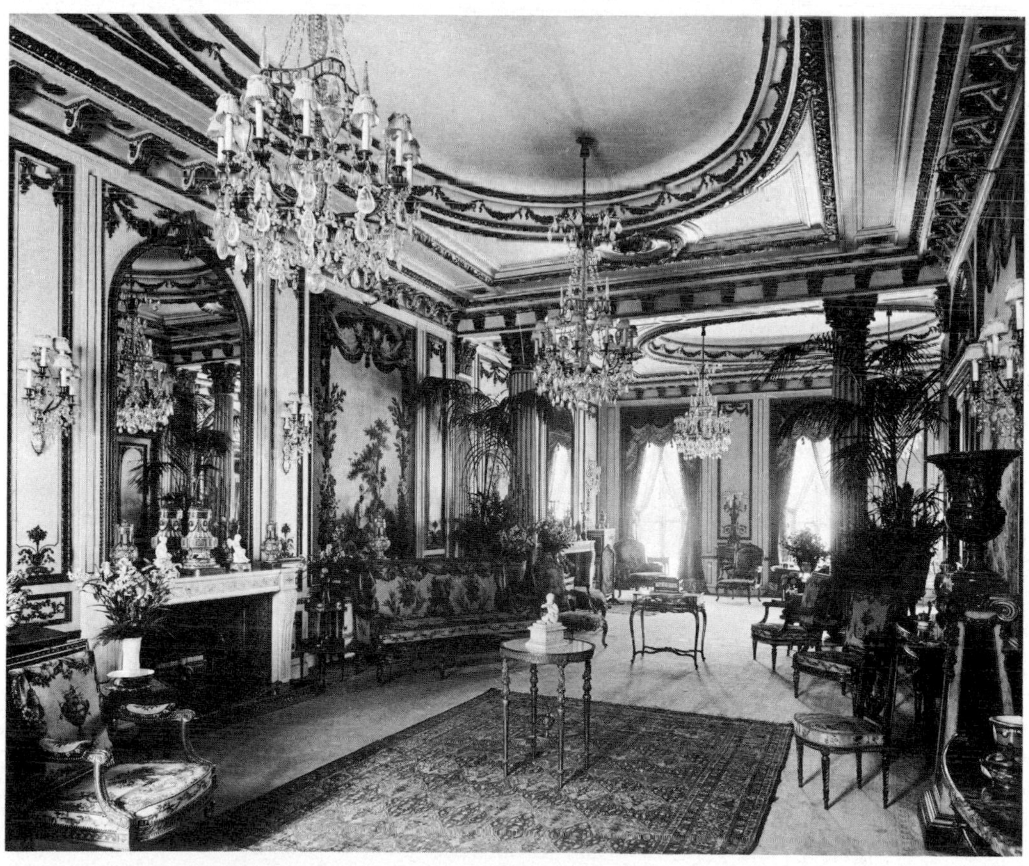

b. No. 26 Grosvenor Square, drawing-room in 1902. Howard and Sons, decorators. *Demolished*

INTERIORS IN THE FRENCH STYLE

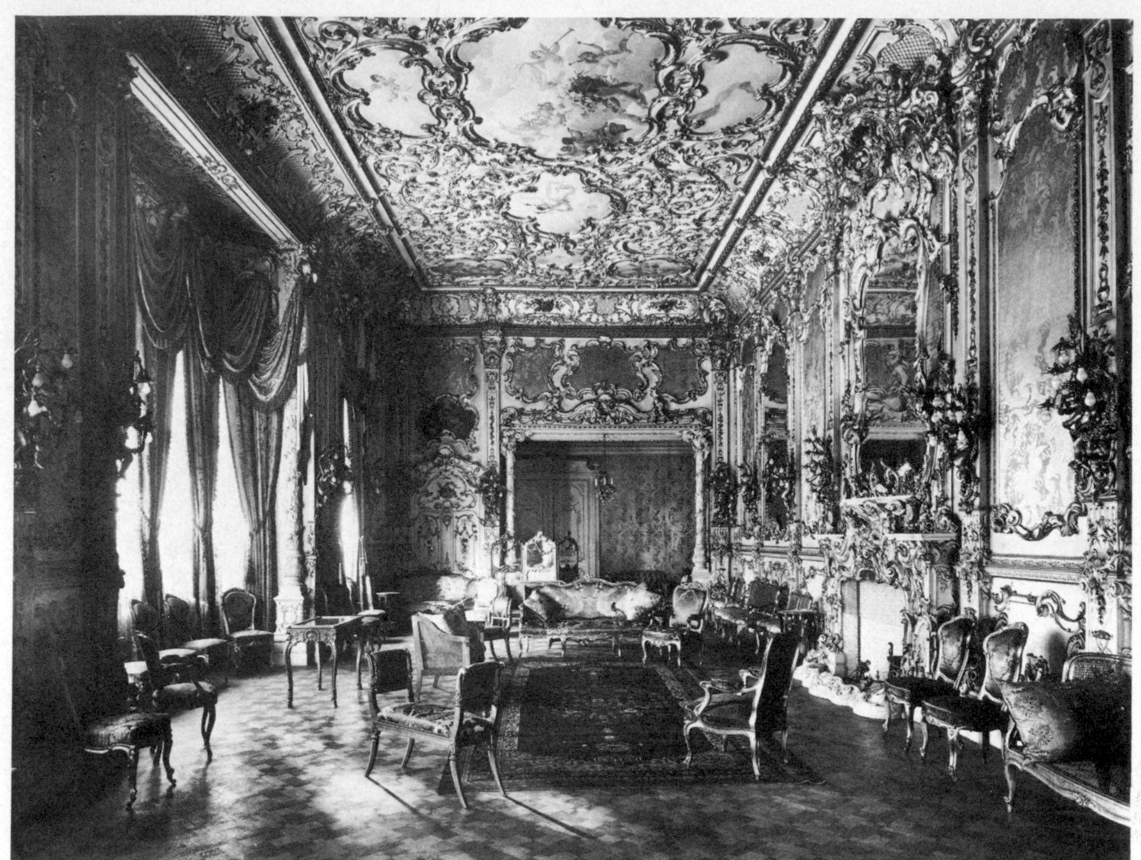

a (*above*). In 1909. Decorators unknown

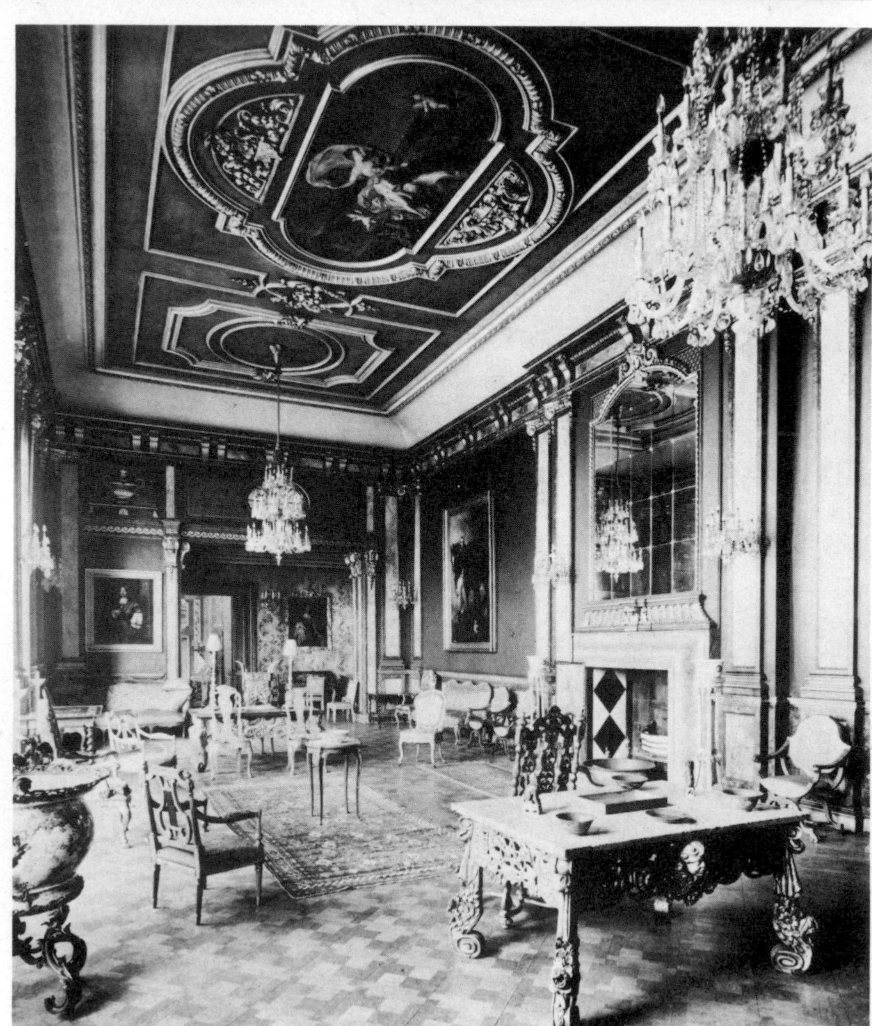

b (*right*). In 1926. Decorations perhaps by Keeble Limited, 1919

No. 41 Grosvenor Square, the Ballroom. *Demolished*

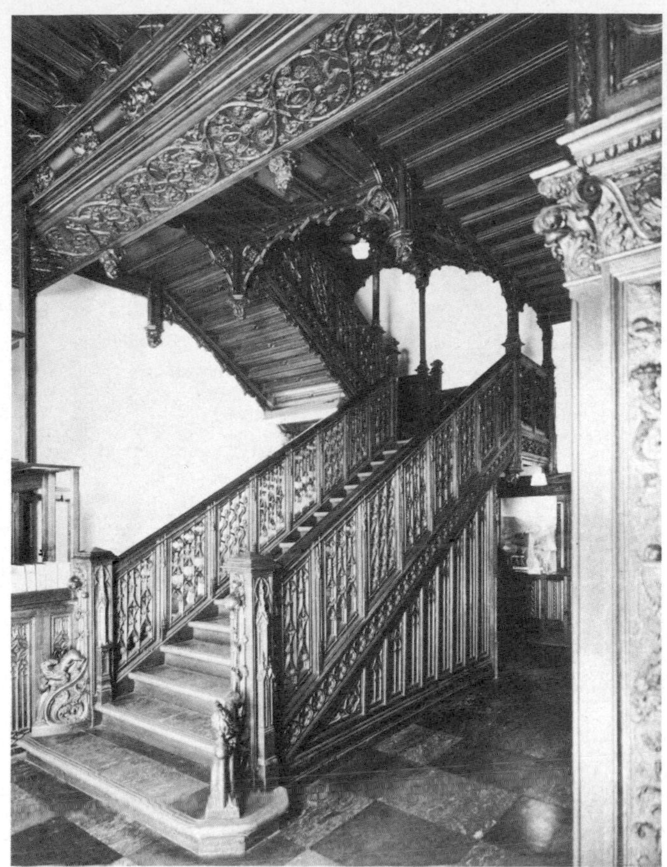

a. No. 46 Grosvenor Street, Gothic staircase in 1970. Blow and Billerey, architects, and L. Buscaylet, decorator, 1910–11

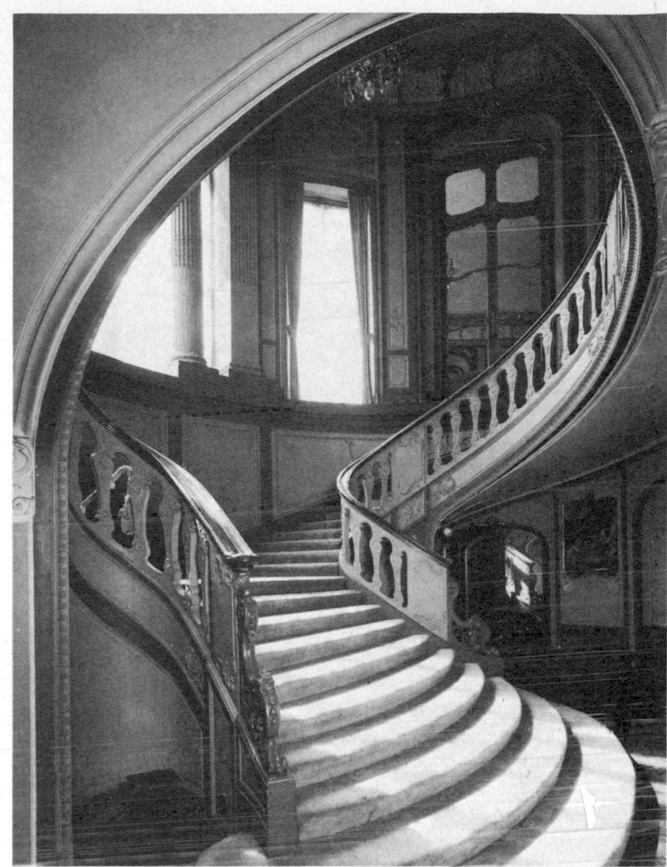

b. Nos. 69–71 (odd) Brook Street, ballroom staircase in 1975. W. O. W. Bouwens van der Boijen and assistants, architects and decorators, *c.* 1890

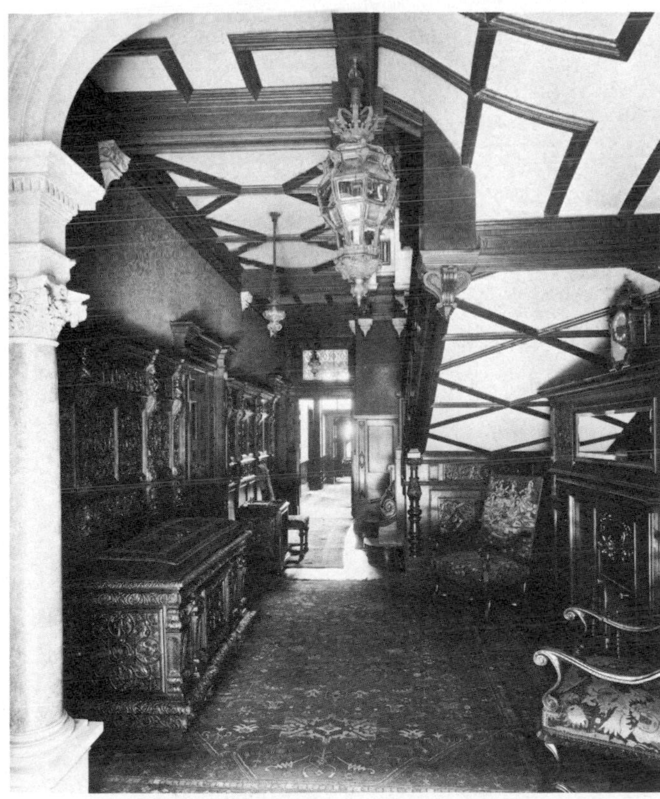

c. No. 24 Upper Brook Street, entrance hall and staircase in 1917. Decorator unknown. *Now simplified*

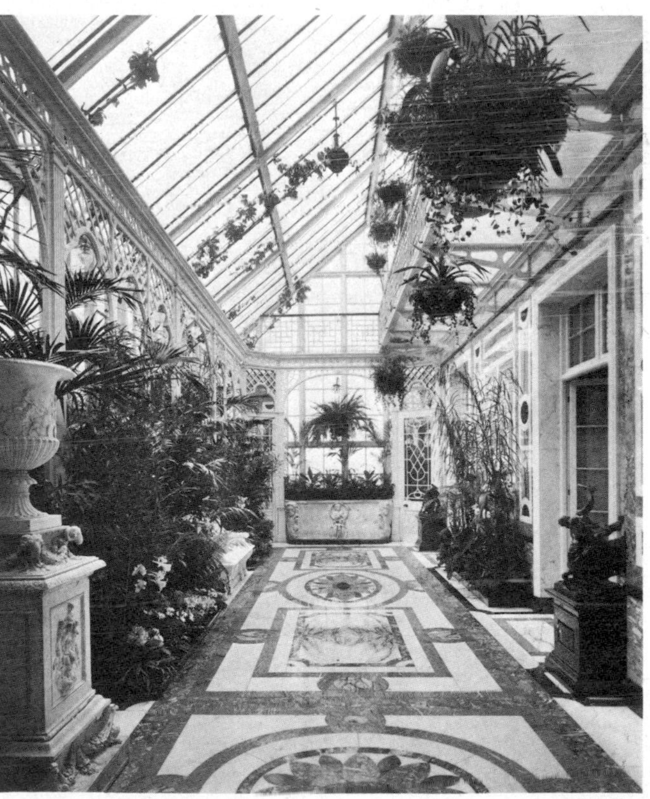

d. No. 45 Grosvenor Square, conservatory in 1897. Charles Mellier and Company, decorators. *Demolished*

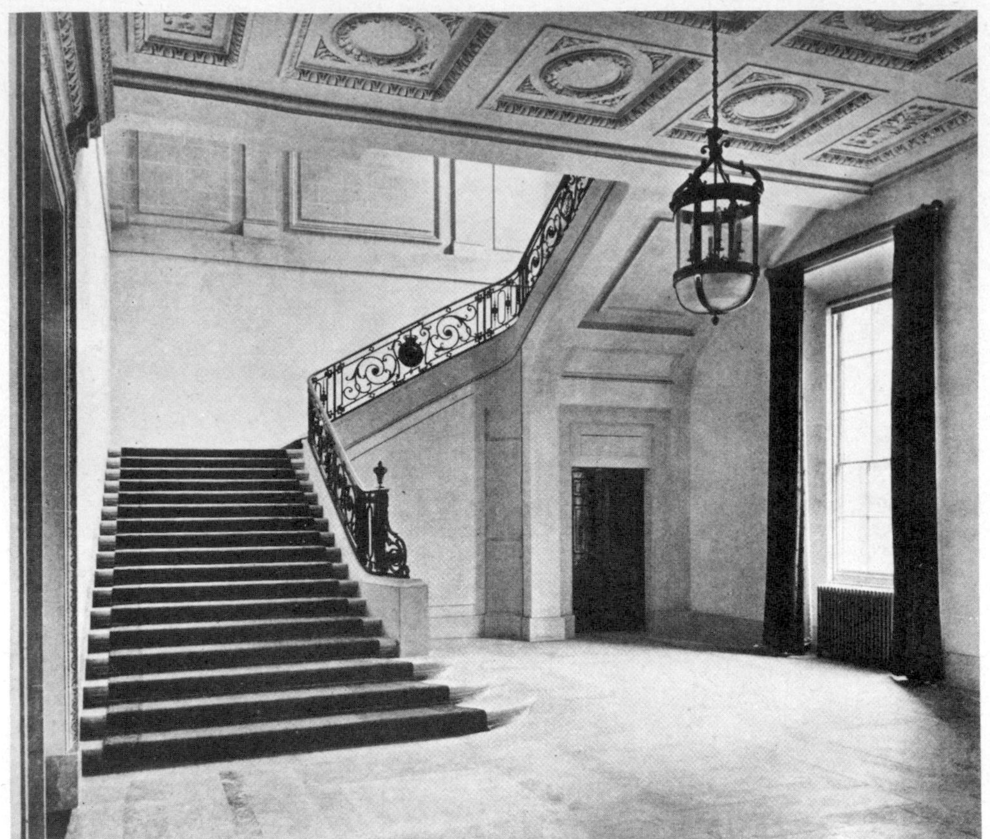

a. Bute House, No. 75 South Audley Street, hall and staircase in 1927. Fernand Billerey, architect, *c*. 1926–7

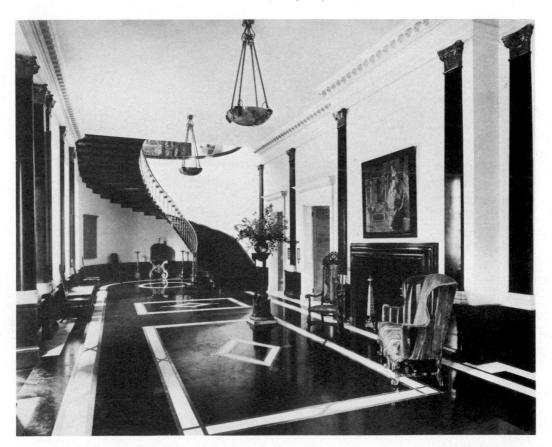

b. No. 38 South Street, hall and staircase in 1924. Wimperis and Simpson, architects, and Harold Peto, decorator, 1919–21

INTER-WAR ENTRANCE HALLS

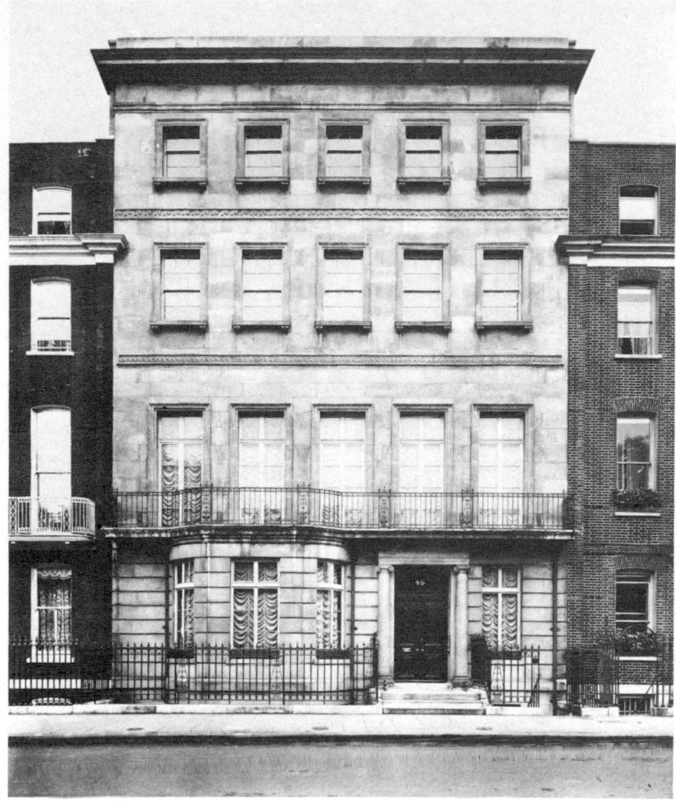

a. No. 45 Grosvenor Square in 1910. Edmund Wimperis and Hubert East, architects of front, 1902. *Demolished*

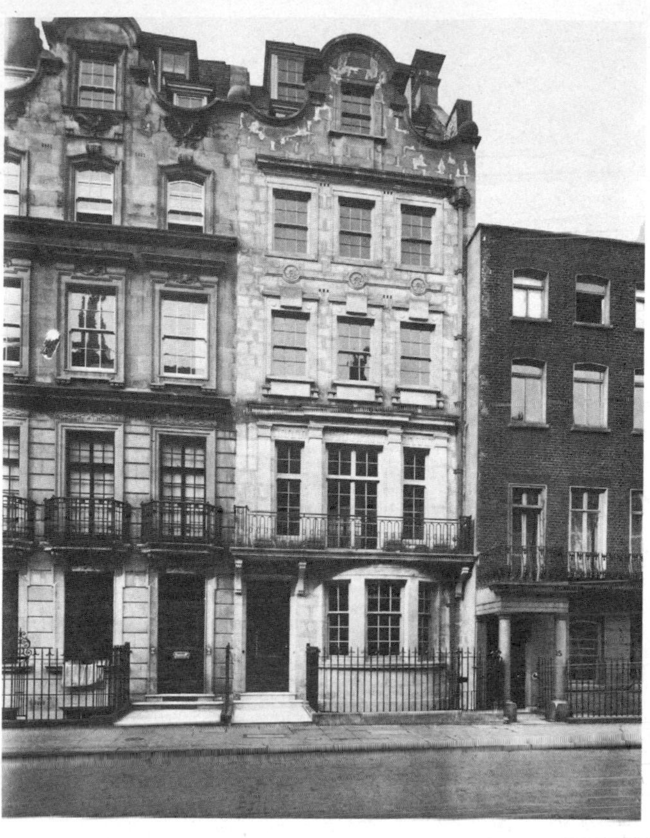

b. Nos. 16 (centre) and 17 (left) Upper Brook Street in 1913. Edmund Wimperis and J. R. Best, architects, 1907–13

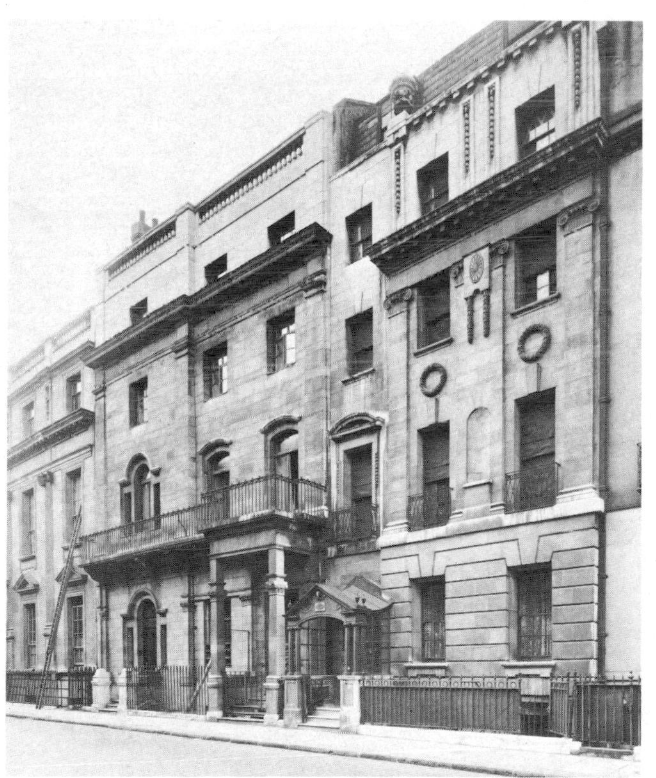

c. Nos. 73 (centre right), 74 (left centre) and 75 (far left) South Audley Street in 1943. Front of No. 73 by Paul Waterhouse (1909), of No. 74 by Balfour and Turner (1908), and of No. 75 by Cyrille J. Corblet (1906–7)

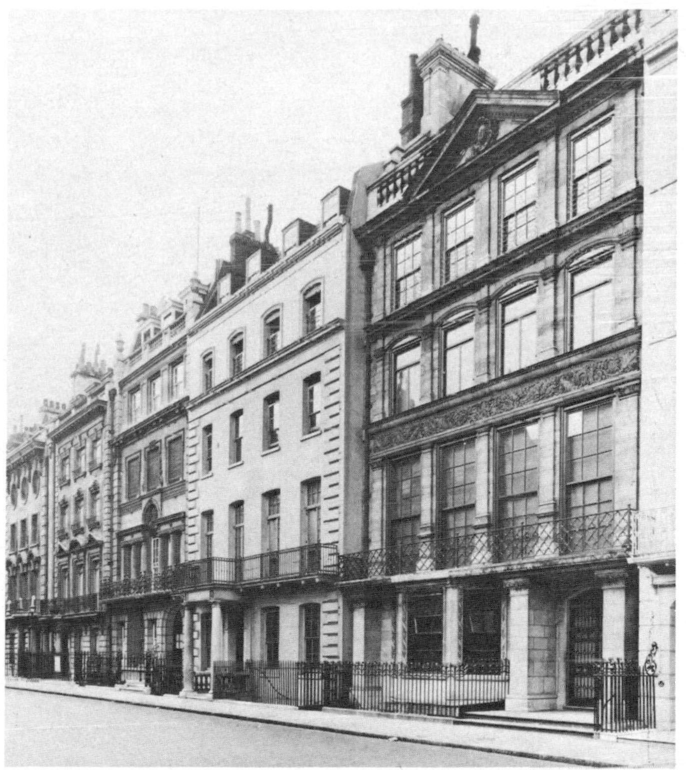

d. Nos. 17–21 (consec.) Upper Grosvenor Street (right to left) in 1927. No. 17 by Balfour and Turner (1906–7); No. 19 by Maurice C. Hulbert (1909–10); No. 20 probably by Boehmer and Gibbs (1909); and No. 21 by Ralph Knott and E. Stone Collins (1908)

Elevations in Stone, 1900–1914

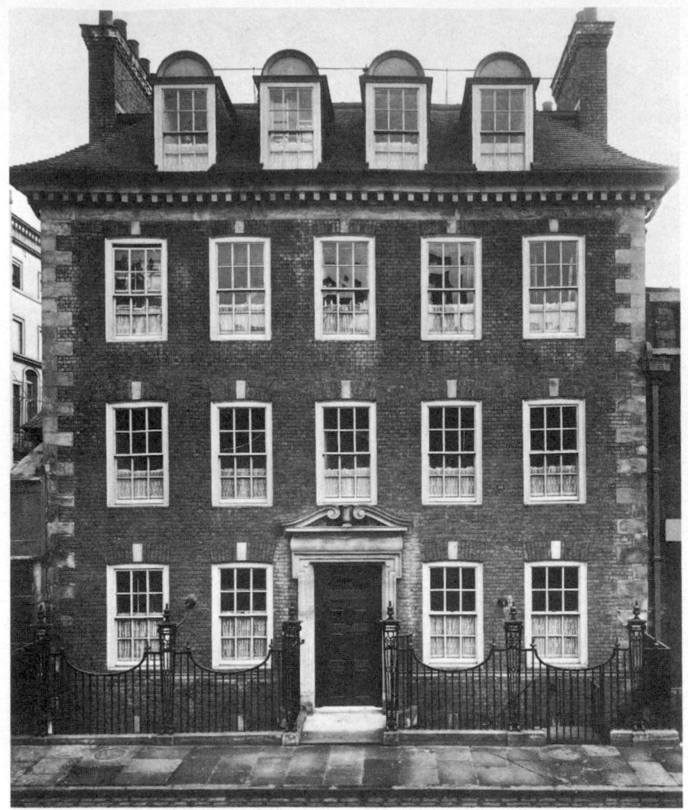

a. No. 28 South Street in 1903. Detmar Blow, architect, 1902–3

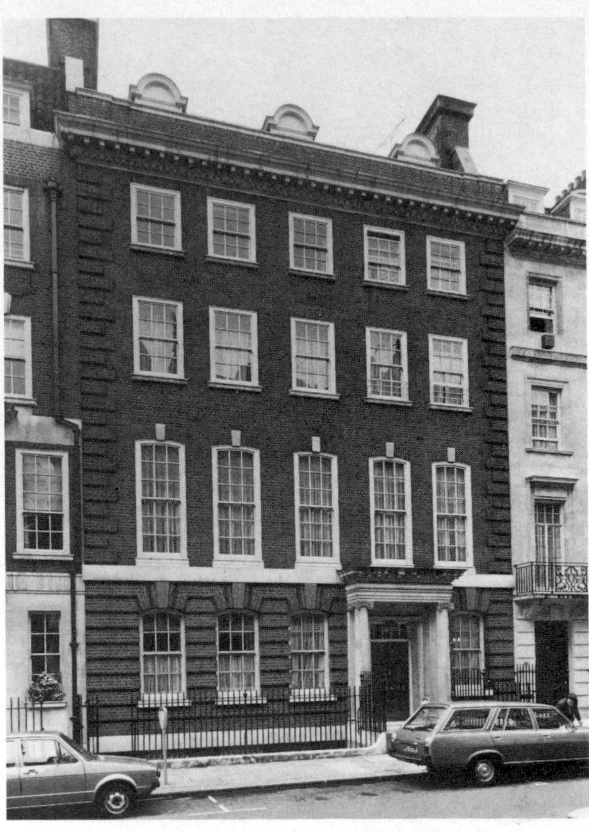

b. No. 46 Green Street in 1976. Wimperis and Simpson, architects, 1913–15

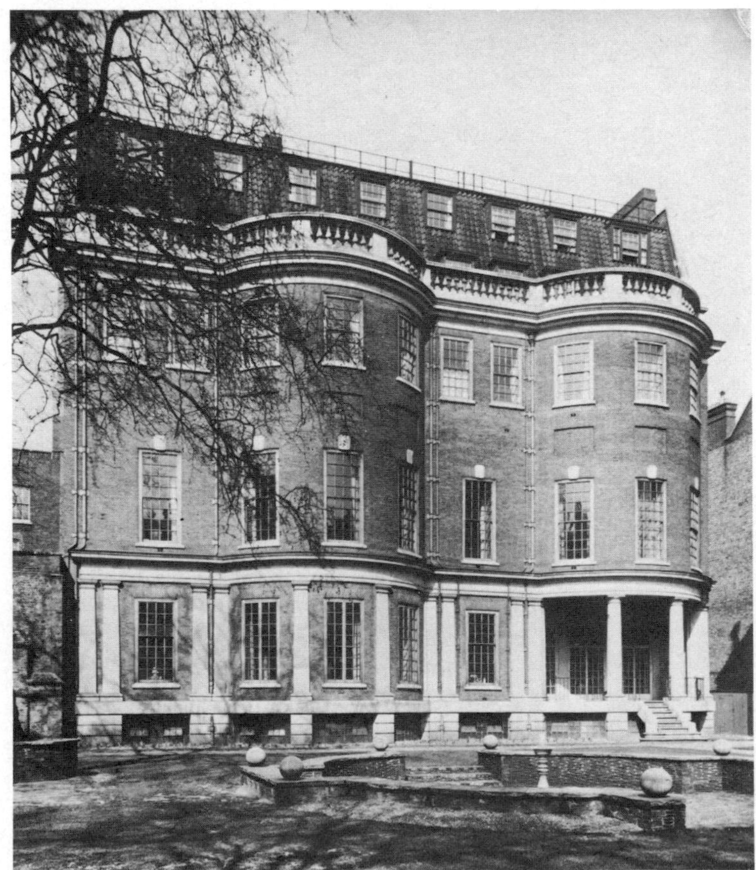

c. No. 38 South Street, rear elevation from South Street garden, in 1924. Wimperis and Simpson, architects, 1919–21

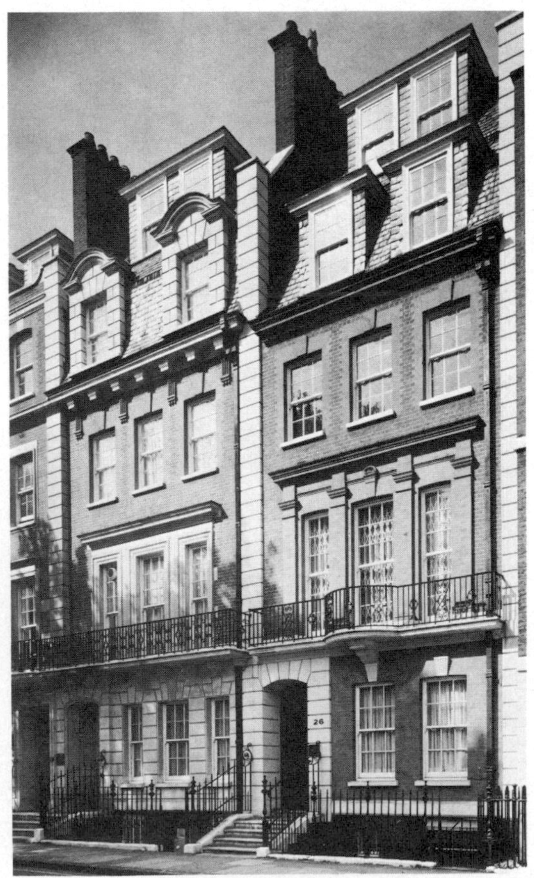

d. Nos. 25 and 26 Gilbert Street in 1974. Maurice C. Hulbert, architect, and Matthews, Rogers and Company, builders, 1910–12

ELEVATIONS IN BRICK, 1900–1920

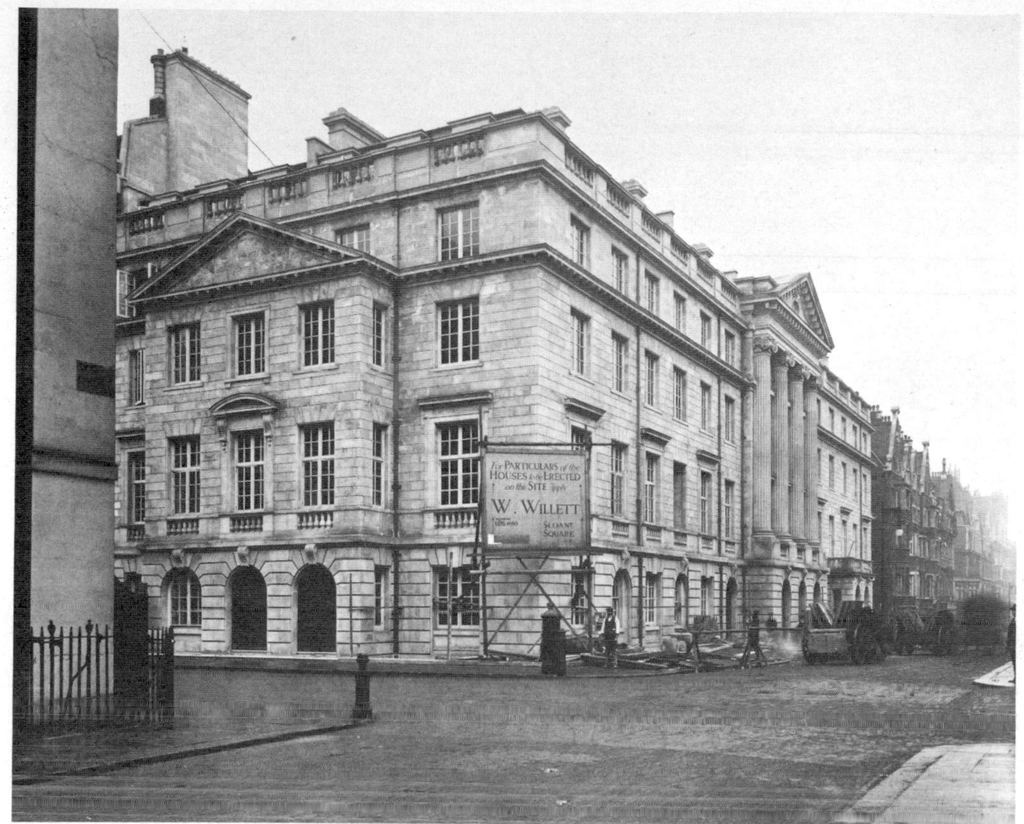

a. Nos. 37 and 38 Upper Grosvenor Street and Nos. 44–50 (even) Park Street, from north-west in 1912. Blow and Billerey, architects, and William Willett, builder, 1911–12

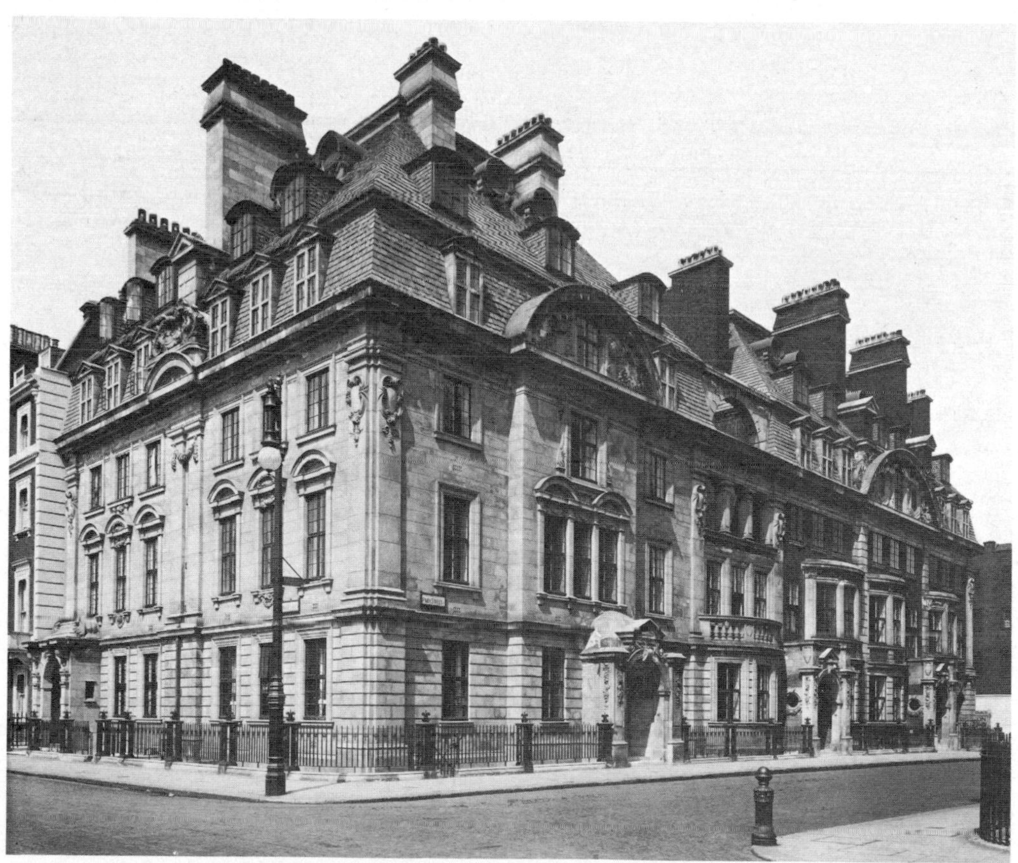

b. Nos. 37–43 (odd) Park Street, from south-east in 1911. W. D. Caröe, architect, and Higgs and Hill, builders, 1908–10

STONE-FRONTED RANGES

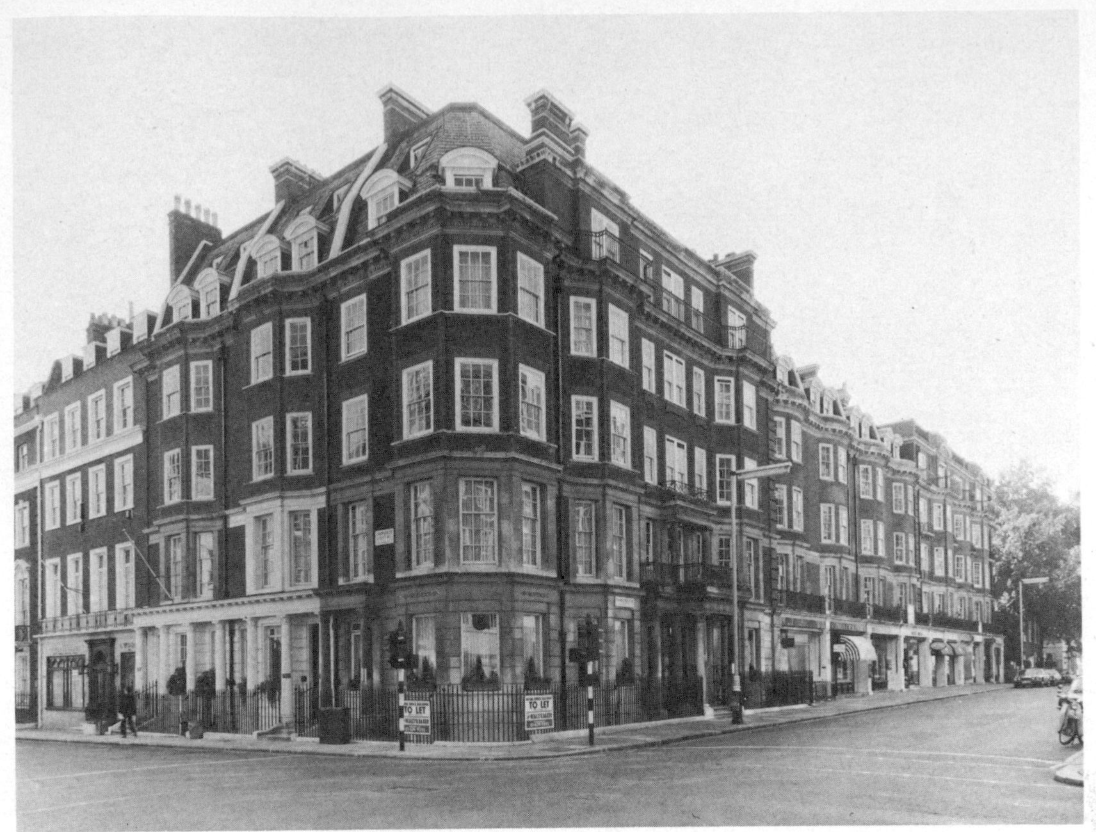

a. Nos. 55–57 (consec.) Grosvenor Street (right to left) and Nos. 4–26 (even) Davies Street (right to left), from north-west in 1976. Wimperis and Best, architects, 1910–12

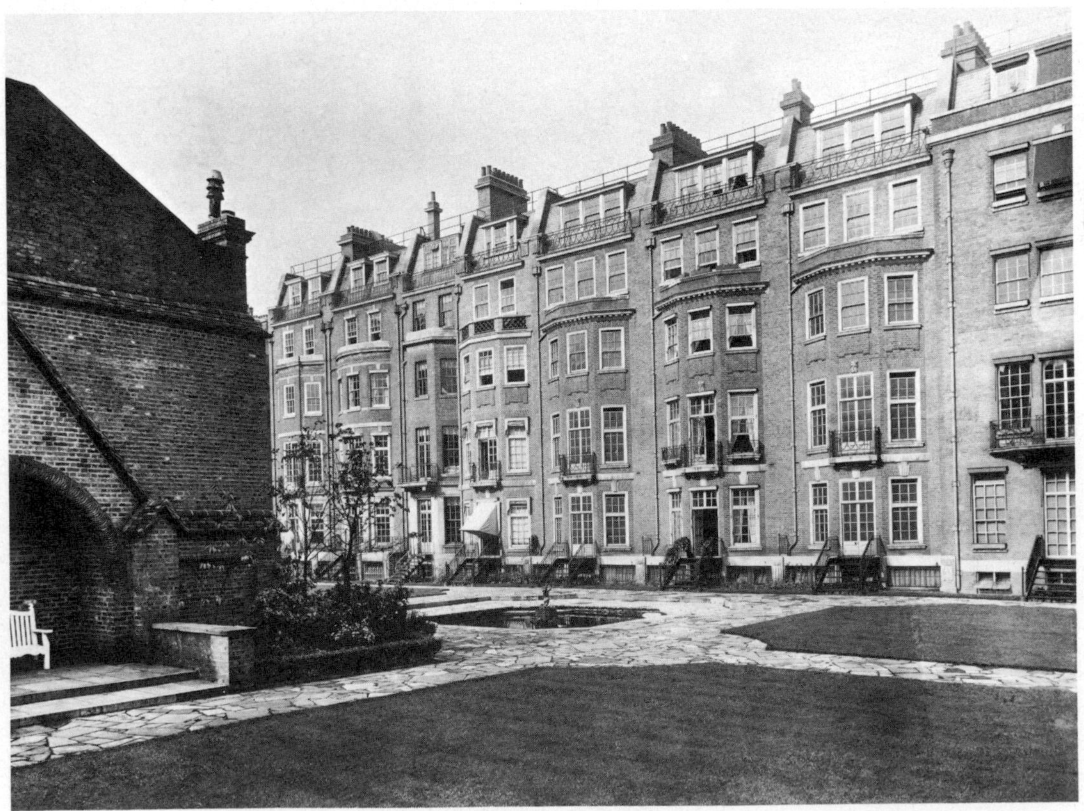

b. Nos. 38–45 (consec.) Green Street (left to right), backs from Green Street garden in 1916. Mostly by Wimperis and Simpson, 1913–16

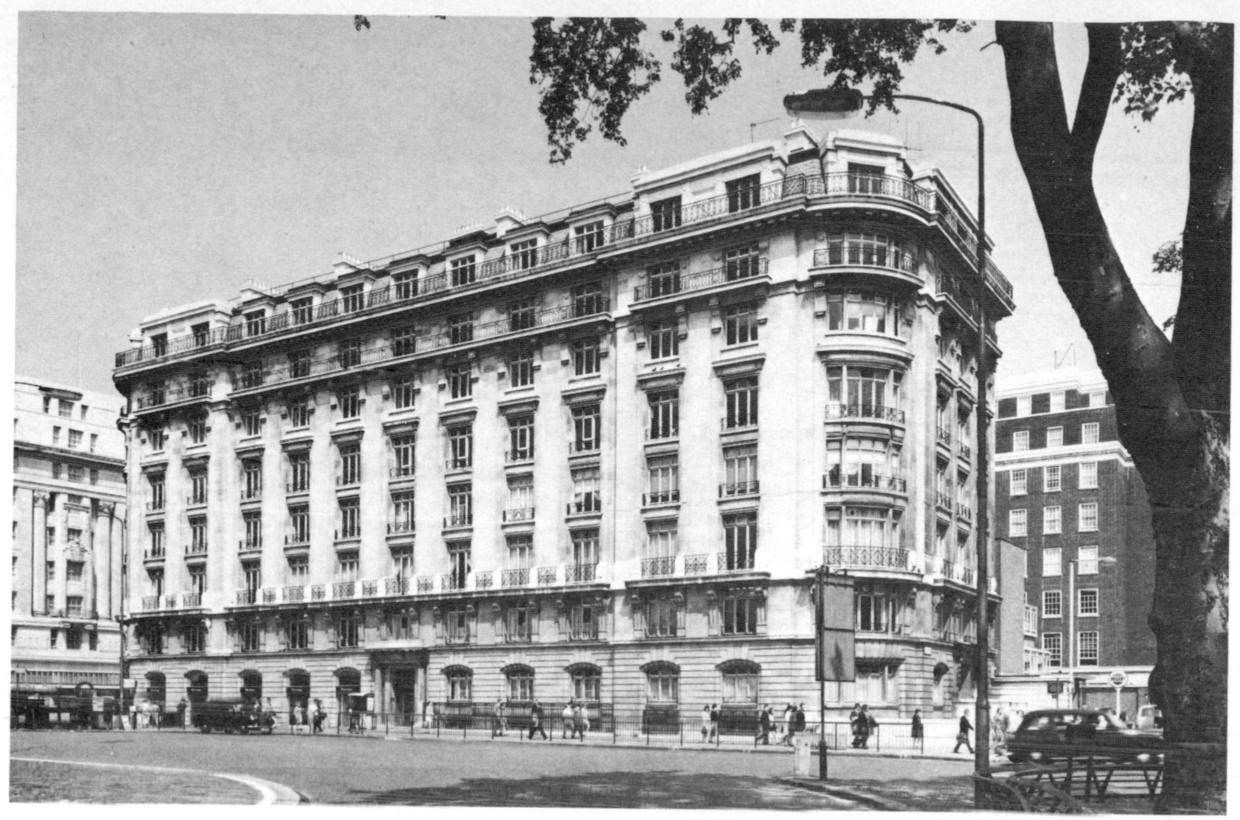

a. Nos. 139–140 Park Lane, from west in 1968. Frank Verity, architect, *c*. 1913–18

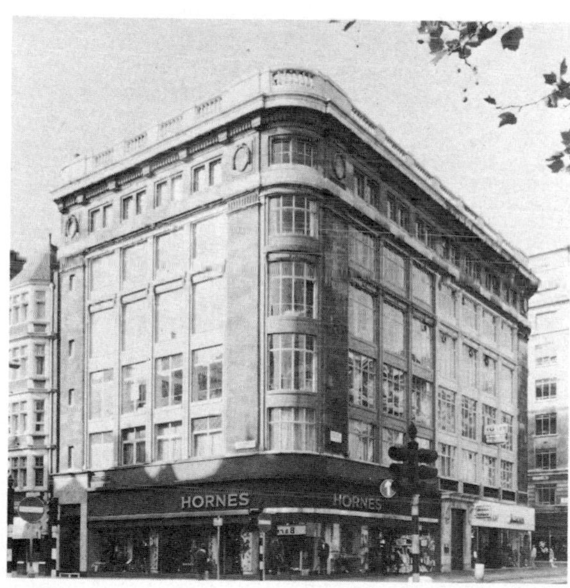

b (*above*). Nos. 415–419 (odd) Oxford Street, from north-east in 1976, showing return front to Duke Street. G. Thrale Jell and Wimperis, Simpson and Guthrie, architects, 1923–35

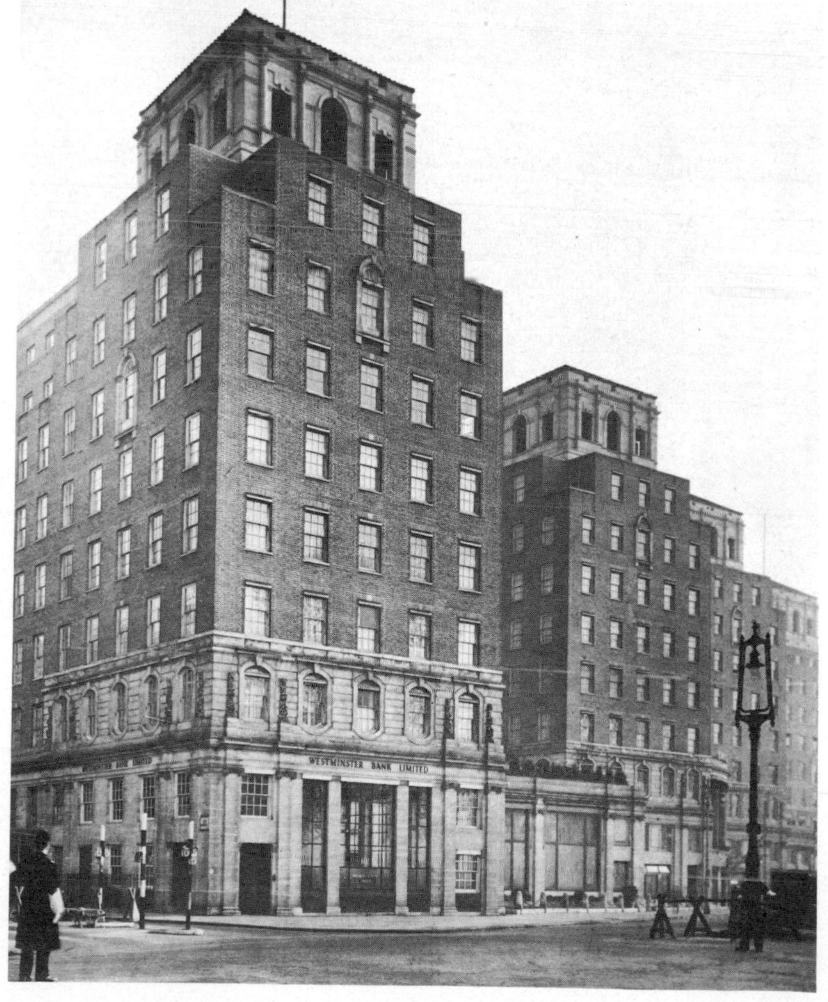

c (*right*). Grosvenor House, Park Lane, from north-west in 1931. Sir Edwin Lutyens and Wimperis, Simpson and Guthrie, architects, 1926–30

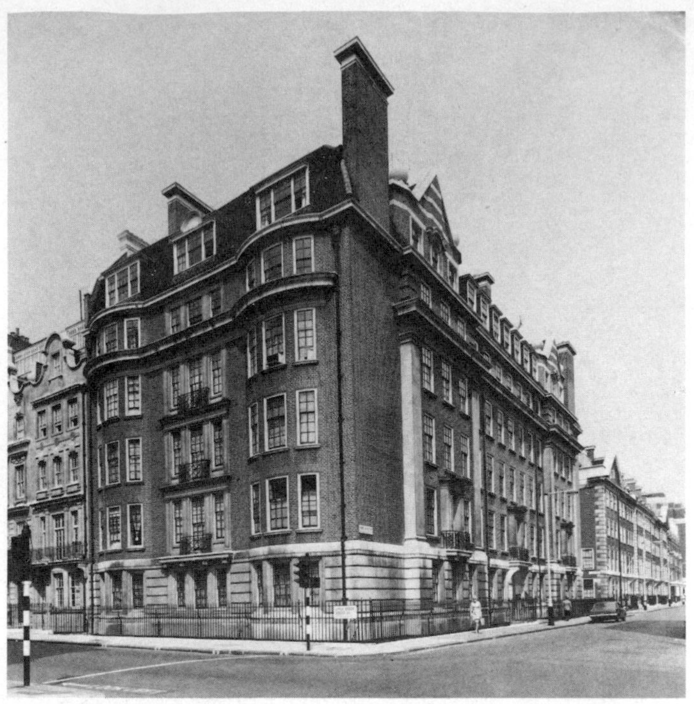

a. Upper Feilde, Upper Brook Street and Park Street, from south-east in 1976. Wimperis and Simpson, architects, 1922–4

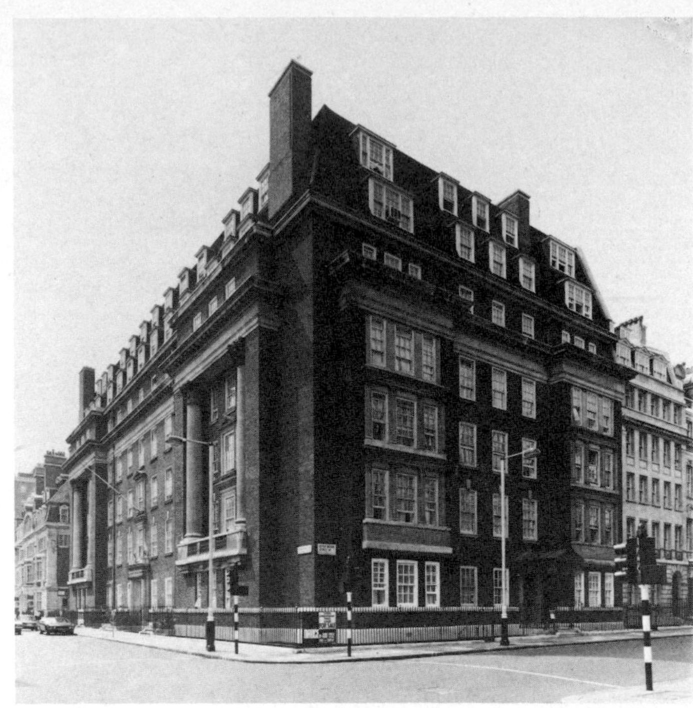

b. Upper Brook Feilde, Upper Brook Street and Park Street, from north-east in 1976. Wimperis, Simpson and Guthrie, architects, 1926–7

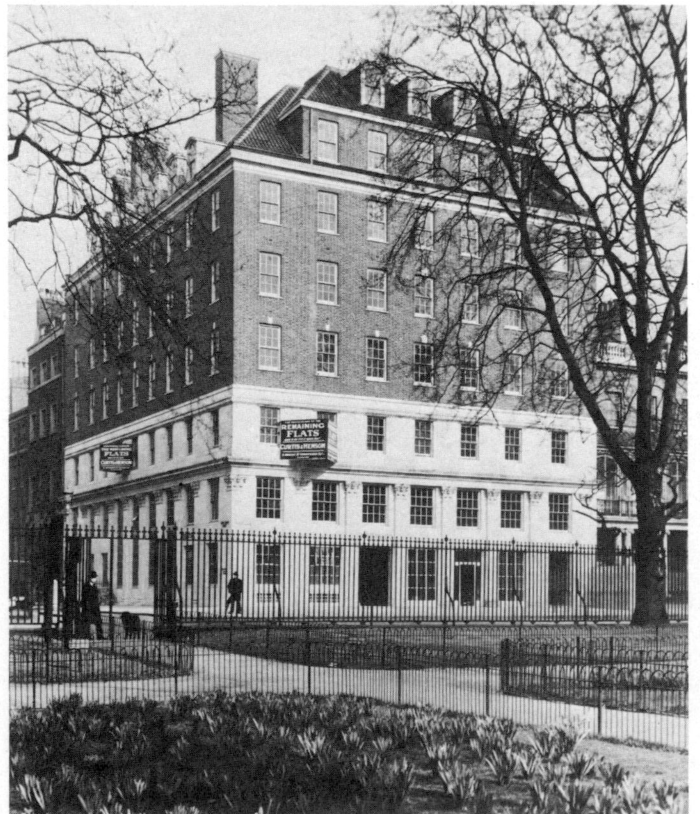

c. Nos. 105–108 (consec.) Park Lane, from west in *c*. 1932. Wimperis, Simpson and Guthrie, architects, 1930–2

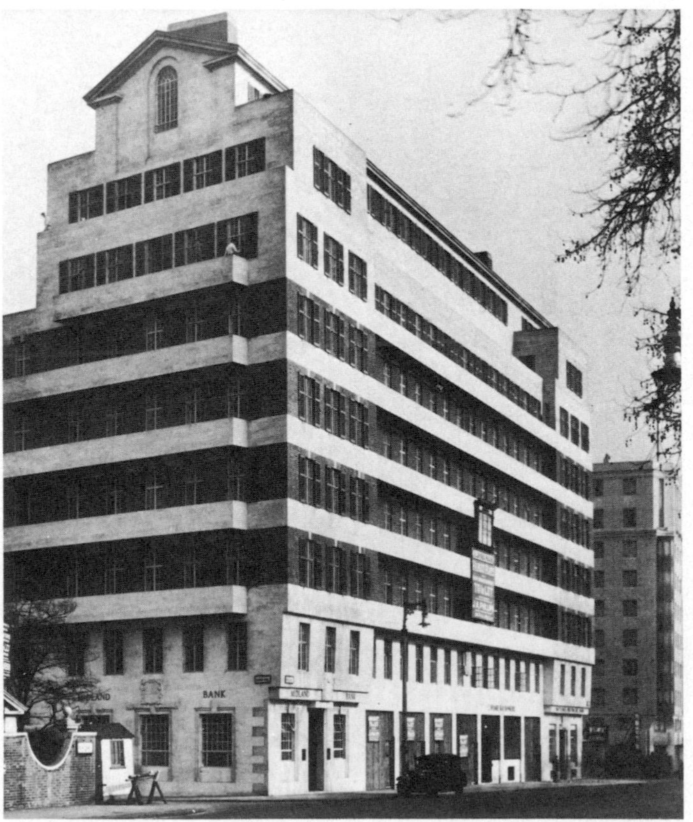

d. Aldford House, Park Lane, from north-west in 1932. George Val Myer and F. J. Watson-Hart, architects, 1930–2

INTER-WAR FLATS

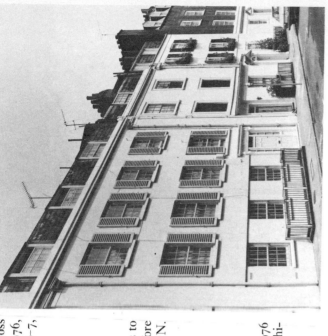

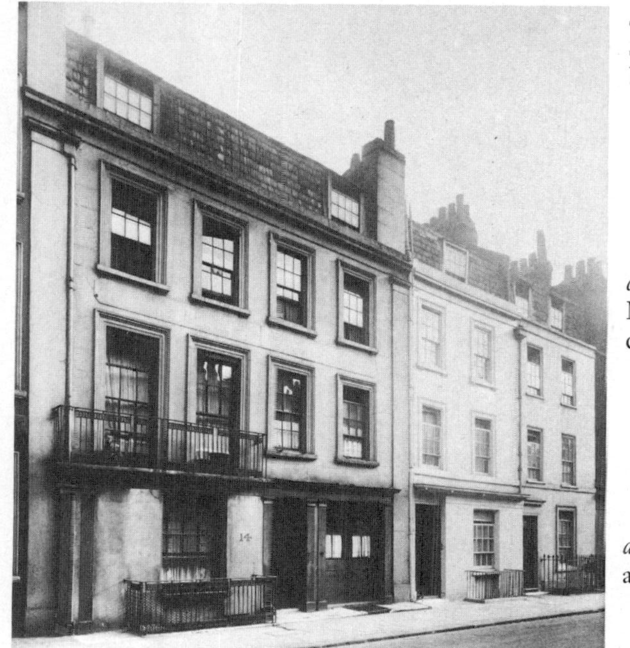

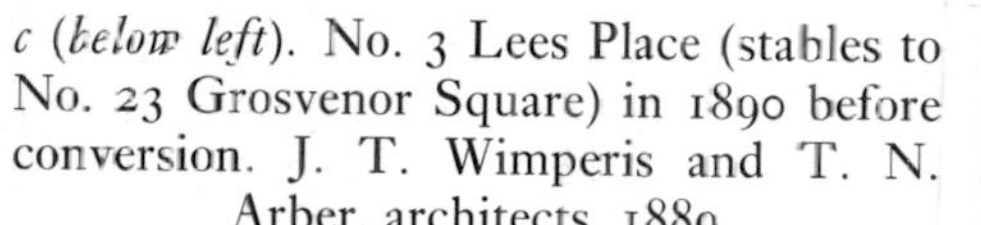

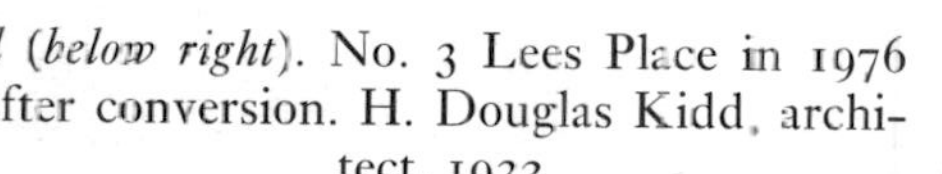

a (*left*), *b* (*right*). Nos. 10–14 (even) Culross Street (right to left), in 1926 and 1976, before and after alterations of 1926–7, mainly by Etchells and Pringle

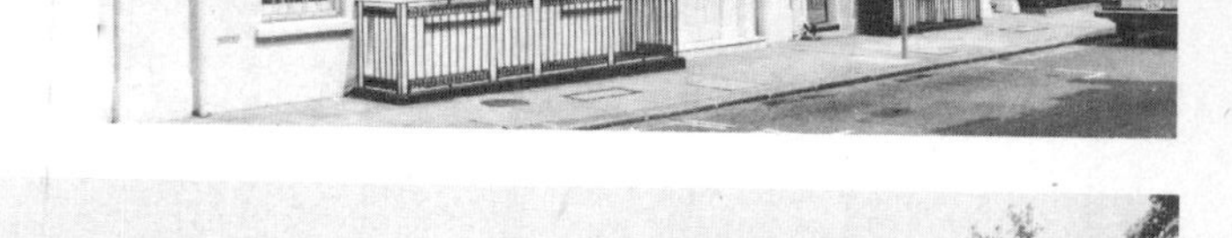

c (*below left*). No. 3 Lees Place (stables to No. 23 Grosvenor Square) in 1890 before conversion. J. T. Wimperis and T. N. Arber, architects, 1889

d (*below right*). No. 3 Lees Place in 1976 after conversion. H. Douglas Kidd, architect, 1932

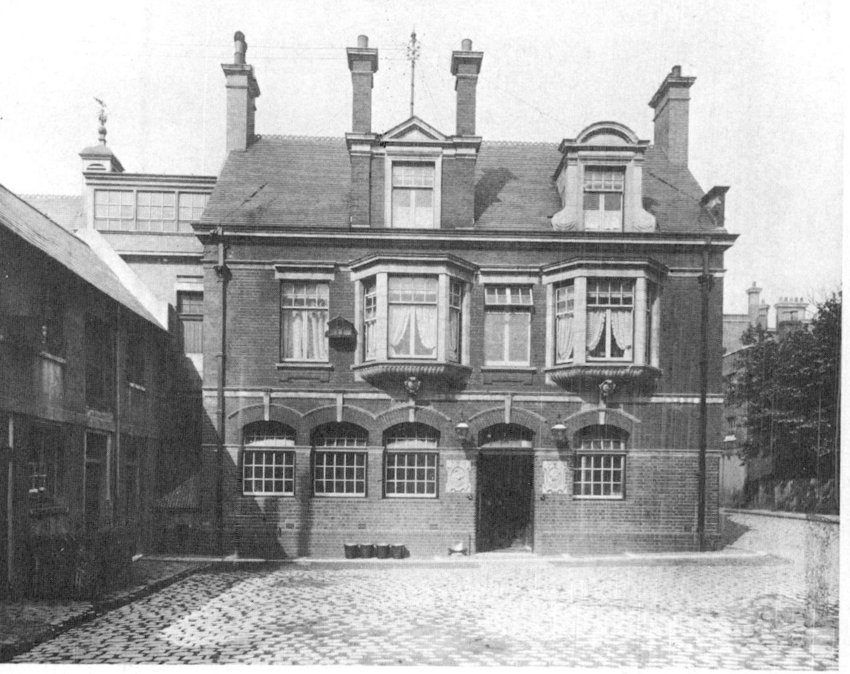

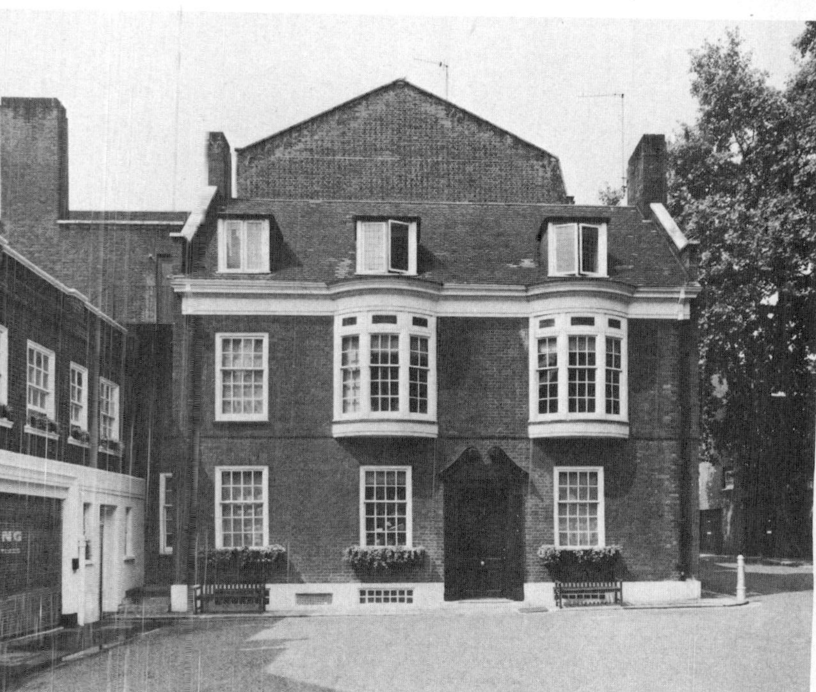

Mews Houses and Conversions

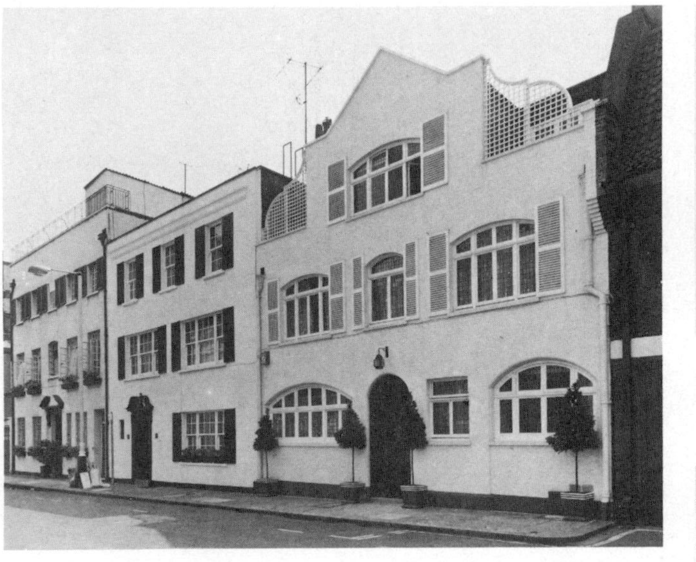

a. Nos. 21–25 (odd) Culross Street (left to right), fronts in 1976. No. 25 by Ernest Cole, 1929

b. Broadbent Street (formerly Little Grosvenor Street), elevations by Etchells and Pringle for proposed conversion of shops, 1927. *Not executed*

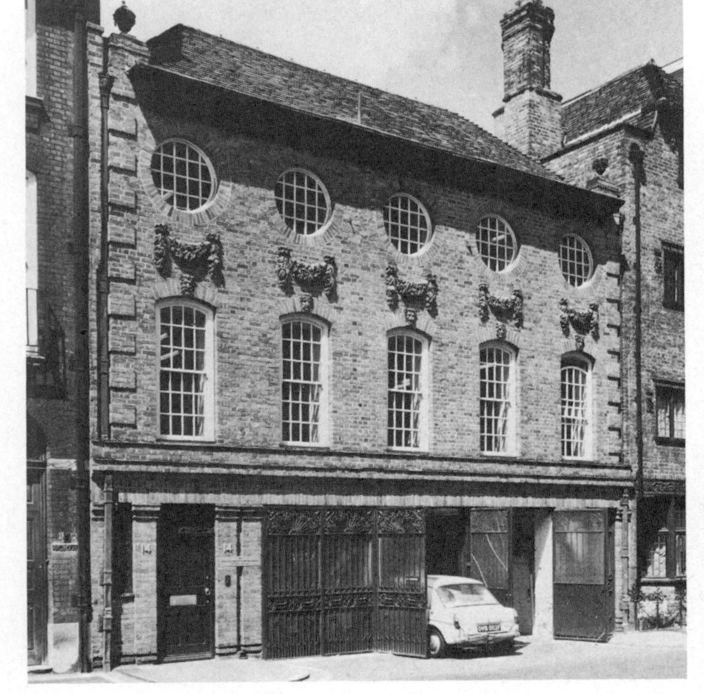

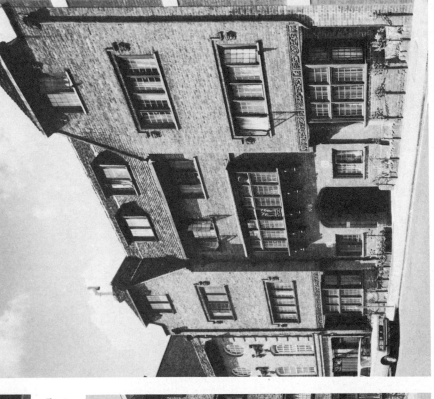

c. Wren House, Nos. 12 and 14 Mount Row, in 1968. T. P. Bennett, architect, 1926–7

d. Tudor House, Nos. 6–10 (even) Mount Row, in 1968. Frederick Etchells, architect, 1929–31

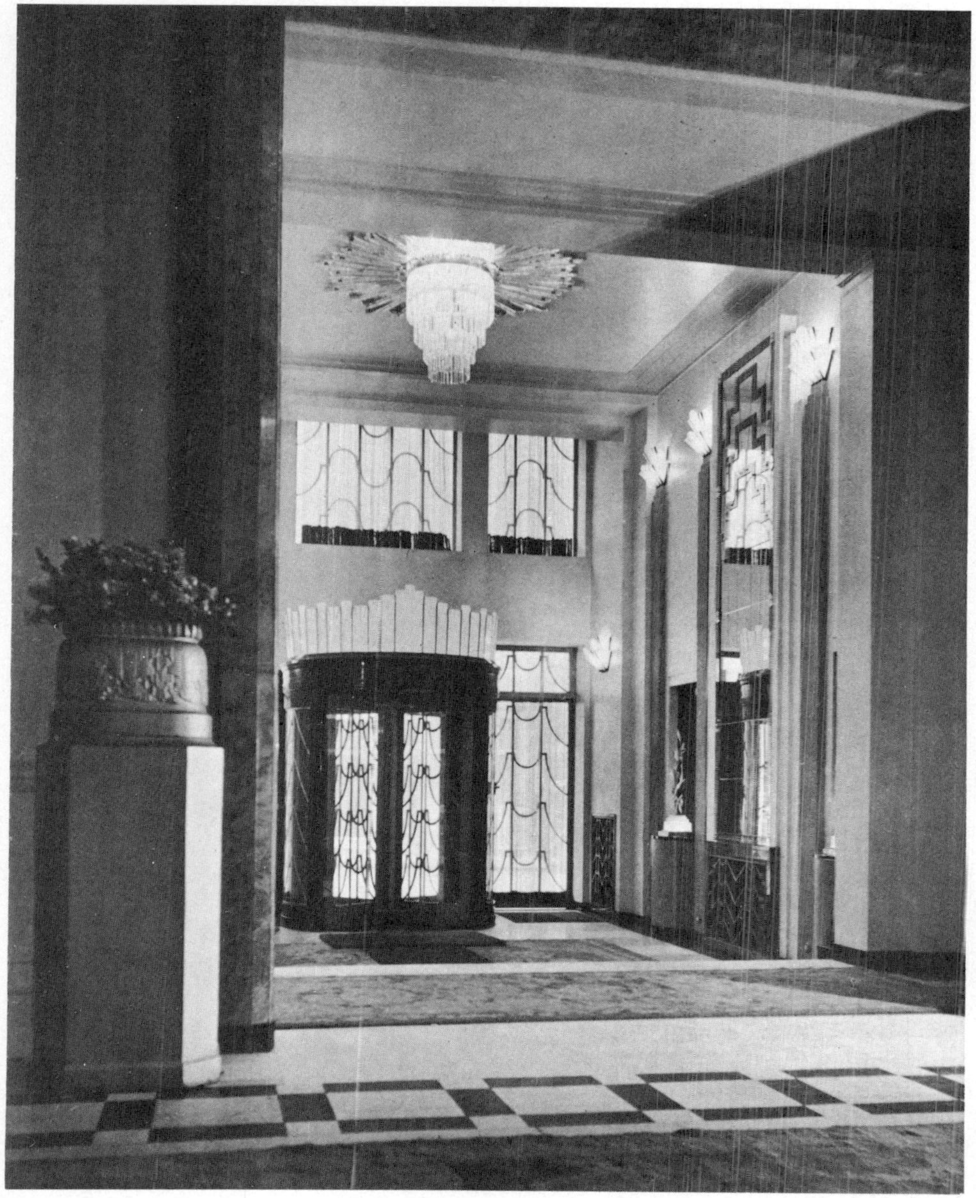

a. Main entrance hall in 1930. Oswald Milne, architect, 1929

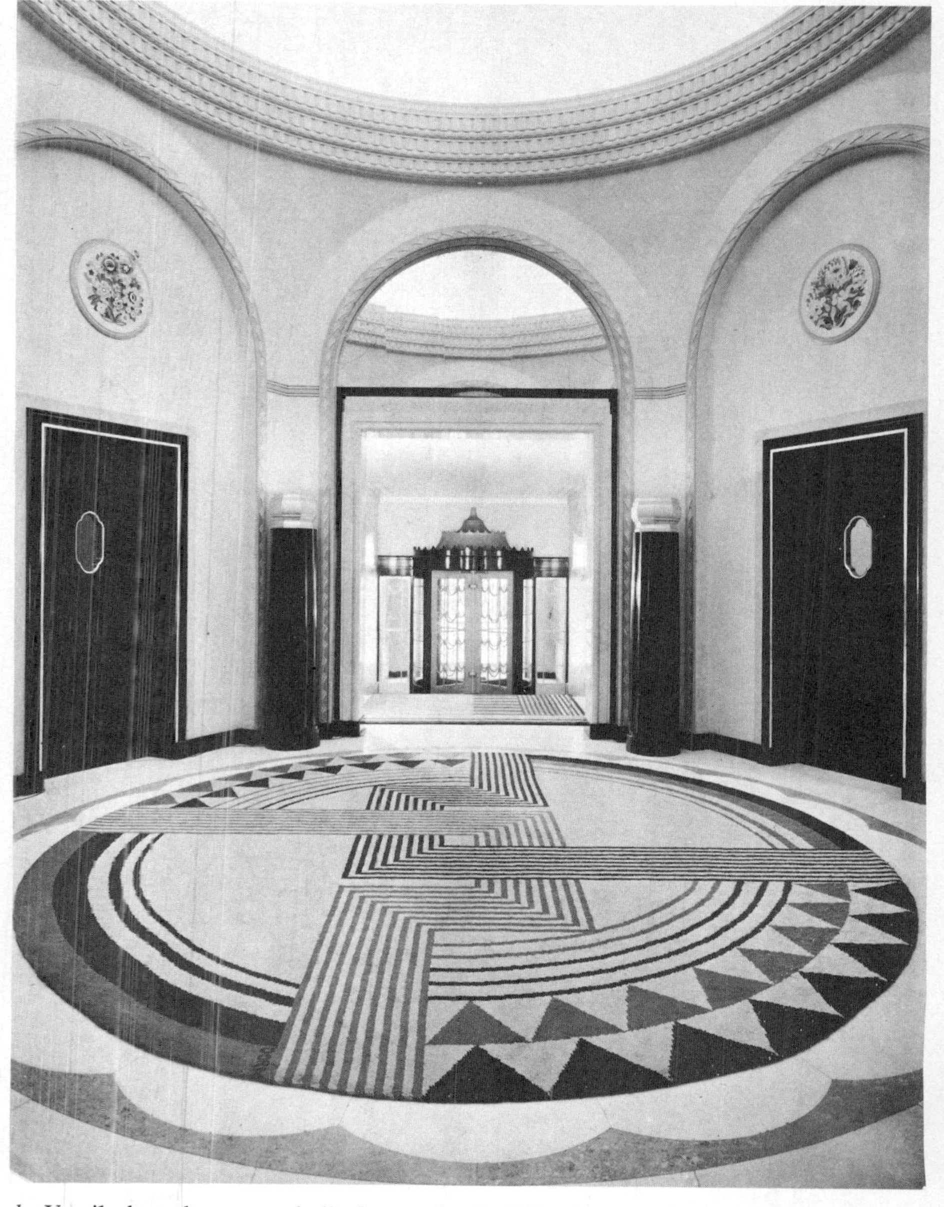

b. Vestibule and entrance hall of extension building in 1932. Oswald Milne, architect, 1930–1

CLARIDGE'S HOTEL, INTERIORS OF 1929–31

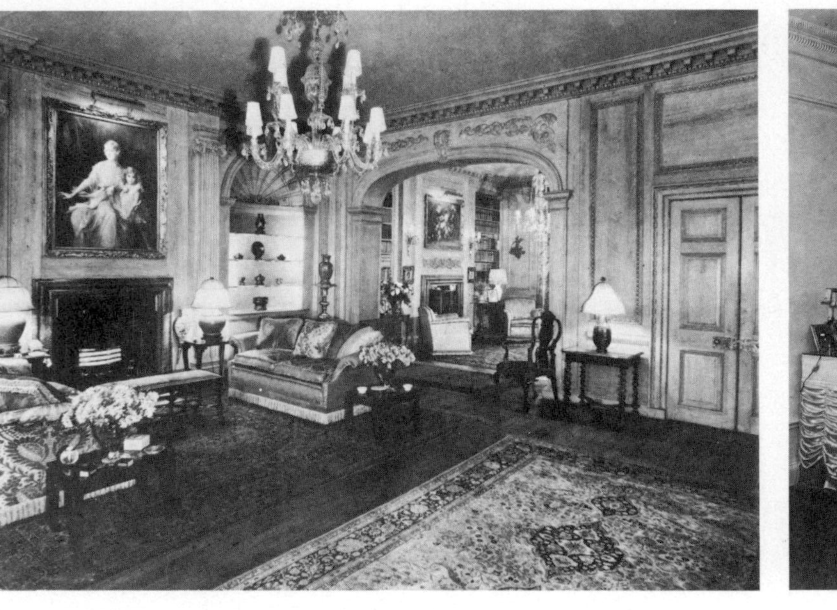

a. No. 25 Upper Brook Street, drawing-room in *c*. 1933. Lenygon and Morant, decorators, 1933

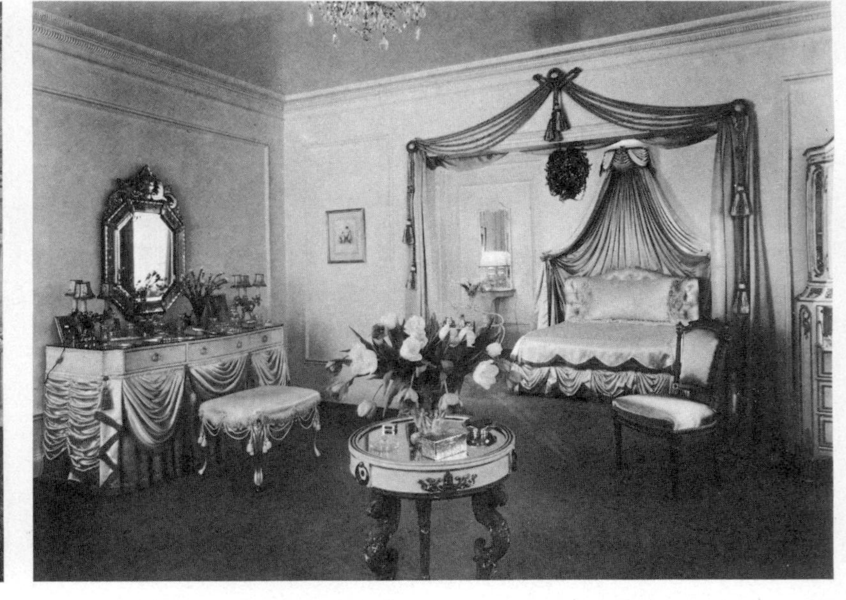

b. No. 42 Upper Brook Street, bedroom of Mrs. F. J. Wolfe's flat in 1939. Decorators unknown

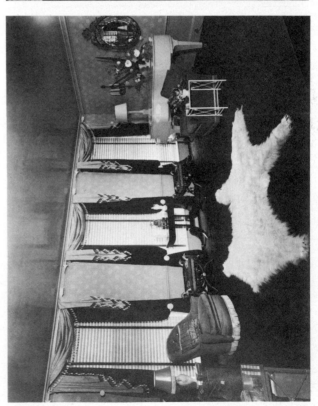

c. No. 25 South Street, sitting-room in 1937. W. Turner Lord and Company, decorators, 1936–7

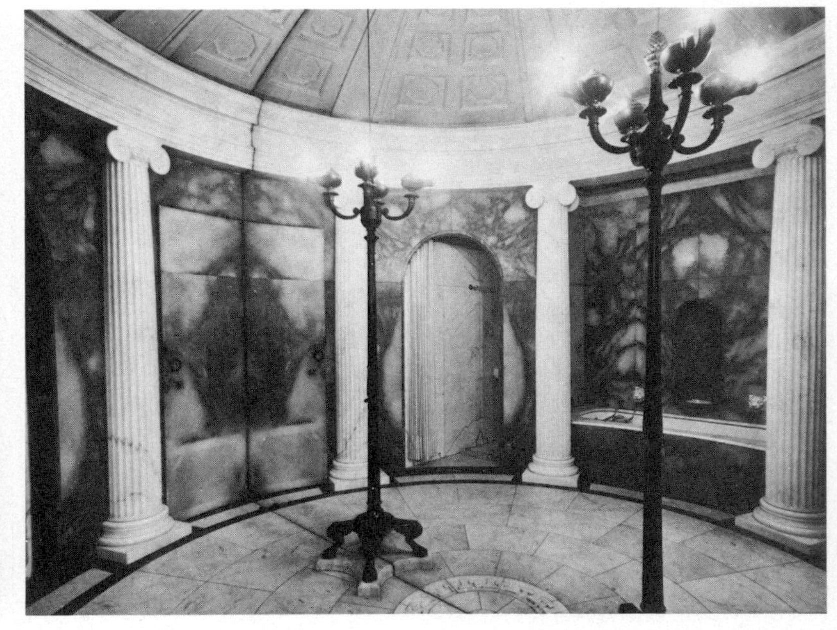

d. No. 12 North Audley Street, bathroom in 1975. Marchesa Malacrida and White Allom and Company, decorators, 1932

INTERIORS OF THE 1930'S

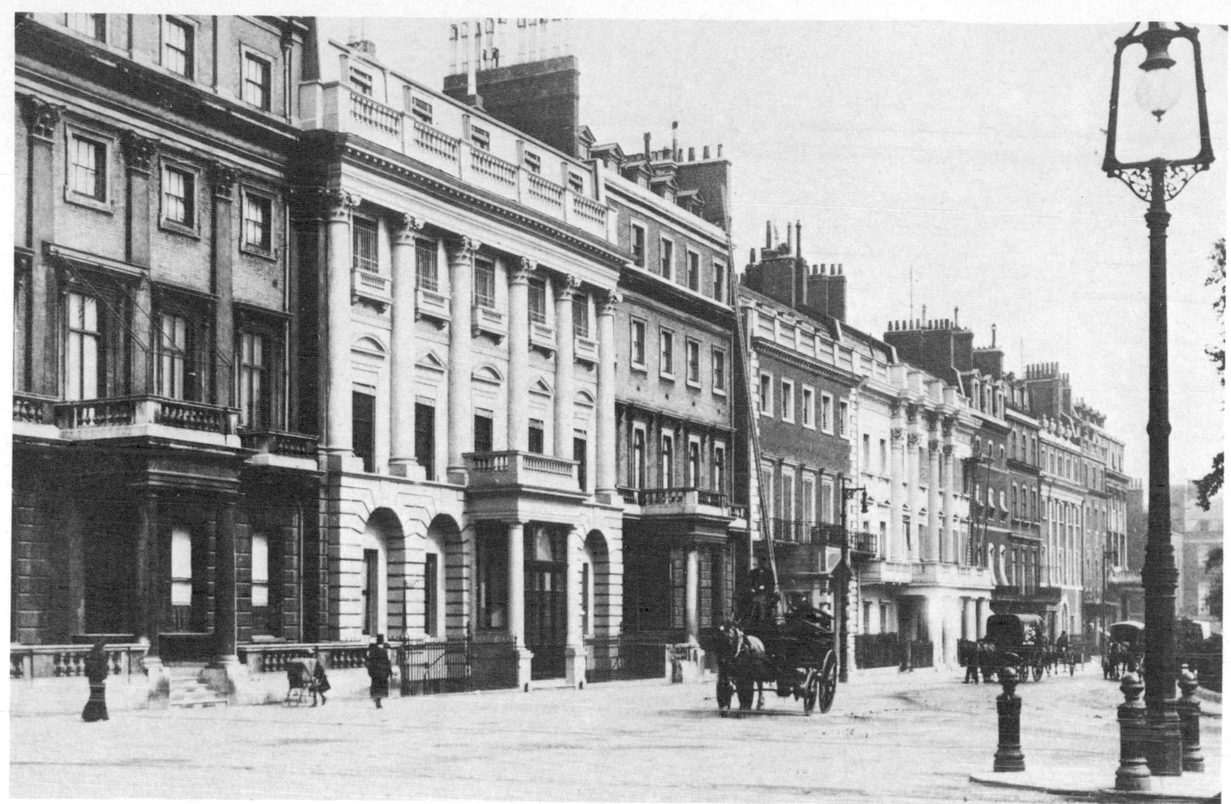

a. North side in *c*. 1910, showing fronts of Nos. 10–20 consec. (right to left). *Demolished*

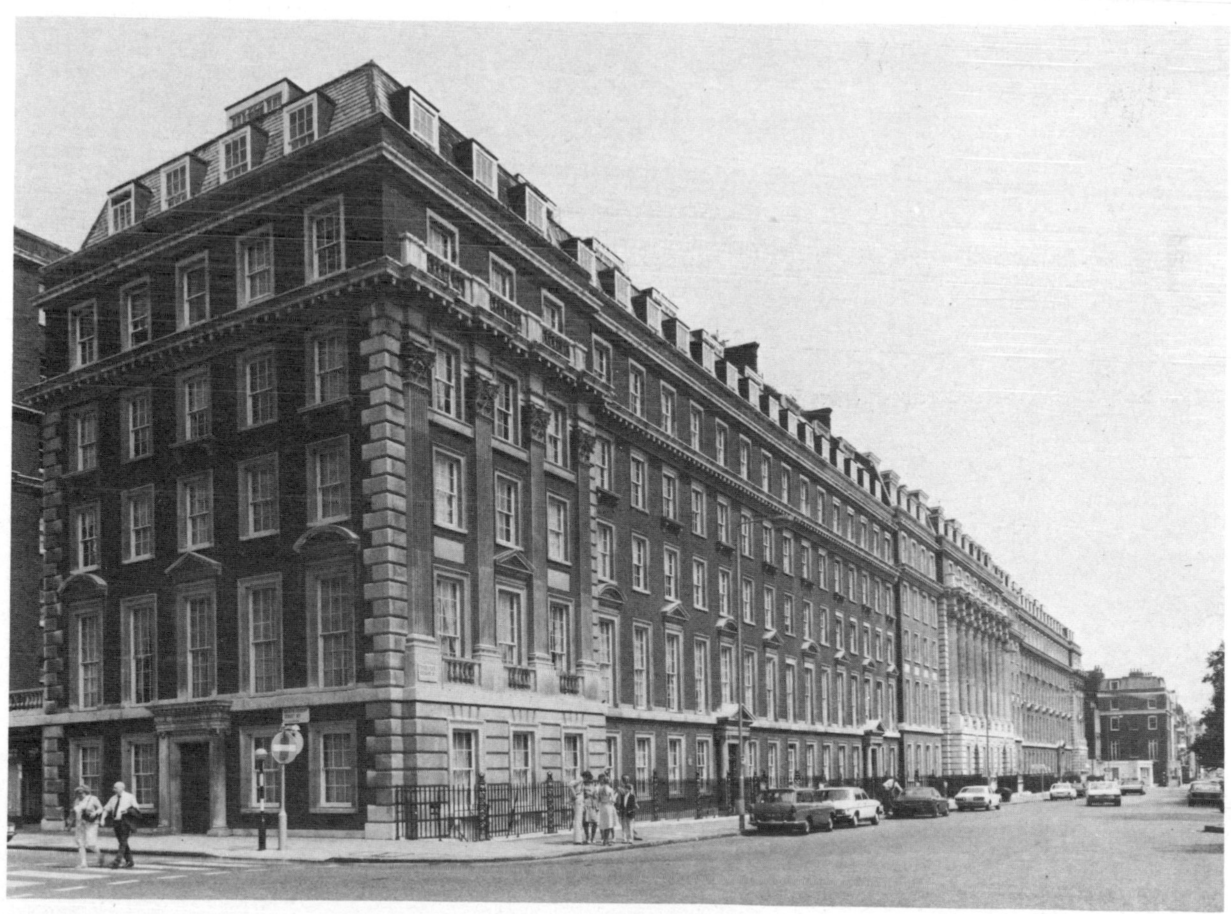

b. North side in 1976, showing fronts of Nos. 10–21 consec. (right to left). Elevations by Fernand Billerey, architect, executed 1933–64

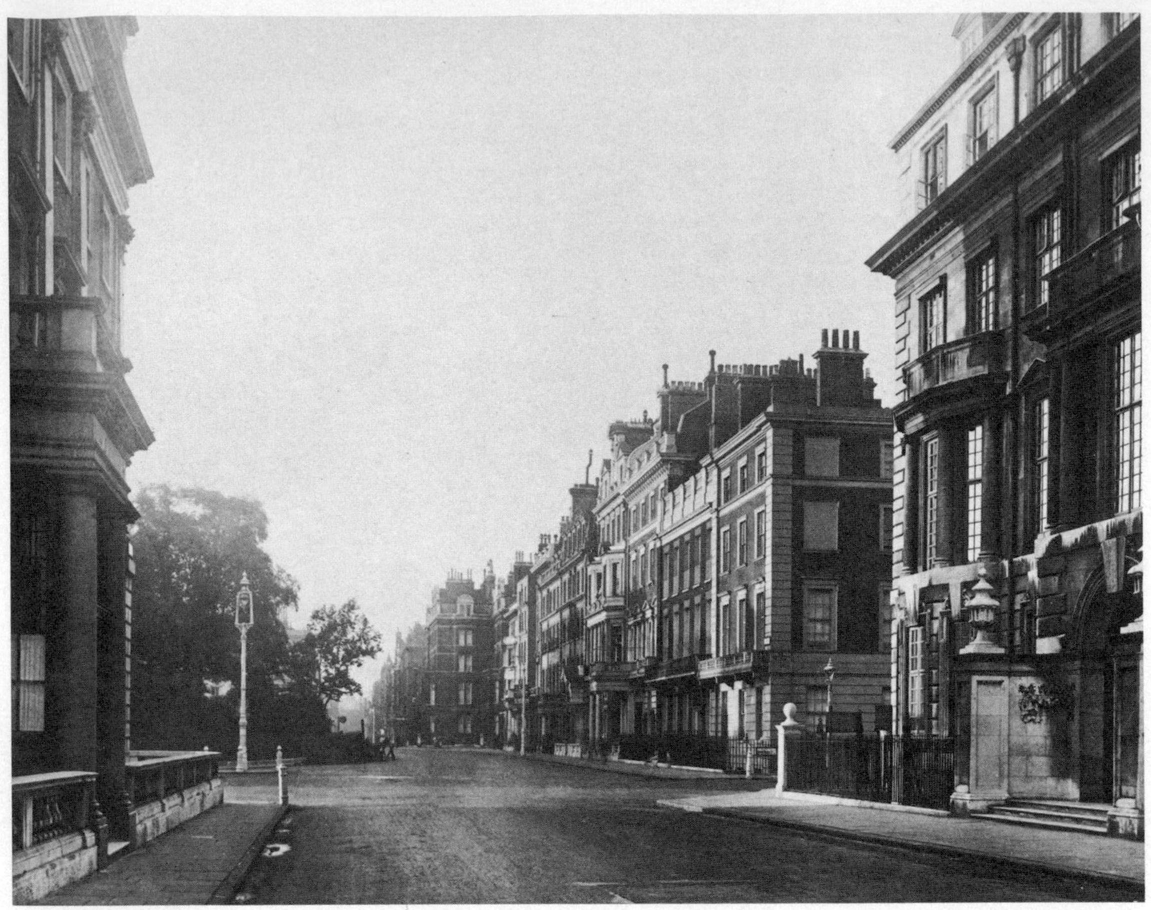

a. West side in *c*. 1930 from North Audley Street, showing No. 21 (extreme left), No. 22 (extreme right), Nos. 24–32 consec. (centre right) and Nos. 33–34 (centre distance). *All demolished except No. 22*

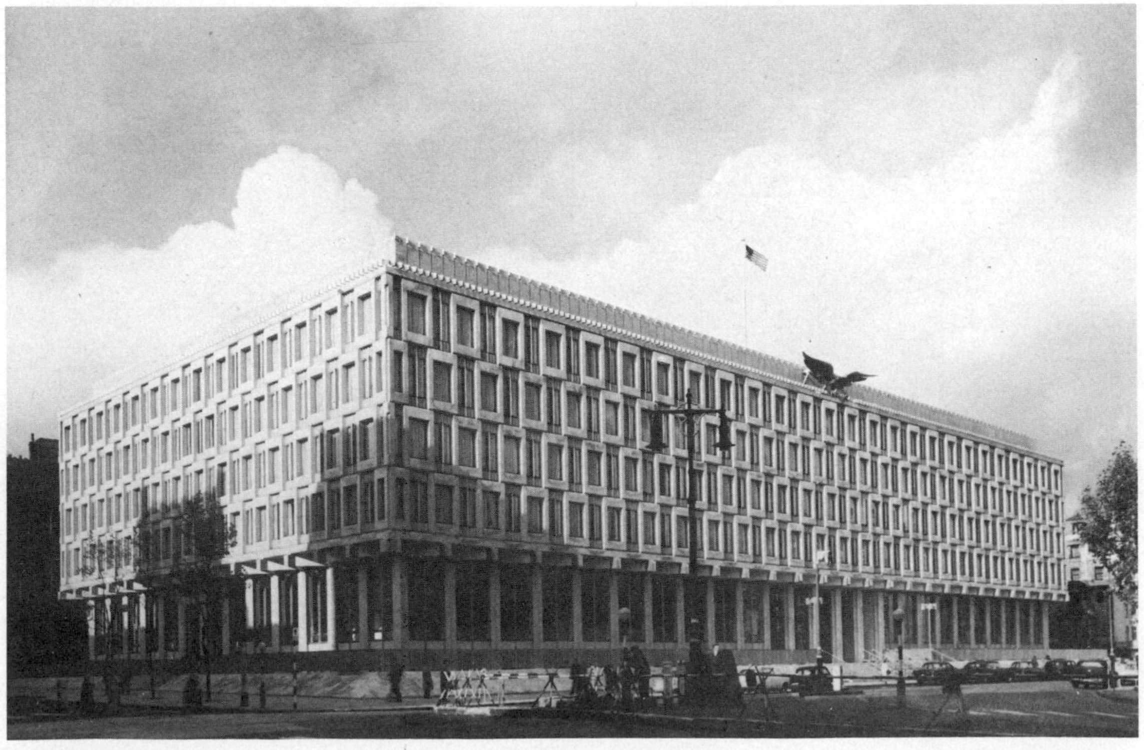

b. West side in 1961 from south-east, showing entrance front and Upper Grosvenor Street front of United States Embassy. Eero Saarinen, architect, 1956–60

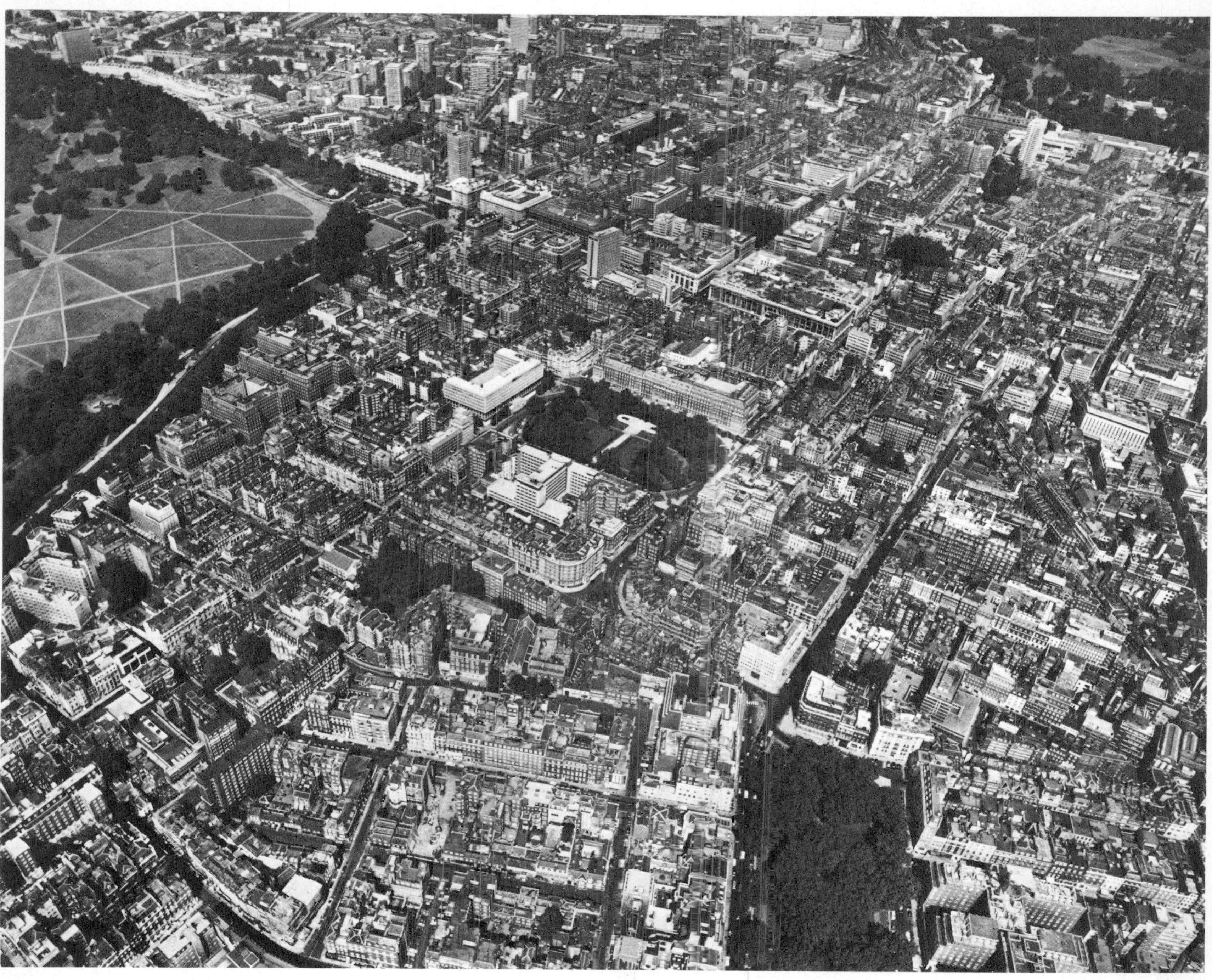

Grosvenor Estate, Mayfair, aerial view from the south-east in 1973. Berkeley Square is in the right foreground, Grosvenor Square in the centre, and Hyde Park at the top left